Child Life and Health

Child Life and Health

Being a fifth edition of the book previously
known as "Child Health and Development"

Fifth Edition

Edited by

Ross G. Mitchell

M.D., F.R.C.P. (Edin.), D.C.H.
Professor of Child Health in the University of Aberdeen

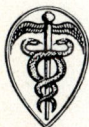

1970

J. & A. Churchill, Gloucester Place, London

CHILD HEALTH AND DEVELOPMENT, First Edition, 1947
  R. W. B. Ellis
  Reprinted, 1949
  Second Edition, 1956
  Third Edition, 1962
  Fourth Edition, 1966

CHILD LIFE AND HEALTH,
  R. G. Mitchell
  Fifth Edition, 1970

I.S.B.N. 0 7000 1478 0

20.4.71

Made in Great Britain at the Pitman Press, Bath

Contributors

E. B. CASTLE, M.A. Emeritus Professor of Education, University of Hull.

F. A. E. CREW, M.D., PH.D., D.SC., F.R.C.P. (EDIN.), F.R.S. Emeritus Professor of Public Health and Social Medicine, University of Edinburgh.

ROBERT CRUICKSHANK, C.B.E., M.D., LL.D., F.R.C.P. (LOND. & EDIN.), D.P.H., F.R.S.E. Emeritus Professor of Bacteriology, University of Edinburgh.

A. J. DALZELL-WARD, M.R.C.S., L.R.C.P., D.P.H., F.R.S.H. Director, Field Services Division, Health Education Council.

IAN DONALD, M.B.E., B.A., M.D., F.R.C.O.G., F.R.C.S. (GLAS.), F.C.O.G. (S.A.). Regius Professor of Midwifery, University of Glasgow.

CECIL M. DRILLIEN, M.D., M.R.C.P. (EDIN.), D.C.H. Lecturer in Child Life and Health, University of Edinburgh.

J. W. FARQUHAR, M.D., F.R.C.P. (EDIN.). Reader in Child Life and Health, University of Edinburgh.

J. D. HOUSTON, B.A. Lecturer in Applied Social Studies, School of Social Study, University of Glasgow.

RAYMOND ILLSLEY, B.A. (OXON.), PH.D. (ABERD.). Director, M.R.C. Medical Sociology Unit, Aberdeen.

T. T. S. INGRAM, M.D., F.R.C.P. (EDIN.), D.C.H. Reader in Child Life and Health, University of Edinburgh.

DENIS MCMAHON, M.A. Director of the Applied Psychology Unit, University of Edinburgh.

JAMES MAXWELL, M.A., M.ED. Principal Lecturer in Psychology, Moray House College of Education, Edinburgh.

SHEENA M. M. MAXWELL, M.A., M.ED. Principal Psychologist, Royal Hospital for Sick Children, Edinburgh.

R. G. MITCHELL, M.D., F.R.C.P. (EDIN.), D.C.H. Professor of Child Health, University of Aberdeen.

J. K. RUSSELL, M.D., F.R.C.O.G. Professor of Obstetrics and Gynaecology, University of Newcastle upon Tyne.

F. H. STONE, M.B., CH.B., F.R.C.P. (GLAS.), M.R.C.P. (LOND.). Consultant in Child Psychiatry, Royal Hospital for Sick Children, Glasgow.

H. P. TAIT, M.D., F.R.C.P. (EDIN.), D.P.H. Principal Medical Officer in charge of Child Health Services, City of Edinburgh.

J. M. TANNER, M.D., D.SC., PH.D., M.R.C.P. (LOND.), D.P.M. Professor of Child Health and Growth, Institute of Child Health, University of London.

A. J. WOOTTON, B.SC. (SOC.) (LOND), M.SC. (ECON.) (LOND.). Research Fellow, Department of Sociology, University of Aberdeen.

DAME EILEEN L. YOUNGHUSBAND, D.B.E., LL.D., J.P. Adviser in Social Work Training, National Institute for Social Work Training.

Preface to the Fifth Edition

The practice of paediatrics concerns the medical care of infants and children, including both the prevention and the treatment of disease. In order to practise clinical paediatrics successfully, the doctor must have a sound knowledge of the healthy child and a broad understanding of children and the environment which shapes them. Departments which teach paediatrics in British universities are not only clinical departments in the medical schools but are also concerned with the wider aspects of child life, and so are closely associated with departments in other faculties, such as sociology, education and psychology. This breadth of interest is not fully conveyed by the short titles 'Child Health' or 'Paediatrics' and some departments have tried to indicate the comprehensive nature of their subject by such titles as 'Child Health and Paediatrics' or, in Edinburgh, 'Child Life and Health'. It seems particularly appropriate to choose the latter as a title for this new edition, since Professor R. W. B. Ellis, the first editor, was professor of Child Life and Health in Edinburgh University. The slight change from the former title of 'Child Health and Development' is also intended to indicate the increasing emphasis on social aspects of child life, though not to suggest that the study of child development is less important. The assessment of development is indeed one of the major tasks of modern paediatrics, but this is encompassed within the general title and its many facets are dealt with by a number of distinguished contributors.

Several short textbooks on the diseases of infancy and childhood are available, as well as longer works of reference. The present volume is complementary to such books, being concerned primarily with the normal child and only describing abnormality where this is necessary to a full understanding of the normal. Thus consideration is given to a few diseases which form an integral part of living for a high proportion of the population, e.g. the respiratory distress syndrome of infants born before term, and to certain categories of abnormality which are so common as almost to constitute a variation of normal, e.g. low birth weight or juvenile delinquency. In addition to describing normal growth and development and the maintenance of health in childhood, this book acquaints the reader with many aspects of child life not dealt with in medical textbooks and with the range of services provided for children by the community. Its purpose is to introduce the junior student to the study of healthy children and their relation to society before he learns about diseases of childhood, and to provide information for the post-graduate which he will not readily acquire during his apprenticeship in clinical practice. I hope that the book will also prove useful to students of sociology and social work and other professions concerned with the young, since they will find gathered together here not only much that relates to childhood from their own spheres but also some of the basic knowledge about normal infants and children which is necessary for all those who work among them professionally.

Though many of the contributors to the fourth edition have again contributed to this, the fifth edition, there are a number of new authors and the whole text has been so thoroughly revised that it is virtually a new book. However, I trust that those many readers who have known and used 'Ellis' since its first appearance in 1947 will recognize an old and valued friend, albeit in new clothing.

Aberdeen, 1970   R. G. M.

Contents

Introduction

Human life is a continuous process of change from conception to death. During the early years the individual is growing and developing but for the greater part of his life he is fully mature and insidiously undergoing the degenerative processes of ageing. The period of development falls naturally into a number of phases— fetal life, infancy, childhood, adolescence—but all are distinguished from adult life by the fact that development is still incomplete. It is this fundamental difference that dictates the need for separate consideration of the young and special provision for their requirements, which are not merely those of a small adult.

The whole process of development from the earliest beginnings to maturity may be looked on as a prelude, a period of preparation for assuming adult status in the community. It must never be forgotten, however, that each phase of development has claims and responsibilities of its own. As Capon (1947) has said "The age of childhood would indeed be dull, insipid and unpromising if those responsible for the management of children thought only of ultimate aims." Indeed, the ultimate aims will be defeated unless each successive phase of development is lived fully, healthily and enjoyably as it is reached.

With new techniques and equipment, the fetus is becoming more accessible to positive benign influences. Protection can be afforded against a variety of harmful agents which may jeopardise survival or interfere with growth, while certain diseases of the fetus can be treated by intra-uterine procedures. Prevention or treatment of maternal disease, regulation of maternal diet and habits such as smoking, early recognition of abnormality and preparation for safe delivery will all help to ensure successful prenatal development. The process of birth itself, though possibly the greatest ordeal that a human being is required to undergo, can be stripped of many of its potential hazards by efficient obstetric and paediatric care, using all the refinements of modern technology.

Following birth, the newborn infant is still supremely helpless and dependent. It will be more than a year before he can even walk securely, feed himself or communicate intelligibly with the surrounding world. Four more years are necessary before he is ready for formal education or can be relied upon to protect himself against common dangers, and he is into the second decade of life before he experiences the rapid spurt of growth and emotional development that occur at puberty. Thus each phase of child life has its own distinctive characteristics and its own reactions to adverse influences, as well as its own social organisation. Any constructive planning of services for children must be based on knowledge of the normal development of the children for whom they are planned. The more extensive this knowledge is, the more likely are the services to fulfil the various purposes for which they are designed.

Individual Variation

Every newly born infant is an individual with a potential determined by his genetic endowment and shaped by his intra-uterine experience. Whether he fulfils that potential depends on the quality of care he receives during the years of dependence, the kind of challenge he encounters and the opportunities which are presented to him. The first few years are of vital importance, for every experience imprints itself indelibly on the child's emergent personality, making impressions which have a lasting effect on his emotional and social development. Each child thus has his own abilities and limitations, which may or may not be considered 'normal' for his age, according to how different they are from accepted standards. The range of normal is wide, however, and shades imperceptibly into the abnormal at either end of the scale, so that standards are often arbitrary and limits difficult to define. Much of medical practice with children is concerned with subnormality, whether it be mental, physical or emotional. The interest of the teaching profession, on the other hand, tends to focus on the supranormal—the child of outstanding performance. Remarkably little attention has been paid in this country to the development of exceptionally gifted children and the extent to which exceptional environmental opportunity is necessary to allow them to achieve what they are capable of. The research of Bartlett (1965) suggests that, in the early stages, the effects of unfavourable environmental influences upon innate potential are damaging in inverse ratio to the degree of a child's intelligence, but much more study of these children is needed.

When we are considering particular children, it is not easy to apply a statistical concept like 'normality', especially in assessing personality and behaviour. Nail-biting, for example, is often stigmatised as an abnormal neurotic habit—and yet can a habit practised by half the child population be considered abnormal? Great caution and experience are necessary, for failure to understand the great diversity of children may lead to a narrow interpretation of normality and a too-ready designation of behaviour as deviant. All concerned with the health and well-being of children should have a sound knowledge of the range of variation acceptable in infancy and childhood. This applies not only to physical development but also to intelligence, personality characteristics and other attributes. Standards must usually be drawn from the population from which the child comes and care must be taken that the child's progress and abilities are not compared with an inappropriate range of normal.

Once this fundamental principle of normal variation has been grasped, we are in a much stronger position to help the individual child. After the requirements common to every child have been considered, we can go on to the special needs of a variety of sub-groups, differentiated on the basis of sex, age, religion, ethnic origin and other criteria as seem appropriate. Then we must think how, within the framework we have erected, each child can be given the opportunity of developing his own capacities to the full. The goal is not only that no child should be hindered by poverty, ignorance, malnutrition or preventable disease from reaching the maximum of which he is inherently capable, but that his environment should actively help in the fulfilment of his potentialities. Equal opportunity for all is an acceptable principle only if we clearly recognize that this means opportunity equally appropriate to each child's needs, not the provision of a single template, for the ideal opportunity for one may prove ill-suited to another. In this country, legislative and other measures have achieved much in the fields of education, medical care for infants and children and help for the underprivileged; a great deal has still to be accomplished, however, if we are to ensure that the administrative machine is always sufficiently adaptable to provide for the needs of each child as a unique person.

The Assessment of Special Needs

When a child has special physical, intellectual, emotional or social needs—or a combination of these—a careful appraisal of all his abilities and disabilities and of the resources of his social environment is required. This should be undertaken jointly by the professions mainly concerned with children—principally paediatrics, education, child psychology and psychiatry, and social work, with others as appropriate. The process is generally known as comprehensive assessment and forms the basis for recommendations about the future management of the child and provision for his needs, with the object of preventing or reducing any handicap caused by his personal or environmental inadequacies and helping him to utilise his inherent capability to the full. Assessment usually extends over a period of time and is not a once-for-all procedure, being repeated at intervals as the child grows and circumstances change. Careful co-ordination of the activities of the professional workers concerned is essential and is achieved by constant inter-communication, both verbal and written, by effective case records and by periodic conferences. The efficient working of an assessment team requires that overall responsibility is delegated to one person, to ensure that final agreement is reached on a plan (often a compromise between conflicting demands) and that the child's parents are not confused by contrary advice and opinions. The work of such a team should be based on an assessment centre where the child can be seen whenever and for as long as necessary and where continuing contact with staff in a day nursery or school setting can give a much deeper insight into the child's personality and potential. The assessment centre is preferably sited in the community rather than in the hospital, since the children are not 'patients' so much as people with various abilities and disabilities. Centres should be organized on a day attendance basis with residential accommodation provided nearby for mothers and children coming from a distance. Because of the costly nature of such provision, there are few assessment centres in Britain at present but an increase is likely in the near future, the pattern varying according to local needs, the availability and interests of trained staff, the geographical location and so on.

This kind of interdisciplinary service is becoming more a feature of child care and will require a change of attitude on the part of all professional workers, who have hitherto tended to work in relative isolation in hospitals, schools and clinics, and who are often unused to sharing responsibility and adapting their activities to the limitations imposed by other needs. A wider and more positive approach to the social, medical and educational difficulties of children and the growing realization that social education rather than criminal proceedings and punishment is appropriate for children in trouble (see Chapter 23) will greatly increase the already unsatisfied demand for comprehensive assessment in the future.

The Quality of Child Life

Throughout most of man's existence, childhood has been a struggle for survival, a time of life overshadowed by disease and the probability of early death. Only the survivors of the first few years were worthy of consideration as members of society and the place accorded to young children was consequently a lowly one. Today, in the greater part of the world, childhood is of short duration and adult responsibilities are assumed early, so that the child can contribute to the family's meagre standard of living. Infection, parasitic disease and hunger are still the stark realities of child life and all other considerations are subordinate to these. In many countries, improving health services, sanitation and food supplies might be expected to raise standards but they are too often overtaxed by rapid increases in population. Progressive urbanisation and the consequent loosening of family ties result in the production of large numbers of unwanted children, who further imperil the ability of the community to provide for them. When the effects of war or large-scale famine are superimposed on such conditions, the loss of child life and the misery of those who survive is incalculable.

By contrast, in that small section of the world's population which is disproportionately wealthy, plentiful food and efficient health services have resulted in a dramatic decline in malnutrition and disease. Whereas formerly large numbers of children suffered from tuberculosis, rheumatism, poliomyelitis, chronic pyogenic infection and many other conditions now mainly of historical importance in Britain, medical treatment today is mainly required for acute transient disease or for the minority of children with congenital malformations. Clinical paediatrics has become more preventive than ever before and is largely concerned with neonatal disorders and their sequelae, with deviations from normal development or behaviour and with the management of the chronically handicapped, all of which require a far greater understanding of the child and his social environment. The modern paediatrician thus has interests very different from those of twenty-five years ago and, incidentally, very different from those of the physician concerned with adults (Joseph and Mac Keith, 1966).

The lives of children freed from the shadow of disease are immeasurably happier and even the handicapped child has much more to look forward to than in former times. It can fairly be said that the present generation of our children is as healthy as any since the world began. Childhood as a period of relative dependence is prolonged in our society, so that excessively early responsibility does not distort maturation and full advantage can be taken of educational opportunity. But there is a darker side to this bright picture. It is a deplorable fact that standards of child welfare in the rich countries often do not equal those of health and nutrition.

Thousands of children have to be looked after by the state, some because they are illegitimate and the parents cannot or will not accept their responsibilities, others because ill-treatment or neglect makes it necessary for the community to take them into care and protection. For every one thus overtly deprived of a normal childhood, there are probably several children whose lives, though materially rich, are impoverished by parental indifference, carelessness or outright cruelty. Child abuse seems to become more frequent as society develops, perhaps because the greater complexity of life throws an increasing strain on youthful parents, who give vent to their emotional turmoil and feelings of inadequacy by ill-treating their children.

The modern child is at the mercy of an urbanised society as well as at risk from adult aggression. Increasing mechanisation brings with it new threats of accidental death or injury. Thus while a child in Britain has today a far smaller chance of dying than he had thirty years ago 'if he dies or is injured at all it is increasingly probable that it will be in some domestic accident' (Backett, 1965). Children come under the influence of television from earliest infancy and few homes in Britain now lack it, with its great potentiality for education but its equal capacity for corruption. Increasingly permissive morality imposes strains on adolescents far greater than their predecessors ever had to contend with. Thus, just as the pattern of child health is rapidly changing, so also is the quality of child life. We cannot yet assess the full impact of violence on television, of the restrictions imposed by high flat dwelling, or of birth control and the contraceptive pill. We cannot know what the child of the future will think about the man in the moon—so long a figment of childish imagination but now a reality—or how he will view the threat of nuclear extinction.

These complex and sometimes unhappy features of child life in the affluent society cannot be ignored by those responsible for the health and education of children, for they impinge on every aspect of their work. With the present rapid sophistication of skills and capabilities, the professions sometimes tend to forget that, in treating or teaching a child, they must take note of the family and the home circumstances if their efforts are to be successful. Yet, over twenty years ago, Sir James Spence said "when I need to understand a child or his illness in order to advise what shall be done for his welfare and treatment, I would hesitate to reach an opinion without a close scrutiny of the parents, without listening to their opinions, and without a knowledge of the conditions in which they live." (Spence, 1949.) For the medical profession in particular, increasing scientific skill must be accompanied by comparable understanding of psychology and sociology, and this has been recognized in the report of the Royal Commission on Medical Education (1968). Doctors and teachers are learning that the social worker is a professional colleague who has at least as much to contribute to the successful rearing of children as they have themselves. Her collaboration as an equal member of the team is essential if the child is to achieve the maximum benefit from health and educational measures. In the past it has too frequently been assumed that the contribution of the social worker is confined to a small under-privileged section of the community and that acceptance of help from this source carried with it a social stigma. Just as medical and educational provision is now made use of as a matter of course and of right, so advice and guidance from the social services should be available to and used by all sections of the community. The increasing complexity of life in an industrial urban community makes such a trend inevitable and there are few who cannot benefit from being shown how to make the most of the opportunities offered by modern society and from professional help with their personal problems. Now that children in Britain are, by and large, healthy and educated, the most pressing need is to ensure that the quality of their lives matches up to the same standards.

R. G. MITCHELL

References

BACKETT, E. M. (1965). *Domestic Accidents*. Geneva: World Health Organization.

BARTLETT, E. M. (1965). Exceptional children. In *Modern Perspectives in Child Psychiatry*. Ed. J. G. Howells. Edinburgh: Oliver and Boyd.

CAPON, N. B. (1947). *The Foundations of Health in Childhood*. London: Nat. Child. Home.

JOSEPH, M. and MAC KEITH, R. C. (1966). *A New Look at Child Health*. London: Pitman.

Report of the Royal Commission on Medical Education (1968). London: H.M.S.O.

SPENCE, J. C. (1949). *The Need for Understanding the Individual as part of the Training and Function of Doctors and Nurses*. London: Nat. Assoc. Mental Health.

PART I

CHILD HEALTH AND DEVELOPMENT

I   Genetical Aspects of Child Health and Development

Characters, Chromosomes and Genes

THE physical development of the individual, throughout its entire course, is controlled by enzymes, proteins that act as catalysts regulating the rate of the chemical processes that are involved. Of enzymes there are many kinds but each kind directly promotes only a very limited range of chemical reactions. Normal development requires that for each event in ontogeny the right kind of enzyme shall be made available in the right amount in the right place and at the right time. The agents that ensure that these conditions shall be fulfilled are the genes in the chromosomes of the cell-nucleus. Though the gene content of every cell-nucleus is the same, not all the genes are active in all of them, some are *repressed*. As a result of differentation, different cell-aggregates come to assume different structural and functional properties and these are reflections of such repression; the genes that are not repressed are those which are involved in the fashioning of the properties of the differentiated cell-aggregate. It seems that there are two main kinds of genes, structural, concerned in the synthesis of proteins and control, regulator or operator genes which, by regulating the activity of the structural genes, control their productivity.

It is thought that there is a network of genetic switches. It is known that included in the protein component of the nucleoprotein of which the chromosomes are compounded are histones and that these in their action repress gene action; they are present in all kinds of cells, save the sperm-cells, and it seems that they repress different genes in different tissues. It is also known that certain hormones such as cortisone, the oestrogens, the androgens and the growth-hormone, stimulate or *de-repress* gene action, counteracting the effects of the histones. The hormones switch gene action on, the histones switch it off. Many enzymes exist in multiple molecular forms, the isoenzymes, and it seems likely that these are also involved in the switch mechanism. It is established that in the developing embryo one tissue exerts a determining influence upon the differentiation of other tissues. This embryonic induction is probably due to the products of genes in one cell diffusing out of that cell and evoking changes in adjacent ones.

In the final analysis it is the genetic constitution of the zygote, the *genotype*, established at the moment of fertilisation, that, working through this switch mechanism and the enzyme, histone and hormone systems, is responsible for the decision that a human ovum shall, as the outcome of development, give rise to a creature equipped with the attributes of *Homo sapiens*, with those of a particular ethnic group of mankind and with those of a particular kindred. Genes must necessarily function in an environment and in the great majority of cases act in conjunction with some specific factor or factors within that environment. Normality of development therefore implies that in the genotype of the zygote there shall be those genes that correspond to, that determine, those *characters*—chemical processes, biochemical properties, structural or functional features, mental traits—that are classified as normal; the absence from the genotype of those genes that correspond to characters that are regarded as abnormal; the presence in the environment of such factors as are either neutral or else conducive to developmental normality and conversely, the absence from the environment of such factors, living and non-living, as in their action, either alone or else in conjunction with that of certain genes, yield abnormality of characterisation.

During cell-division each gene replicates itself, producing, in the vast majority of instances, an exact copy of itself. In this way replicas of the original chromosomes are created. But this copying process does not invariably yield a gene that is identical with that from which it arose; *mutation*, a specific alteration of the internal organisation of the gene, can occur to yield a new form of the original one. The two genes, the old and the new, the unmutated and the mutated, constitute a pair of *alleles*. These affect the same developmental processes of the same tissue or organ but because of the differences in their internal organisation and therefore in their action they yield different end-results, the mutated gene leading to the production of a new, mutant or 'abnormal' character. A gene, mutating, can give rise to more than one mutant allele, there can be a whole series of such and these, together with the original gene from which they arose, constitute a *multiple allelomorphic series*. An example of such a series is provided by the genes on which the ABO blood-groups rest.

If mutation occurs in the germ-track of an individual during gametogenesis, its effects will not be displayed by the individual concerned but by his or her descendants. It is this gametic mutation that provided novelty of characterisation in great variety during the evolution of the species. These novelties were exposed to the selective forces in the intra-uterine, physico-climatic and social environments, being appraised, rejected or encouraged according to whether or not they increased the biological fitness of the individual (as measured by the number of offspring that reached the reproductive age). The present characterisation (and therefore the underlying genotype) of mankind, within which there is a wide range of variation, is the product of a very long and severe process of selection during which very many mutant forms have been tested and during which a high degree of harmony between the *phenotypes*, the characterisations, of the different ethnic groups and the differing conditions of the various habitats which have accommodated them has become established.

Thus it is that as a general rule mutant characters that have appeared during the later stages of man's evolution have to be classified as disadvantageous or even pathological for the reason that they disturb, more or less, this equilibrium and yield defect and derangement that can range from the merely inconvenient to the completely disabling. There are hundreds of known genes that in their action, either alone or else in conjunction with some environmental factor, yield gross, pathological abnormality in characterisation. If such a gene is present in the genetic endowment an infant receives from its parent or parents, its healthiness is seriously endangered or even destroyed.

A character can be *monogenic* in origin, being based upon a single major gene with large effects; it can be *polygenic*, multifactorial, based upon a number of genes which in their actions are additive; or it can be *genetico-environmental*, a genetic inclination to develop in a particular way being reinforced by an environmental encouragement to do so.

Most of the genes in the genotype of an individual are such as have been received from related individuals of a previous generation. But *fresh* or recurrent mutation is constantly occurring and this can neither be foreseen nor prevented (in individuals who are not exposed to the action of mutagenic agencies in industry or elsewhere). All genes are prone to mutation, some far more than others. In man the general mutation-rate is about 1–100 mutations per million gametes per generation. The transmission of an undesirable gene from one generation to its successor can only be blocked, for the present, by non-propagation on the part of the individual known to possess it. It does not follow that because a particular gene corresponding to an abnormal condition is present in the genotype of an individual this abnormality will be displayed by that individual; the phenomena of *dominance*, *recessivity*, *penetrance*, *expressivity* and *sex-limitation* and the question as to whether or not the co-operation of some specific environmental factor is necessary before the gene in question can exert its action, all bear upon this matter.

The chromosome number characteristic of *Homo sapiens* is 46 or 23 pairs. Of these, 22 pairs, the *autosomes*, are common to both sexes. In respect of the remaining pair, the *sex-chromosomes*, the sexes differ. In the female there are two X-chromosomes, in the male there is one X associated with a smaller Y-chromosome. The two members of each autosomal pair are *homologous*, having the same series of loci in linear order along their lengths. Only part of the X and part of the Y are homologous so that of the sex-chromosomes there are homologous and non-homologous or differential segments. Each gene has its own particular locus in a particular chromosome. Genes resident in the differential segment of the X must necessarily be present in the single dose in the XY male who must be *hemizygous* for them. Genes resident in the differential segment of the Y-chromosome must necessarily be restricted to the male line, passing from father to son, *holandric* inheritance.

The human chromosome complex, as it now exists, has been fashioned by the process of chromosome formation during which independent genes came to be congregated into groups as a consequence of chromosome fragmentation and union, during which new gene associations came into being. There was much *deletion* in which, following breakage, a part of a chromosome was lost during cell-division; *translocation* in which a chromosome, or a part of one, following breakage, became attached to the end of another chromosome; and *inversion* in which two synchronous breaks in the length of a chromosome were followed by a 180 degree inversion of the broken segment and subsequent re-incorporation into the chromosome concerned. During the formation of the human chromosome complex, thoroughly tested and found to be satisfactory, the genes that in their action are female-determining became mainly congregated in the X-chromosome while the male-determining genes became spread among the autosomes and especially concentrated in the Y.

The most remarkable feature of cell-division is the precision with which the chromosomal (genic) material is distributed. In mitosis the chromosomal content of the daughter-cells is identical with that of the mother-cell that gave them origin. In meiosis there is a reduction of the chromosome number to one-half, this reduced or *haploid* (*n*) number consisting of one member of each of the chromosome pairs. In fertilisation the two haploid sets are brought together, one from each of the parents, and the *diploid* (*2n*) number that is characteristic of the species is reconstituted. But mitosis and meiosis occur so frequently and the mechanism of chromosome distribution is so very delicate and intricate that it is not surprising that from time to time mishap occurs. A daughter-chromosome, moving towards the forming nucleus of a daughter-cell, can lag behind the rest and so fail to become incorporated in that nucleus (*anaphase lagging*). When the two daughter-chromosomes should separate, disjoin, to pass into the forming nuclei of the two daughter-cells, they can fail to do so with the result that both of them pass together into one of these nuclei while the other nucleus fails to receive this particular chromosome (*non-disjunction*). Should this occur during gametogenesis it could yield gametes with two chromosomes of a kind and gametes lacking this chromosome altogether. Should these gametes then unite with those of the opposite kind (with spermatozoa if they are ova), each with the normal haploid number of chromosomes, two forms of zygotes would result, one with three chromosomes of a kind instead of the normal two (*trisomic* for this particular chromosome) and others with only one (*monosomic* for this particular chromosome). Such *aneuploidy*, (having more or fewer than an exact multiple of the haploid number), means the addition or subtraction of genes and a more or less profound disturbance of the genic balance leading to consequent abnormality in characterisation. Maldistribution of this kind is accidental and can neither be foreseen nor prevented though the transmission of a translocation can be blocked by non-propagation on the part of an individual known to possess it.

Autosomal dominant genes

Autosomal major genes, corresponding to abnormalities of development and affecting the health of the individual, that are dominant over their alleles that correspond to normality. (While many authorities prefer to limit the use of the term dominant to the description of a character, for reasons of convenience it is applied, herein, to both the character and to the gene which underlies it.)

Examples of frequencies of such conditions in the population

Retinitis pigmentosa (all forms)	1 in 5,000
Achondroplasia	1 in 10,000
Retinoblastoma	1 in 33,000
Epiloia (irregular in its transmission)	1 in 50,000
Osteogenesis imperfecta (irregular)	1 in 50,000

A gene possessing this property of dominance produces its effects when present only in the single dose; the character based upon it is displayed by the *heterozygote* (Dd). (The heterozygote has both the dominant and recessive alleles of a pair or two different members of a multiple allelomorphic series.) A pedigree that relates to such a character shows that, as a general rule, every affected individual has one affected parent. All the individuals in such a pedigree that are unaffected, that do not display the abnormality, are *homozygous* for the normal recessive allele of the gene in question (dd). (Homozygous = carrying two either of the dominant or of the recessive genes of a pair of alleles or carrying identical genes of a series of multiple alleles). As a general rule these autosomal major dominant genes do not give rise to serious defect, most of the pathological conditions based upon them are relatively innocuous and are such as can be repaired or cured, e.g. polydactyly and congenital cataract, but to this generalisation there are many notable exceptions, such as those listed above.

This property of dominance is very variable in respect of the degree to which it is displayed. For example, polydactyly can range from a small wart-like nodule on the side of the hand to a complete extra digit. Sometimes the condition based upon such an autosomal major dominant gene is not exhibited by an individual known to possess the gene, since this is transmitted to the individual's offspring who display the condition, the character 'skips a generation' in its transmission from parent to offspring. The ability of a gene to gain expression, its *penetrance*, is affected by the action of other genes in the genotype with the result that while in some gene associations it gains expression, in others it fails to do so. This penetrance is also affected by the conditions that exist in the internal physiological environment in which it finds itself.

Not uncommonly it is found that a child displaying an autosomal monogenic dominant abnormality has parents both of whom are without it. Furthermore, it is found that when the pedigree is examined there is no trace of this particular abnormality in it. In such cases penetrance is not involved, they are instances of fresh mutation occurring in the germ-track of one of the parents of the affected infant.

Some autosomal major dominant genes yield characterisations that are so abnormal as to be incompatible with continued life; they are *lethal*. When this is so the gene in question cannot be transmitted from one generation to the next and any new example of the condition must therefore be the result of fresh mutation. For example, in epiloia it is found that not more than about half of the affected children have affected relatives. If the frequency of epiloia in the general population is to remain more or less constant, as it does, fresh mutation must be responsible for about 50 per cent of the cases. Many disadvantageous genes result, either directly or indirectly, in a lowering of the biological fitness of those who display the abnormalities based upon them. It is usual for such as are seriously disabled by defect or derangement of genetic origin to have fewer offspring than does a comparable group of 'normals'. An equilibrium becomes established, the rate at which elimination of a particular gene from the population through a lowered reproductive rate occurs is balanced by the rate at which fresh mutations involving this gene are fed into the population.

The cure or repair of an abnormality of genetic origin must and will remain the aim of medicine but such therapy in no way touches the responsible gene or genes so that the abnormality will still be handed on. In those instances in which such repair or cure results in the raising of the reproductive fitness of an individual it can lead to an increase of the *genetic load* that must be carried by that population (the numbers of disadvantageous genes in the constitution of the population).

Autosomal recessive genes

Autosomal major genes, corresponding to abnormalities of development and affecting the health of the individual, that are recessive to their alleles that correspond to normality. (The term recessive is applied, herein, to both gene and character.)

Examples of frequencies of such conditions in the population

Deafmutism	1 in 3,000
Exomphalos	1 in 3,000
Albinism	1 in 10,000–20,000
Phenylketonuria	1 in 10,000–20,000
Microcephaly	1 in 25,000–50,000
Amaurotic family idiocy, juvenile form	1 in 40,000
Fructosuria	1 in 130,000
Pseudoxanthoma elasticum	1 in 160,000
Amaurotic family idiocy, infantile form	1 in 250,000
Alkaptonuria	1 in 1,000,000

The term recessive indicates that in the heterozygote, possessing a dominant gene in one chromosome of a homologous pair and the corresponding recessive allele in the other, the latter fails to gain expression; that a gene can find expression only when present in the genotype in duplicate (dd), one member of the pair having been received by the zygote from each of the parents who, in the great majority of instances, are themselves heterozygotes (Dd) and who therefore do not display the condition based upon the gene. In the heterozygous condition a recessive gene can remain hidden for many generations and so can find itself in a wide variety of genotypes. Any individual who displays an autosomal monogenic recessive character is homozygous for the corresponding gene (dd). In a pedigree all those who display the alternative dominant 'normal' character are either homozygous for the dominant allele of this recessive gene (DD) or else are heterozygous for it (Dd). These heterozygotes (Dd), carriers of a recessive gene, greatly outnumber the individuals who are homozygous for it (dd) and are affected.

It has been estimated that everybody in the population is heterozygous for three to eight autosomal recessive genes corresponding to defect or derangement. But because there are so very many such genes in the human genotype, mutated and unmutated, it is most unlikely that two individuals heterozygous for the same undesirable recessive gene will marry and reproduce and even should they do so it is to be expected that such children as are born to them will very commonly be either homozygous normals or else heterozygous carriers. But near relatives, such as first cousins, are far more likely to possess the same autosomal recessive gene, derived from a common ancestor, than are unrelated individuals. In fact the chance that first cousins will be heterozygous for the same autosomal recessive gene is 1 in 8. The rarer the abnormality the more likely it is that the parents of an affected child are first cousins. In cystic fibrosis (fibrocystic disease of the pancreas), the commonest genetically caused disease in man, about 1 in every 2,000 infants born is homozygous for the autosomal recessive gene that is the cause of the condition and so suffers from the disease. This means that about 1 in every 22 individuals in the population is a carrier of this gene. The chances of two such carriers, themselves unaffected, meeting, marrying and reproducing, being completely unaware of the hidden danger, are very considerable. At the other end of the scale is alkaptonuria. About 1 in every million individuals in the population suffers from this disease and this frequency means that about 1 in every 500 in the population is a carrier of the gene. Of the parents of an alkaptonuric infant about one-third are first cousins whereas in cystic fibrosis the frequency of consanguinity among the parents of affected children is only a little higher than in the general population (about 0·5 per cent).

Alkaptonuria, fructosuria and phenylketonuria are examples of 'inborn errors of metabolism' and belong to the field of biochemical genetics. They are conditions, genetically caused, that indicate in the clearest possible fashion the nature of gene action and illustrate the role of the enzymes in metabolism. For example, phenylalanine, an aminoacid component of protein-containing foodstuffs, is broken down in a series of steps each one of which requires the action of a particular enzyme. The steps are as follows:

		The enzyme concerned
1.	phenylalanine to tyrosine	L-phenylalanine hydroxylase
2.	tyrosine to *p*-hydroxyphenylpyruvate	tyrosine transaminase
3.	*p*-hydroxyphenylpyruvate to homogentisate	*p*-hydroxyphenylpyruvic acid oxidase
4.	homogentisate to maleylacetoacetate	homogentisic acid oxidase
5.	maleylacetoacetate to fumarylacetoacetate	maleylacetoacetic acid isomerase
6.	fumarylacetoacetate to fumarate + acetoacetate	fumarylacetoacetic acid hydrolase

A genetic block in step 1, due to a deficiency or lack of the enzyme L-phenylalanine hydroxylase, results in phenylketonuria. A genetic block resulting in deficiency or absence of the enzyme *p*-hydroxyphenylpyruvic acid oxidase is the cause of that very rare condition tyrosinosis. Absence or deficiency of the enzyme homogentisic acid oxidase results in alkaptonuria. The enzyme dehalogenase, acting upon tyrosine, is involved in the production of the thyroid hormones and a deficiency of this enzyme leads to goitrous cretinism. The enzyme tyrosinase, acting upon tyrosine, is responsible for the production of melanin and a deficiency of this enzyme is a cause of albinism.

Other examples of these inborn errors of metabolism, similarly based upon autosomal recessive genes which cause a deficiency or absence of specific enzymes, are:

The condition	*The enzyme concerned*
Acatalasaemia (acatalasia)	catalase
Congenital hyperbilirubinaemia	glucuronyl transferase
Cystathioninuria	cystathioninine cleavage enzyme
Galactosaemia	galactose-1-phosphate uridyl transferase
Glycogen storage disease (*a*)	glucose-6-phosphatase
(*b*)	amylo-1:6-glucosidase
(*c*)	amylo-(1:4 → 1:6) transglucosidase
Hypophosphatasia	alkaline phosphatase
Methaemoglobinaemia (a form of)	diaphorase 1. methaemoglobin reductase
Suxamethonium sensitivity	serum cholinesterase (pseudo-cholinesterase)

The last of these conditions is of unusual interest and falls into the field of pharmacogenetics. The presence of this gene (in duplicate) is revealed only when the drug suxamethonium is used as a muscle relaxant in anaesthesia when a fatal apnoea is liable to develop. The gene is a very common one, about 1 in every 2,000 in the population being homozygous for it.

Sex-linked genes

Mutant recessive genes, corresponding to monogenic abnormalities of development and affecting the health of the individual, that are resident in the differential segment of the X-chromosome. (Sex-linkage. X-linkage.)

More than 50 such genes have been identified, those for classical haemophilia, Christmas disease, red-green colour blindness, one form of ichthyosis vulgaris, one form of the Duchenne type of muscular dystrophy, nephrogenic diabetes insipidus and red blood corpuscle deficiency of glucose-6-phosphate dehydrogenase can serve as examples. The mode of inheritance of the characters based upon these X-borne genes is necessarily different from that of an autosomal monogenic recessive for the reason that the male, having but one X-chromosome, is constitutionally hemizygous. He can possess but one gene of a pair and this will gain expression even if it is a recessive since there can be no dominant allele associated with it. Dominance, recessivity, homozygous and heterozygous are terms that are inapplicable. In the female with two Xs a gene can be a dominant or a recessive just as with autosomal genes. Most of the known X-borne genes are recessive in the female and she can be a carrier whereas the male cannot.

The characteristic feature of this sex-linked mode of inheritance is that an affected male cannot pass the gene on to his sons but only to and through his daughters who will be carriers and who will pass it on to some of their sons who will display the character. The recessive abnormalities based upon genes in the differential segment of the X-chromosome have a higher frequency in the male for the reason that he needs but one such gene to display the character whereas the female needs two, one from each parent. It is for this reason that the haemophiliac female is so rare and that while 8 in every 100 males in the general population are red-green colour blind only about 1 woman in every 200 is similarly affected. The rate of elimination of a gene such as that for haemophilia is quite considerable for the fertility of the haemophiliac is much reduced. Possibly the life of the average haemophilia gene is not more than three generations and not less than a quarter of all the cases of this condition existing at any one time are due to fresh mutation.

Quite a number of autosomal abnormalities also have a higher frequency in the male, though for a different reason. Cleft lip, with or without cleft palate, is twice as common among male infants, pyloric stenosis five times as common. On the other hand, anencephaly is three times as common among female infants and congenital dislocation of the hip six times as common. The penetrance of a gene is certainly affected by the sex of the individual for maleness and femaleness are two different physiological environments which include factors that affect gene action.

A few sex-linked dominant genes are known, e.g. those for vitamin-D-resistant rickets and for the Xg blood-group system. Since such a gene is resident in the differential segment of the X-chromosome, an affected male, (XD)Y, cannot transmit it to his sons but only to and through his daughters who will be affected heterozygotes (XD)(Xd). An affected heterozygous female, on the other hand, can transmit the gene, and therefore the character, to both sons and daughters.

So far only one gene has been located in the differential segment of the Y-chromosome—hairy ear-rims—and this is of no interest in the present context.

Identification of the Heterozygote

When the abnormality is a common and a serious one it is of considerable importance to recognise the carriers of autosomal recessive, non-penetrant autosomal dominant and sex-linked recessive genes, to distinguish these from such as do not possess the gene. When a double dose of a gene has a different effect from that of a single dose, when dominance is not complete, when the mode of inheritance is *intermediate*, the heterozygote has a character all its own.

The homozygous recessive	*The heterozygous recessive*
Afibrinogenaemia	Fibrinogenopenia
Anophthalmia	small eyeballs
Friedreich's ataxia	Pes cavus, absent tendon reflexes
Laurence-Moon-Biedl syndrome	Obesity, skeletal abnormalities
Myopia, severe degree	Myopia, mild degree
Sickle-cell anaemia	Sickle-cell trait
Thalassaemia major (Cooley's anaemia)	Thalassaemia minor
Xanthomatosis	Hypercholesterolaemia
Xeroderma pigmentosum	excessive freckling

Sickle-cell anaemia and trait and thalassaemia major and minor are examples of *balanced polymorphism* (the occurrence in a population of two or more genetically determined forms in frequencies such that the rarest of them could not be maintained by mutation alone). In certain areas of the world about 1 in every 25 children has sickle-cell anaemia, a very fatal disease so that the rate of elimination of the gene is relatively enormous. A mutation-rate high enough to compensate for a loss of this magnitude is inconceivable. About 1 in 3 in the general population is a carrier and has the sickle-cell trait which is relatively harmless. In the countries bordering the Mediterranean, thalassaemia is prevalent. In certain townships of northern Italy about 1 in every 5 of the population has thalassaemia minor, the majority of them suffering no ill effects. It can be expected, therefore, that about 1 in every 100 children born in these townships is doomed to die from the effects of Cooley's anaemia. The explanation of these astonishing observations is to be found in the fact that such genes as these *in the single dose* confer great advantages upon their possessors. In the case of thalassaemia the heterozygotes are very resistant during infancy and childhood to the prevalent falciparum malaria; they therefore survive to reproduce and disperse the gene and so balance the loss of the gene through the death of the homozygotes.

In a number of instances in which the carrier is not to be distinguished phenotypically from the homozygous unaffected, biochemical tests have been devised for the recognition of the heterozygote. For example, in acatalasia the carrier has an intermediate level of blood catalase; in phenylketonuria the fasting plasma phenylalanine level of the carrier is, on the average, higher than in those without this gene, also a large dose of phenylalanine is followed by a rise in the level of plasma phenylalanine greater than in those without this gene; in cystinuria there are excreted in the urine of the heterozygote moderate quantities of cystine and lysine but no arginine or ornithine; in galactosaemia the carrier can be identified by a distinctive degree of galactose tolerance; in the classical type of Duchenne muscular dystrophy the carrier tends to have a raised value of creatine kinase in the blood in the mild and in the severe sex-linked forms but not in the autosomal recessive form. In nephrogenic diabetes insipidus the carrier is unable to produce a normally concentrated urine; in classical haemophilia and in Christmas disease the heterozygote can often be detected by the value of anti-haemophilic globulin.

Polygenic (Multifactorial) and Partly Genetic Abnormalities

Very many of the 'normal' characters and most defects, derangements and disorders are of this kind. Stature, finger-print ridge patterns, body-build, birthweight, general intelligence, mental subnormality, disease resistance and susceptibility, major malformations of the central nervous system, congenital pyloric stenosis, spina bifida, Hirschsprung's disease, schizophrenia, diabetes mellitus, and benign essential hypertension are all examples of such. In their causation there is a genetic element, usually consisting of several genes, the effects of which are additive, and an environmental element that consists of some specific factor

or factors that in their action permit or encourage gene action. The relative importance of the two elements varies widely. Mendelian ratios cannot be fitted to the
mode of inheritance of such characters but from large scale investigations, twin
studies, pooled pedigrees and the like, it is possible to demonstrate that there is a
genetic element in aetiology and to compute the probability that relatives of an
affected individual will display the same character.

The Same Abnormality caused by Different Genes: Mimicry

Muscular dystrophy can be an autosomal recessive in some instances, a sex-
linked recessive in others. Of retinitis pigmentosa there are three distinct genetic
forms, an autosomal dominant, an autosomal recessive and a sex-linked recessive:
that this is so should not be surprising since the condition can be due to an abnormality of the retina, of the lens or of the whole optical apparatus. The dystrophic form of epidermolysis bullosa is an autosomal dominant as is also the simple
form of this disease, but the severe dystrophic form is an autosomal recessive and
in addition there is a very rare form that is a sex-linked recessive. Of ichthyosis
vulgaris there is an autosomal recessive form and a sex-linked recessive form. If
during the development and differentiation of a tissue or organ several developmental processes are involved, different genes affecting different processes could
easily yield the same end-result.

Because a particular abnormality has been shown to be genetically caused in
other instances it does not follow that this is so in a case being examined. The
impress of a particular environmental factor upon a developmental process can
produce an exact simulation of an abnormality that in many an instance is undoubtedly genetically based. For example, deafmutism, in about 50 per cent of
instances, is certainly genetic in origin, being an autosomal monogenic recessive
(it seems probable that there is more than one genetic form of this condition). In
the remaining 50 per cent of cases the condition is a consequence of disease, e.g.
meningitis, and is an acquisition, a *phenocopy*, a mimic. So it is that the mating
deafmute × deafmute, if one of the partners happens to be of the genetic kind and
the other of the acquired kind, can give none but unaffected carriers of the recessive
gene.

The Risks of Recurrence

The risk that another affected child will be born to parents who have already
produced one with a particular abnormality is high only in the case of the monogenic characters, the autosomal dominant, the autosomal recessive and the sex-
linked recessive; it is very much lower in the case of the polygenic and genetico-
environmental abnormality in which the recognition of the genetic element in
causation is far more difficult. In the case of the monogenic abnormalities the risk
can be stated with considerable confidence; with the polygenic and genetico-
environmental ones the probability has to be estimated in empirical terms and a
deep and wide knowledge of the relevant medical genetic literature is a prime
requirement.

In the case of an autosomal monogenic dominant abnormality, completely expressed, the risk is 50 per cent, it being assumed that one of the parents is an affected heterozygote, which is practically certain if the condition is a rare one. If both parents are unaffected, the abnormality of the affected infant being the result of a fresh mutation occurring in the germ-track of one of the parents, it is very unlikely that another child born to the same parents will be similarly affected. Once a child displaying a clearly autosomal monogenic recessive condition has been born to two unaffected parents, it is quite certain that each of the parents is a heterozygote and the risk of recurrence is therefore 25 per cent. In the case of a sex-linked monogenic recessive the risk that a brother of the affected male child will display the same condition and that a sister will be a carrier is 50 per cent, these predictions being based upon the assumption that the affected male child received the responsible recessive gene in the X-chromosome that came from his carrier mother.

As examples of the risk in cases of abnormalities of polygenic and genetico-environmental origin, the following can be cited. The risk of recurrence in spina bifida is 5 per cent; in anencephaly 5 per cent; in cleft lip with or without cleft palate, 4 per cent; in cleft palate about 1 in 80, with one parent with the same condition about 1 in 6, with both parents unaffected but with an affected relative, about 1 in 10; in congenital dislocation of the hip, 1 in 15 for a sister, 1 in 100 for a brother of an affected female (risks higher for sibs of an affected male); in pyloric stenosis 1 in 12 for a brother, 1 in 20 for a sister; in club-foot about 1 in 50; in lowgrade mental subnormality 1 in 25.

Maldistribution of Chromosomal Material as a cause of Abnormality in Characterisation

The human chromosomes differ among themselves in size and in respect of the position of the centromere in the length of the chromosome. They fall into seven

TABLE I

*Classification of the Chromosomes**

Group	Size and position of the centromere	Ideogram number	Number in each group male	female
I or A.	largest: median and sub-median	1–3	6	6
II or B.	large: sub-median	4 and 5	4	4
III or C.	medium: sub-median	6–12 + X	15	16
IV or D.	medium: sub-terminal	13–15	6	6
V or E.	small: median and sub-median	16–18	6	6
VI or F.	smallest: median	19 and 20	4	4
VII or G.	smallest: sub-terminal	21 and 22 + Y	5	4
			46	46

* For the study of the size, shape and number of the chromosomes a variety of tissues can be used; skin, bone marrow and peripheral blood are preferred. In the case of blood the leucocytes

size-groups ranging from the largest in group I or A to the smallest in group VII or G. In the metacentric chromosome the centromere is near its middle, in the acrocentric it is near an end and in the telocentric it is terminal. Intermediate positions of the centromere are sub-medial and sub-terminal.

Chromosome anomalies can be either numerical or structural. Autosomal anomalies have been reported in a wide variety of clinical conditions but for the most part these associations are inconstant. This is not so, however, in the case of the following:

Autosomal Numerical and Structural Anomalies associated with Specific Clinical Syndromes

Trisomy D	Patau's syndrome
Trisomy E	Edwards' syndrome
Trisomy G	Down's syndrome
Translocation 13–15/21–22	Down's syndrome
Translocation 21/21	Down's syndrome
Translocation 22/22	Down's syndrome

Deletion short arm of a group B chromosome (5?) Cri du chat syndrome
Deletion long arm of a group G chromosome (21?) Anti-mongolism
Deletion long arm of a group G chromosome (21?) Chronic granulocytic leukaemia.

Patau's syndrome has a frequency of about 1 in every 4,000 births. It is lethal, the infant living only a few hours and most examples of this condition die *in utero*. Its cause is non-disjunction involving one of the chromosomes of size-group D. About 1 in every 3,000–4,000 infants display the stigmata of Edwards' syndrome. Early death is the rule. The cause of the condition is non-disjunction involving one of the chromosomes of size-group E.

Once in every 600–700 livebirths an infant with Down's syndrome (mongolism) is encountered. Since the vast majority of these do not survive to reproduce, most instances of this condition, must arise *de novo*. This must be true also of Edwards' and Patau's syndromes. In the great majority of cases of Down's

---

are separated from the rest and added to a small volume of nutrient medium containing phyto-haemagglutinin which stimulates the leucocytes to divide. The cells are then cultured for about three days. Then a small quantity of colchicine is added. This has the property of preventing the formation of the spindle and halts mitosis at the stage of metaphase when the chromosomes are most clearly defined. Next, hypotonic saline solution is added and this causes the cells to swell so that the chromosomes become spread out. The cells are then transferred to a microscopic slide, fixed and stained and the preparation is then photographed. An enlargement is made and the individual chromosomes are cut out, arranged in pairs in descending order of size and numbered 1 to 22. Of the two sex-chromosomes, the X is of the same size as the members of group C and the Y of the same size as the members of group G. It is not at all easy to distinguish between individual chromosomes belonging to the same size group but it is possible to distinguish between any two size groups. The resulting arrangement is the *karyotype* and a diagrammatic representation of a karyotype is an ideogram. In the karyotype the chromosomes are seen to have begun to divide longitudinally and the two chromatids are still joined at a single point, the centromere. When this centromere is sub-terminal or acrocentric the chromosome is divided into a long and a short arm

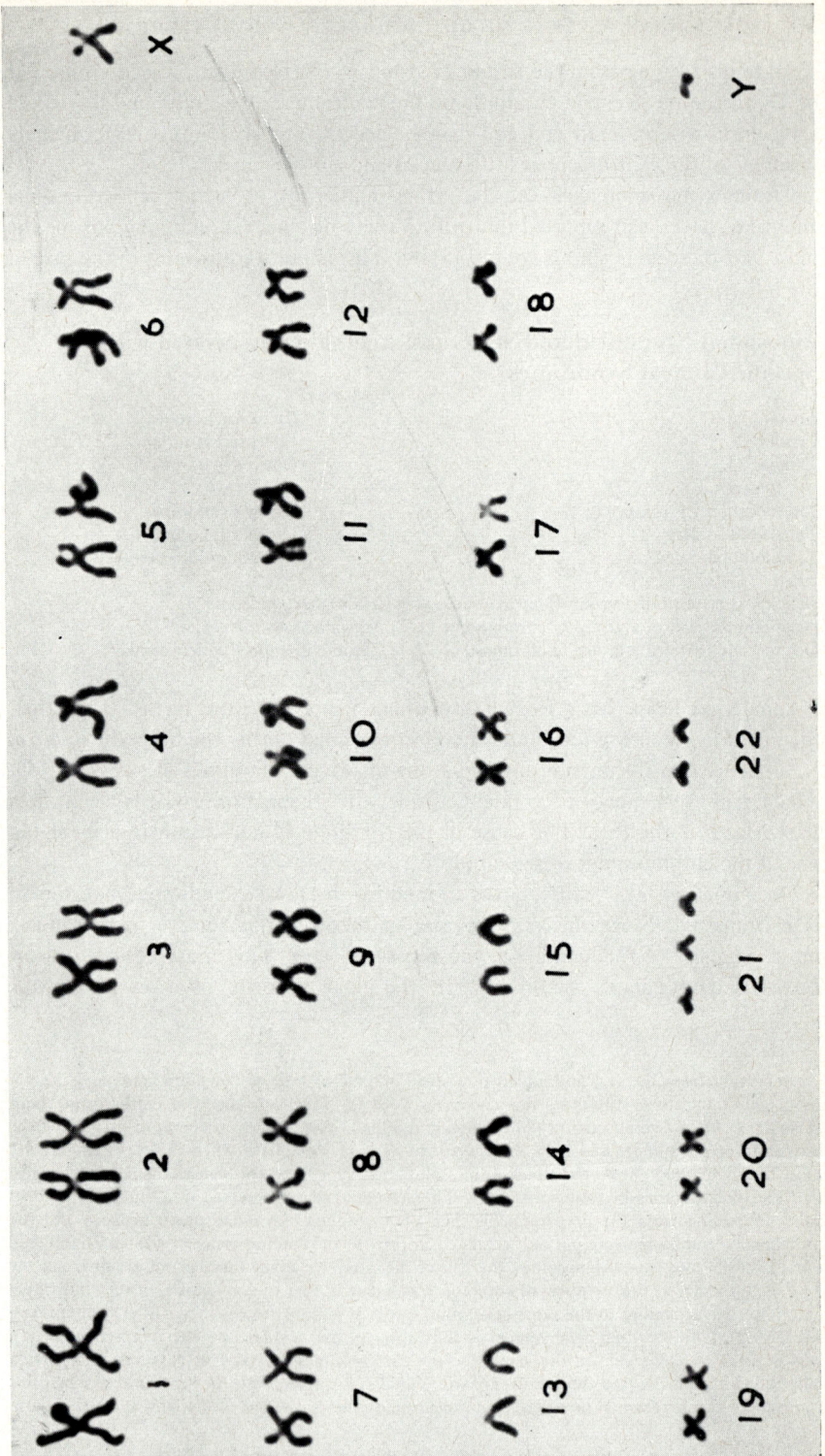

FIG. 1. Karyotype of a Human Male with Mongolism. Trisomy for chromosome 21.

syndrome the karyotype shows 47 chromosomes, there being three of one of size-group G, most probably 21, the result of non-disjunction. The ova produced by a woman with this condition are of two kinds, one with two 21s and the other with only one. These ova being fertilised by spermatozoa with the normal single 21 can give rise to infants with trisomy 21 or with the normal number of chromosomes including a pair of 21s. It is possible for one of a pair of identical twins to be triso-mic for 21 while the other is not, should non-disjunction occur at an early cleavage stage in the one and not in the other.

The cause of non-disjunction is not known as yet but the age of the mother, and therefore the age of the ovum, is certainly a factor that is involved. At the age of 25 the risk of producing an affected child is about 1 in 2,000; at the age of 35, 1 in 200; and at 40 and over it is 1 in 40. These estimates relate to women who have not had a child with Down's syndrome and in whose pedigrees there is no trace of this condition. But non-disjunction is not the only chromosome aberration that is associated with Down's syndrome for in women under 35 years of age an age-independent anomaly, translocation, is also a cause, though a less frequent one, of this condition. It is usually the female parent who has this translocation; the rare male with such an anomaly, for reasons as yet unknown, very seldom has affected offspring. The parent with the translocation, though possessing the normal number of chromosomes, 46, is found to have one or other of these translocations, 13–15/21–22, 21/21 or 21/22 so that one of the chromosomes is really a double one. If it is the mother that has the translocation the risk that any particular pregnancy will yield a child with Down's syndrome is 1 in 3, should the translocation be either the 13–15/21–22 (the D/G) or the 21/22 kind. But if it happens to be a 21/21 translocation, fortunately a very rare anomaly, then all her offspring will display the stigmata of this condition.

Unusual dermal ridge patterns are often found in these instances of trisomy but they are not specific for any one of them. They can be very helpful in diagnosis, however.

In infants with multiple congenital abnormalities a ring chromosome is some-times found. The ring is formed when a deletion occurs at both ends of a chromo-some, the ends thereafter becoming stuck to each other. Such ring formation has been described for several of the autosomes and also for the X. In chronic granulo-cytic leukaemia an abnormal chromosome, the Philadelphia or Ph[1] chromosome, has been observed in the blood and marrow cells. It is a very small chromosome that replaces one of those of size-group G and at first was thought to be derived from the Y. It is now thought to be a deletion of the long arm of one of the G group chromosomes. It is found only in individuals with this form of leukaemia but whether it is the cause or an effect of this condition is not yet decided.

Anomalies of the Sex-Chromosomes associated with Specific Clinical Entities

Non-disjunction of the X-chromosome during meiosis in the female can occur at the first division of the oocyte, at the second division or at both divisions. If it occurs at the first or second the mature ova will come to have either two Xs or else none at all. If it occurs at both divisions there can be ova with three or four Xs. In the male non-disjunction at the first division yields spermatozoa with the XY sex-chromosome constitution and spermatozoa with no sex-chromosome at all (O); at the second division XX, XY and O spermatozoa and at both divisions XXY, XYY, XXYY, X, Y and O spermatozoa.

Meiosis   *in the female*   *in the male*

Normality
Germ-cell   XX   XY

1st division: daughter-cells   X   X   X   Y

2nd division: mature gametes   X   X   X   X   X   X   Y   Y

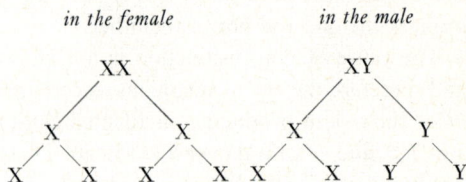

Non-disjunction: 1st division
Germ-cell   XX   XY

1st division: daughter-cells   XX   O   XY   O

2nd division: mature gametes   XX   XX O   O   XY   XY O   O

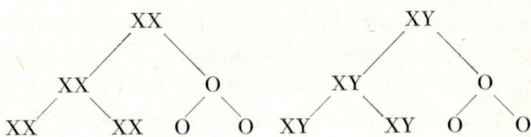

Non-disjunction: 2nd division
Germ-cell   XX   XY

1st division: daughter-cells   X   X   X   X

2nd division: daughter-cells   XX   O XX   O XX   O YY   O

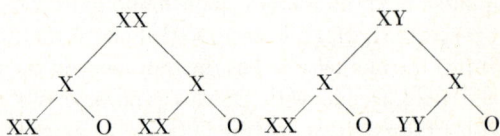

Non-disjunction: both divisions
Germ-cell   XX   XY

1st division: daughter-cells   XX   O   XY   O

2nd division: mature gametes   XXX   X O   O   XXY   Y   O   O
                                XXXX   O   XYY   X
                                                      XXYY O

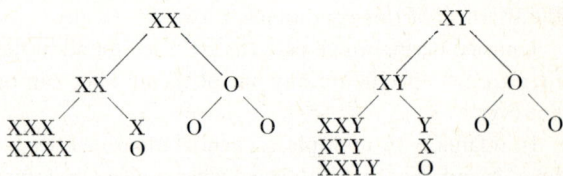

When such non-disjunctional ova and spermatozoa are available it becomes possible for a wide variety of karyotypes to appear among the zygotes resulting from fertilisation. Meiotic non-disjunction should yield an individual composed of cells all with the same abnormal number of chromosomes. Mitotic non-disjunction occurring at the first cleavage division of the fertilised ovum yields two kinds of cells, one with one chromosome fewer than the normal number and the other with one chromosome more than this. If it occurs at a later division it will give rise to three cell-lines, one with the normal number of chromosomes, 46, one with one fewer than this, 45, and one with one more, 47. Individuals whose bodies are composed of cells derived from two or more cell-lines are *mosaics*.

A mosaic can arise in another way, far less common than non-disjunction. An XX/XY mosaic can result from the fertilisation of a binucleated ovum by two different spermatozoa, one with an X and the other with a Y-chromosome. It is important to distinguish between a mosaic and a *chimaera*. In both there is more than one population of cells but whereas in the mosaic they are both of the same

| *Mitotic non-disjunction of the X-chromosome at the 1st division* | *At a later division* |

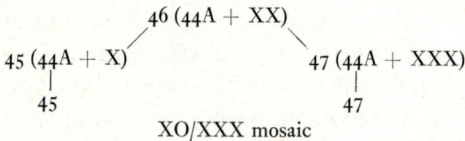

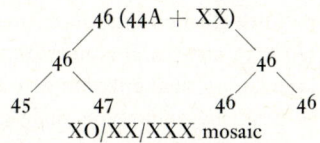

$$46\ (44A + XX)$$

$$45\ (44A + X) \qquad\qquad 47\ (44A + XXX)$$

$$45 \qquad\qquad\qquad 47$$

XO/XXX mosaic

$$46\ (44A + XX)$$

$$46 \qquad\qquad\qquad 46$$

$$45 \quad 47 \qquad\qquad 46 \quad 46$$

XO/XX/XXX mosaic

genetic origin, in a chimaera they are not, the two kinds of cells, differing in respect of their chromosome content, being derived from two different individuals. Human chimaeras have resulted from an exchange of cells across the placenta between fraternal twins *in utero*. In such chimaeras, as in identical twins, skin grafts can successfully be exchanged.

Abnormality in respect of the number of X-chromosomes can be detected by the use of the sex-chromatin and the drumstick tests. Lying just beneath the nuclear membrane in about 50 per cent of somatic cells in the female, e.g. the epithelial cells in a buccal smear or in the debris of the amniotic fluid, a Feulgen-positive particle, the sex-chromatin particle or Barr body, is to be found. This particle is absent from cells from tissues from a male. When it is present the individual is said to be chromatin-positive ($+$), when it is not present, chromatin-negative ($-$). The lobed nuclei of polymorph leucocytes from the female have, in a small proportion of instances, projections ('drumsticks') which are not found in similar cells from the male.

The number of sex-chromatin particles is one less than the number of X-chromosomes in the nuclei of the cells of the individual so that the XY male has none and the XX female has one per cell. It is now accepted that this particle, in the mouse, the cat, the human subject and possibly in all mammals, represents an X-chromosome that is genetically inactive and much condensed. According to what is known as the Lyon hypothesis there occurs at an early stage of embryogenesis a random inactivation of one (or of part of one) of the two X-chromosomes and all the descendants of the cell with the inert X maintain this inactivity of the same X. The result is that the female is a mosaic consisting of two cell-populations. In one of these one X is active and the other rests; in the second of these cell-lines the latter X is active and the other one is inert so that when the two differ in respect of the genes they carry this phenomenon of mosaicism can be observed. In ocular albinism, for example, the iris and fundus of the affected hemizygous male are completely lacking in pigment whereas in the heterozygous female there is a mosaic pattern of pigmentation, some areas being pigmented, others not.

Since it is the rule that an XY zygote follows the developmental path that ends in a male-type phenotype and that an XX zygote comes to assume the characterisation of a female, the chromatin-particle and the drumstick tests can be used with confidence for the identification of the sex of an individual when, for any reason, doubt concerning this exists. The sex-chromatin particle can be identified in interphase but not dividing nuclei in cells from the majority of tissues from the female body.

Sex-dimorphism

Since chromosome anomalies of this kind are so closely and so regularly associated with structural abnormality of the gonads, of the external genitalia and of the accessory sexual apparatus, it is necessary to state what, in this particular context, is meant by phenotypic male and female. The term phenotypic merely means that the physical attributes of the individual are male-like or female-like, that the individual has the general appearance of a male or of a female, having regard to such features as body-build, stature, distribution of hair and the like. It is also desirable to give precise definitions to such terms as sex, male, female, intersex and hermaphrodite.

Sex is the term used to define the division of the individuals of a species into the two more or less contrasted forms known respectively as male and female, the two sexes. Male is the term used to define that sex which is equipped for the production of male-type gametes, female that applied to the sex that is equipped for the production of female-type gametes. In the higher forms of life the two types of gametes are physiologically and structurally different, the female-type being characteristically relatively large, food-laden and passive while the male-type is relatively small, lean and motile. The gametes are the products of the gonads, of the male-type testis and of the female-type ovary. In a species such as our own in which the two sexes can readily be distinguished by differences in characterisation, this sex-dimorphism can be broken down into differences in (i) the sex-chromosome constitution, (ii) the structure and physiology of the gonads, (iii) the anatomy of the accessory sexual apparatus of glands and associated ducts that are concerned with the transference of the gametes from the gonads to the site of fertilisation, (iv) the anatomy of the external genitalia and (v) a number and variety of cutaneous, skeletal, physiological and psychological features, the secondary sexual characters, not exercised in sexual congress but playing their parts in courtship and, in the case of the female, in the post-natal care of the young.

Maleness, the state associated with the production of male-type gametes and femaleness, that associated with the elaboration of female-type gametes, can co-exist in one and the same individual. Such an individual, possessing the equipment necessary for the production of both kinds of gametes, either at the same time or at different times, is an hermaphrodite. In unisexual species, in which the individual is either a male or else a female and produces only one form of gamete, male-type or female-type, hermaphroditism is abnormality. Normality in respect of maleness and femaleness in the unisexual species is a reflection of the condition of congruence between all the five classes of sex-dimorphic characters listed above. When all of them are male-type or when all of them are female-type, normality exists. Intersexuality, essentially, is the condition of incongruity between these five sets of characters, e.g. a male-type sex-chromosome constitution and a female-type gonadal structure or external genitalia or with a mixture of male-type and female-type structures of the accessory sexual apparatus. About 3 in every 1,000 babies born display some grade of intersexuality. Hermaphroditism in a unisexual species is regarded by some as being a high-grade form of intersexuality.

The basic cause of the sex-dimorphism that distinguishes male from female is the difference between two distinct genetic constitutions. In these there are many genes that are particularly concerned with the determination of sex, some being female-determining, others male-determining. The latter have become congregated in the Y-chromosome and the autosomes, the former in the X-chromosome. In the XY zygote the male-determining genes are in effective excess of the female-determining, whereas in the XX zygote the female-determining genes are in effective excess. The quantitative difference between these two kinds of sex-determining genes decides which kind of internal physiological environment shall become established within the developing embryo, one of maleness or one of femaleness. As the embryo evolves the precursors of the gonads are laid down. To begin with they are completely undifferentiated but soon come to consist of two parts, a cortex and a medulla, the former being the forerunner of the ovary, the latter having a specific potentiality for becoming a testis. In the male-type internal environment the growth and differentiation of the medulla are encouraged and those of the cortex inhibited; in the female-type of internal environment the differentiation of the cortex into an ovary is promoted.

When the gonads have become differentiated and endocrinologically functional they assume control of the differentiation of the rest of the sexual and reproductive equipment. A zygote becomes equipped with a male-type characterisation because it was, in the beginning, an XY zygote in which the male-determining forces were paramount with the result that the gonads became testes, functionally active. A zygote becomes equipped with the female-type characterisation because, in the beginning, it was an XX zygote in which there was no Y-chromosome and in the absence of this particular chromosome, it is generally agreed, the developmental path that is followed is one that ends in a neutral or female-type characterisation. So, because the zygote is an XX zygote, the female-determining genes are able to direct the differentiation of the primordial gonads into ovaries and these, becoming endocrinologically functional, play their part in the control of the differentiation of the rest of the sexual and reproductive equipment.

Abnormality of Sexual Characterisation

It follows that abnormality of the sexual characterisation can result from (a) disturbance of the genic equilibrium between the male-determining and the female-determining genes by gene mutation or aneuploidy; (b) delay in the elaboration of those forces that control the differentiation of the embryonic gonads and (c) a lack of response on the part of those tissues that are components of the accessory sexual apparatus and genitalia to the endocrine stimulus provided by the differentiated gonads.

It is established that hormonal stimuli other than those provided by the differentiated gonads can profoundly affect the processes of sex-differentiation. An XX zygote can be diverted, in its development, in a male-type direction by the androgenic activity on the part of a hormonally active tumour, such as an arrhenoblastoma, in the mother. Hormone therapy of the pregnant mother, involving testosterone proprionate, methyl testosterone and the like, can masculinise the XX fetus whose ovaries will remain unaffected but there can be a fusion of the labia and a much enlarged clitoris with a penile urethra. In the adreno-genital syndrome the external appearance and general physique of an XX zygote are masculinised by the action of androgens secreted by the enlarged adrenal cortex. This hyperplasia of the adrenal cortex and this increased production of androgens are the consequences of deficient cortical function, taking the form of an inadequate synthesis of cortisol. The ultimate cause of this syndrome would seem to be an autosomal recessive gene that in its action causes a deficiency of certain cortical enzymes that are necessary for the synthesis of cortisol. The degree of masculinisation is determined by the time during ontogeny at which the increase in androgen production reaches the threshold level at which differentiation will proceed in the male direction. In the XY zygote the effect of the increase in androgen production is a precocious puberty.

Already about 50 different combinations and permutations of the X- and Y-chromosomes have been recorded and doubtless there are many more to come; they range from a singleton, $44A + XO$, to as many as 15 sex-chromosomes in the triple mosaic $44A + XXXY/XXXXY/XXXXXY$. The clinical features associated with these sex-chromosome aberrations vary very greatly. They can roughly be divided into four groups, (i) those that are, as far as can be discerned, near-normal or normal male-type or female-type characterisations, (ii) those in which imperfection in a male-type or female-type phenotype exists, (iii) those in which there is a degree of incongruity among he sex-dimorphic characters, in which intersexuality exists and (iv) those in which imperfect ambisexuality, hermaphroditism, exists.

Examples of unusual sex-chromosome numbers and combinations that have been encountered are:

in the phenotypic male, XX, XXY, XYY, XXYY, XXXY, XXXXY, XXXYY, XY/XX, XY/XXY, XO/XXY, XO/XXY.
in the phenotypic female, XO, XY, XXX, XXXX, XXXXX, XO/XY, XO/XX, XO/XXX, XO/XYY, XO/XX/XXX.
in the 'hermaphrodite', XX, XX/XY, XO/XY, XX/XXX, XX/XXY/XXYYY.

The phenotypic male with the XX sex-chromosome constitution, chromatin-positive, is rare and may well be either an XXY male in whom the Y was lost at an early cleavage division after male-type differentiation had already become established, or else an XX/XXY mosaic in which the second of these cell-lines had not been identified. Other instances may be the result of crossing-over between the homologous segments of the X and the Y during spermatogenesis in the male parent who then contributed to an XX zygote an X which was in part Y-chromosomal material.

Chromatin-positive phenotypic males with sex-chromosome constitutions ranging from XXY to XXXXY, together with various forms of mosaicism, of which the commonest is XY/XXY, are usually found in such as display the stigmata of Klinefelter's syndrome. Of those with the XXY constitution, 25 per cent are mentally subnormal; those with the XXYY or XXXY are invariably subnormal; such as are XXXXY have testicular hypoplasia and are mentally gravely subnormal while those with the XXXYY, XY/XX, XY/XXY, XO/XXY, XX/XXY, XO/XYY, XXXY/XXXXY and XXXY/XXXXY/XXXXXY constitutions show very variable clinical features. Klinefelter's syndrome is a condition of imperfection of the sex-equipment in the male. Eighty per cent of the cases are chromatin-positive, have a male-type phenotype, have atrophic and azoospermic testes and may or may not develop gynaecomastia at the time of puberty. The XYY (and the XXYY) males have so far been encountered mainly in maximum security hospitals. Typically they are well above average height, mentally retarded and aggressive. But since it is not yet known how frequently this sex-chromosome constitution with its extra Y occurs in the general population, it cannot be concluded that such a constitution predetermines that the individual possessing it shall display an anti-social behaviour pattern.

In the phenotypic female the following chromosome constitutions have been found in association with Turner's syndrome (complete primary agonadism) XO, XO/XX, XO/XY, XO/XXX, XO/XYY, XO/XX/XXX. The majority of cases are chromatin-negative females of short stature with ovarian dysgenesis or aplasia. In the place of the ovaries are streaks of whitish tissue; the rest of the sex-equipment is of the female (or neutral) type and remains infantile in proportions at puberty. A few cases of Turner's syndrome have been found to be chromatin-positive and to have the normal number of chromosomes, 46, but one of the Xs is considerably larger than is usual and this enlargement is the result of a duplication of its long arm; its short arm is missing. This *isochromosome* results from the transverse division of the centromere instead of the normal longitudinal division. The XXX and XXXX phenotypic females can either be normal in every way or else suffer from primary or secondary amenorrhoea. Turner's syndrome is a condition of imperfection in the female.

There are two kinds of phenotypic female with the XY constitution. The first consists of individuals who are noticeably tall and eunuchoid with external genitalia of the female pattern and with a uterus but no gonads. Since in the experimental animal it is established that the removal of the embryonic ovary does not prevent the assumption of the female-type accessory sexual apparatus and external genitalia, whereas the removal of the embryonic testes blocks differentiation in the male direction so that the accessory sexual apparatus and external genitalia come to be of the neutral or female-type, it is accepted that these individuals with this gonadal dysgenesis are grossly imperfect males because, for reasons as yet unknown, the embryonic gonads failed to become testes in an XY zygote.

The second kind of phenotypic female with the XY sex-chromosome constitution is characterised by female-type external genitalia, normal breasts but no uterus and by the presence of testes. This is the condition known as testicular feminisation and most probably is genetically caused, the gene responsible being either a sex-linked recessive or else an autosomal dominant that, in its action, causes a metabolic block in the production of the masculinising evocator substances produced by the medulla of the primordial gonad or alternatively renders the tissues of the developing genital apparatus unresponsive to the action of these substances. The condition is one of imperfection in the male.

These phenotypic females with the male-type sex-chromosome constitution raise the question as to whether or not they are instances of incomplete sex-reversal, of the transformation of a male into a female. The same question presented itself when the phenotypic male with the XX constitution was first described. Complete sex-reversal does occur and can be experimentally induced in animals other than man so that this question has to be examined. The notion that incongruence between the sex-chromosome constitution and the rest of the sex-dimorphic characters constitutes partial or complete sex-reversal stems directly from the invention of the terms nuclear sex, chromosomal sex, gonadal sex, apparent (or phenotypic) sex, psychological sex and social sex and their extensive use in medical literature. These terms, useful though they may be, can be very misleading. Maleness and femaleness and hermaphroditism are characterisations of complete individuals and not of their component cells or organs and organ-systems. An XY zygote at the moment of fertilisation is not a male; it is a zygote that is so endowed genetically that, if all goes well during development and differentiation, from it there will arise an individual that will display the characterisation that is typical of the male, it has the potentialities of becoming a male. All that is meant by nuclear sex is the presence or absence of the sex-chromatin-particle; chromosomal sex is merely an easy way of indicating the sex-chromosome constitution of the karyotype, XY or XX; gonadal sex is merely an imprecise way of stating that the gonads have the structure of testes or of ovaries, male-type and female-type respectively; social sex is the term used to define the opinion of other people concerning the sex of a particular individual. A perfectly normal (physically) female can masquerade as a male and be accepted by society as such; a male child with indeterminate external genitalia can be thought to be a girl and raised as such only later to be found to be an imperfect male.

Pseudohermaphroditism

Of the intersexual condition known as pseudohermaphroditism there are two forms, a male form in which the individual has a male-type phenotype, is chromatin-negative and has testes while the rest of the sex-equipment shows a degree of feminisation, and a female form in which the individual has the female-type phenotype, is chromatin-positive and has two ovaries while the rest of the sex-equipment shows a degree of masculinisation. The male pseudohermaphrodite is an imperfect male in whom the masculinising stimulus normally provided by the differentiated testes is either deficient or lacking altogether so that the accessory sexual apparatus and external genitalia pursued an uncontrolled differentiation to assume the neutral or female pattern. The cause of female pseudohermaphroditism is usually congenital adrenal hyperplasia in a female. In both male and female forms genetic factors would seem to be involved.

True Hermaphroditism

The essential feature of the condition known as 'true hermaphroditism' is the presence in one and the same individual of both testicular and ovarian tissues (not necessarily perfect in either structure or function). There is a wide range of variation in the general appearance of these individuals, ranging from the masculine to the feminine and an equally wide range in the anatomy of the external genitalia from the almost completely male-type to the almost completely female-type. Some of them are chromatin-positive, others chromatin-negative. The sex-chromosome constitution is also very varied. The gonads can be one ovary and one testis, an ovary and an ovo-testis or two ovo-testes. In view of the wide range of variation it is indeed difficult to find any one explanation that could cover all the recorded cases. Since it is thought that testicular material can only develop if there is a Y-chromosome present in the karyotype it would seem that the hermaphrodite should be an XY/XX mosaic. Some are but others are XY or XX. In several of the recorded cases the gonadic tissues are so ill-developed that it is reasonable to wonder if the condition is really one of 'true hermaphroditism'. The fault is surely to be found in the genic control of the differentiation of the embryonic gonads. Normally either the medulla or the cortex is encouraged to pursue its development, in the hermaphrodite there seems to be neither encouragement nor inhibition so that both medulla and cortex flourish and provide both testicular and ovarian tissues. Possibly genetic factors are responsible for the disturbance of the quantitative relationship of the male-determining and female-determining genes, neither of these sets of genes being in effective excess throughout the whole period of time during which the differentiation of the gonads proceeds.

When all these sex-chromosome aberrations and the clinical conditions associated with them are reviewed, it becomes possible to arrive at a number of conclusions concerning them. If one component of a mosaic is XO the phenotype is Turner-like; if one component of a mosaic has one or more Xs additional to the normal XY, the phenotype is Klinefelter-like; if a mosaic contains both the XO and the Klinefelter-determining component, the XO element dominates and the phenotype is Turner-like. Two sex-chromosomes are necessary for the development of a normal gonad and if one of these is a Y the embryonic gonads become testes, but if there is more than one X associated with this Y the development of the testis remains imperfect. The YO constitution has not so far been encountered and probably does not exist for the reason that it is incompatible with continued life. Though as a general rule such conditions as trisomy of an autosome, loss of a part, if not of the whole, of an autosome and the addition of several sex-chromosomes lead to abnormality of characterisation, they are not lethal.

Estimated Frequencies of Genetic and Genetico-environmental Abnormalities

Stevenson (1963) gives the following figures for the frequencies in liveborn infants of certain groups of abnormalities which are either present at birth or become manifest later.

	Frequencies per 1,000 births
Malformations of complex genetic and environmental aetiology	20
Malformations due to single major genes	5
Disorders associated with chromosome aberrations	4
Single gene traits determining disease	8
Erythroblastosis	4
Common disorders with genetic components in their aetiology	10
	51

Stevenson, Carr, and Hall and Källen, among others, have studied the frequencies of these chromosome aberrations among abortuses. They found that they were, for the most part, the same as those encountered in the liveborn infant but had higher frequencies, with the exception of polyploidy (a multiple of the haploid number, $3n$, for example) which is exceedingly rare in the liveborn infant. Stevenson, in a report to the Vth World Congress on Gynaecology and Obstetrics, dealt with 1,000 spontaneous abortions.

Aberration	Frequency
XO	20 per cent
Polyploidies	22 ,, ,,
Trisomy 16–18 size group chromosome	14 ,, ,,
Trisomy 21–22 size-group chromosome	12 ,, ,,
Mosaics for aneuploidies	7 ,, ,,
Trisomy 13–15 size-group chromosome	6 ,, ,,
Structural changes in the chromosomes	6 ,, ,,
Trisomy 1–3 size-group chromosome	5 ,, ,,
Trisomy in other chromosome size-groups	5 ,, ,,
XXY or XYY	3 ,, ,,

Because of the higher frequencies of these abnormalities in those dying in the perinatal period and earlier, it is reasonable to conclude that while certain of them are the causes of death *in utero* they all lower the viability of the infant before and after birth.

Conclusion

As morbidity and mortality from all causes decreases as a consequence of expanding control over the environmental causes, the role of the genetic causes becomes increasingly high-lighted. Preventive action against diseases of environmental origin will certainly continue to be successful and the time is coming when similar action against defects, derangements and disorders of genetic origin will be called for. For the present the power to prevent and to cure these is very limited but, as biochemistry continues to make its contributions to medicine, the efficiency of therapy will certainly enlarge. In so far as those abnormalities which are genetico-environmental in origin are concerned, it is most likely that it will always remain easier to bring the environmental element in causation under control and when this has been done the genetic element is rendered impotent.

The genes and the chromosome aberrations that are responsible for so much suffering and distress constitute a challenge that cannot possibly be disregarded. At present it can be met only in the genetic counselling clinic. There can be no doubt, however, that in the future, possibly not very remote, the knowledge that is being forged with such amazing speed in the field of molecular biology will be transmuted into the power of controlling the sequences and arrangements within the deoxyribonucleic acid molecule. The time will surely come when it will be possible to identify certain of the abnormalities of genetic and cytogenetic origin in the fetus and to remedy them before birth and to prevent the development of certain kinds of abnormality in the unborn child by the treatment of the pregnant mother. These things will come to pass for the need for them is so strong and so urgent. As knowledge expands, the power of medicine to prevent and to cure will become enlarged and the ethical aspects of medical intervention will assume an ever-increasing importance. In the meantime it must suffice to prepare for the future, for the time when genetical therapy will take its place alongside genetical diagnosis and prognosis as an integral part of medical education and practice.

F. A. E. CREW

References

ARMSTRONG, C. N. and MARSHALL, A. J. (1964) (Ed.). *Intersexuality in Vertebrates, Including Man*. London: Academic Press.

BLYTH, H. and CARTER, C. O. (1969). *A Guide to Genetic Prognosis in Paediatrics*. London: Spastics International Med. Publ.

CARR, D. H. (1963). Chromosome studies in abortuses and stillborn infants. *Lancet*, 2, 603.

CARTER, C. O. (1969). *An ABC of Medical Genetics*. London: Lancet.

COURT BROWN, W. M. *et al.* (1964). Abnormalities of the sex-chromosome complex in man. *Med. Res. Counc. Spec. Rpt*. 305. London.

—— (1967). *Human Population Cytogenetics*. Amsterdam, North Holland Publ. Co.

CREW, F. A. E. (1968). *Sex Determination*. 4th ed. London: Methuen.

DARLINGTON, C. D. (1958). *Evolution of Genetic Systems*. Edinburgh: Oliver and Boyd.

EMERY, A. E. H. (1968). *Elements of Medical Genetics*. Edinburgh: Livingstone.

HALL, B. and KÄLLEN, B. (1964). Chromosome studies in abortuses and stillborn infants. *Lancet*, 1, 110.

HAMERTON, J. L. (1962). *Chromosomes in Medicine*. Little Club Clinic No. 5. London: Spastics Society/Heinemann.

HARRIS, H. (1966). *Human Biochemical Genetics*. 2nd ed. Cambridge: Univ. Press.

HSIA, D. YI-YUNG (1968). *Human Developmental Genetics*. Chicago: Year Book Med. Publ.

McKUSICK, V. A. (1964). *Human Genetics*. New Jersey: Prentice-Hall.

—— (1966). *Mendelian Inheritance in Man: Catalog of Autosomal Dominant, Autosomal Recessive and X-linked Phenotypes*. London: Heinemann.

OVERZIER, C. (1963). (Ed.). *Intersexuality*. London: Acad. Press.
PAPAZIAN, H. P. (1967). *Modern Genetics*. London: Weidenfeld and Nicolson.
ROBERTS, J. A. FRASER (1970). *An Introduction to Medical Genetics*. 5th ed. London: Oxf. Univ. Press.
STEVENSON, A. C. (1963). (Ed.). Human genetics. *Brit. Med. Bull.*, **17**, 3.

2   Prenatal Development

ALL living creatures are the product of their heredity and their environment. This statement is so obvious that it is easy to overlook the commonplace miracle of man's normal development in all its functional and structural complexity.

A faulty genetic endowment is responsible for hereditary defects but often congenital abnormalities result from 'a flaw, localised in space and time in some aspect of the ontogenetic pattern for which some environmental factor, acting upon a particular process of development, is to blame'. (Wyburn, 1953).

Earliest Stages of Development

Three main periods of prenatal development have been described by Hamilton, Boyd and Mossman (1962):

1. From the time of fertilisation to the full implantation of the blastocyst, but before the establishment of an intra-embryonic circulation, that is to say, up to a gestational age of 21 days.
2. From the beginning of the fourth week to the end of the eighth week, during which all the main organs and systems are differentiated.
3. From the end of the eighth week until delivery, a period of quantitative rather than qualitative change. This is the period of growth rather than new development.

Human ova are only likely to be fertilised within about the first 12 hours of ovulation but spermatozoa may retain their ability up to 48 hours after their emission. The ovum takes 4 or 5 days to reach the uterine cavity after ovulation and starts to embed in the uterine decidua about the sixth day. Rock and Hertig (1948) studied very early human ova and embryos in hysterectomy specimens and found that the embryo is at the eight-cell stage within 3 days of fertilisation. The embryo now enters the blastocyst stage and by the tenth day it is fully embedded in the endometrium, its diameter by now being about half a millimetre. By the fourteenth day the amniotic sac has enveloped the ectoderm and trophoblastic masses on the surface, which, having opened up the capillary network within the endometrium, now form lacunae and are bathed and nourished by maternal blood. These early villi soon receive their mesoblastic core and by the sixteenth day a system of branching villi is developing.

We have been much interested in studying by sonar the levels of nidation of the ovum in very early pregnancy, but it is not until between 3 and 4 weeks after ovulation and fertilisation that a gestation sac can be seen by this means (Donald, 1965, 1967, 1968a and b) (Fig. 2). The normal situation is very high up in the uterus. One would expect those apparently implanting low in the uterine cavity to develop placenta praevia in later pregnancy but our experience hitherto suggests that these cases are followed by abortion. It is possible that more mid-cavity as

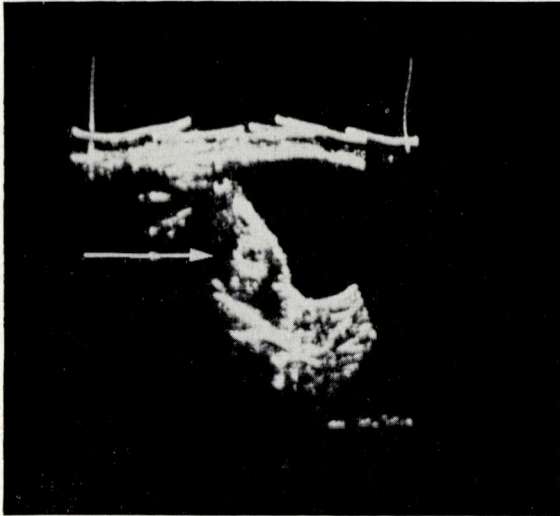

FIG. 2. Six weeks' amenorrhoea. Gestation sac in utero
(arrow). Longitudinal section. Cranialwards to left.

distinct from high-cavity implantations are precursors to placenta praevia but we have not yet established this point beyond doubt.

Blighted Ovum

Rock and Hertig commented that 12 out of the 26 embryos which they had studied as above were already clearly blighted in one respect or another. It has to be noted, however, that this high figure may be the result of indications for which the hysterectomy was done, which in themselves may have constituted an unfavourable environment. Nevertheless the wastage in fetal life which occurs at this time is greater than at any subsequent period. Ultrasonograms are useful not only in showing the level of nidation of the gestation sac but also in indicating maturity which can be very easily assessed at this stage by the size of the sac and the rate of enlargement in the normal case (Donald, 1967, 1968a and b). The blighted ovum, however, shows either no such clean ring appearance within the uterus but rather a more blotchy mass, or else a ring which fails to grow at the proper rate. This method has a good deal of promise in studying the very early development of the fetus in prenatal life (Donald, 1969).

Further Early Growth

By the ninth week of menstrual age of the pregnancy, i.e. 7 weeks from the time of fertilisation in a normal 28 day menstrual cycle, a small dot may appear

within this ring representing the fetal body (Fig. 3). Between the tenth and
eleventh weeks, the uterine cavity is completely filled by the enlarging gestation
sac, after which the echoes become difficult to interpret because of their multiplicity.
Usually by the thirteenth week, however, the fetal head can be separately identified
by the demonstration of the midline echoes, presumably from the falx cerebri.

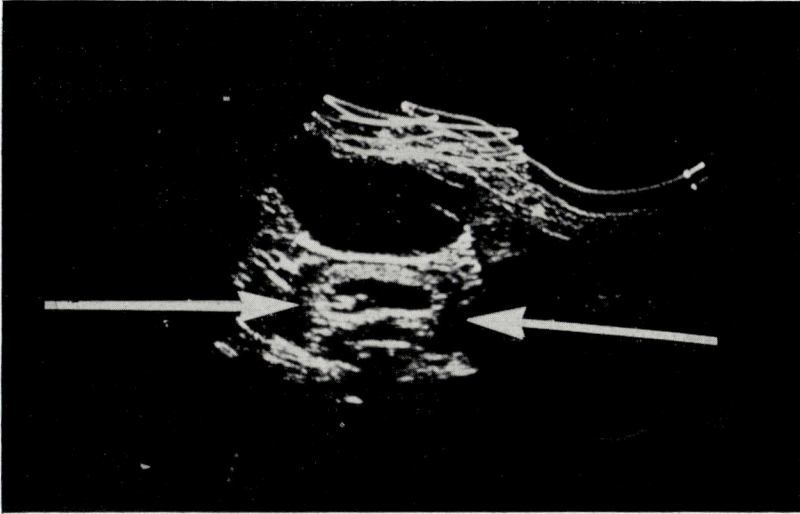

FIG. 3. Nine weeks' amenorrhoea. Fetal body visible within
gestation sac. Transverse section.

The fetal heart beat can be detected by the ultrasonic Doppler effect with ease
at the thirteenth week, usually at the twelfth week and occasionally at the eleventh
week of gestation (menstrual age).

The embryo enters upon the second stage of its development having survived
the first 3 weeks. By now its size and volume have become too great for subsistence
to be maintained by the diffusion of materials through its surface and there is a
growing need for a circulatory system to distribute to its different parts the materials for further development. This involves the need for blood as a vehicle, the
development of vessels in which it is to travel and the mechanical force of a pump
in the form of a heart in order to distribute the materials. Already by the eighteenth
day blood islands and vessel rudiments are present in the chorion and its villi, as
well as the body stalk, yolk sac and embryo itself. At 21 days a circulation of sorts
is established between the embryo and the early vessels within the villi.

The Placenta as an Organ of Nutrition and Excretion

It was once thought that maternal and fetal circulations flowed by counter
current in opposite directions in order to increase the efficiency of the gradients of
gaseous transfer, as occurs in rabbits, but this has not been substantiated in the
human.

There are several possible different mechanisms by which the placenta is believed to transfer gases, electrolytes, antibodies, nutrient substances and excretory products, some simple and some too complex to be yet understood.

Simple diffusion applies to the interchange of respiratory gases, oxygen and carbon dioxide, and the more simple electrolytes. This is sometimes referred to

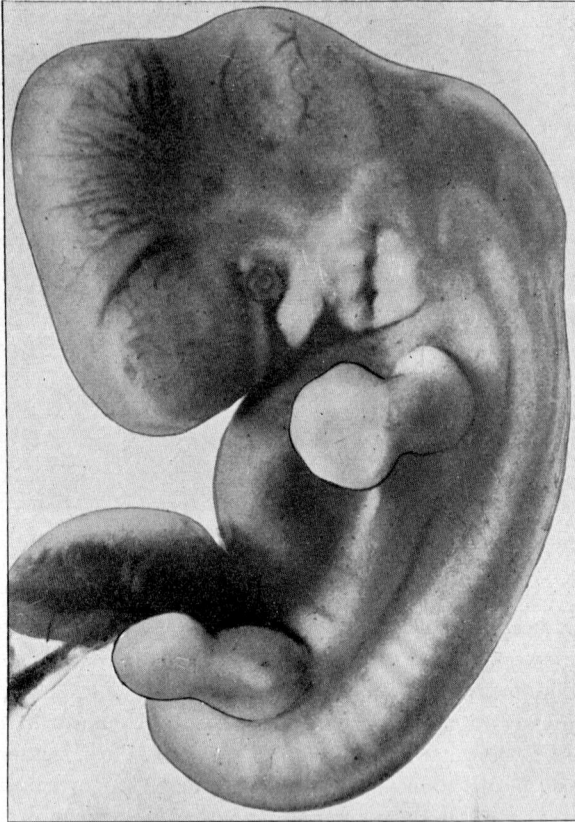

FIG. 4. Human embryo of about five and a half weeks showing the primary curve of the spine in the mesenchyme stage when cartilage is appearing in the vertebrae and ossification has not yet occurred (No. 801 in Professor J. P. Hill's collection at University College, London. Harris, H. A., 1943. *Proc. Roy. Soc. Med.*, 36, 300).

as a 'downhill' mechanism which operates until chemical equilibrium is established on either side of the membrane. The mechanism of 'facilitated diffusion' applies to slightly more complex molecules such as glucose in which some energy is expended by the placenta in transferring this substance. A more active transport mechanism has to be invoked to explain the movement of a substance 'uphill, against an electrochemical gradient and here the intervention of an enzyme pathway is usually postulated. It is thought that amino acids in their transfer across the placenta from mother to fetus require this mechanism. Really large molecules such as proteins, gamma globulins, invoke a process of pinocytosis in which the substances are engulfed in amoeboid fashion and transported across the so-called placental barrier.

The placenta is such a good excretory organ for the fetus that there is no need, during intra-uterine life, for an efficient genito-urinary system. In fact, a baby may be born alive at term with bilateral renal agenesis or a complete obstruction to urinary outflow. Compared with other special organs the development of the kidney from the metanephros occurs relatively late in embryonic life and only begins in the fifth week. Increasing numbers of glomeruli develop up to the time at which the fetus reaches a weight of about $5\frac{1}{2}$ lb. or 2,500 g. (Potter, 1961), and furthermore if an infant is born before that size is reached, glomerular formation continues for a time after birth. Nevertheless, even the very immature kidney is capable of secreting a dilute urine fairly early on and urine can be found in the bladder at 16 weeks' gestation.

The fetus is known to excrete urine into the liquor amnii and oligohydramnios may result from renal agenesis or from congenital obstruction to urinary outflow. The extent to which fetal urine contributes to the quantity of liquor amnii is not known, but urea can be detected in the liquor even before the sixteenth week. The lobulated fetal form of the kidney persists long after renal development is otherwise complete, i.e. about 36 weeks, and may persist for some weeks after birth. The ability of the kidneys to concentrate urine, and indeed to demonstrate a full excretory functional capacity, is not achieved until some time after birth.

The above brief summary of events may help to explain at least some of the difficulties which the immature infant may have in controlling its own fluid and electrolyte balance after birth.

Adverse Environmental Factors and their Effects on Prenatal Development

Until recently it was assumed that antenatal care which was in all respects obstetrically adequate for the mother was also automatically all that could be expected for the child in utero. When, therefore, malformations cropped up they were accepted with sorry fatalism. But there is now increasing evidence that the child may be injured by agents which are fairly innocuous to the mother and that, in those children who survive, many diseases of childhood originate in prenatal life (Warkany, 1957). This modern concept of fetal medicine puts a new responsibility on present and future generations of obstetricians who must increasingly recognise the interests of two patients instead of one (Gairdner, 1968).

In a prospective study in Birmingham of 57,000 children from birth, an incidence of congenital defects was found of 17·3 per thousand at the age of a fortnight and 23 per thousand at the age of 5 years (McKeown and Record, 1960). It was also noted that the frequency of congenital malformations had doubled in Scotland in the previous decade (McKeown, 1961). A fifth of all these affected children died at birth and only a half reached the age of 5 years. Other sources tell a similar tale. For instance in a pamphlet on malformations issued by the Ministry of Health (1963), it is reckoned that some abnormality was present in more than 1 per cent of children surviving to the age of a year. Twenty per cent of stillbirths were found to be deformed; likewise over a fifth of spontaneous abortions are associated with chromosomal aberration (Carr, 1967). Conversely about 15 per cent of cases of congenital abnormality are stillborn and a further 30 per cent die in the first 12 months. About half survive to over the age of 5 years. In rough figures it can be reckoned that about one in every 50 babies is born malformed in some degree.

It is now clear that healthy prenatal development can be interfered with even before conception (see Chap. 1). Nevertheless adverse genetic effects must to some extent be capable of being modified by environment since in cases of mono-chorionic, so-called identical twins it is possible for one child to have a congenital defect which is not matched by the other, for example in Down's syndrome, and yet their genetic endowment must have been the same originally. It would be a mistake, therefore, to divide fetal handicaps into cast-iron categories of those due to genetic and those due to environmental factors. Bacsich (1964) classified abnormalities into three main groups: 10 per cent are due to genetic factors and traceable in the family history, 10 per cent are due to some chromosomal aberration and the vast majority, namely 80 per cent, are due to some extraneous teratogenic factor. Anatomically he classifies them under the following headings:

1. Arrestation, resulting in either failure of differentiation or failure of development.
2. Failures of fusion, for example cleft palate and spina bifida.
3. Failures of the normal and expected atrophy with the persistence of some structure for which there is no further use in adult life. Such lesions concern particularly the heart and the urogenital organs.
4. Failures of canalisation, particularly in the gut and Mullerian system.
5. Failures of migration, for example imperfect descent of the testicle.
6. Duplication of structures, for example ureters, digits, etc.
7. The abnormal hypertrophy of a given organ.

In addition to this formidable list, Bacsich went on to point out that metabolism itself is controlled by a mosaic of enzymes which are under genetic control. Defect in a specific enzyme system may produce aberrations of molecular structure or inadequate synthesis of an essential protein, or the accumulation of a metabolite. These inborn errors of metabolism are usually inherited as Mendelian recessive characters.

From conception onwards until the completion of organ differentiation at the end of the third month, fetal development is exposed to teratogenic hazards of which the best recognised are certain viruses (which readily traverse the placenta), hypoxia, changes of temperature, toxins, ionising radiations, hypervitaminosis A, and certain hormones. The list grows with the years. The resulting defect depends not only upon the teratogenic insult and the severity thereof but its exact timing for selection of the vulnerable organ at that particular moment of differentiation. For example, whatever may be the genetic aetiology of anencephaly several adverse environmental factors must also operate, such as the time of year—pregnancies conceived in early summer having a much higher incidence than those conceived at other times. Anencephaly is reckoned to be 30 times more common in families previously so affected and the writer has experience of an unfortunate patient who had 3 consecutive anencephalic monsters. Nevertheless, it is considered that some factor operates about the sixteenth day of gestation and certainly not after the twenty-sixth day (Giroud, 1960). This would be equivalent to gastrulation time in rats and mice. Anencephaly would appear to be particularly common in the Irish race and it has been suggested that exposure to influenza virus may be a factor (Green, 1964).

Congenital abnormalities can be experimentally produced in animals by means which have not yet been satisfactorily demonstrated in humans, for example, the absence of trace elements or excessive or deficient amounts of certain vitamins. In pregnant sows hypovitaminosis A produces absence of eyes and cleft palate in piglets. This is a subject in which species difference makes it very difficult to make direct inferences.

The effect of drugs administered in early pregnancy came sharply to notice with the thalidomide catastrophe. Here was a drug which had been amply tested out on animals and had already had wide use as a sedative in elderly and depressed patients without ill effect. This apparently harmless drug first appeared in Western Germany in 1954, but it was not until 1958 that the first baby victim was recognised, suffering from absence of upper and lower limbs. More cases in West Germany were then reported; 34 newborn affected infants were presented at a paediatric meeting in Dusseldorf at about this time, and it was Lenz of Hamburg who drew attention to the possible association of thalidomide and phocomelia and associated lesions of the ears and gastrointestinal tract. It further appeared that a single dose was capable of producing such deformity, provided that it was taken between the thirty-seventh and fiftieth day since the onset of the last menstrual period. Nearer home a similar disaster overtook a number of pregnant women and their babies and there was quite a crop in a small town, namely Stirling, where thalidomide had come to be prescribed in early pregnancy, and reports began to grow in number (Speirs, 1962).

Ever since the thalidomide disaster a very thorough witch hunt has been maintained to incriminate a whole variety of drugs as possible teratogenic agents. The affinity of the tetracyclines, for example, for bone and growing teeth which they discolour, particularly the first dentition, are striking examples but more often than not the suspicion of damage by all manner of drugs given in early pregnancy has not been substantiated.

Drugs used in the treatment of thyrotoxicosis such as thiouracil and the iodides may produce fetal goitre, but this is more a compensatory phenomenon which remits spontaneously after the child is born. Cortisone and the adrenal steroids have, in a number of cases, been held responsible for cleft palate by interfering with fusion in embryonic development, but these cases are in a minority of the many receiving this type of treatment.

In the list given by Apgar (1964) of medications and the changes produced, or alleged to be produced by them, damage would appear to be more commonly inflicted either in the form of abortion or premature birth or as some metabolic disorder such as, for example, hyperbilirubinaemia from Vitamin K analogues, masculinisation from oral progestogens or fetal haemorrhage from anticoagulants of the dicoumarol class, but not the striking and hideous structural deformities of phocomelia caused by thalidomide. Many abnormalities such as microcephaly, hydrocephaly, cardiac malformations and limb distortions may be due to different sets of causes both genetic and environmental. All of us, therefore, live with the uneasy feeling that thalidomide is not alone as a teratogenic drug and that other environmental factors may be operating in our midst in producing defects which are common and less shatteringly obvious than the limb defects which brought the effects of thalidomide so quickly to light. If, as is commonly recognised, about 5 per cent of all children surviving at the age of one year are found to have some congenital defect, one has reason indeed to wonder what may be going on in our midst, especially when practically every woman in the Western world exposes herself to several drugs of one sort or another in the course of her pregnancy and these must include the pesticides used in agriculture, to say nothing of the more commonly used drugs like acetylsalicylic acid, antihistamines, tranquillisers, anti-emetics and purgative drugs.

It is even possible that a crop of drugs will be found that can counteract the harmful effects which other drugs may be producing in unborn children but, in spite of a very lively awareness on the part of the profession, the science of fetal pharmacology has not yet come upon us.

It is clear, as Bacsich has summed up, that drugs in general are not important factors in congenital malformations and, in fact, very few drugs have been observed to be teratogenic in spite of general watchfulness.

The reason for prescribing a drug, for example for bleeding, etc., may be more important in its effects on the fetus than the drug itself. For an agent to have teratogenic properties it must have some specific relationship to the metabolic and homeostatic needs of the embryo at the time of administration (Mellin, 1964). Furthermore, susceptibility even at such a time may itself be determined by genotype.

Significant amounts of irradiation if given early enough in pregnancy may kill the fetus, a little later may deform it through microcephaly and later still may increase its chances of developing leukaemia or some other form of malignant disease in childhood.

The importance of episodes of severe hypoxia in early pregnancy is often over-looked, especially where abortion following intra-uterine fetal death is not thereby provoked. Instances are provided by attempts at suicide by carbon monoxide poisoning or barbiturates. Ingalls (1960) cited 3 instances of ectromelia caused by this means.

It is certain that endocrine disorders may influence prenatal development and latent endocrinopathies such as pre-diabetes are already regarded as causing an increased incidence of fetal abnormality. In frank diabetes the increased incidence of abnormality has been long recognised and Pedersen *et al.* (1964) in Denmark noted the rate was 3 times as high in diabetics at 6·4 per cent as in controls, but they further remarked that the incidence was highest where there were vascular complications as well.

Virus Infections in Early Pregnancy

It is when we come to consider the effects of viruses on the developing embryo that the most striking advances in our knowledge to date are apparent.

In clinical medicine infections are usually identified by the nature of the tissue response evoked, that is to say, by the varieties of the physical signs of inflammation, including leucocytosis, but in the case of the very early fetus, for example before the tenth week, these responses cannot be made. Instead either the fetus dies or the rapidly differentiating organs suffer some aberration in their development. Leucocytosis is not possible in the very early fetus and Potter stated that the first signs of abnormal collections of leucocytes are to be found in the pulmonary tree as late as the sixteenth to the eighteenth week (before alveolar development).

The role of virus infections came suddenly to notice with Gregg's observations in 1941 in Australia. He noted in 78 cases of congenital cataract (which was usually bilateral and frequently associated with microphthalmia) that there was a history of maternal rubella during the first 2 months of pregnancy in all but 10 cases. This important finding has since led to an intensive search for possible effects of other virus infections on the early human embryo.

A number of viruses are damaging to the fetus, mainly by producing abortion (Evans and Brown, 1963): rubella and cytomegalovirus are the two whose teratogenic properties have so far been most fully documented, the role of the other viruses being less certain. The latter may indeed infect the child without necessarily producing a congenital abnormality, or may cause abortion, or fetal death; for example, the viruses of herpes simplex and some of the exanthemata, although it must be remembered that hyperpyrexia in itself can produce intra-uterine death.

Rubella. The rubella virus is transmitted straight through to the fetus very easily and can be isolated from fetal tissues and antibody levels can be assayed. Furthermore the infection may persist for some months after birth. An infection acquired by the mother, even in the second half of pregnancy, may therefore be transmitted to her fetus but the incidence of specific malformations is related to the time of viral attack, amounting to almost half in the first month of pregnancy, about a quarter in the second month and about 7 per cent in the third month. Whether the eyes, the heart, the organs of hearing or the brain are most likely to be involved, is to some extent determined by the precise stage of development involving organs at their most susceptible state. The fact that a woman does not herself demonstrate a clear clinical picture of rubella does not protect her child, nor will the prophylactic administration of gammaglobulin, although it may suppress the usual clinical manifestations in the mother. Since there may be some doubt about the diagnosis of rubella in early pregnancy, it is fortunate that recently it has become possible to assay antibody levels in the maternal serum and where these are very high, or show a rapid rise, a recent infection can be postulated, whereas in other cases a more steady level without a rise in titre within a fortnight would indicate that the patient had already contracted the infection earlier in her life and was now immune and her child therefore safe.

The prospective survey instituted by the Ministry of Health has been summarised by Manson *et al.* (1960) in which some hundreds of affected cases were matched by controls, and it would appear from this that not only is the death rate in utero and up to the age of 2 years more than doubled when rubella is contracted by the mother within the first 12 weeks but the abnormality rate is also raised; in the case of congenital heart disease to approximately 20-fold, cataract 100-fold, deafness more than 30 times and mental subnormality about quadrupled.

The eyes, the ears and the heart are particularly susceptible. In the case of the first, the lens starts to develop at the beginning of the second month as an area of thickened ectoderm and new fibres are formed peripherally throughout early life. It is the innermost portions of the lens which are affected by rubella in utero, resulting in cataract. Other congenital abnormalities of the eyes, such as congenital glaucoma due to failure of the canal of Schlemm to develop and congenital coloboma due to failure of the choroidal fissure to close, are less characteristic effects of this disease, although microphthalmia is common. The period of vulnerability of the organs of hearing is slightly later than in the case of the ocular structures. Although by the end of the second month the face is complete, including the appearance of the external ear, and all the essential parts of the inner ear are being differentiated, the organs of Corti, which are the end-organs of hearing, are vulnerable during the third month and the middle ear structures likewise. Potter drew attention to the fact that eye and ear defects are unusual in the same baby, presumably due to the fact that their periods of vulnerability do not overlap, so that whereas eye defects occur when rubella develops within the second month of pregnancy, ear defects tend to occur a bit later when the infection occurs late in the second or early in the third month. The structures of the middle ear develop about the same time as the organ of Corti and are likewise vulnerable.

The cardiac lesions most commonly produced by maternal rubella are, according to Campbell (1961), patent ductus (58 per cent), ventricular septal defect (18 per cent), atrial septal defect, pulmonary vascular stenosis and Fallot's tetralogy (each 6 per cent). Mental retardation and microcephaly are fortunately less common.

Rubella is only truly teratogenic in early pregnancy and infection in utero in late pregnancy does not result in a malformed baby at birth. The infant may however show signs of infection and excrete virus.

Rubella and cytomegalovirus disease produce a true viraemia, whereas toxoplasmosis and syphilis, for example, have to get into the fetal system by destructive degrees, affecting placenta and liver first. Medearis (1964) pointed out that the fetal handicaps in a viral infection consist of a slower or very indifferent immuno-globulin response, poor macrophage mobilisation, and diminished interferon synthesis and that a relatively greater number of tissues possess specific receptor sites for the action of a virus. There are also less effective barriers, for example, between blood and brain.

The proportion of congenital malformations caused by rubella and all the viral infections is reckoned to be less than 10 per cent. Nevertheless the present en-thusiasm of parents to get their daughters infected with rubella before they reach marriageable age may be all very well for their own families but may inadvertently expose others in early pregnancy with whom they come in contact.

Cytomegalic inclusion disease. Cytomegalic inclusion disease, caused by the human cytomegalovirus (H.C.M.V.), produces a clinically inapparent infection in the mother. Fortunately the majority of women have already been infected before pregnancy (as in the case of toxoplasmosis) otherwise the infection would be more common in the fetus. It is noteworthy, however, that the risks here are most common after the fifth month of pregnancy and in an active infection both the mother and fetus have the same virus. The disease in the human fetus is characterised by inclusions within the cells of infected organs, the cells themselves being much enlarged in the process. Cases of congenital infection may demonstrate microcephaly, liver and splenic enlargement, thrombocytopoenic purpura, cerebral disorders and sometimes encephalitis; the kidneys are commonly infected and the virus may be isolated from the urine. Mental retardation is also a sequel. Focal lesions in the central nervous system are demonstrated by inco-ordination and spasticity. Immunity acquired at the time prevents the affection of subsequent babies.

Diet

Although adequate, or more than adequate, diet is all-important for the well-being of the pregnant woman, the fetus is less readily affected by deficiencies in maternal nutrition. It is, after all, the complete parasite and helps itself to the best of all that is going, if necessary at the expense of its mother. All this is certainly true of the first half of pregnancy, but rather less so in the second half.

Barcroft observed in sheep that it made little difference to the weight of the fetus whether the diet were severely restricted or not for the first 90 days out of the 144 days of the sheep's pregnancy, but that diet became more important during the latter part. As far as birth-weight goes, the human fetus is likewise susceptible, but the fetal weight at term is unlikely to be seriously affected by dietary deficiencies unless malnutrition is extreme and the maternal calorie intake is consistently less than 1,900 calories a day. It might be pointed out, however, that birth-weight is by no means the only factor to consider and that the baby's vigour is of more import-ance to its healthy survival than its size. The poorer classes of society, who are for that reason less well nourished than the more well-to-do, were shown by Baird (1945) to have a higher prematurity rate, so that the factor of gestational age comes into considerations of birth-weight in relation to diet.

The rate at which the fetus acquires and retains nourishment from its mother progressively increases *pari passu* with its maturity and growth so that its demands may not be fully met within the last 12 weeks of pregnancy and in the case of vitamins and minerals it may go short if the maternal stocks of these substances are very low. Because both the uptake and the needs of the fetus are greater in the last weeks of pregnancy it will be readily seen why prematurely born infants have a greater liability to develop rickets.

It is generally assumed that outside the range of a healthy maternal dietary intake any environmental influence upon the baby detracts from rather than adds to its natural endowment at birth. Even such a trivial and neurotic habit as smoking on the part of the mother, as is well known, produces significantly smaller babies (Herriot *et al.*, 1962) and this cannot be accounted for by the fact that the less educated social classes have less self-control in the curtailment of this dirty habit, so that the difference in birth weights is not purely sociological.

Two mineral elements, namely iron and calcium, deserve special mention here. During pregnancy the mother develops a positive calcium balance of about 50 g. and maternal nutritional deficiencies in calcium and vitamin D are now believed to affect the child's subsequent dental health more than the child's own diet later and likewise the seeds of rickets are often sown in utero. With regard to iron, quite apart from the well-known tendency of the pregnant woman to develop an iron-deficiency anaemia, the fetus itself has to lay down iron stores and the maternal diet, to meet the needs of both mother and fetus, should not contain less than 15 to 20 mg. of iron a day.

The fetus of a woman who suffers from anaemia usually has a normal haemoglobin level at birth but some months later it may show a tendency towards an iron-deficiency anaemia due to a previous deficient storage of this substance, a lack of which will not be made good during neonatal life since milk is an inadequate source of iron.

At birth a normal infant contains about 350 mg. of iron, rather less than half being laid in store, particularly in the liver, during the last three months of pregnancy. The effects of a deficient iron storage are only manifest some weeks after birth, since erythropoiesis greatly diminishes after the child is born and haemolysis adds to the stores of iron.

Shortly after birth, even in the normal case, the baby's blood-sugar may be 40 mg. per cent or even less, and lower still in the infant of low birth weight (see p. 100). Sudden attacks of hypoglycaemia may be a cause of symptoms at the age of one or two days and may be manifested by sudden and unexplained collapse of the baby. This is now increasingly recognised and the response to the intravenous injection of glucose is dramatic. It is difficult to explain why these attacks should occur out of the blue, but the exhaustion of glycogen stores in labour and as the result of hypoxia may be a possible cause.

Landmarks in Fetal Development

Gestational age in early pregnancy is most readily, though roughly, estimated by a measurement of crown-rump length and a simple rule is that given by Hamil-ton, Boyd and Mossman as follows: At 35 days the C.R. length is 5 mm. and from 35 to 55 days of gestation the C.R. length increases by 1 mm. a day and thereafter by about 1·5 mm. daily. At least half of the baby's birth-weight is gained within the last 12 weeks (Fig. 5).

The early landmarks of development are detailed in the table of correlated human development in Arey's Developmental Anatomy (1965), but it is in the

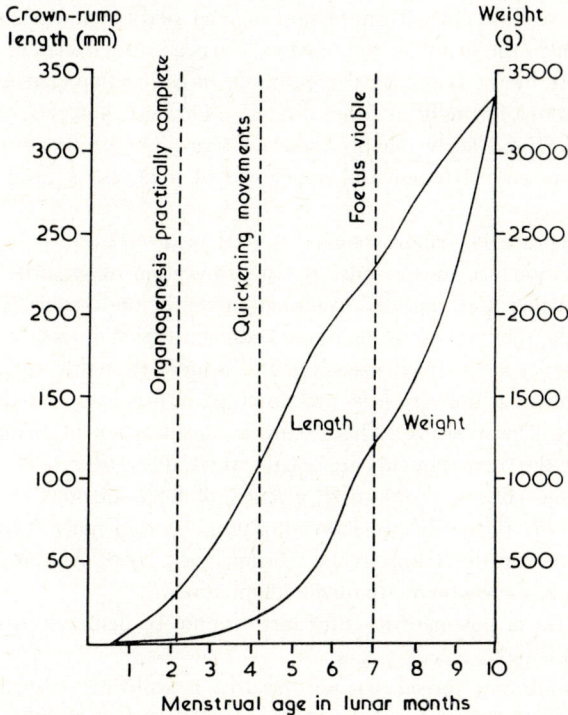

FIG. 5. Diagrammatic representation of fetal growth in relation to menstrual age (from various data).

second half of pregnancy that the landmarks are less certain but clinically more important. Meconium is present at the beginning of the second half of pregnancy and consists of lanugo hairs and cornified squames which have been swallowed, the desquamated cells of the intestine and the secretions of liver, pancreas and succus entericus.

At the twenty-eighth week of gestation lanugo begins to disappear from the face and the nails are well formed and by the thirty-second week the face is clear of lanugo. At this stage the umbilicus is below the mid-point of the total fetal length and subcutaneous fat is very scanty. A baby so prematurely born has consequently a very unstable temperature control, aggravated further by deficient sweating, a large surface area relative to volume and less muscular activity with which to generate heat and furthermore is liable to overswings of temperature in attempting to adjust itself to its environment. At the thirty-sixth week lanugo begins to disappear from the body and the subcutaneous fat increases in amount. At about this time the insertion of the umbilical cord will be found to be approximately at the mid-point of the baby's total length.

The estimation of maturity, however, is particularly important while the child is still in utero. The clinical impression of fetal size is notoriously liable to be mistaken even in the hands of the most experienced obstetrician and attempts to gauge maturity by the radiological appearance of ossification centres may involve an error of up to a fortnight in either direction. Of these, however, the ossification centre of the cuboid fairly reliably indicates term. The centres around the knee joint, i.e. lower end of femur and upper end of tibia, are a little less constant (Fig. 6.)

We have repeatedly demonstrated that fetal biparietal cephalometry by ultrasonic mensuration provides a more reliable indication of maturity than of fetal weight and furthermore repeated examination can be undertaken without known hazard (Donald, 1967, 1968a: Donald and Abdulla, 1967: Willocks et al., 1964, 1967). In our experience a biparietal measurement in utero exceeding 9·8 cm. definitely indicates maturity at the very least and anything in excess of 10·1 cm. is evidence that the fetus is postmature. This excludes consideration of hydrocephalus, of course, where the measurements are usually very large—over 11 to 13 cm.

Where amniocentesis is indicated, a study of fetal squames so obtained and stained with Nile Blue sulphate showing a proportion of more than half staining orange indicates maturity (Brosens and Gordon, 1965, 1966). As a means of diagnosing maturity, however, there are obvious limitations.

The diagnosis of postmaturity after birth cannot be definitely sustained unless the total fetal length exceeds 54 cm.

Most of us are now agreed that postmaturity is associated with mounting fetal hypoxia and this adverse trend is even more pronounced in other asphyxiating conditions, for example, pre-eclamptic toxaemia and hypertensive states.

After delivery there comes a halt to the rapid increase in erythropoiesis which preceded it so that by the second week of life no extramedullary sites of blood formation remain and erythropoiesis is wholly confined to the bone marrow. In premature birth, because of the immaturity of the liver, prothrombin levels may be lower than later so that the infant has consequently an increased tendency to haemorrhagic disease.

At birth the baby is endowed with far more haemoglobin and red cells than it needs for the immediate present but the iron made available by the physiological haemolysis which follows birth is stored to meet the iron famine which is likely to result from a purely milk diet. The extra blood therefore which can be saved by late tying of the cord at birth, though not needed at the moment, may come in useful later on as a source of storage iron.

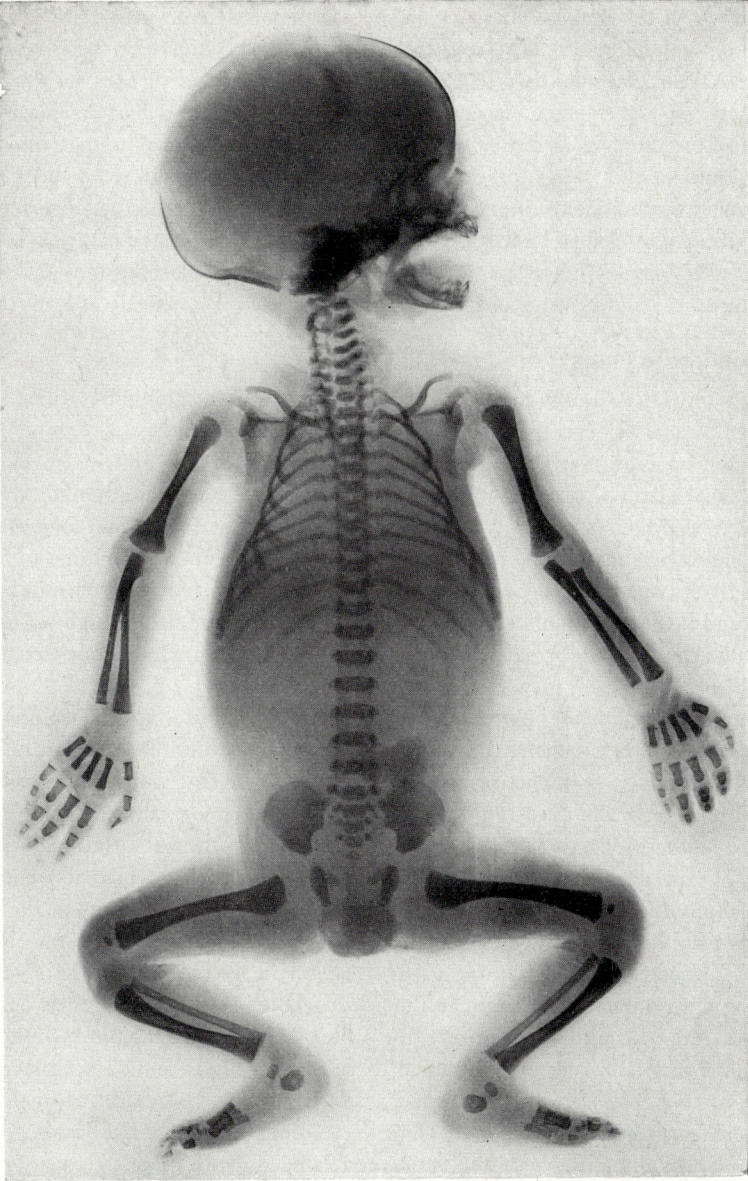

FIG. 6. Radiograph of newborn infant at term. The centre of ossification in the distal epiphysis of the femur appears about 2 weeks before term (Professor H. A. Harris).

Transmission of Disease and Immunity during Prenatal life

A variety of antigens and infecting agents may cross from mother to fetus, either through an intact placenta or where the placental barrier has first been damaged. In the case of micro-organisms, as distinct from viruses, for example those of syphilis, tuberculosis and malaria, the placenta must first be affected, so that the term 'placental barrier' is not wholly inappropriate. Viruses, on the other hand, traverse the intact placenta very easily so that babies may be born with the manifestations of an active infection. Much will depend, of course, upon the availability of the virus; for example, the writer has encountered two cases of active and acute poliomyelitis complicating labour, yet in neither instance was the baby affected, presumably because the virus is quickly fixed in the maternal central nervous system in preference to overflowing across the placenta into the fetus. On the other hand measles and mumps can occur at or very shortly after birth.

Antibodies in Fetus

The fetus has an endowment of sorts with immunoglobulins which may appear by one of several possible mechanisms. It may synthesise some of these itself during intra-uterine life although this capacity is poor and improves with gestational age. The placenta itself may take part in the synthesis although this has not yet been conclusively demonstrated. In the case of lower molecular weight antibodies there may be a direct transfer across the placenta from mother to fetus. Actual cells capable of producing antibodies may be transferred from mother to fetus and finally, as in horses, antibodies may be richly supplied through colostrum although this is not supposed to be a human capability of any consequence (Evans and Brown, 1963).

Immunoglobulins are to be found in the fetal circulation from the beginning of the second half of pregnancy onwards in increasing amount. The premature baby is thus handicapped in this respect in its resistance to infections. The γG class of antibodies are the most important in human immunology and fortunately this class is most readily transferred from mother to fetus; the baby thus at its birth enjoys a fair degree of passive immunity from the diseases which its mother's own immunity responses have conquered. Indeed the concentrations in the fetal serum may exceed those in the maternal at birth. The effect, however, is not always beneficial as for example in Rh. haemolytic disease where the so-called blocking, incomplete or albumin antibodies cross the placenta and do their damage whereas the γM saline or complete antibodies do not. Any γM or γA immuno-globulins in fetal serum are presumed to be of fetal origin and varying levels of γM (but not γA) have been detected as different stages of maturity in infants delivered prematurely or aborted (Jones, 1969). In this series the levels, unlike those of γG globulins, were not however related directly to gestational age but demonstrated a fetal response to a direct immunological stimulus operating in utero.

Intra-uterine immunity mechanisms in fetal life differ from the inflammatory responses with antibody formation which occur after birth. The fetus learns in utero to accept potentially antigenic proteins, including those of its own tissues, without producing a hostile response. Failure of this latter mechanism may be responsible for the development of auto-immune disease in later life.

Obstetrical Complications and Prenatal Development

Considering the number of conditions to which the flesh of the pregnant woman is heir, it is surprising how well protected the fetus remains in utero and, provided it escapes intra-uterine death, how rarely its development is retarded or set awry by obstetrical complications. Certain maternal conditions, of course, kill it outright, for example any acute febrile illness of the mother associated with hyperpyrexia, serious degrees of abruptio of the placenta, or profound maternal asphyxia, as, for instance, in badly administered anaesthesia. Even traumatic accidents to the mother have to be gross in order to affect the child in its well-cushioned intra-amniotic existence. Certain conditions, however, commonly interrupt the comfortable and undisturbed life of the fetus by favouring the onset of premature labour, including severe degrees of cardiac disability, renal deficiencies, hydramnios, large fibroids and malnutrition. Development, however, is more often abnormal in uniovular twins and in fetuses of elderly primigravidae, the latter being particularly liable to mongolism (see Chapter 1). In placenta praevia, Macafee (1945) showed a 3·4 per cent incidence of fetal abnormality.

Of all the general diseases of the mother, diabetes mellitus is one of the most important and interesting in its effects upon the fetus. Of the babies perishing, about one-third die in utero and more than half succumb in the neonatal period. The pregnant diabetic patient is also liable to suffer the additional risks of pre-eclamptic toxaemia and coma and in many of the cases there are sound indications for the premature induction of labour, or the performance of elective Caesarean section before the thirty-seventh week of pregnancy. It takes a nicely balanced judgment to decide between the mounting risks of intra-uterine death if pregnancy is allowed to continue too long and the greater risks of neonatal death from prematurity if intervention is undertaken too soon. Added to all this, the incidence of fetal abnormality in diabetic pregnancy is higher than normal.

Hydramnios is also associated with defects in fetal development but this is more often an effect than a cause as, for example, in anencephaly and oesophageal atresia where riddance of excessive quantities of liquor amnii cannot be achieved by swallowing and ingestion. To exclude the latter at birth, it is now routine practice to pass an oesophageal catheter in all cases of hydramnios. Oligohydramnios, on the other hand, may mechanically restrict the normal development of the limbs, particularly the feet.

Our knowledge of factors during intra-uterine life which may handicap the subsequent development of the child is not as great as it is of actual perinatal mortality, especially since the massive nation-wide survey undertaken by the National Birthday Trust (Butler and Bonham, 1963) and there is a natural tendency to extrapolate from the causes of perinatal death to subsequent handicap in the surviving child, which may be misleading. When one comes to consider the causes of handicap it is necessary to look further afield than merely obstetrical causes and Sheridan (1962) divided babies at risk of handicap into five main groups:

1. Background group—family and social history.
2. Prenatal—disorders of early and late pregnancy.

3. Perinatal group, whether premature or not.
4. Postnatal.
5. Symptomatic group in which mental or physical retardation or some major defect comes to light in childhood.

The obstetrician is therefore only concerned with Groups 2 and 3, and these factors are listed as follows:

Unfavourable Obstetric Factors

Low birth weight
Hypertension
Rh. with antibodies
Acute infections
Threatened abortion
Antepartum haemorrhage of any variety
Postmaturity—over 42 weeks
Diabetes and thyrotoxicosis
Twins and hydramnios
Difficulties in labour
   Malpresentation
   Forceps and caesarean section
   Fetal distress

Often obstetrical factors are superimposed upon bad social and genetic antecedents and Drillien (1964), for example, considered that it was unlikely that obstetric complications apart from low birth weight could account for the mental retardation or neurological disorder in many of the cases which she considered but she thought that an obstetrical complication might constitute an added insult to an already damaged central nervous system. When dealing with the subject of neonatal hyperbilirubinaemia, it is likewise uncertain to what extent high serum bilirubin alone may be responsible for damaging intellectual development and Illingworth (1963), doubted if this factor operated unless associated with the full picture of kernicterus.

It will thus be seen from these examples that the modern study of factors which may interfere with prenatal development now ranges far and wide on an ever-increasing scale.

Fetal Growth Retardation

The assessment of intra-uterine clinical wellbeing is extremely difficult on clinical grounds alone (Donald, 1968b). The fetus lives behind a veritable 'iron curtain' and it is hard indeed to know when there is danger of it outrunning its placental reserve. The matter is important since not only may the baby die in utero but, if born alive, may suffer handicap both mental and physical, one striking example of which is the cerebral damage resulting from neonatal hypoglycaemia if not promptly spotted and corrected. Many conditions like chronic renal inadequacy, pre-eclamptic toxaemia sometimes, diabetes and certain hypertensive states may be responsible for the condition but even more striking is its appearance as a recurrent phenomenon in successive pregnancies without obvious discernible cause and completely unrelated to social grading. As the Perinatal Survey carried out in the United Kingdom showed, one third of all babies weighing less than 2,500 g. are not born prematurely but are retarded in growth (Butler and Bonham, 1963). In fact in comparing them with infants whose low weight is simply due to the premature interruption of pregnancy, they are at a considerable disadvantage. Whatever the aetiology, it would appear that the placenta nourishes the growing fetus inadequately so that the baby is scraggy with poor subcutaneous fat although the brain is developed in accordance with gestational age, as are also the lungs. The liability to meconium inhalation because of intra-uterine fetal distress is common and the liver reserves in glycogen are poor so that there is reduced resistance to the vicissitudes of birth including bouts of hypoxia and consequently of hypoglycaemia due to glycolysis (Shelley, 1961, 1969: Stafford and Weatherall, 1960). Ischaemia of the placental site would appear to be the main aetiological factor (Wigglesworth, 1966).

Since the clinical assessment of fetal growth is so notoriously inadequate, obstetricians are increasingly interesting themselves in more objective assessments of placental function such as the capacity of the placenta to produce oestriol in maternal urine and ultrasonic measurement studies of fetal growth (Klopper, 1963, 1968: Willocks *et al.*, 1964, 1967).

Of all hormone assays the estimation of oestriol in 24-hour or 48-hour collections of urine from the mother provide the best index of feto-placental viability and impending or actual fetal death are commonly preceded by a significant drop in these levels. It is one of the functions of the placenta to convert the precursor substance dehydroisoandrosterone, which originates in the fetal adrenal cortex, into oestriol. The anencephalic fetus because of defective pituitary stimulation of fetal adrenal cortical development produces very little of this material; therefore the oestriol excretion levels are extremely low in anencephaly (Frandsen and Stakemann, 1961). The range of normal excretion is fairly wide but increases throughout the length of pregnancy. A single spot reading is therefore useless and what is required is an oestriol excretion plotted curve.

Klopper (1968) pointed out some of the pitfalls of assessing placental function on the basis of oestriol excretion estimations, even though these are serially calculated. Although quite a good index may be provided in cases of growth retardation, fetal death, pre-eclamptic toxaemia and antepartum haemorrhage, he questions their value in diabetic pregnancy and finds them useless in Rh haemolytic disease.

There is a good deal of overlap between what is normal and abnormal in oestriol excretion but Coyle's figures, which we use, indicate extreme likelihood of intra-uterine death with an excretion rate of less than 3 mg. of oestriol per 24 hours, as term approaches.

In a small series of babies followed up following pregnancies with low oestriol rates, Wallace and Michie (1966) found that only 8 out of 14 were completely normal, 2 were seriously handicapped neurologically and were mentally retarded

3

and the rest had less serious but nevertheless significant neurological or be-havioural defects.

It is our practice to combine oestriol excretion curves with serial measurements of the biparietal growth of the fetus. Where this growth rate is defective or con-firms a clinical diagnosis of underdeveloped fetus for the period of gestation, coupled with low excretion levels, the danger of intra-uterine death and a small poorly grown fetus can be recognised in advance. Timely intervention in the form of interrupting the pregnancy may remove the underdeveloped baby from its unhealthy environment and give it a better chance of survival in a properly equipped and staffed paediatric unit where the hazards of mental retardation associated with neonatal hypoglycaemia, to which these babies are prone, can be largely forestalled. Where placental efficiency is being undermined by pre-eclamptic toxaemia or diabetes or other hypertensive states, these combined techniques can contribute much to clinical judgment.

Fetal electrocardiography has been under intensive investigation for many years but the subject remains difficult to the ordinary clinician. Likewise studies of fetal heart rate changes by advanced methods of computing small but significant changes in heart rate as a means of foretelling which baby is in intra-uterine jeopardy are still under assessment.

Inspecting the forewaters through an amnioscope as advised by Säling may indicate meconium in the liquor even before the onset of labour and is useful in postmaturity and where fears may be entertained of fetal hypoxia. But an occasional inspection of this sort may not give adequate warning of disaster and may have to be repeated every 2 or 3 days. In this state of mind one might as well induce labour! Once the membranes have been ruptured fetal blood sampling as described by Säling becomes quite a useful method of gauging the biochemical wellbeing of the fetus, sometimes indicating that there is no need to terminate labour by untimely caesarean section and in others indicating peril which clinical examina-tion had not so far suggested.

Fetal Circulation

The accompanying diagram (Fig. 7) illustrates the ingenious mechanism whereby the fetus not only receives its oxygen and nourishment and gets rid of its waste products through the placenta, but can adapt itself with a minimum number of alterations to extra-uterine life.

Oxygenated blood coming from the placenta via the umbilical vein travels by the ductus venosus to the inferior vena cava and some of it filters through the liver to mingle with the circulation supplied to this organ through the hepatic arteries and the portal vein. From the inferior vena cava it reaches the right atrium. Three-quarters of this blood is thereupon diverted through the foramen ovale into the left side of the heart and only a quarter proceeds into the right ventricle. The blood which traverses the foramen ovale enters the left atrium and is passed into the left ventricle from which, still retaining most of its oxygen supply from the placenta, it is pumped directly to the head and neck and upper extremities. The blood returning from the head enters the right atrium via the superior vena cava and is passed straight on into the right ventricle, there to mingle with the fraction coming from the inferior vena cava. Both ventricles pump equally. A small quantity of the blood from the right ventricle, containing an even smaller quantity of

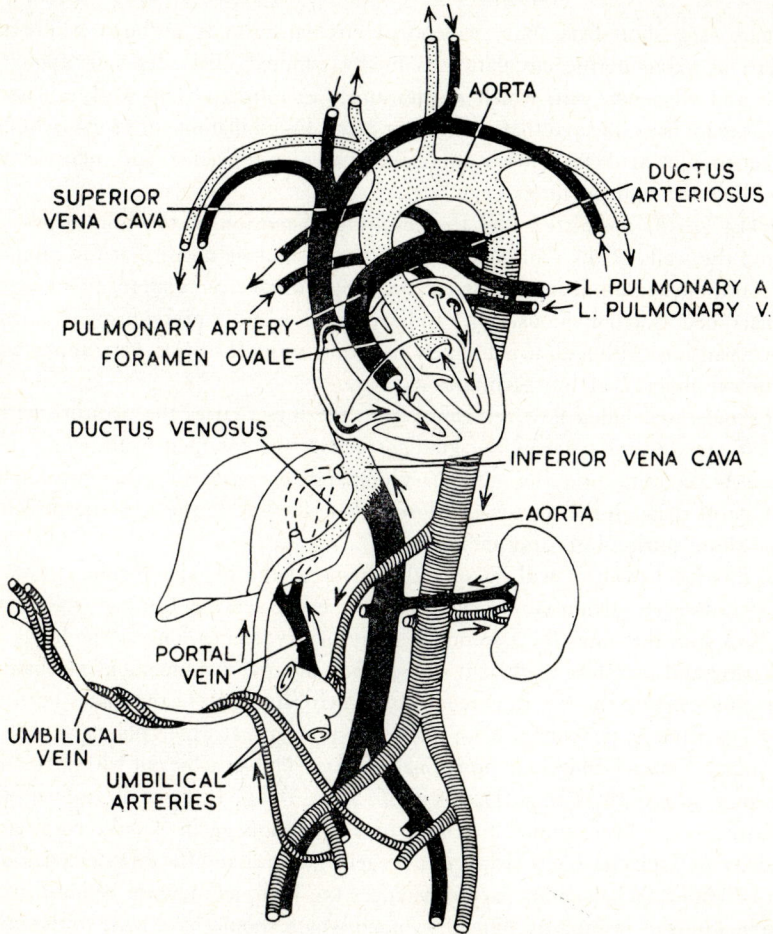

NORMAL CIRCULATION IN THE FETUS

FIG. 7. The normal circulation in the fetus. Vessels containing blood with high oxygen saturation are shown white; stippled, shaded and black areas indicate decreasing degrees of oxygen saturation (Re-drawn from *Seminar Int.*, 1953, 8).

oxygenated blood from the inferior vena cava, goes to the lungs via the pulmonary arteries, but the majority is shunted from the pulmonary system through the ductus arteriosus into the aorta distal to the vessels supplying the head and neck and upper extremities. This blood has lost most of its oxygen and, although a certain amount goes to the lower trunk and lower extremities, the majority is pumped down the umbilical arteries to the placenta. It will be seen therefore that the brain and liver get the best of the available supplies of oxygenated blood.

Circulatory Changes at Birth

There is a short-lived but transitional circulatory state at birth before the pattern of extra-uterine circulation is finally adopted. This depends upon the speed and efficiency with which respiration is established. The work of Dawes and his team has indicated that, in the first place, lung inflation with a gas, whether spontaneous or artificial, lowers pulmonary vascular resistance and increases the blood flow through the lungs.

Jäykkä (1958) postulated that the resulting distension of the lung capillaries erected the walls of the crumpled sac-like alveoli and he noted that the capillary bed is not opened up in areas of atelectatic lungs. Furthermore he regards a patent capillary bed as synonymous with capillary erection and a prerequisite of normal lung expansion. Although it is unlikely that this, in itself, causes very appreciable aeration it almost certainly facilitates it.

The increased blood flow returning from the lungs raises the pressure within the left atrium and reverses the gradient across the foramen ovale which now closes. At the same time the pulmonary demands encourage a temporary left-to-right shunt through the ductus arteriosus, that is to say in the opposite direction to the shunt during intra-uterine life.

By this mechanism it will be seen that some of the blood returning from the lungs via the left atrium is now pumped by the left ventricle through the ductus and back into the lungs for a second helping of oxygen. As long as the lungs are atelectatic and therefore inefficient oxygenating organs, this ingenious mechanism helps to accelerate the rise in percentage oxygen saturation of the blood until the level rises from 60 per cent at birth to over 90 per cent, at which point the walls of the ductus contract and cause functional closure. This is achieved within the first hour or two in normal cases (Dawes et al., 1953, 1954). In cases of asphyxia this mechanism has been shown to come into operation again should respiratory difficulty or asphyxia recur (Lind and Wegelius, 1954) and the foramen ovale and ductus reopen. When pulmonary resistances are high, as they are believed to be in some kinds of respiratory difficulty, blood which should have gone to the lungs is now shunted from right to left through the ductus into the aorta as in intra-uterine existence. A vicious circle is set up, less blood returns to the left atrium which suffers a pressure drop and the foramen ovale reopens. This is believed to be one of the mechanisms in 'blue' or cyanotic attacks after birth.

It will be seen then that the initiation of respiration is of paramount importance in bringing about the neonatal circulatory readjustments and no important circulatory changes have been observed before the first breath (Jäykkä, 1958).

Resistance to Hypoxia

Where asphyxia complicates the birth process, Mott (1961) showed that survival depends on the stores of glycogen within the heart muscle of the fetus. Fetal brain does not store glycogen to any extent and it depends upon glucose for its metabolism which may under certain circumstances be largely anaerobic. This glucose has to be efficiently circulated to the brain and this in its turn will depend upon efficient cardiac activity. One of the worst signs in neonatal asphyxia is a slowness, irregularity and feebleness of the cardiac impulse and glycogen metabolism would appear to play a very dominant role in maintaining cardiac activity. The liver stores of glycogen have been shown by Shelley (1961) to increase very rapidly towards term, but these stores are rapidly depleted in the presence of hypoxia, and Stafford and Weatherall (1960) indicated that it may take many hours to replace them after they have been thus depleted. Chronic hypoxic conditions are therefore more dangerous than acute episodes, which often occur late in the second stage of labour and from which recovery is rapid whatever the method of resuscitation employed.

The asphyxiated baby can survive for a remarkably long time on anaerobic glycolysis. When oxygen supplies are deficient there is a rise, as a result of this mechanism, in the ratio of reduced to oxidised nicotinamide adenosine dinucleotide (NAD) and the ratio of lactate to pyruvate in the blood, which is determined by the lactate dehydrogenase system (LDH) working within the cells, is likewise related (Derom, 1964). This lactate/pyruvate ratio is the same in tissue cells and blood because of ready diffusion. When the ratio is significantly increased due to excess lactate a measure of the degree of anaerobic glycolysis taking place is furnished. Derom (1964) studied these ratios in relation to the fetus at birth. Labour increases both the lactate and pyruvate levels within the mother and, as in muscular exercise, the lactate increase predominates. But Derom showed by comparison with the ratio in fetal blood that the fetus, at least in normal labour, did not itself produce lactate by having to resort to anaerobic metabolism; in fact any excess lactate in a baby following a normal delivery simply reflects the state within the mother. The baby, however, at birth must now metabolise the excess lactate itself by acquiring oxygen by hyperventilation. All babies are born with a metabolic acidosis to which may be superadded a respiratory acidosis, the elimination of both of which depends upon the adequate initiation of respiration.

Intra-uterine Preparation for Respiration

The functional development of the central nervous system proceeds from below upwards, starting at the lower part of the medulla. It is incorrect to think of the respiratory centre as an anatomical point. In fact, it extends longitudinally in the hind-brain. Barcroft (1946) showed that the lowest part of this centre, which develops first, has a very crude respiratory function and can initiate only gasping movements. As the respiratory centre develops, however, its function becomes more refined and now a respiratory rhythm can be evoked, though the movements are associated with other somatic muscular movements, for example of the head and neck. As the development of this centre proceeds higher still, the respiratory rhythmical movements become separated from associated and irrelevant somatic muscular movements. Both the last two mentioned types of respiratory activity can be initiated by sensory stimuli. As development proceeds still further the highest portion of the respiratory centre comes into play, whose effect is one of inhibition, so that respiratory movements can only be initiated by severe stimuli, including those of asphyxia.

Prolonged respiratory activity in utero is pointless and it will therefore be seen that in later pregnancy the fetus, thanks to the inhibitory effect of the highest part of the respiratory centre, will not continually engage in respiratory movements except from time to time in response to appropriate stimuli. Before the onset of labour, these stimuli are most likely to be chemical, but after labour starts sensory stimuli also begin to operate. The baby therefore is progressively woken up during normal labour to start breathing. Obviously prolonged labour with, for example, infected liquor and mounting asphyxia, will encourage deep inspiratory movements before birth, so that in these unfortunate cases the child may be born with an already established pneumonia contracted intranatally.

The presence of liquor amnii within the lungs at birth is physiological, but the amount is normally not great and is in no way harmful since it is very rapidly absorbed, provided always that the pulmonary circulation at birth is efficiently established. In cases of prematurity and fetal shock (white asphyxia) this very necessary proviso may not obtain; in fact, a stagnant pulmonary circulation may account for much of the respiratory difficulty which is sometimes encountered.

Not only does the fetus rehearse the efforts of respiration in utero but as term approaches the surface tension properties within the lung are now recognised to alter. Reference has often been made in the past to the difficulty in expanding lungs in the newborn due to the moist cohesion of the alveolar walls. Many of us have considered that the difficulty was fundamentally mechanical and made worse by prematurity with a poor thoracic cage which yielded by recession to the respiratory efforts which the newborn baby might find itself having to make to overcome these resistances to aeration (Donald, 1954: Donald et al., 1958).

There is more to the onset of breathing, however, than simply a bellows activity on the part of the lung and as gestation proceeds the lungs accumulate increasing quantities of a lipo-protein substance within the alveoli, now called surfactant (see also p. 63). Where this substance is deficient the alveoli have high surface tensions and the difficulty in opening them up is consequently greater. This interesting material cannot be found within the fetal lung before about the twenty-fourth week, a time at which aeration is impossible anyway. Prematurity therefore provides yet another handicap in this respect to successful pulmonary aeration.

Establishment of Respiration at Birth

Five necessary conditions must be present for respiration to become satisfactorily established:

1. A functionally active and competent respiratory centre.
2. A clear airway.
3. Adequate respiratory movements.

4. A suitable atmosphere.
5. An adequate circulation to the vital centres.

A baby's arrival into this world must come as a rude sensory shock. At once, afferent stimuli from the skin and joints, reinforced by mild hypoxia, crowd in upon the child's central nervous system. The carotid sinus, too, reacts as a receptor organ to chemical as well as pressor stimuli and is sensitive to rising carbon dioxide concentrations. Provided therefore that the respiratory centre is not already damaged or depressed, it is bound to react. The baby that has even half a chance to breathe at birth will usually take it, and it is very doubtful if immaturity of the respiratory centre is in itself responsible for failure to breathe after birth (Potter, 1961).

The activity of the respiratory centre may, of course, be depressed by antecedent anoxia during labour, howsoever caused, by raised intracranial pressure including intracranial bleeding and by the persistent action of narcotic and analgesic drugs given to the mother.

The inhibition of respiratory centre activity, which has developed in later pregnancy, is removed at birth by the magnitude of the sensory and chemical stimuli which reach it. If, on the other hand, this centre is depressed at birth, it takes more than sensory stimuli to start rhythmical breathing and mounting asphyxia evokes a more primitive type of respiratory activity, for example, the gasp. If, now, the baby is lucky enough to absorb enough oxygen with such a gasp it is possible that the rhythm-controlling centre may be revived. The chemo-receptors within the carotid sinus play a part in initiating gasps when the respiratory centre itself is severely handicapped provided that the sinus itself is not too severely depressed.

Asphyxia mounts with lengthening delay in establishing respiration, so that the very centres called upon to initiate breathing become less and less capable of doing so. A vicious circle is consequently set up and before long the damage becomes irreversible and death ensues. Animal fetuses can withstand complete oxygen starvation for about 10 times as long as adult animals. The safety margin is not so large in the human, but it is nevertheless considerable and periods up to 10 minutes are compatible with recovery, although the extent to which the higher intellectual centres of the brain may be damaged has not yet been fully determined. The ability of the fetus to withstand anoxia at birth diminishes within the first day or two.

With regard to the remainder of the conditions which must be necessary at birth in order to establish respiration, the patency of the air passages is too obvious to need further comment. Respiratory movements may be inadequate to ventilate the lungs in the child suffering from severe fetal shock or prematurity. In the latter instance, the softness of the thoracic cage often provides insufficient mechanical purchase for the action of the diaphragm so that, in atelectasis, the well-known clinical signs of recession of the chest wall can be observed in the child's unrewarding attempts to overcome the moist cohesion of its alveolar walls and the internal resistances of the lung structure.

The lungs can only be opened up by the exercise of intrathoracic pressure changes. Initially these pressures are very great and, using a method of intra-oesophageal pressure electromanometry, pressure swings up to 90 cm. of water, of which the purely negative component commonly exceeded 40 cm. of water, have been recorded (Donald *et al.*, 1958). In fact no appreciable lung inflation is regarded as possible with anything less than a negative intrathoracic pressure of 20 to 40 cm. of water (Karlberg, 1960). This is indeed a great effort and compares with the maximum inspiratory effort of which an adult is capable, namely 95 cm. of water. It will be seen therefore how difficult it must be for the premature, narcotised, or shocked infant to achieve a flying start to respiration (Donald, 1954).

The rapidity with which the alveoli may open up and the lungs expand is inversely proportional to the degree of prematurity. Nevertheless, radiographic studies of the lungs have shown that, even in quite severe degrees of prematurity, a satisfactory state of aeration can be demonstrated, at least radiologically, within the first 2 hours of life (Donald and Steiner, 1953) although it is probable that, in these cases, histological evidence of full aeration will not be apparent for several days.

The measurement of intrathoracic pressures upon which the writer, amongst others, has been engaged serves to indicate two things; firstly, the vigour with which the child is trying to expand its lungs and, secondly, a measure of its great need in this respect. Once the lungs have expanded these fierce pressure swings are no longer necessary. On the other hand the child who is centrally depressed may never make much of an effort from the start. It has also been noted by others that the sick infant, suffering from respiratory distress, requires to exert itself 2 to 5 times as greatly as the normal child (Karlberg *et al.*, 1954).

The lungs, particularly those affected by atelectasis, show evidence of acute infection more often than any other organ at birth. It is reasonable to suppose that this infection gains access by the upper air passages, for example, from the inhalation of infected liquor amnii rather than through the cord blood, since otherwise the liver would be the first organ to show such evidences.

To establish respiration is one thing but to maintain it is another and, particularly in the case of the premature infant, failure in the second respect is common. The differential diagnosis with which the clinician may then be faced is formidable indeed.

A normal and uninterrupted intra-uterine development, culminating in an uncomplicated delivery at term, is the surest defence against a situation which modern obstetrics must increasingly seek to prevent. The life and health of the unborn and newly born child are more at hazard than at any time in later childhood.

IAN DONALD

REFERENCES

APGAR, V. (1964). Drugs in pregnancy. *J. Amer. med. Ass.*, **190**, 840.
AREY, L. B. (1965). *Developmental Anatomy*. 7th ed. Philadelphia and London: Saunders.

BACSICH, P. (1964). Congenital malformations. *Philosophical Jl.*, **1**, 62.

BAIRD, D. (1945). Influence of social and economic factors on stillbirths and neonatal deaths. *J. Obstet. Gynaec. Brit. Emp.*, **52**, 217.

BARCROFT, J. (1946). *Researches on Prenatal Life.* Oxford: Blackwell.

BEARD, R. W. and MORRIS, E. D. (1965). Foetal and maternal acid-base balance during normal labour. *J. Obstet. Gynaec. Brit. Comm.*, **72**, 496.

BRAMBELL, W. F. R., HEMMINGS, W. A. and HENDERSON, M. (1951). *Antibodies and Embryos.* London: Athlone Press.

BROSENS, I. and GORDON, H. (1965). The cytological diagnosis of ruptured membranes using Nile blue sulphate staining. *J. Obstet. Gynaec. Brit. Comm.*, **72**, 342.

—— —— (1966). The estimation of maturity by cytological examination of the liquor amnii. *J. Obstet. Gynaec. Brit. Comm.*, **73**, 88.

BUTLER, N. R. and BONHAM, D. G. (1963). *Perinatal Mortality.* Edinburgh: Livingstone.

CAMPBELL, M. (1961). Place of maternal rubella in the aetiology of congenital heart disease. *Brit. med. J.*, **1**, 691.

CARR, D. H. (1967). Chromosome anomalies as a cause of spontaneous abortion. *Amer. J. Obstet. Gynaec.*, **97**, 283.

COYLE, M. G., GREIG, M. and WALKER, J. (1962). Blood progesterone and urinary pregnanediol and oestrogens in foetal death from severe pre-eclampsia. *Lancet*, **2**, 275.

DAWES, G. S., MOTT, J. C., WIDDICOMBE, J. G. and WYATT, D. G. (1953). Changes in lungs of the newborn lamb. *J. Physiol.*, **121**, 141.

—— —— —— (1954). The foetal circulation in the lamb. *J. Physiol.*, **126**, 563.

DEROM, R. (1964). Anaerobic metabolism in the human foetus. *Amer. J. Obstet. Gynec.*, **89**, 241.

DONALD, I. (1954). Atelectasis neonatorum. *J. Obstet. Gynaec. Brit. Emp.*, **61**, 725.

—— (1965). Ultrasonic echo sounding in obstetrical and gynaecological diagnosis. *Amer. J. Obstet. Gynec.*, **93**, 935.

—— (1967). Diagnostic ultrasonic echo sounding in obstetrics and gynaecology. *Trans. Coll. of Physicians, Surgeons and Gynaecologists of South Africa.* Vol. II, No. 2, p. 61.

—— (1968a). Ultrasonics in Obstetrics. *Brit. Med. Bull.*, **24**, 71.

—— (1968b). Obstetric aspects of preventive medicine in the perinatal period. *Proc. 5th International Congress of Hygiene and Preventive Medicine (Rome).* Vol. I, Part II, p. 675.

—— (1969). Sonar as a method of studying prenatal development. *J. Pediat.*, **75**, 326.

—— and ABDULLA, U. (1967). Ultrasonics in obstetrics and gynaecology. *Brit. J. Radiol.*, **40**, 604.

—— and BROWN, T. G. (1961). Demonstration of tissue interfaces within the body by ultrasonic echo sounding. *Brit. J. Radiol.*, **34**, 539.

—— KERR, M. M. and MACDONALD, I. R. (1958). Respiratory phenomena in the newborn. *Scot. med. J.*, **3**, 151.

—— and STEINER, R. E. (1953). Radiography in diagnosis of hyaline membrane. *Lancet*, **2**, 846.

DRILLIEN, C. M. (1964). *The Growth and Development of the Prematurely born Infant.* Edinburgh: Livingstone.

EVANS, T. N. and BROWN, G. C. (1963). Congenital anomalies and virus infections *Amer. J. Obstet. Gynec.*, **87**, 749.

FRANDSEN, V. A. and STAKEMANN, G. (1961). The site of production of oestrogenic hormones in human pregnancy. *Acta Endocrinol.*, **38**, 383.

GAIRDNER, D. (1968). Fetal medicine—who is to practise it? *J. Obstet. Gynaec. Brit. Comm.*, **75**, 1223.

GIROUD, A. (1960). Chromosomal abnormality and congenital malformations. *Ciba Symposium.* London: Churchill.

GREEN, C. R. (1964). The frequency of mal-development in man. *Amer. J. Obstet. Gynec.*, **90**, 994.

GREGG, H. M. (1941). Congenital cataract following german measles in the mother. *Trans. Ophthal. Soc. Austral.*, **3**, 35.

HAMILTON, W. J., BOYD, J. D. and MOSSMAN, H. W. (1962). *Human Embryology*. 3rd ed. Cambridge: Heffer.

HERRIOT, A., BILLEWICZ, W. Z. and HYTTEN, F. E. (1962). Cigarette smoking in pregnancy. *Lancet*, **1**, 771.

ILLINGWORTH, R. S. (1963). *The Development of the Infant and the Young Child*. 2nd ed. Edinburgh: Livingstone.

INGALLS, T. H. (1960). Environmental factors in causation of congenital abnormalities. *Ciba Symposium*. London: Churchill.

JÄYKKÄ, S. (1958). Capillary erection and the structural appearance of fetal and neonatal lungs. *Acta Paediat.*, **47**, 484.

JONES, W. R. (1969). Immunoglobulins in fetal serum. *J. Obstet. Gynaec. Brit. Comm.*, **76**, 41.

KARLBERG, P. (1960). The adaptive changes in the immediate postnatal period, with particular reference to respiration. *J. Pediat.*, **56**, 585.

—— COOK, C. D., O'BRIEN, D., CHERRY, R. B. and SMITH, C. A. (1954). Studies of respiratory physiology in the newborn infant. *Acta Paediat.*, **43**, Suppl. 100.

KLOPPER, A. (1963). *Research on Steroids*. Rome: Tipografia Poliglotta Vaticana.

—— (1968). The assessment of feto-placental function by estriol assay. *Obstet. Gynec. Survey*, **23**, 813.

LIND, J. and WEGELIUS, C. (1954). Human fetal circulation. *Cold Spring Harbour Symposia Quant. Biol.*, **19**, 109.

MACAFEE, C. H. G. (1945). Placenta Praevia—A study of 174 cases. *J. Obstet. Gynaec. Brit. Emp.*, **52**, 313.

MANSON, M. M., LOGAN, W. P. D. and LUZ, R. M. (1960). Rubella and other virus infections in pregnancy. *Min. of Health Reports on Public Health and Medical Subjects*, No. 101.

McKEOWN, T. (1961) *in* Conference on Foetal Abnormality. *Brit. med. J.*, **1**, 1102.

—— and RECORD, R. G. (1960). Congenital malformations. *Ciba Symposium*. London: Churchill.

MEDEARIS, D. N. (1964). Viral infections during pregnancy and abnormal human development. *Amer. J. Obstet. Gynec.*, **90**, 1140.

MELLIN, G. W. (1964). Drugs in the first trimester of pregnancy. *Amer. J. Obstet. Gynec.*, **90**, 1169.

MINISTRY OF HEALTH, (1963). *Report on Congenital Malformations*. Prepared by Standing Medical Advisory Committee. London: H.M.S.O.

MORRIS, E. D. and BEARD, R. W. (1965). The rationale and technique of foetal blood sampling and amnioscopy. *J. Obstet. Gynaec. Brit. Comm.*, **72**, 489.

MOTT, J. C. (1961). The ability of young mammals to withstand total oxygen lack. *Brit. med. Bull.*, **17**, 144.

PEDERSEN, L. M., TYGSTRUP, I. and PEDERSEN, J. (1964). Congenital malformations in newborn infants of diabetic women. *Lancet*, **1**, 1124.

POTTER, E. L. (1961). *Pathology of the Fetus and the Newborn Infant*. 2nd ed. Chicago: Year Book Publ.

ROCK, J. and HERTIG, A. T. (1948). Human conceptions during first two weeks of gestation. *Amer. J. Obstet. Gynec.*, **55**, 6.

RYAN, K. J. (1958). Conversion of $\Delta 5$ androstene, 3β, 16α, 17β-triol to estriol by human placenta. *Endocrinology*, **63**, 392.

SÄLING, E. quoted by Beard and Morris and Morris and Beard (q.v.)

SHELLEY, H. J. (1961). Glycogen reserves and their changes at birth and in anoxia. *Brit. med. Bull.*, **17**, 137.

—— (1969). The metabolic response of the fetus to hypoxia. *J. Obstet. Gynaec. Brit. Comm.*, **76**, 1.

SHERIDAN, M. D. (1962). Infants at risk of handicapping conditions. *Monthly Bull. Min. of Hlth.*, **21**, 238.

SPEIRS, A. L. (1962). Thalidomide and congenital abnormalities. *Lancet*, **1**. 303.

STAFFORD, A. and WEATHERALL, J. A. C. (1960). The survival of young rats in nitrogen. *J. Physiol.*, **153**, 457.

WALLACE, S. J. and MICHIE, E. A. (1966). A follow-up of infants born to mothers with low oestriol excretion during pregnancy. *Lancet*, **2**, 560.

WARKANY, J. (1957). Congenital malformations and pediatrics. *Pediatrics*, **19**, 725.

WIGGLESWORTH, J. S. (1966). Foetal growth retardation. *Brit. med. Bull.*, **22**, 13.

WILLOCKS, J., DONALD, I., DUGGAN, T. C. and DAY, N. (1964). Foetal cephalometry by ultrasound. *J. Obstet. Gynaec. Brit. Comm.*, **71**, 11.

—— —— CAMPBELL, S. and DUNSMORE, I. R. (1967). Intrauterine growth assessed by ultrasonic foetal cephalometry. *J. Obstet. Gynaec. Brit. Comm.*, **74**, 639.

WYBURN, G. M. (1953). Congenital defects of anterior abdominal wall. *Brit. J. Surg.*, **40**, 553.

3   The Newborn Infant

Birth normally occurs when fetal development with all its intricate anatomical and biochemical inter-relationships reaches a point at which the extra-uterine environment offers significant advantages. At term, a gestational age of 40 weeks, the baby is a unique mixture of helplessness and capacity for survival. The transformation from the life of an aquatic parasite to separate existence in air is dramatic and it is accompanied by radical and sudden changes in every system and in the physiological relationships between systems. Survival and health depend upon their successful establishment. Truly independent living, of course, is achieved only gradually over the years to maturity and in the newborn period the infant's susceptibility to such common dangers as chilling, starvation, dehydration, assault and infection place him entirely at the mercy of those entrusted with his care. Yet, in spite of this frailty, he can survive undamaged a degree of oxygen lack which would prove lethal to an athlete while he can withstand major illnesses and surgery in a way which belies his appearance.

The period during which an infant is regarded for statistical purposes as 'newborn' is the first month after birth and deaths during this time are classified as neonatal deaths. (Some authors, in referring to the neonatal period, however, confine themselves to the first 14 days of life or to the lying-in period, particularly when considering perinatal mortality, that is the combined fetal wastage from stillbirth and death during the early neonatal period.)

Whilst we are concerned here primarily with normal development rather than with mortality and morbidity, an appreciation of the physiology of the normal newborn infant is essential if deviations from the normal are to be recognised early and adequately treated. The purpose of this chapter is to provide an outline of current knowledge upon which his care can be based.

Methods evolved for the evaluation of maturity are discussed by Drillien on page 94 and Ingram describes the behavioural characteristics of the normal newborn infant in pages 212 to 221.

Weight

Birth weight varies quite widely in babies judged to have a gestational age of 40 weeks and it is influenced by such variables as social class, height, weight, parity and smoking habits of the mother, the existence of toxaemia or diabetes mellitus and the sex of the child. It also varies between races but this is at least partly dependent upon the state of maternal nutrition. Tables and graphs of expected weight are available from different countries, *e.g.* Battaglia and Lubchenco (1967) for the United States and Ghosh and Daga (1967) for India. The former also provide the anticipated fetal mortality at different weights and maturities. British figures are available from Neligan (1965a), Butler (1965) and Thomson, Billewicz and Hytten (1968). The latter provide detailed tables which display smoothed percentile values of birth weight for all pregnancies at various gestational ages and then again for each sex both with regard to first pregnancies and second or subsequent pregnancies. In general big mothers produce heavier babies, first babies are smaller than subsequent ones, and male infants are heavier than females. Thus in Figure 8

Percentiles of Birthweight for Gestation.

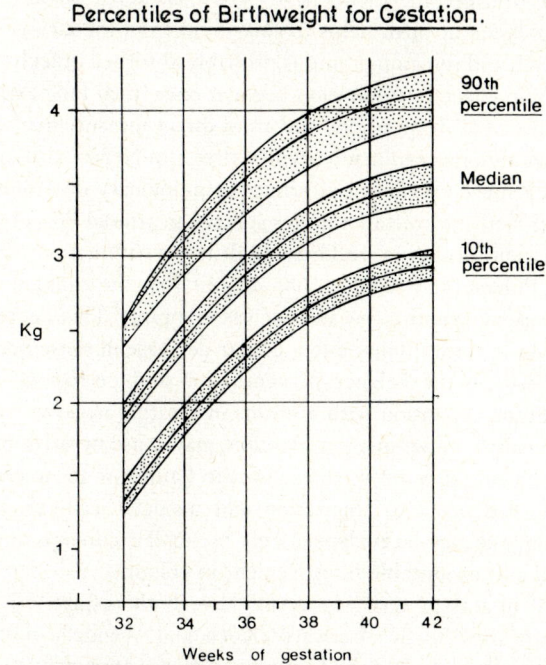

Fig. 8. Percentiles of birthweight for gestation (reproduced with permission from Thomson, Billewicz and Hytten, 1968, J. Obst. Gynaec. Brit. Comm., 75, 903).

percentiles of birth weight for gestation are shown, the central line in each curve being the percentile for all cases irrespective of sex or parity. The lower boundary of each curve is the percentile for female first births and the upper boundary is that for male second or subsequent births.

It has for long been accepted that normal mature newborn babies lose about 7 per cent of birth weight in the first few days and that this is made good by the end of the first week (Farquhar and Sklaroff, 1958). This was correctly attributed to fluid and meconium loss at a time when the breast was yielding only small quantities of colostrum. The current habit in developed industrial societies of meeting in full the demands of the newborn by providing cow's milk in one or other form from birth is accompanied by a change in the body weight behaviour in the first week. Many babies actually gain weight from the first day of life and the others may maintain their weight over the week or make good a relatively small loss. Babies who are ill, of course, may fail to preserve fluid and caloric balance and consequently lose 10 per cent or more of birth weight.

Respiration

The prenatal preparations for respiration, its control, the resistance of unexpanded lung tissue and the cohesion of the fetal lung surfaces, along with the forces available to overcome them, have been considered already in Chapter 2. Thoracic compression at birth helps to clear fluid from the airway in preparation for the first breath and remaining fluid is probably absorbed quickly by the alveolar capillaries. Should effective respiration begin at once, then lung expansion may be achieved within several respirations and from direct measurement of the arterial-alveolar pressure differences for nitrogen Nourse and Nelson (1969) conclude that normal infants achieve excellent uniformity of pulmonary distribution of gas and blood soon after birth and within minutes achieve an arterial PO_2 of 70–80 mm. Hg with 80–90 per cent saturation, reaching adult levels within hours or days. Studies by Thibeault, Poblete and Auld (1968) suggest that the thoracic gas volume is greater than normal, possibly because of gas trapping. This decreases and lung volume improves in term infants but a similar decrease in those born prematurely is thought to disturb the balance of ventilation and perfusion. This could be improved by aiding expansion with a means of creating negative pressure around the chest. The baby's initial inspiratory effort may cause negative pressures in the chest of up to 60 cm. of water settling down to figures of 20–30 cm. Between the extremes of normal onset of respiration and neonatal asphyxia there are such gentler beginnings as may be evidenced only by small excursions of the alae nasi or abdominal wall and by suitable improvement in colour.

Even normal infants at term, however, have both respiratory and metabolic acidosis at birth and shortly afterward (Koch and Wendell, 1968). Lactic acid concentration increases during the first few moments after delivery but decreases quickly thereafter approaching normal adult levels by approximately 24 hours. The respiratory acidosis is generally corrected within an hour of delivery. Judged by PO_2 intrapulmonary gas exchange in the newborn may be less effective than it is in later life but this may be due in part to varying degrees of right to left shunting. Data referring to acid-base determinations in prematurely born infants in the first 2 months of life have been provided by Malan, Evans and Heese (1966).

Experiments using small animals (Dawes, 1968) have shown that asphyxiation leads first to a short burst of increased respiration which is followed by primary apnoea lasting a few minutes. This gives way to a longer period of gasping respiration which is terminated by a clearly recognisable 'last gasp' after which the animal makes no further respiratory effort (secondary apnoea). The duration of gasping respiration up to the last gasp is estimated by Dawes to lie somewhere between that of newborn monkeys (8 minutes) and rabbits (10 minutes). Animals may be resuscitated by intermittent positive pressure respiration up to the last gasp and for a short time afterwards, but the last gasp is the herald of death which advances quickly during subsequent minutes. The duration of primary apnoea may be extended by pentobarbitone or pethidine (Campbell, Milligan and Talner, 1968) and may be difficult to distinguish therefore from secondary apnoea.

Intermittent positive pressure respiration given at any point up to the last gasp is likely to resuscitate the baby but thereafter his response will depend on the duration of secondary apnoea. If recovery does take place it will be apparent in an acceleration of heart rate followed by spontaneous gasping which will gradually give way to rhythmic respiration.

It is assumed that the human newborn behaves similarly and because there may be some difficulty in distinguishing primary from secondary apnoea and because the integrity of the central nervous system is likely to suffer directly with the duration of severe oxygen lack, the practice of intubating apnoeic infants and using intermittent positive pressure respiration has greatly increased. The time taken to establish spontaneous respiration may be a guide to the severity of the anoxic insult. Resistance to anoxia is certainly greater in the newborn, perhaps because of anaerobic metabolism and because the relative simplicity of immature tissue may be associated with reduced demand for oxygen and substrate. Survival, however, depends on circulation and this in turn involves the adequacy of cardiac glycogen (Shelley, 1964).

Other work on experimental animals has shown that survival may be increased by maintaining plasma pH with sodium bicarbonate and by giving intravenous glucose (Dawes, Mott and Stafford, 1960). The severity of anoxic effect has been expressed as a score (0–10) by Apgar (1953) who allots points to the heart rate, respiration, colour, muscle tone and reflex irritability of babies one minute after delivery (Table 2).

TABLE 2

Sign	Score		
	0	1	2
Heart rate	Absent	Under 100/min.	Over 100/min.
Respiratory effort	Absent	Weak, irregular	Strong, regular
Muscle tone	Limp	Some flexion	Active movements
Reflex response to stimulation	None	Weak movements	Cry
Colour	Blue or pale	Body pink, extremities blue	Completely pink

Resuscitative measures should have a physiological basis. Thus a clear nasal and laryngo-tracheo-bronchial airway is a prerequisite of success and care should be taken to maintain body heat although cooling has been employed under both

experimental and clinical conditions (Miller *et al.*, 1964). Positive pressure inter-
mittently applied to mimic respiration and within the pressure limits attainable by
the newborn is the most effective measure and is best carried out by tracheal intu-
bation. Inflation of the newborn's lungs at appropriate pressures increases the
magnitude of his own effort and may lead to improved alveolar expansion. Established respiration has a normal frequency of 25–50 each minute but may be irregular
in rhythm or puntuated by short periods of apnoea. Although these irregularities
may be corrected by giving oxygen this need not be done if the infant appears to
be well otherwise. Scattered moist sounds may be heard throughout the chest
during the first few hours but otherwise the careful examination of the chest yields
the normal or abnormal physical findings of infancy. Some degree of costal
recession is permissible in babies of low birth weight.

Circulation

The major circulatory readjustments which accompany the change from
intra-uterine to extra-uterine life continue to be the object of much investigation.
The umbilical arteries usually cease pulsating within 5 minutes but in some infants
pulsation continues considerably longer and along with a very high umbilical
venous pressure it may persist for hours in the presence of even moderate degrees
of respiratory distress, so that release of cord occlusion may be accompanied by
profuse bleeding (Desmond *et al.*, 1959). The relationship of the umbilical arteries
to those supplying the sciatic nerves should be remembered, as the accidental injection of such materials as nikethamide into the former may result in sciatic paralysis
and sometimes cutaneous gangrene of the ipsilateral buttock (Hudson *et al.*, 1950).
They can, however, be catheterised soon after birth and used to provide blood
specimens on which to measure arterial pressure and blood gas tensions.

Although the umbilical vein usually remains functionally patent for some
minutes only in order to permit drainage from the placenta it can be catheterised
without difficulty during the first week of life and is therefore available for late
exchange transfusion in such conditions as hyperbilirubinaemia. The hazards of
prolonged catheterisation have been recognised and should be avoided if possible
(Cochran, Davis and Smith, 1968).

The wall of the ductus venosus contains little muscle and it possesses no
sphincter. Functional closure at birth seems to depend upon a fall in portal sinus
pressure, retracting and narrowing its origin so that it is no longer an open vessel
although intermittent shunting through it may continue for a few days. Organic
closure is probably completed in the third week (Meyer and Lind, 1966a). As a
result of this closure the vessel no longer transmits arterialised blood to the liver
from the umbilical vein. This chiefly affects the left lobe which previously received
preferential treatment and it now grows more slowly than the right. As portal
blood flow increases it is directed more to the right lobe and this difference in blood
supply between right and left may be clearly distinguished in some cases at autopsy
(Gruenwald, 1949; Emery, 1952; Meyer and Lind, 1966b).

With termination of the placental circulation a sharp rise occurs in peripheral resistance and simultaneously expansion of the lungs increases their vascular bed so that pulmonary resistance falls. The resulting increased pressure in the left heart and decreased pressure in the right cause functional closure of the flap valve covering the foramen ovale and any subsequent shunt through it in the normal human newborn is thought to be very small. Functional closure of the ductus arteriosus, however, may be delayed for some time. At least some of those cardiac murmurs which can frequently be detected soon after birth have been attributed by Burnard (1958) to deferred closure but could be caused by mitral regurgitation secondary to asphyxia and cardiac dilatation (Burnard, 1963). A right to left shunt has been demonstrated during the first hour (James, 1961) but thereafter the evidence favours a flow from left to right (Adams and Lind, 1957; James and Rowe, 1957; Jegier et al., 1964). Shunting through the foramen ovale is confined to the first 24 hours (James et al., 1961). The balance of pressure within the ductus is likely to be delicate during the first few hours but evidence of shunting through it may be detected up to one week after birth (Jegier et al., 1964). Closure may be favoured by oxygen and pressor amines and opposed by hypoxia. The frequency with which cardiac murmurs are recorded at this age depends upon the skill of the observer and the frequency of auscultation, but only the minority persist and are associated with congenital heart disease whereas some severe malformations are quite unassociated with neonatal cardiac murmurs (Benson et al., 1961).

The heart is relatively large at birth and a greatest permissible transverse diameter on X-ray of 5·7 cm. is a preferable measurement of size than is the cardiothoracic ratio (Smith, 1959). The size varies somewhat in the first few hours, particularly in the presence of respiratory distress (Burnard, 1959) or of changes in blood volume (Wallgren et al., 1964), and may do so for some days, but progressive disproportionate increase during the newborn period generally indicates a malformation. The normal heart rate varies quite widely but tends to stabilise between 120 and 130 each minute after the first few hours when it may be a little higher. The electrocardiographic pattern in the first few months of life shows right ventricular preponderance; occasional extra systoles or variability of the T-waves need not be abnormal.

The practical value of recording the blood pressure of the newborn has lain in the diagnosis of aortic coarctation. Recent studies, however, have called attention to variations in individual blood pressure readings during the first few hours and days and possibly significant differences in the mean blood pressures of certain groups. Thus Ashworth and Neligan (1959) found that the systolic blood pressure at birth ranged from 62–116 mm. of mercury and that it fell to 44–74 mm. in a few hours if the umbilical cord were clamped early, or rather later if clamping had been delayed. It then rose during the second day and slowly throughout the first week. Lower means were recorded in infants suffering from respiratory distress syndrome and in those who were delivered by caesarean section. The simple and effective sphygmomanometer designed by Ashworth, Neligan and Rogers (1959) occludes the brachial artery by means of a 2·5 cm. cuff. On gradually releasing this the return of radial pulsation is picked up by a second cuff which indicates the point by transmitting the wave to a drop of xylol in a capillary column. A 4 cm. cuff has been gaining in popularity (Young, 1961) and a simple cot-side electronic oscillometer capable of measuring both systolic and diastolic pressures has been described by Nelson (1968).

Deferred clamping of the umbilical cord assures the baby of a considerable placental transfusion (De Marsh *et al.*, 1942; Gunther, 1957) especially if the cord is uninterrupted until respiration has begun (Redmund, Isana and Ingall, 1965). The effect of delayed clamping correlates well with the venous haematocrit and with blood volume (Usher *et al.*, 1963). The problem has been well reviewed by Moss and Monset-Couchard (1967) who expressed the view that delayed clamping of the cord was not a vital issue for well babies at term but could be important in mature babies showing signs of cerebral depression, and who also believed that it could possibly be critical in achieving the survival of small prematurely born infants who may find great difficulty in filling the pulmonary circulation at the expense of the systemic one and who may then do neither well. They conclude that there is insufficient evidence at present to justify early clamping in order to prevent erythrocytaemia and jaundice. The relationship between early clamping of the cord and the development of the respiratory distress syndrome has aroused much interest and has produced no firm conclusion. In 1969 Philip *et al.* presented good evidence that babies who have had fetal distress in labour have unexpectedly low residual volumes of blood in the placenta when compared with controls. They have suggested that the fetus in distress in some way recalls to its circulation before birth all the blood available to it and that this may be the mechanism underlying neonatal erythrocytaemia or transient tachypnoea of the newborn. The whole truth about placental transfusion remains elusive and is of lesser importance as the baby ages, Lanzkowsky (1960) having already shown that although placental transfused infants have significantly higher haemoglobins than those submitted to early clamping of the cord, this difference had disappeared by the age of 3 months. Spontaneous variations in blood volume and haematocrit may occur in individual newborn infants during the first few hours but quite contrary findings have been reported by Gairdner *et al.*, (1958) and Sisson and Whalen (1960). The former attributed decreased blood volume and increased haematocrit to loss of protein, water and salts from the vascular compartment, while Sisson and Whalen suggested that an increased volume results from the postnatal release of blood temporarily sequestrated in reservoirs.

Vasomotor tone exists from birth although immaturity of control may explain the harlequin colour changes (Neligan and Strang, 1952) which may sometimes be seen in newborn infants, particularly if they are immature. The attacks are of short duration and are characterised by a striking difference in the colour of the two longitudinal halves of the body. They occur mostly on the third and fourth days of life. Peripheral stagnation and cyanosis are common on the first day and should not be misinterpreted as necessarily implying congenital heart disease. The capillary network of the newborn infant is less well developed than that of the adult (Arajärvi, 1953). Capillary resistance is low at birth (Walker and Balf, 1954) and increases over the first week. Prematurely born infants have a lower initial capillary resistance but it increases from birth in the same way and even among term babies the resistance increases with birth weight. The authors found no variation with sex or season and the capillary resistance appears to be uninfluenced by the mode of delivery, the giving of vitamin K or the presence or absence of jaundice. They concluded that the maturity of the capillary bed at birth is of primary importance in determining capillary resistance. This decreasing resistance with immaturity may explain the greater permeability of the small blood vessels of newborn babies as a result of which water, salts and protein can escape more readily from the vascular compartment so causing the firm oedema which may develop after birth in certain circumstances.

Idiopathic Respiratory Distress Syndrome

Because the pulmonary hyaline membrane associated with respiratory distress is responsible for at least half the deaths occurring among prematurely born babies, this syndrome which is fully described in most textbooks of paediatrics or obstetrics remains the object of intensive research. Although the aetiology is still rather obscure, it seems to involve immaturity in one or more systems and to be closely linked with some still unrecognised prenatal disturbance. Placental blood transfusion is claimed to have some prophylactic value (Bound et al., 1962) and a means of ensuring this in babies delivered by caesarean section, a group which is at increased risk, has been described by Secher and Karlberg (1962). Distressed infants may also show oedema of the limbs but the pulmonary membrane which contains fibrin is chiefly found in the terminal bronchioles and alveoli. Present opinion probably still favours atelectasis as being the primary pathological lesion (Gruenwald, 1952; Gairdner, 1965) and all other changes including the cardiovascular ones as secondary to it. Deficiency of surfactant, a lipoprotein which reduces surface tension within the lung and so facilitates the separation of cohesive surfaces (Avery and Mead, 1959), not only makes expansion difficult but makes it unstable so that it collapses again on expiration (Gruenwald, 1964). Reynolds et al. (1968) conclude that surfactant deficiency is the crucial factor in causing respiratory distress syndrome. They suggest that synthesis may be defective not only because of immaturity but because it has been damaged by prenatal or intrapartum asphyxia. Prematurely born infants are also deficient in fibrinolytic activators (Lieberman, 1959; Quie and Wannamaker, 1960; Ambrus et al., 1965) and may have abnormal difficulty in removing the hyaline material.

A significant increase in diameter of pulmonary lymphatics is claimed by Lauweryns et al. (1968), and Lauweryns (1968), using an injection technique in neonatal deaths, found that the pulmonary veins and venules in the lungs were easy to fill but many small muscular arteries and most pulmonary arterioles could not be filled. This is taken to indicate pulmonary ischaemia and that respiratory distress syndrome is not only a failure of ventilation but also of perfusion. According to Russell and Cotton (1968) lung perfusion and a decrease in right to left shunting may be affected by giving intravenous bicarbonate. A similar effect is claimed for the amine buffer THAM (Gupta *et al.*, 1967).

Distressed infants have a severe uncompensated respiratory acidosis during the early hours of life and evidence of a metabolic acidosis, a rising potassium and excessive tissue breakdown also exists. Usher (1961) found that the severity of the acidosis correlates closely with the prognosis and he recommended a regimen in which the acidosis and hyperkalaemia are controlled from birth by intravenous sodium bicarbonate and glucose. Such treatment, which has been effectively modified by Hutchison *et al.* (1962; 1964), does not affect the primary respiratory process but improves survival rate. Until the body is able to remove the hyaline membrane, mechanical ventilators seem to offer some solution to the problem. Earlier attempts involved the use of muscle relaxants with poor results and ventilators now exist which can impose a respiratory rhythm on the baby or follow his own efforts if these are satisfactory. The subject has been well reviewed by Tunstall *et al.* (1968). In such a difficult field in which so many variables exist, it is not surprising that, technical skill aside, widely different views exist about its value. Thus those who ventilate early are likely to have a better survival rate than those who use it only when the battle is almost lost. On the other hand babies who might otherwise survive may die on the ventilator unless it is skilfully used. An attempt to deal with the membrane by intravenous fibrolysin has been unsuccessful (Gomez and Graven, 1964).

These possibilities, and there are others, serve to illustrate the importance of neonatal physiology as well as of disturbed function.

Heat Regulation

The naked fetus is launched at birth into a world which may differ from his previous one by 10–15°C (18–27°F). His relatively large surface area and his limited capacity to produce heat make cooling very easy and the less mature he is the more serious the problem becomes because not only are the above factors exaggerated but also he has even less fat to insulate him. The pace of heat loss also depends on humidity and cooling draughts which flow over the baby. Contrary to the opinion held some years ago that a reduced body temperature might benefit the newborn by reducing the metabolic rate when he might well be having respiratory difficulties, it has now been shown that cooling increases metabolism and oxygen need as the infant attempts to maintain body heat. The harmful effects of this upon the newborn child (Silverman *et al.*, 1958) and upon the erythroblastic one during exchange transfusion (Hey *et al.*, 1969) have been stressed, while other authors have shown the benefit of maintaining babies of low birth weight at appropriate temperatures (Jolly *et al.*, 1962; Silverman and Agate, 1964; Buetow and Klein, 1964; Day *et al.*, 1964).

The newborn human infant, unlike the newborn animal, has no fur, no nest and no litter-mates to keep him warm and he is less active. Heat production must take place without shivering because the human newborn is largely unable to do this. Much of the experimental work on heat production in the newborn has been conducted necessarily on small animals, *e.g.* by Smith (1961), Smith and Hock (1963), Dawkins and Hull (1963), Hein and Hull (1966). These studies have focused attention on brown fat as a principal source of heat at this age, the heat probably being generated locally in response to catechol amines. The subject has been well reviewed by Hull (1966) and by Dawes (1968). According to Aherne and Hull (1966) the human newborn also has a thin sheet of brown fat around the neck, between the scapulae, behind the sternum and round the kidneys and adrenals. The fat content declines during the first few days of life, presumably in response to the cooler environment. The intravenous infusion of noradrenaline into newborn humans is associated with an increase in oxygen consumption and a fall in respiratory quotient to 0·75 (Karlberg *et al.*, 1965) and Silverman *et al.* (1964) believe that the nape of the neck in human newborns remains moderately warm when the babies are exposed to a cool environment. In such babies the plasma glycerol concentration doubles but there is no significant rise in plasma free fatty acids, suggesting that the human infant probably burns fat within brown adipose tissue rather than releasing free fatty acids to be burned elsewhere (Dawkins and Scopes, 1965; Scopes, 1966). The range of environmental temperature within which newborn babies must be kept if they are not to increase oxygen consumption has been well recorded at various ages and for differing weights and maturities by Scopes and Ahmed (1966a). The same authors were able to show that hypoxia in a newborn baby impairs or abolishes his ability to achieve a metabolic response to cooling (Scopes and Ahmed, 1966b). The reasons why babies with neonatal asphyxia often have subnormal temperatures should now be clear.

The modern incubator has been designed with a view to providing the best environmental temperature for the immature or sick baby. Even then Hey and Mount (1967) have shown that small newborn babies kept in an incubator at 34°C must increase their oxygen consumption by 25 per cent if they are to maintain body temperature at 37°C in a room at 20°C. The authors had no easy solution to this problem and Pribylova (1968) found little significant difference between clad and naked infants in incubators. A reduction in humidity may increase heat loss but Hey and Maurice (1968) have shown that this depends on environmental temperature, a temperature reduction significantly increasing the effect of lowering humidity. The limitations of incubators to maintain the requisite temperature and humidity have been demonstrated by Bardell *et al.* (1968).

When hypothermic the baby feels cold, is often reddish in colour, is inactive and shows at first oedema and then progressive solidifying of the subcutaneous tissue (sclerema). Recovery is possible but rewarming is fraught with such dangers as pulmonary haemorrhage. For these reasons the greatest care should be taken to protect the newborn from chilling. Temperatures in hospital should be recorded once daily with individual thermometers, and in the case of infants of low birth weight these should read down to 29·5°C (85°F).

Fever in the newborn is more difficult to understand but about the third day of life it is so common in term babies that it is called 'dehydration fever'. In hospital nurseries it does seem to be commoner when environmental temperature is high or when the baby is wrapped in too many clothes. Lighter clothing and extra fluid by mouth are usually enough to restore temperature to normal, but a careful search for infection is an essential prerequisite of treatment.

Blood

The observations of different authors on the blood during the neonatal period vary widely, average normal values being given by Gairdner *et al.* (1952). The haemoglobin in cord blood varies between 13 and 18 g./100 ml. and is higher in capillary blood (14–22 g./100 ml.). These high values depend to some extent on the source of the specimen and the age in hours of the baby but may also depend on the erythropoietin level in response to low arterial oxygen tension.

The haemoglobin value falls gradually during the first month of life and continues to do so during early infancy. Approximately 85 per cent is of fetal type at term but prematurely born babies have more. Such haemoglobin resists alkaline denaturation, remaining pink in the presence of sodium hydroxide, and this fact has been used to distinguish fetal from maternal blood in the mother should fetus-to-mother transfusion be suspected, in antepartum vaginal bleeding when signs of fetal distress develop and in the vomitus or stools of newborn babies in whom haemorrhagic disease is suspected. The packed cell volume, the mean corpuscular volume, the total white cell count and the percentage of neutrophils also diminish rapidly after birth and immature red cells which are present on the first day of life disappear from the peripheral blood. Indeed the life span of the red cell is almost certainly shorter at this age (Garby *et al.*, 1964). The haematocrit is believed to be a good guide to blood viscosity and exceptionally high haematocrit values, as for example after placental transfusion, or more particularly in the infant of a diabetic mother, may distress the infant and make reduction of the haemoglobin desirable by a carefully calculated exchange of donor plasma for the baby's blood. There is some evidence (Vanier and Tyas, 1967) that prematurely born infants may become folate deficient by the age of 3 months and that the resulting anaemia responds well to folic acid. The range of the eosinophil polymorph value has been found to be above that of normal adults and shows considerable day-to-day variation (Farquhar, 1954; 1955). The reticulocytes increase during the first few hours and then fall progressively. The fragility of the red cells at birth may be normal or slightly increased.

The prothrombin level of the newborn infant falls progressively over the first 3 days of life and rises to normal during the subsequent 3 to 4 days. This period of hypoprothrombinaemia (and resultant prolonged clotting time) is in fact coincidental with the age at which the signs of haemorrhagic disease of the newborn appear, and vitamin K has been used in attempts to prevent it. Success was reported earlier by Lehmann (1944) and Dyggve (1950) but Hay *et al.* (1951) found that administration of the vitamin to a large series of pregnant women before delivery failed to influence the incidence of haemorrhagic disease. This condition may in fact result from a number of abnormalities, and Smith (1959) expresses the view that the failure of vitamin K to prevent all haemorrhagic disease of the new-born is not surprising.

Attention has been called by Edson *et al.* (1968) to the severe defibrination syndrome which may be caused in the newborn child by abruptio placentae. Interest has recently been generated in fibrin degradation products as evidence of intravascular coagulation. Normal values are given by Bonifaci *et al.* (1968) and by Uttley *et al.* (1969). Evidence of disseminated intravascular coagulation in severely ill newborn infants has been presented by Hathaway *et al.* (1969).

Jaundice

Physiological jaundice is detectable clinically on the second or third day of life in the majority of newborn infants, is normally associated with relatively low serum levels of bilirubin, and clears gradually in one week although it may persist for longer. As in haemolytic disease of the newborn the circulating bilirubin is mostly in unconjugated (indirectly reacting) form. It is derived from the contents of the fetal macrocytes which are removed progressively after birth. It should be linked in the liver with uridine diphosphoglucuronic acid under the influence of glucuronyl transferase, an enzyme the activity of which increases with maturity but which may still be deficient at term. Thus in the absence of adequate enzyme action the unconjugated bilirubin levels rise and anything which serves to increase red cell breakdown will increase the hyperbilirubinaemia. The haemolysis of rhesus iso-immunisation is the obvious example of this but other causes exist and only some of them can be explained at present. An inherited deficiency of the red cell enzyme glucose-6-phosphate dehydrogenase has been recognised, and the factors which precipitate haemolysis are known (Doxiadis *et al.*, 1961; Larizza *et al.*, 1960). Circulating unconjugated bilirubin may be harmless to the brain so long as it is bound to albumin (Odell, 1959) but should the serum albumin level be low, as in the infant born before term, or should some drug be given which competes favourably with bilirubin for the albumin molecule, such as the sulphonamides, indirect bilirubin may be released to move into tissue from the vascular space and it may then produce cerebral damage.

Exposure of affected babies to blue light (phototherapy) may help to break down unconjugated bilirubin in the skin and so help reduce the serum level of bilirubin (Cremer *et al.*, 1958; Broughton *et al.*, 1965; Lucey *et al.*, 1968).

Trolle (1968a) reported that neonatal jaundice was less common in babies whose mothers had had phenobarbitone in pregnancy than where the mothers had not. This led to such further studies as those of Trolle (1968b) and of Yeung and Field (1969). These were mostly favourable to the idea of using phenobarbitone for this purpose, although Walker *et al.* (1969) have sounded a note of caution. The present position has been recently reviewed in the *Lancet* (1969a).

Metabolism

Digestion, like respiration, starts as the placental circulation ends but it need not and should not do so as abruptly. The gut is designed to deal with a specific food at first but it can digest the milks of other species although they are likelier to cause upset if unwisely used (Oppé and Redstone, 1968). During the first few days, when the mother's breasts secrete colostrum, the baby derives most of his energy from carbohydrate stores but his respiratory quotient (Benedict and Talbot, 1915) soon indicates a change to the use of fat. The altered nature of infant feeding in the industrialised West from routine breast feeding to almost routine bottle feeding has certainly assured the infant of more fluid and more calories during the first few days than used to be possible. By analogy with other species (Shelley, 1961) the human newborn is thought to have high liver and heart glycogen concentrations and a fair amount also in muscle. Although these reserves fall rapidly (Shelley, 1964) they can be conserved by maintaining the infant's body heat. Glucose derived from the mother is regarded by Shelley (1968) as the main source of energy for the fetus and as the principal substrate for fat and glycogen. The rapid use of it by the fetus at a time when gluconeogenesis is still rather shaky may explain the brief excursions into asymptomatic hypoglycaemia which are relatively common-place (Griffiths, 1968; Farquhar and Isles, 1968). Some babies who have survived an abnormal prenatal environment such as that due to placental insufficiency may convulse while others, born to diabetic mothers, may be undisturbed (Neligan, 1965b; Farquhar, 1965a, 1965b). Poor glycogen reserves, asphyxia and exposure to cold may contribute but do not entirely explain this biochemical disorder (Campbell et al., 1967), while the duration of profound hypoglycaemia is certainly important. The glucose tolerance of newborns is poor by adult standards (Baird and Farquhar, 1962; Von Euler et al., 1964) and the response to glucagon is rela-tively poor in babies delivered by caesarean section (Cornblath et al., 1961).

The total serum protein is rather lower than in adults but the deficiency does not seem to be responsible for neonatal oedema and it probably requires no treatment. A rise in non-protein nitrogen and some increase in the circulating amino acid level may be regarded as normal during the first few days. The plasma amino acid levels of term babies differ little from normal but the range is wider in those born before term in whom abnormally high levels of tyrosine in particular may persist for some time and may make necessary repeat examination of blood specimens for phenylalanine and tyrosine in population screening for phenylke-tonuria. Data on normal levels of immunoglobulins in neonatal blood have been provided by Thom et al. (1967).

The plasma prothrombin level may be low but fibrinogen levels are normal.

Lipids seem not to cross from mother to baby in significant amounts during pregnancy and levels in cord blood serum at birth are much lower than in maternal serum (Zee, 1968). Fetal levels of free fatty acids, although lower, seem to bear a relationship to maternal levels in labour. Glycerol seems not to pass from mother to fetus but ketones do and may provide, after glucose, a reserve of energy (Sabata et al., 1968). Stores, however, are adequate and the lipid blood level rises quickly after delivery (Rafstedt, 1955; Zee, 1968) as the baby 'lives off his hump' while awaiting adequate calories by mouth. Indeed hypoglycaemia may stimulate the formation of active endogenous lipoprotein lipase and the release from store of free fatty acids (Gürson and Etili, 1968). Glycerol when injected intravenously is removed most rapidly in light-for-dates babies, takes longer in normal term babies, accelerates during the first few weeks of life and in all cases is associated with a rise in blood glucose (Wolf et al., 1968). It seems likely that the lipid stores, including brown fat, are made by the fetus as a source of energy on which to draw when carbohydrate is being spared or is exhausted.

Serum phosphorus levels tend to rise and calcium to fall during the first week of life, changes which are commonly attributed to endocrine immaturity—a 'physiological' hypoparathyroidism—and to the greater phosphate content of cow's milk when compared with that of humans. This has been demonstrated again by Oppé and Redstone (1968) while Southgate et al. (1969) believe that the unabsorbed fat of various cow's milk preparations may interfere profoundly with the absorption of calcium. Neonatal hypocalcaemia is certainly commoner than was thought some years ago and may present as irritability or even convulsions: it may be commoner after instrumental delivery or in the newborn of diabetic mothers (Gittleman et al., 1956, 1959; Craig and Buchanan, 1958). Although Bajpai et al. (1966) found no appreciable change in serum magnesium levels during the first week of life in relatively small series of breast and bottle fed babies, hypomagnesaemia is quite a common finding in neonatal tetany and convulsions which then respond to careful injection of magnesium sulphate.

In development of such complexity, incomplete as it is at birth, it would be surprising if all enzyme functions involved were perfect. Some, such as glucuronyl transferase and the pulmonary surface active agent, are quite commonly inadequate and others whose deficiency is of genetic origin may declare their absence then, e.g. glucose-6-phosphate dehydrogenase, or later as in phenylketonuria.

Renal Function

Urine is secreted by the fetal kidney by the fourth month and micturition at the time of birth is common. This prenatal secretion may in the presence of congenital obstructions result in hydronephrosis even before the baby is born, while the absence of function as in renal agenesis is associated with oligohydramnios. The placenta probably undertakes most of the work, however, until delivery when, even at term, the kidney is functionally immature. The assessment of renal efficiency is difficult and, as McCance (1959) points out, such tests as the glomerular filtration rate and urea clearance, which are expressed in terms of millilitres of extracellular fluid passing through the glomeruli or cleared of urea per minute, can no more be used to compare the newborn and the adult than they can to compare the fieldmouse and the elephant. Corrections for weight, surface area and body water have all been used and make difficult the comparison of published series. The newborn infant's kidney, however, is less able to clear water, salt and urea than is the adult's and it may have difficulty in conserving water but is nevertheless effective in maintaining a relatively stable state, particularly when the baby's food and fluid needs are correctly and adequately met. Growth is the biochemical stabiliser, mopping up nitrogen and minerals, and human breast milk best meets its needs while stressful delivery, asphyxia, starvation or exposure to cold increase tissue breakdown, interfere with growth and upset homeostasis. Similarly, an abnormal mineral load in an artificial diet may upset growth and stability. A relatively small increase in the salt content of a milk formula, for example, may by reason of the large volumes of fluid taken by babies result in their ingesting proportionately more salt than a normal adult would do, with the consequent development of loss of appetite, lethargy and oedema (McCance and Widdowson, 1957).

The neonatal kidney may be regarded, therefore, as adequate under normal conditions but inadequate to meet abnormal loads, and intravenous therapy which can be of great value must be employed with caution. The risk of accidental over-loading has been much reduced in recent years by the development of improved recipient equipment designed for infants.

Urinary osmolality has been used as a measure of dehydration in the newborn (Davis *et al.*, 1966). The normal limits of the cell count in neonatal urine have been established by Silver *et al.* (1967).

Endocrine System

The developing fetus is exposed to both maternal and endogenous endocrine secretions (Deanesly, 1961) which influence permanent and temporary changes in morphology. At birth the female external genitalia are congested, the labia minora and clitoris are prominent, and to the mucoid vaginal discharge there may be added in occasional cases a little endometrial bleeding. The vaginal mucosa is hypertrophied and contains glycogen but begins to desquamate within the first few days. The uterus is enlarged but involutes from birth. The epithelium of the male utricle, prostatic urethra and prostatic glands may show squamous metaplasia. Breast milk is secreted by most mature and a good many immature infants of both sexes (Fig. 9) but gradually decreases after the newborn period although it may persist for months in some cases.

According to Laron *et al.* (1967) growth hormone levels in babies at birth are from 2 to 4 times greater than the growth hormone levels in their mothers. This has been interpreted as evidence of growth hormone secretion by the baby at this time.

The adrenal glands of the newborn are much larger in proportion to body weight than at any other age. This is due almost entirely to the large fetal zone of cortex which involutes from birth independent of maturity and the function of which remains obscure (Tähkä, 1951). According to Migeon (1959) cortisol can cross the placental barrier from mother to fetus and possibly also in the reverse direction. The maternal levels already raised by pregnancy rise further during labour, while the response to caesarean section is less immediate. In consequence cortisol levels are higher after vaginal than after abdominal delivery. The newborn does not lack corticosteroids during the first few days at least, but they are in part of maternal origin, and because of a deficiency of catabolic enzyme action their half life is prolonged. Migeon believes that differences in the metabolism of steroids at this age may lead to the erroneous interpretation of urinary steroid levels. The urinary output of 17-hydroxy-corticosteroids in prematurely born infants is thought to be less than in term babies during the first week but this difference then disappears (Cranny and Cranny, 1960). The nature of the adrenal steroids found in the pooled urine of newborns has been described by Birchall *et al.* (1961) while the ability of

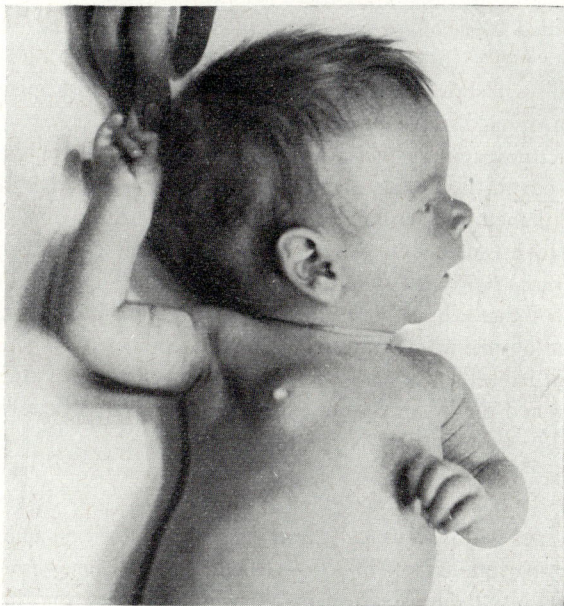

FIG. 9. Breast enlargement in the newborn, showing secretion of milk.

the newborn adrenal cortex to react to stress has been reviewed recently by Cathro *et al.* (1969). Their own contribution in this field showed the wide range of urinary steroids possible: normal and 'premature' infants on average showed a significant response to stress in the first few days whereas 'dysmature' babies did not. The adrenal medulla of the newborn infant contains much less pressor amines than do the organs of Zuckerkandl. Both structures produce noradrenaline almost entirely at this age. West *et al.* (1953) were of the opinion that the organs of Zuckerkandl secrete this potent pressor substance in order to maintain vascular tone at a developmental stage when the adrenal medulla and the sympathetic nervous system are still immature. The urinary output of 3-methoxy-4-hydroxy-mandelic acid, a major metabolite of noradrenaline and adrenaline, increases when the newborn is exposed to lower environmental temperatures (Sandler *et al.*, 1961), although this may not be so when the mother is diabetic, and the adrenal medulla would seem then to be exhausted (Stern *et al.*, 1968).

The histology of the thyroid gland suggests the existence of heightened activity before birth and a further powerful stimulus to activity at or about birth, decreasing from the third or fourth day (Sclare, 1956). Thyroxine can probably pass the placental barrier in each direction so that the maternal and umbilical cord levels of butyl-extractable iodine are very similar. Following delivery the maternal level changes little but a striking rise in the baby can be interpreted as representing the release to the circulation of a considerable quantity of thyroid hormone (Pickering *et al.*, 1958; Chadd *et al.*, 1968). Further evidence of normal or increased function has been provided by Spafford *et al.* (1960), Marks (1965) and Malkasian and Tauxe (1965).

The possibility of brief functional hypoparathyroidism (Kaplan, 1942) has already been mentioned in relation to neonatal tetany.

In the endocrine pancreas the ratio of alpha to beta cells in the newborn is normally 1 : 1, but in the infants of diabetic mothers, presumably in response to some maternal diabetogenic stimulus, the beta cells increase both in number and size, and the pancreas of such babies is able to produce much more insulin than is normally the case (Baird and Farquhar, 1962). A further study on gestational diabetics showed that while their babies produced significantly higher levels of insulin than did normal newborns a few minutes after an intravenous injection of glucose, normal babies had a high late response about an hour after the glucose had been given and they then became normoglycaemic more rapidly (Isles *et al.*, 1968).

Immunity

The fetus brings with him as a gift from his mother a certain amount of partial or complete passive immunity to infectious diseases. Thus he may have considerable temporary immunity to measles and poliomyelitis provided that his mother has had them or has been immunised against them. This will dictate the time at which active immunisation can be attempted. On the other hand he may already have been the victim of infection in prenatal life (syphilis, toxoplasmosis, rubella) and at birth he is immediately vulnerable to infection by staphylococci and gram negative bacilli. Normal values of immunoglobulins for umbilical cord plasma are given by Thom *et al.* (1967). Data on immunoglobulin levels in a number of pathological states have also been provided by McKay *et al.* (1967, 1968). Raised levels of IgM after prenatal rubella have been found in only 18 per cent of affected babies by McCracken *et al.* (1969).

Iatrogenic Disease

Clinical experience has recently revealed that drugs which are well tolerated by older children and adults may be dangerous to the fetus when they 'leak across' the placenta from the mother or when they are given to the infant or accidentally come into contact with him after birth. The disastrous effects of thalidomide on the development of the fetal limbs and other structures have intensified research in this field. The androgens (Grumbach and Ducharme, 1960), the androgenic progestagens (Moncrieff, 1958; Wilkins, 1960), and occasionally the synthetic oestrogens (Bongiovanni *et al.*, 1959) may cause masculinisation of the female fetus if given to the mother in early pregnancy. The goitrogenic effect upon the fetus of antithyroid drugs given to the thyrotoxic mother and occasionally of iodides given to the asthmatic or bronchitic one are well known (Wilkins, 1957). The uncritical administration of intravenous infusions to labouring women may cause marked changes in tonicity and sodium concentration in the fetus (Battaglia *et al.*, 1960), and it is possible that dietary restriction of the mother or her treatment with powerful diuretic agents may also do so. Hexamethonium bromide given for maternal hypertension has produced paralytic ileus in the baby (Hallum and Hatchuel, 1954) but is no longer used. Anaesthetic and analgesic agents may seriously depress the fetal respiratory centre while wild excitation may appear in newborn infants of heroin addicts. The use of succinylcholine as an aid to anaesthesia may cause prolonged apnoea in sensitive babies (Kaufman *et al.*, 1960), and skin contact with unlaundered marking ink may produce severe methaemoglobinaemia (Ramsey and Harvey, 1959). The use of sulphonamides in neonatal infections is associated with an increased risk of kernicterus (Silverman *et al.*, 1956) and their use in the newborn or in the pregnant woman at term should be avoided. Both aspirin and caffeine sodium benzoate, like sulphafurazole, may *in vitro* split unconjugated bilirubin from the albumin molecule (Odell, 1959) but in the doses used are unlikely to release serious amounts of it. Chloramphenicol is poorly conjugated and excreted by the newborn (Nyhan, 1961) and should no longer be used in the newborn except perhaps in the treatment of neonatal gram negative meningitis or in countries where other antibiotics are unavailable.

The Care of the Newborn

In addition to those features of good antenatal care which are designed to promote normal intra-uterine development and uncomplicated delivery, wise preparation of the mother will include not only education about the advisability of breast feeding and preparation for it but also a short course of mothercraft. This latter should comprise lessons on elementary hygiene, feeding and bathing the baby, and the management of simple infantile disorders. Guidance should be given also in the preparation of the layette.

Reception

At birth the infant's eyelids may be cleansed with pledgets of cotton wool, but the custom of instilling 1 per cent silver nitrate has been discontinued in communities where antenatal care is adequate and hospital delivery common. Babies delivered in their homes may have sulphacetamide instilled or such other preparations as may be ordered by the local supervising authority, but in hospital it is better to await, diagnose and treat energetically any conjunctivitis that may develop. Should local opinion favour delay in clamping the cord until the contracting uterus has effected a placental transfusion of blood, then it may be deferred until eye toilet is complete. It is not always advisable to wait until pulsation of the cord has ceased since the duration of pulsation is very variable and long delay may lead to chilling of the infant. Pulsation may in fact continue for some considerable time after the cord has been cut. After clamping, it should be firmly ligatured and divided. Only a very small quantity of blood should ooze from the cut end and if oozing continues the cord must be religatured. It is essential to keep a careful watch on it throughout the first week since any recurrence of oozing indicates either that the ligature has become insecure or that the infant is suffering from haemorrhagic disease or sepsis. The danger of poor ligation has been greatly reduced by the use of disposable plastic clamps or by means of elastic bands (Neligan et al., 1964). The dying cord tissue provides an ideal pabulum for bacteria and in certain circumstances it may provide the portal through which common pyogenic bacteria and the toxins of tetanus gain entry. Present practice inclines to exposure of the occluded cord rather than to covering it with powder, a dressing and binder.

The squeeze exerted on the baby's thorax during vaginal delivery assists in the expulsion of fluid from the airway, but the fear that he may be drowned by such secretions often excites such unnecessary fervour over pharyngeal aspiration that harm may result. In most cases positional drainage will be all that is required and this may be done before the cord is cut by laying him on his back on a mobile resuscitation trolley. Fluid can then drain freely from the lungs and the chest can expand readily. It is always advisable to have available equipment by means of which fluid can be sucked out of the oropharynx if necessary. This may be simply a small soft rubber catheter attached to a glass 'trap' (Fraser, 1951) but there are advantages in having multiple sterile catheters and a mechanical source of suction, the negative pressure of which can be controlled and which not only frees the nurse from the unpleasant and even hazardous task of sucking but removes the danger to the child of a nurse who also blows through the catheter. Suction is more frequently required after caesarean section.

Even a normal labour exposes the infant to appreciable stress and the greatest care must be taken to avoid chilling and rough handling after birth. The infant should be wrapped in a warm sterile towel as soon as practicable; there is no urgency about the ritual cleansing unless infection of the maternal passages is suspected.

The cot should be very simple but should be so constructed as to make handling easy. It should avoid having surfaces which cannot be cleaned and should be capable of carrying with it articles such as thermometers personal to the baby. Fig. 10 illustrates the type of cot used at the Simpson Memorial Maternity Pavilion in Edinburgh. At home a carry-cot will suffice for much of the first year and is also very useful if the baby is taken visiting. The dangers of hot-water bottles and of electric heating pads are so great that they should be avoided wherever possible.

General Examination

The presence of hydramnios may already have suggested the possibility of congenital abnormality of the fetus (Moya et al., 1960). The umbilical cord should be examined at birth for the presence of a single umbilical artery. Although uncommon it may be associated with congenital malformation (Van Leeuwen et al., 1967). Shortly after birth the infant should be thoroughly examined in a good light. Any congenital anomaly such as club foot or cleft palate and any evidence of birth injury should be noted. The heart must be carefully examined and the femoral pulses should always be felt in order to exclude aortic coarctation. It is most important to make certain that the orifices are patent and that the infant passes

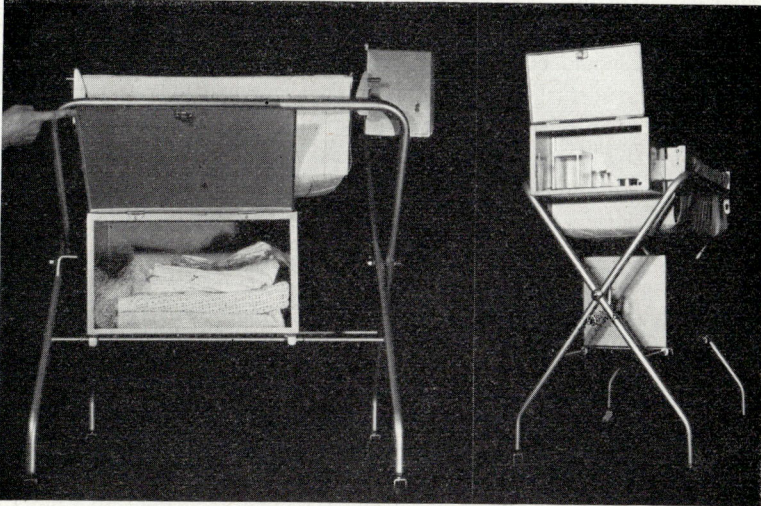

Fig. 10. A cot suitable for the rooming-in of baby with mother. The large locker contains clothing, blankets and napkins: the small one has a thermometer, skin applications and other items for the infant's own use.

urine and meconium during the first 24 hours. The abdomen should be palpated to make sure that the bladder is not distended and that there are no masses such as abnormal kidneys or tumours. The presence of a pilonidal depression at the base of the spine is not of clinical importance unless it leads to a true sinus, but care should be taken to exclude epidermal sinuses higher over the spine. The genitalia and inguinal regions should be examined to exclude hernia, hydrocele, maldescent of the testicles or adhesions of the labia. Birthmarks should be noted. If either parent has Mongolian or Negro blood it should be remembered that 'Mongolian blue spots' may be present on the buttocks or sacral area and are apt to be mistaken for ecchymoses.

The prepuce is commonly adherent to the glans and is not fully retractile at birth. In a high proportion of cases it will become retractile later. The circumcision of newborn infants is often recommended much too lightly and the case against it has been fully reviewed by Gairdner (1949) and Weiss (1964). The report of the first year of the Newcastle 'thousand family' survey (Spence et al., 1954) showed that 11 per cent of the boys were circumcised, and of these circumcisions no fewer than 22 per cent were complicated, usually by haemorrhage and infection. In no case should the infant be circumcised during the first 8 days of life, because of the physiological hypoprothrombinaemia of that period, or when jaundice is present. One of the few medical grounds for circumcision of the newborn, as distinct from the demands of religion or fashion, is the presence of a preputial orifice so small as to cause obstruction and ballooning of the prepuce during micturition. This condition is rare.

The breast enlargement which may accompany the common secretory activity of male and female infants requires no treatment and attempts to express the milk only predispose to mastitis. Congenital dislocation of the hip may be diagnosed at this age and it should be looked for routinely as early treatment will be more effective and less disturbing to the child. The knees can normally be abducted more than 45° from the midline and limitation of this should arouse suspicion. When testing, the hips are flexed to 90°. Each thigh is gripped firmly from the back so that the examiner's thumbs lie on the medial aspect and can abduct the thigh while his fingers lie just behind the femoral head and can lift it forward. By alternately abducting and adducting at the hip joint distinct 'clunks' may be felt as the dislocated or unstable femoral head enters and leaves the acetabulum. Good results are obtained when dislocation is recognised and treated early (Dickerson, 1968).

Head. The occipito-frontal circumference of the head should be measured within 24 hours of birth. This may be easily and cheaply done using disposable paper tapes stamped in centimetres.* Serial circumferences may then be entered on a suitable skull circumference chart (Farquhar, 1961). Head-moulding, which is normally present at birth except in elective caesarean deliveries and a proportion of easy breech extractions, varies in degree from minimal distortion of the skull to overriding of the sutures. Unless it is accompanied by intracranial damage it has no permanent effect and moulding tends to become less obvious during the first week of life. The presence of a caput succedaneum, or oedematous area over the part of the head which has presented during a prolonged labour, is often observed at birth, and in the case of a face presentation may be associated with great discoloration. This normally disappears rapidly, leaving no permanent disability.

A *cephalhaematoma*, or large fluctuant swelling, limited by the suture lines and due to the presence of blood under the periosteum, may appear on the second or third day after birth It is due partly to local trauma, but is also probably related to hypoprothrombinaemia, though not commonly associated with other evidence of haemorrhage. If uncomplicated, it is of no serious significance and calcification and absorption will occur spontaneously. Since calcification starts at the margin, a calcifying haematoma is sometimes mistaken for a depressed fracture.

The *anterior fontanelle* is readily palpable at birth and varies greatly in size. It is normally pulsatile, but if it is found to be tense or bulging when the infant is at rest, intracranial haemorrhage or hydrocephalus should be suspected. The sutures are often more easily palpable than in the older infant, and one or more of the 5 other fontanelles present at birth may often be identified clinically. The

---

* These tapes are obtainable from Messrs T. Lyon & Co. Ltd., Letterpress and Lithographic Printers, 142a–148 London Road, Liverpool 3.

face and neck may provide the diagnosis of one of the trisomic chromosomal disorders such as Down's syndrome.

Trunk. Although the thoracic cage is relatively soft and flexible during the newborn period, and the respiratory excursion is slight, it should be possible to detect inequality of movement or deformity of the ribs, *e.g.* due to fracture. The abdomen appears relatively large in the newborn infant and moves freely with respiration. The liver edge is normally palpable one or more finger-breadths below the costal margin, but the spleen is not felt unless it is pathologically enlarged.

The umbilical cord rapidly becomes white or semi-translucent in colour after it has been tied, and shrivels during the time that it remains attached. Separation normally occurs spontaneously about 7 days after birth, but the cord may remain attached considerably longer in prematurely born infants. When the cord has separated, the umbilicus should be dry. Any stickiness or bleeding of the umbilicus is a danger signal as it suggests the presence of infection.

Skin. The skin of the infant at birth is usually erythematous and normally shows no appreciable jaundice. The pinkness tends to fade during the first few days of life and during this time icteric tinting appears. The term infant is well supplied with subcutaneous fat, and the skin is elastic; the nails extend slightly beyond the nail-beds; lanugo is usually slight in amount, though there is a variable amount of soft, silky hair on the scalp. Occasionally infants are born with a thick mass of dark hair of coarser texture. This tends to fall out during the sixth or seventh week of life and to be replaced by the more typical fine silky hair of early infancy. Milia on the face are commonly seen, and small naevi on the frontal and occipital regions are so frequent as to be popularly known as 'marks of the stork's beak'.

Any rash occurring during the neonatal period should be carefully noted and the cause sought, *e.g.* staphylococcal infection, congenital syphilis, or maternal scabies.

Hearing. Response of the newborn to hearing may be helpful in assessing the gestational age of the baby (Graziani *et al.*, 1968) and may just possibly be used to predict mental ability (O'Doherty, 1968).

Metabolic Screening

Microbiological and biochemical tests for such inborn metabolic diseases as phenylketonuria are now available and are widely used in some parts of Britain (Consultant Paediatricians and Medical Officers of Health of the S.E. Scotland Hospital Region, 1968) and in much of the United States. Care must always be taken to diagnose with absolute certainty as many positive cases and diseases as possible at lowest cost and at no risk to the patient or distress to the parents. Screening programmes are currently built around phenylketonuria but the programme is likely to continue so that doctors must try to exercise some control over the disease or witness its possible increase in the community.

4

Accommodation and the Prevention of Cross-Infection

Wherever the baby is nursed his cot should be screened from draughts and a stable room temperature of about 20°C (68°F) maintained. Babies born at home must also be protected from fluctuations in room temperature and overheating is as liable to cause distress as chilling. The advantages to the mother of institutional delivery at least for the first baby are generally felt to outweigh the possible disadvantages, but the extent to which this faith is justified depends largely on the standards of the hospital available. Where the mother is given every opportunity of learning the care of her own infant she should derive full benefit from the skilled nursing and rest which are now seldom equally possible in the home. The common disadvantages of hospital, however, lie in the impersonal and often hurried institutional atmosphere, such monopoly of the baby by overworked nursing staff that his mother may gain little experience in infant care during her stay, and the addition of nocturnal interruptions to busy days. There is also the ever present risk of cross-infection with antibiotic-resistant bacteria. Staphylococcus aureus and the gram negative bacilli offer a continuing threat although the contribution of each seems to vary from time to time. Thus the staphylococcus *seems* to have been mastered in many hospitals in recent years although experienced clinicians remain alert to the possibility of an unexpected counter-attack. The gram negative bacilli constitute the greater danger at present for a variety of reasons and must be assiduously sought after by bacteriological screening routines which must include, among other things, the culture of blood and of clean and immediately plated urine samples. The number of newborn babies who die because of infection is much lower than it was before antimicrobial substances became available, but there may not have been much change in mortality in recent years. Furthermore, the ease with which communication happens in this age group makes obligatory a much simpler but time-consuming and expensive routine.

Infecting organisms may spread from baby to environment, from environment to baby, and between babies. The agitation of dust by cleaning, bedmaking, and excessive traffic in an overcrowded unit may result in a heavy staphylococcal fall-out which may be reduced by coating the floors with dust-trapping preparations, wet cleaning, piped vacuum cleaning from a central department, the sterilisation of cotton blankets, the provision of suitable bins for the disposal of soiled articles and the strict limitation of hospital population. The hospital staff are of fundamental importance because, colonised as they may be by resistant organisms, they make intimate contact with the newborn by means of hands, upper respiratory tracts, clothing and possibly their hidden septic lesions. These dangers should in theory be reducible by decreasing the number of contacts between babies and staff, by strict discipline in hand-washing and personal hygiene with regard to bathing and all clothing, by replacing personal handkerchiefs with tissues and providing means for their disposal, and by maintaining such an adequate ratio of staff to patients that efficiency can be maintained. This will make necessary the provision of adequate numbers of wash-hand basins with wrist- or foot-operated taps, continuous roller or disposable towels, antiseptic hand creams, and the frequent re-education of both medical and nursing staff in barrier techniques.

Infection may be spread from baby to baby and by using for all infants such communal points of indirect contact as changing tables, weighing machines, communal ointments, hair brushes, towels and baths. Some of these can be avoided altogether, contact with others can be much reduced in frequency, and precautions can be taken to reduce the bacterial population of tables and weighing scale pans by using plastic rather than cloth coverings and by mopping them with a bactericidal detergent between babies. The care of the baby's skin is an important measure in reducing infection. It may be cleansed with a good baby soap but hexachlorophane may be very effective in reducing the incidence of staphylococcal sepsis. Present experience suggests that although hexachlorophane is effective in reducing the concentration of staphylococci, its greater use has been associated with increasing coliform infection, although proof of a causal relationship is unavailable. Portable and easily sterilised baths are useful for cot-side bathing in the mother's room, but routine cleansing of the napkin area may be carried out in the cot. In the case of feeble infants and where there is much vernix caseosa, cleansing is best carried out with warm olive oil. Chilling must be avoided. After the skin has been washed and gently patted dry, the flexures should be dusted with a good baby talc. The nails should be kept short and clean to prevent infection from scratching. Adequate provision must be made for the isolation of both suspect and established infections, and an agreed policy designed to control the use of anti-biotics is very desirable.

Elaborate air filtration plants may create an erroneous sense of security unless they are known to be efficient and to be regularly serviced. Even then they are of little value if the clean air provided is later contaminated by careless staff.

Crusading zeal and success or disillusionment and despair often surround the practice of keeping the baby in a cot beside his mother by day and night (Fig. 11) and making her responsible for nursing him. In theory this should eliminate many sources of infection in a central nursery suite and should give the mother valuable supervised practice in handling him.

In practice, however, mothers may tolerate, often with some difficulty, the crying of their own baby in hospital but may find utterly exhausting the many nocturnal disturbances caused by the babies of fellow patients. This may lead in turn to inappropriate heavy sedation of mothers as well as to transfer of babies back to the central nursery and the collapse of the cross-infection barriers which rooming-in provides.

Experience suggests that, short of the ideal hospital design and the ratio of nursing staff to patients which few possess, the prevention of cross-infection depends on disciplined and dedicated staff.

Care of the Infant of Low Birth Weight

The difficulties of establishing respiration become greater with decreasing maturity and birth weight of the baby. The cause of the premature birth may itself have a depressing effect on the respiratory centres while a softer chest cage and deficient surfactant material are major problems. The need for skilful resuscitative measures should therefore be anticipated at all premature births and provision should be made where possible for the treatment of the idiopathic respiratory

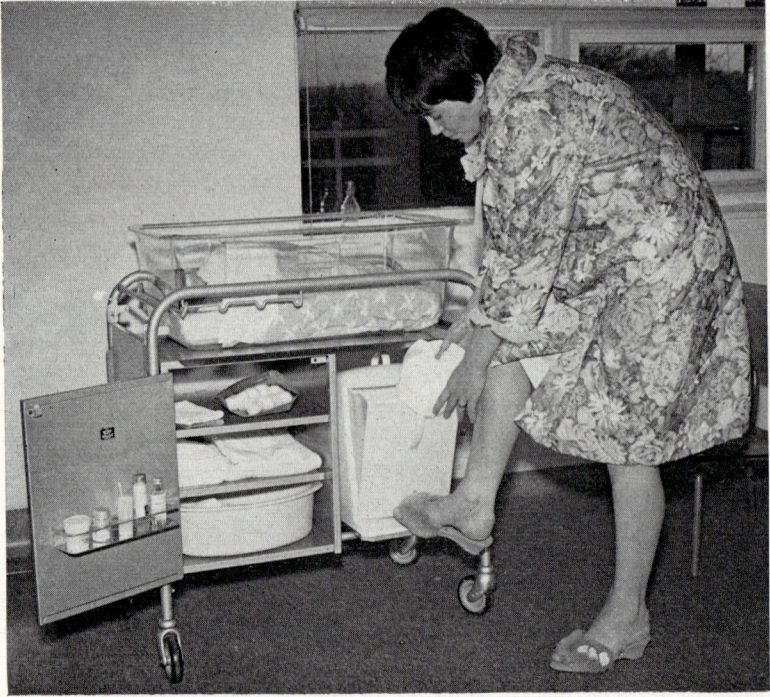

FIG. 11. Mother attending to her baby in a maternity hospital.

distress syndrome. Oxygen is used in as high a concentration as is needed to relieve cyanosis and the baby is in no danger of developing retrolental fibroplasia, so long as discretion is exercised. At least one make of baby incubator now incorporates a conspicuous indicator that a higher than usual concentration of oxygen is likely to exist and it is wise also regularly to record the concentration measured by a simple oximeter. The danger of blindness from retrolental fibroplasia must not be forgotten, however, and there is no place for the prolonged use of oxygen as a routine part of care. The other components of treatment for respiratory distress syndrome include correction of acidosis, the provision of water and glucose and the giving of antimicrobials and perhaps mechanical assistance to respiration, but these matters are dealt with in text-books on diseases of the newborn.

The importance of preserving body heat has been stressed already and one of the most important functions of an incubator is to provide a personal environment for the infant while his nurse can be comfortable in hers. A modern incubator should also filter the incoming air in such a way as to reduce the danger of infection but again it is no substitute for good staff. Incubators may be quite beyond the financial resources of many lands where other public health matters are of greater importance. Yet excellent results in the management of small infants are being obtained in Asia and Africa even where the outside temperature falls to freezing-point. Simple draught-free cots or boxes may be fly-screened with gauze, and the temperature may be maintained by the use of stoves, or cooling may be facilitated by fans and screens.

The feeding of larger babies (2 to 2·5 kg. body weight) creates a problem only if the baby is ill in some way, *e.g.* respiratory distress, when an attempt must be made to meet in part the baby's need by intravenous infusion. The feeding of smaller babies remains a controversial subject. Objections to early feeding were often based in the past on a failure to distinguish clearly between small babies with and without respiratory distress syndrome so that distressed breathing and apnoeic spells were attributed to the inhalation of feeds; a fact which was sometimes demonstrable (Wharton and Bower, 1965). On the other hand hyperbilirubinaemia and hypoglycaemia may be attributed to delay in feeding (*Lancet*, 1969b) so that on balance some special care units in the past decade have sought so to improve their techniques that the advantages of early feeding clearly outweigh the hazards. The smaller the baby the likelier is tube-feeding to be necessary, and there is a general move toward the use of fine plastic catheters which are passed through the nose and which require only infrequent changing. Once in the correct position these help to conserve the baby's energy and the nurse's time, and they are probably safer than tubes which need to be passed for each feed.

In a study reported by Barrie (1968) all newborn infants fed by nasogastric tube regurgitated milk into the lower half of the oesophagus and in consequence developed a variety of respiratory disturbances. This observation has been shared by others but it must depend to some extent on the number and skill of staff in the special care unit. Hughes-Davis (1968) has suggested that regurgitation is reduced if babies are nursed prone and with a head upward tilt. A comparison of early intravenous and oral feeding of very small infants has been reported by Mamunes *et al.* (1969). Little separated the two groups except that there were fewer low blood glucose levels in the group fed intravenously at first. Even the nature of the feed formula is controversial although lactose seems to present no problem (Jarrett and Holman, 1966) and not all fat may be absorbed. Amino acids, however, may not all be metabolised at normal pace so that phenylalanine and tyrosine may so increase in the blood that an inborn error may be suspected. Were neonatal tetany always the result of temporary hypoparathyroidism, it might be expected more often in immature babies but this seems seldom to be so even when milk is reconstituted near to full strength. Small babies graduate to and larger ones start with feeding bottles according to their ability to suck without tiring.

Older babies will certainly be fed according to appetite and should have supplements of iron and vitamins at the age of one month. The early anaemia of prematurely born infants can be striking and is not preventable by iron alone. In a study of folic acid status in such babies Vanier and Tyas (1967) found that the majority showed some evidence of folate deficiency by the age of 2–3 months and that some of these had marked haemopoietic response to folic acid. Later in the first year iron is required. The infant of low birth weight should also have 400 i.u. daily of vitamin D. Such small babies are more susceptible to infection in the newborn period and, perhaps because of nutritional deficiency or environmental circumstances, may remain so during the first few years. In the unlikely event of a small newborn infant needing chloramphenicol, the dose should not exceed 20 mg./kg. body weight in the first week of life.

J. W. FARQUHAR

References

ADAMS, F. H. and LIND, J. (1957). Physiologic studies on the cardiovascular status of normal newborn infants. *Pediatrics*, **19**, 431.

AHERNE, W. and HULL, D. (1966). Brown adipose tissue and heat production in the newborn infant. *J. Path. Bact.*, **91**, 223.

AMBRUS, C. M., WEINTRAUB, D. H., NISWANDER, K. R. and AMBRUS, J. L. (1965). Studies on hyaline membrane disease. *Pediatrics*, **35**, 91.

APGAR, V. (1953). Proposal for a new method of evaluation of the newborn infant. *Curr. Res. Anes. Analg.*, **32**, 260.

ARAJÄRVI, T. (1953). Microscopic investigation into the capillaries of the newborn, especially premature infants. Helsinki.

ASHWORTH, A. M. and NELIGAN, G. A. (1959). Changes in systolic blood-pressure of normal babies during the first 24 hours of life. *Lancet*, **1**, 804.

—— —— and ROGERS, J. F. (1959). Sphygmomanometer for the newborn. *Lancet*, **1**, 801.

AVERY, M. E. and MEAD, J. (1959). Surface properties in relation to atelectasis and hyaline membrane disease. *Amer. J. Dis. Child.*, **97**, 517.

BAIRD, J. D. and FARQUHAR, J. W. (1962). Insulin-secreting capacity in newborn infants of normal and diabetic women. *Lancet*, **1**, 71.

BAJPAI, P. C., SUGDEN, D., RAMOS, A. and STERN, L. (1966). Serum magnesium levels in the newborn and older child. *Arch. Dis. Childh.*, **41**, 424.

BARDELL, E., FREEMAN, J. and HEY, E. N. (1968). Relative humidity in incubators. *Arch. Dis. Childh.*, **43**, 172.

BARRIE, H. (1968). Effect of feeding on gastric and oesophageal pressures in the newborn. *Lancet*, **2**, 1158.

BATTAGLIA, F., PRYSTOWSKY, H., SMISSON, C., HELLEGERS, A. and BRUNS, P. (1960). Fetal blood studies. *Pediatrics*, **25**, 2.

—— and LUBCHENCO, L. O. (1967). A practical classification of newborn infants by weight and gestational age. *J. Pediat.*, **71**, 159.

BENEDICT, F. G. and TALBOT, F. B. (1915). The physiology of the newborn infant. Character and amount of the katabolism. Washington: Carnegie Inst. Pub. No. 233.

BENSON, P. F., BONHAM CARTER, R. E. and SMELLIE, J. M. (1961). Transient and intermittent systolic murmurs in newborn infants. *Lancet*, **1**, 627.

BIRCHALL, K., CATHRO, D. M., FORSYTH, C. C. and MITCHELL, F. L. (1961). Separation and estimation of adrenal steroids in the urine of newborn infants. *Lancet*, **1**, 26.

BONGIOVANNI, A. M., DI GEORGE, A. M. and GRUMBACH, M. M. (1959). Masculinization of the female infant associated with estrogenic therapy. *J. clin. Endocrinol. Metab.*, **19**, 1004.

BONIFACI, E., BAGGIO, P. and GRAVINA, E. (1968). Demonstration of split products of fibrinogen in the blood of normal newborns. *Biol. Neonat.*, **12**, 29.

BOUND, J. P., HARVEY, P. W. and BAGSHAW, H. B. (1962). Prevention of pulmonary syndrome of the newborn. *Lancet*, **1**, 1200.

BROUGHTON, P. M. G., ROSSITER, E. J. R., WARREN, C. B. M., GOULIS, G. and LORD, P. S. (1965). Effect of blue light on hyperbilirubinaemia. *Arch. Dis. Childh.*, **40**, 666.

BUETOW, K. C. and KLEIN, S. W. (1964). Effect of maintenance of normal skin temperature on survival of infants of low birth weight. *Pediatrics*, **34**, 163.

BURNARD, E. D. (1958). A murmur from the ductus arteriosus in the newborn baby. *Brit. med. J.*, **1**, 806.

—— (1959). Changes in heart size in the dyspnoeic newborn baby. *Brit. med. J.*, **1**, 1495.

—— (1963). in *Modern Trends in Reproductive Physiology*. Ed. H. M. Carey. London: Butterworth.

BUTLER, N. (1965). in *Gestational Age, Size and Maturity*. Ed. M. Dawkins and W. G. MacGregor. *Clinics in Developmental Medicine No. 19*. London: Spastics Society/ Heinemann.

CAMPBELL, A. G. M., MILLIGAN, J. E. and TALNER, N. S. (1968). Studies of anoxia and resuscitation in newborn rabbits. *J. Pediat.*, **72**, 518.

CAMPBELL, M. A., FERGUSON, I. C., HUTCHISON, J. H. and KERR, M. M. (1967). Diagnosis and treatment of hypoglycaemia in the newborn. *Arch. Dis. Childh.*, **42**, 353.

CATHRO, D. M., FORSYTH, C. C. and CAMERON, J. (1969). Adrenocortical response to stress in newborn infants. *Arch. Dis. Childh.*, **44**, 88.

CHADD, M. A., DAVIES, D. F. and GRAY, O. P. (1968). Protein-bound iodine in premature infants. *Arch. Dis. Childh.*, **43**, 217.

COCHRAN, W. D., DAVIS, H. T. and SMITH, C. A. (1968). Umbilical artery catheterization. *Pediatrics*, **42**, 769.

Consultant Paediatricians and Medical Officers of Health of the S.E. Scotland Hospital Region (1968). Population screening by Guthrie test for phenylketonuria in South East Scotland. *Brit. med. J.*, **1**, 674.

CORNBLATH, M., NICOLOPOULOS, D., GANZON, A. F., LEVIN, E. Y., GORDON, M. H. and GORDON, H. H. (1961). Studies of carbohydrate metabolism in the newborn infant. *Pediatrics*, **28**, 592.

CRAIG, W. S. and BUCHANAN, M. F. G. (1958). Hypocalcaemic tetany developing within 36 hours of birth. *Arch. Dis. Childh.*, **33**, 505.

CRANNY, R. L. and CRANNY, C. L. (1960). The creatinine excretion and urine volume of premature infants. *Amer. J. Dis. Child.*, **99**, 507.

CREMER, R. J., PERRYMAN, P. W. and RICHARDS, D. H. (1958). Influence of light on the hyperbilirubinaemia of infants. *Lancet*, **1**, 1094.

DAVIS, J. A., HARVEY, D. R. and STEVENS, J. F. (1966). Osmolality as a measure of dehydration in the neonatal period. *Arch. Dis. Childh.*, **41**, 448.

DAWES, G. S. (1968). *Foetal and Neonatal Physiology*. Chicago: Year Book Med. Publ. Inc.

—— MOTT, J. C. and STAFFORD, A. (1960). Prolongation of survival in the anoxic foetal lamb. *J. Physiol.*, **153**, 16P.

DAWKINS, M. J. R. and HULL, D. (1963). Brown fat and the response of the newborn rabbit to cold. *J. Physiol.*, **169**, 101P.

—— and SCOPES, J. W. (1965). Non-shivering thermogenesis and brown adipose tissue in the human newborn infant. *Nature*, **206**, 201.

DAY, R. L., CALIGUIRI, L., KAMENSKI, C. and EHRLICH, F. (1964). Body temperature and survival of premature infants. *Pediatrics*, **34**, 171.

DEANESLY, R. (1961). Foetal endocrinology. *Brit. med. Bull.*, **17**, 91.

DEMARSH, Q. B., WINDLE, W. F. and ALT, H. L. (1942). Blood volume of newborn infant in relation to early and late clamping of umbilical cord. *Amer. J. Dis. Child.*, **63**, 1123.

DESMOND, M. M., KAY, J. L. and MEGARITY, A. L. (1959). The phases of transitional distress occurring in neonates in association with prolonged postnatal umbilical cord pulsations. *J. Pediat.*, **55**, 131.

DICKERSON, R. C. (1968). Congenital subluxation of the hip. *Pediatrics*, **41**, 977.

DOXIADIS, S. A., FESSAS, Ph. and VALAES, T. (1961). Glucose 6-dehydrogenase deficiency. *Lancet*, **1**, 297.

DYGGVE, H. (1950). Proc. 6th Int. Congress of Pediatrics.

EDSON, J. R., BLAESE, R. M., WHITE, J. G. and KRIVIT, W. (1968). Defibrination syndrome in the infant. *J. Pediat.*, **72**, 342.

EMERY, J. L. (1952). Degenerative changes in the left lobe of the liver in the newborn. *Arch. Dis. Childh.*, **27**, 558.

FARQUHAR, J. W. (1954). Control of the blood sugar level in the neonatal period. *Arch. Dis. Childh.*, **29**, 519.

—— (1955). The evaluation of the eosinopenic response to corticotrophin and cortisone in the newborn infant. *Arch. Dis. Childh.*, **30**, 133.

—— (1961). Measurement of the occipitofrontal circumference in children. *Lancet*, **2**, 779.

—— (1965a). In *Recent Advances in Paediatrics*, 3rd edit., Ed. D. Gairdner, London: Churchill.

—— (1965b). Metabolic changes in the infant of the diabetic mother. *Pediat. Clin. N. Amer.*, **12**, 743.

—— and SKLAROFF, S. A. (1958). The post-natal weight loss of babies born to diabetic and non-diabetic women. *Arch. Dis. Childh.*, **33**, 323.

—— and ISLES, T. E. (1968). Hypoglycaemia in newborn infants of normal and diabetic mothers. *South African med. J.*, **42**, 237.

FRASER, M. S. (1951). Mucus catheters. *Brit. med. J.*, **1**, 165.

GAIRDNER, D. (1949). The fate of the foreskin. *Brit. med. J.*, **2**, 1433.

—— (1965). In *Recent Advances in Paediatrics*, 3rd edit., Ed. D. Gairdner. London: Churchill.

—— MARKS, J. and ROSCOE, J. D. (1952). Blood formation in infancy. *Arch. Dis. Childh.*, **27**, 128 and 214.

—— —— —— and BRETTELL, R. O. (1958). The fluid shift from the vascular compartment immediately after birth. *Arch. Dis. Childh.*, **33**, 489.

GARBY, L., SJÖLIN, S. and VUILLE, J. -C. (1964). Studies on erythro-kinetics in infancy. *Acta paediat.*, **53**, 165.

GHOSH, S. and DAGA, S. (1967). Comparison of gestational age and weight as standards of prematurity. *J. Pediat.*, **71**, 173.

GITTLEMAN, I. F., PINCUS, J. B., SCHMERZLER, E. and SAITO, M. (1956). Hypocalcaemia occurring on the first day of life in mature and premature infants. *Pediatrics*, **18**, 721.

—— —— —— and ANNECCHIARICO, F. (1959). Diabetes mellitus or the pre-diabetic state in the mother and the neonate. *Amer. J. Dis. Child.*, **98**, 342.

GOMEZ, M. F. and GRAVEN, S. N. (1964). The use of fibrinolysin in the treatment of respiratory distress syndrome. *Pediatrics*, **34**, 877.

GRAZIANI, L. J., WEITZMAN, E. D. and VELASCO, M. S. A. (1968). Neurologic maturation and auditory evoked responses in low birth weight infants. *Pediatrics*, **41**, 483.

GRIFFITHS, A. D. (1968). Association of hypoglycaemia with symptoms in the newborn. *Arch. Dis. Childh.*, **43**, 688.

GRUENWALD, P. (1949). Degenerative changes in right half of liver resulting from intra-uterine anoxia. *Amer. J. clin. Path.*, **19**, 801.

—— (1952). In *Pulmonary Hyaline Membranes*. Report of Fifth M. and R. Pediatric Research Conference, Columbus, Ohio.

—— (1964). The course of the respiratory distress syndrome of newborn infants. *Acta paediat.*, **53**, 470.

GRUMBACH, M. M. and DUCHARME, J. R. (1960). The effects of androgens on fetal sexual development. *Fertility and Sterility*, 11, 157.

GUNTHER, M. (1957). The transfer of blood between baby and placenta in the minutes after birth. *Lancet*, 1, 1277.

GUPTA, J. M., DAHLENBURG, G. W. and DAVIS, J. A. (1967). Effects of THAM in respiratory distress syndrome. *Arch. Dis. Childh.*, 42, 416.

GÜRSON, C. T. and ETILI, L. (1968). Plasma lipoprotein lipase, FFA and glucose in newborns. *Arch. Dis. Childh.*, 43, 679.

HALLUM, J. L. and HATCHUEL, W. L. F. (1954). Paralytic ileus in a newborn baby. *Arch. Dis. Childh.*, 29, 354.

HATHAWAY, W. E., MULL, M. M. and PECHET, G. S. (1969). Disseminated intravascular coagulation in the newborn. *Pediatrics*, 43, 233.

HAY, J. D., HUDSON, F. P. and RODGERS, T. F. (1951). Vitamin K in the prevention of haemorrhagic disease in the newborn. *Lancet*, 1, 423.

HEIM, T. and HULL, D. (1966). Brown adipose tissue. *J. Physiol.*, 186, 42.

HEY, E. N. and MOUNT, L. E. (1967). Heat losses from babies in incubators. *Arch. Dis. Childh.*, 42, 75.

—— and MAURICE, N. P. (1968). Effect of humidity on production and loss of heat in the newborn baby. *Arch. Dis. Childh.*, 43, 166.

—— KOHLINSKY, S. and O'CONNELL, B. (1969). Heat losses from babies during exchange transfusion. *Lancet*, 1, 335.

HUDSON, F. P., McCANDLESS, A. and O'MALLEY, A. G. (1950). Sciatic paralysis in newborn infants. *Brit. med. J.*, 1, 223.

HUGHES-DAVIS, T. H. (1968). Feeding the newborn. *Lancet*, 2, 1241.

HULL, D. (1966). The structure and function of brown adipose tissue. *Brit. med. Bull.*, 22, 92.

HUTCHISON, J. H., KERR, M. M., McPHAIL, F. M., DOUGLAS, T. A., SMITH, G., NORMAN, J. N. and BATES, E. H. (1962). Studies in the treatment of the pulmonary syndrome of the newborn. *Lancet*, 2, 465.

—— —— DOUGLAS, T. A., INALL, J. A. and CROSBIE, J. C. (1964). A therapeutic approach in 100 cases of the respiratory distress syndrome. *Pediatrics*, 33, 956.

ISLES, T. E., DICKSON, M. and FARQUHAR, J. W. (1968). Glucose tolerance and plasma insulin in newborn infants of diabetic mothers. *Pediat. Res.*, 2, 198.

JAMES, L. S. (1961). Ross Conference on Pediatric Research, No. 37.

—— and ROWE, R. D. (1957). Pulmonary arterial pressures and hypoxia. *J. Pediat.*, 51, 5.

—— BURNARD, E. D. and ROWE, R. D. (1961). Abnormal shunting through the foramen ovale after birth. *Amer. J. Dis. Childh.*, 102, 550.

JARRETT, E. C. and HOLMAN, G. H. (1966). Lactose absorption in the premature infant. *Arch. Dis. Childh.*, 41, 525.

JEGIER, W., BLANKENSHIP, W., LIND, J. and KITCHIN, A. (1964). The changing circulatory pattern of the newborn infant. *Acta paediat.*, 53, 541.

JOLLY, H., MOLYNEUX, P. and NEWELL, D. J. (1962). A controlled study of the effect of temperature on premature babies. *J. Pediat.*, 60, 889.

KAPLAN, E. (1942). The parathyroid gland in infancy. *Arch. Path.*, 34, 1042.

KARLBERG, P., MOORE, R. E. and OLIVER, T. K. (1965). Thermogenic and cardiovascular responses of the newborn baby to noradrenaline. *Acta paediat.*, 54, 225.

KAUFMAN, L., LEHMANN, H. and SILK, E. (1960). Suxamethonium apnoea in an infant. *Brit. med. J.*, 1, 166.

KOCH, G. and WENDELL, H. (1968). Adjustment of arterial blood gases and acid base. *Biol. Neonat.*, 12, 136.

LANCET (1969a). *Phenobarbitone and Dicophane in Jaundice.* 2, 144.

—— (1969b). *Blood-sugars in the Newborn.* 1, 1199.

LANZKOWSKY, P. (1960). Effect of early and late clamping of umbilical cord on infant's haemoglobin level. *Brit. Med. J.*, **2**, 1777.

LARIZZA, P., BRUNETTI, P. and GRIGNANI, F. (1960). Enzyme deficient haemolytic anaemia. *Lancet*, **1**, 601.

LARON, Z., MANNHEIMER, S., NITZMAN, M. and GOLDMAN, J. (1967). Growth hormone, glucose and FFA levels in mothers and infants. *Arch. Dis. Childh.*, **42**, 24.

LAUWERYNS, J. M. (1968). The pulmonary venous vasculature in neonatal hyaline membrane disease. *Science*, **160**, 190.

—— CLAESENS, ST. and BOUSSAUW, L. (1968). The pulmonary lymphatics in neonatal hyaline membrane disease. *Pediatrics*, **41**, 917.

LEHMANN, J. (1944). Vitamin K as a prophylactic. *Lancet*, **1**, 493.

LIEBERMAN, J. (1959). Clinical syndromes associated with deficient lung fibrinolytic activity. *New Eng. J. Med.*, **260**, 619.

LUCEY, J., FERREIRO, M. and HEWITT, J. (1968). Prevention of hyperbilirubinaemia by phototherapy. *Pediatrics*, **41**, 1047.

McCANCE, R. A. (1959). The maintenance of stability in the newly born. *Arch. Dis. Childh.*, **34**, 361.

—— and WIDDOWSON, E. M. (1957). Hypertonic expansion of the extracellular fluids. *Acta paediat.*, **46**, 337.

McCRACKEN, G. H., CHEN, T. C., HARDY, J. B. and TZAN, N. (1969). Serum immunoglobulin levels in newborn infants. *J. Pediat.*, **74**, 383.

McKAY, E., THOM, H. and GRAY, D. (1967). Immunoglobulins in umbilical cord plasma II. *Arch. Dis. Childh.*, **42**, 264.

—— THOM, H. and GRAY, D. (1968). Immunoglobulins in umbilical cord plasma III. *Arch. Dis. Childh.*, **43**, 161.

MALAN, A. F., EVANS, A. and HEESE, H. de V. (1966). Acid-base determinations in normal premature infants. *Arch. Dis. Childh.*, **41**, 678.

MALKASIAN, G. D. and TAUXE, W. N. (1965). Uptake of L-triiodothyronine-131-I by erythrocytes during pregnancy. *J. clin. Endocrinol. Metab.*, **25**, 923.

MAMUNES, P., BADEN, M., BASS, J. W. and NELSON, J. (1969). Early intravenous feeding of the low birth weight neonate. *Pediatrics*, **43**, 241.

MARKS, J. F. (1965). Free thyroxine index in the newborn. *J. clin. Endocrinol. Metab.*, **25**, 852.

MEYER, W. W. and LIND, J. (1966a). The ductus venosus and the mechanism of its closure. *Arch. Dis. Childh.*, **41**, 597.

—— —— (1966b). Postnatal changes in the portal circulation. *Arch. Dis. Childh.*, **41**, 606.

MIGEON, C. (1959). Cortisol production and metabolism in the neonate. *J. Pediat.*, **55**, 280.

MILLER, J. A., MILLER, F. S. and WESTIN, B. (1964). Hypothermia in the treatment of asphyxia neonatorum. *Biol. Neonat.*, **6**, 148.

MONCRIEFF, A. (1958). Non-adrenal female pseudohermaphroditism associated with hormone administration in pregnancy. *Lancet*, **2**, 267.

MOSS, A. J. and MONSET-COUCHARD, M. (1967). Placental transfusion. *Pediatrics*, **40**, 109.

MOYA, F., APGAR, V., JAMES, L. S. and BERRIEN, C. (1960). Hydramnios and congenital anomalies. *J. Amer. med. Ass.*, **173**, 1552.

NELIGAN, G. A. (1965a). In *Gestational Age, Size and Maturity*. Ed. M. Dawkins and W. G MacGregor, *Clinics in Developmental Medicine, No. 19*. London: Spastics Society/ Heinemann.

—— (1965b). In *Recent Advances in Paediatrics*, 3rd ed. Ed. D. Gairdner. London: Churchill.

—— and STRANG, L. B. (1952). A harlequin colour change in the newborn. *Lancet*, **2**. 1005.

—— PARKIN, J. M. and PAUL, C. (1964). The use of an elastic band to prevent haemorrhage from the umbilical cord. *Arch. Dis. Childh.*, **39**, 630.

NELSON, N. M. (1968). On the indirect determination of systolic and diastolic blood pressure in the newborn infant. *Pediatrics*, **42**, 934.

NOURSE, C. H. and NELSON, N. M. (1969). Uniformity of ventilation in the newborn infant. *Pediatrics*, **43**, 226.

NYHAN, W. L. (1961). Toxicity of drugs in the neonatal period. *J. Pediat*, **59**, 1.

ODELL, G. B. (1959). The dissociation of bilirubin from albumin and its clinical implications. *J. Pediat.*, **55**, 268.

O'DOHERTY, N. (1968). A hearing test applicable to the crying newborn infant. *Develop. Med. Child Neurol.*, **10**, 380.

OPPE, T. E. and REDSTONE, D. (1968). Calcium and phosphorous levels in healthy newborn infants given various types of milk. *Lancet*, **1**, 1045.

PHILIP, A. G. S., YEE, A. B., ROSY, M., SURTI, N., TSAMTSOURIS, A. and INGALL, D. (1969). Placental transfusion as an intrauterine phenomenon. *Brit. med. J.*, **2**, 11.

PICKERING, D. E., KONTAXIS, N. E., BENSON, R. C. and MEECHAM, R. J. (1958). Thyroid function in the perinatal period. *Amer. J. Dis. Child.*, **95**, 616.

PRIBYLOVA, H. (1968). The importance of thermoreceptive regions for the chemical thermoregulation of the newborn. *Biol. Neonat.*, **12**, 13.

QUIE, P. G. and WANNAMAKER, L. W. (1960). The plasminogen-plasmin system of newborn infants. *Amer. J. Dis. Child.*, **100**, 836.

RAFSTEDT, S. (1955). Studies on serum lipids and lipoproteins in infancy and childhood. *Acta paediat.*, Suppl. 102.

RAMSAY, D. H. E. and HARVEY, C. C. (1959). Marking-ink poisoning. *Lancet*, **1**, 910.

REDMOND, A., ISANA, S. and INGALL, D. (1965). Relation of onset of respiration to placental transfusion. *Lancet*, **1**, 283.

REYNOLDS, E. C. R., ROBERTSON, N. R. C. and WIGGLESWORTH, J. S. (1968). Hyaline membrane disease, respiratory distress and surfactant deficiency. *Pediatrics*, **42**, 758.

RUSSELL, G. and COTTON, E. K. (1968). Sodium bicarbonate and oxygen in respiratory distress syndrome. *Pediatrics*, **41**, 1063.

SABATA, V., WOLF, H. and LAUSMANN, S. (1968). Role of FFA, glycerol, ketone bodies and glucose in energy metabolism of the mother and fetus. *Biol. Neonat.*, **13**, 7.

SANDLER, M., RUTHVEN, C. R. J., NORMAND, I. C. S. and MOORE, R. E. (1961). Environmental temperature and urinary excretion of 3-methoxy-4-hydroxymandelic acid in the newborn. *Lancet*, **1**, 485.

SCLARE, G. (1956). The histological structure of the thyroid in the newborn. *Scot. med. J.*, **1**, 251.

SCOPES, J. W. (1966). Metabolic rate and temperature control in the human baby. *Brit. med. Bull.*, **22**, 88.

—— and AHMED, I. (1966a). Range of critical temperatures in sick and premature newborn babies. *Arch. Dis. Childh.*, **41**, 417.

—— —— (1966b). Indirect assessment of oxygen requirements in newborn babies. *Arch. Dis. Childh.*, **41**, 25.

SECHER, O. and KARLBERG, P. (1962). Placental blood transfusion. *Lancet*, **1**, 1203.

SHELLEY, H. J. (1961). Glycogen reserves and their changes at birth and in anoxia. *Brit. med. Bull.*, **17**, 137.

—— (1964). Carbohydrate reserves in the newborn infant. *Brit. med. J.*, **1**, 273.

—— (1968). Carbohydrate metabolism in the fetus and newly born. *Develop. Med. Child Neurol.*, **10**, 675.

SILVER, H., DREVER, J. C. and DOUGLAS, D. M. (1967). Cells in the urine of newborn infants. *Arch. Dis. Childh.*, **42**, 598.

SILVERMAN, W. A., ANDERSEN, D. H., BLANC, W. A. and CROZIER, D. N. (1956). Mortality and kernicterus in prematures. *Pediatrics*, **18**, 614.

—— FERTIG, J. W. and BERGER, A. P. (1958). Influence of the thermal environment on the survival of newly born premature infants. *Pediatrics*, **22**, 876.

—— and AGATE, F. J. (1964). Variation in cold resistance among small newborn infants. *Biol. Neonat.*, **6**, 113.

—— ZAMELIS, A., SINCLAIR, J. C. and AGATE, F. J. (1964). Warm nape of the newborn. *Pediatrics*, **33**, 984.

SISSON, T. R. C. and WHALEN, L. E. (1960). The blood volume of infants. *J. Pediat.*, **56**, 43.

SMITH, C. A. (1959). *The Physiology of the Newborn Infant*, 3rd edit. Oxford: Blackwell.

SMITH, R. E. (1961). Thermogenic activity of the hibernating gland in the cold-acclimated rat. *Physiologist*, **4**, 113.

—— and HOCK, R. J. (1963). Brown fat. *Science*, **140**, 199.

SOUTHGATE, D. A. T., WIDDOWSON, E. M., SMITS, B. J., COOKE, W. T., WALKER, C. H. M. and MATHERS, N. P. (1969). Absorption and excretion of calcium and fat by young infants. *Lancet*, **1**, 487.

SPAFFORD, N. R., CARR, E. A., LOWREY, G. H. and BEIERWALTES, W. H. (1960). I[131] labelled triiodothyronine erythrocyte uptake of mothers and newborn infants. *Amer. J. Dis. Child.*, **100**, 844.

SPENCE, J., WALTON, W. S., MILLER, F. J. W. and COURT, S. D. M. (1954). A *Thousand Families in Newcastle-upon-Tyne*. London: Nuffield Foundation.

STERN, L. S., RAMOS, A. and LEDUC, J. (1968). Urinary catecholamine excretion in infants of diabetic mothers. *Pediatrics*, **42**, 598.

TÄHKA, H. (1951). On the weight and structure of the adrenal glands. *Acta paediat.*, **40**, Suppl. 81.

THIBEAULT, D. W., POBLETE, E. and AULD, P. A. M. (1968). Alveolar-arterial O_2 and CO_2 in relation to neonatal lung volume. *Pediatrics*, **41**, 574.

THOM, H., McKAY, E. and GRAY, D. (1967). Immunoglobulins in umbilical cord plasma I. *Arch. Dis. Childh.*, **42**, 259.

THOMSON, A. M., BILLEWICZ, W. Z. and HYTTEN, F. E. (1968). The assessment of fetal growth. *J. Obstet. Gynaec. Brit. Comm.*, **75**, 903.

TROLLE, D. (1968a). Phenobarbitone and neonatal icterus. *Lancet*, **1**, 251.

—— (1968b). Decrease of total serum bilirubin concentration in newborn infants after phenobarbitone treatment. *Lancet*, **2**, 705.

TUNSTALL, M. E., CATER, J. I., THOMSON, J. S. and MITCHELL, R. G. (1968). Ventilating the lungs of newborn infants for prolonged periods. *Arch. Dis. Childh.*, **43**, 486.

USHER, R. (1961). The respiratory distress syndrome of prematurity. *Pediat. Clin. N. Amer.*, **8**, 525.

—— SHEPHARD, M. and LIND, J. (1963). The blood volume of the newborn infant and placental transfusion. *Acta paediat.*, **52**, 497.

UTTLEY, W. S., ALLEN, A. G. E. and CASH, J. D. (1969). Fibrin/fibrinogen degradation products in sera of normal infants and children. *Arch. Dis. Childh.*, **44**, 761.

VANIER, T. M. and TYAS, T. F. (1967). Folic acid status in premature infants. *Arch. Dis. Childh.*, **42**, 57.

VAN LEEUWEN, G., BEHRINGER, B. and GLENN, L. (1967). Single umbilical artery. *J. Pediat.*, **71**, 103.

VON EULER, U., LARSSON, Y. and PERSSON, B. (1964). Glucose tolerance in the neonatal period and during the first six months of life. *Arch. Dis. Childh.*, **39**, 393.

WALKER, C. H. M. and BALF, C. L. (1954). Capillary resistance studies. *J. Obstet. Gynaec. Brit. Emp.*, **61**, 1.

WALKER, W., HUGHES, M. I. and BARTON, M. (1969). Barbiturate and hyperbilirubinaemia of prematurity. *Lancet*, **1**, 548.

WALLGREN, G., BARR, M. and RUDHE, U. (1964). Haemodynamic studies of induced acute hypo- and hyper-volaemia. *Acta paediat.*, **53**, 1.

WEISS, C. (1964). Routine non-ritual circumcision in infancy. *Clin. Pediat.*, **3**, 560.

WEST, G. B., SHEPHERD, D. M., HUNTER, R. B. and MACGREGOR, A. R. (1953). The function of the organs of Zuckerkandl. *Clin. Sci.*, **12**, 317.

WHARTON, B. A. and BOWER, B. D. (1965). Immediate or later feeding for premature babies? *Lancet*, **2**, 769.

WILKINS, L. (1957). *The Diagnosis and Treatment of Endocrine Disorders in Childhood and Adolescence.* Oxford: Blackwell.

—— (1960). Masculinization of female fetus due to use of orally given progestins. *J. Amer. med. Ass.*, **172**, 1028.

WOLF, H., MELICHAR, V. and MICHAELIS, R. (1968). Elimination of intravenously administered glycerol from the blood of newborns. *Biol. Neonat.*, **12**, 162.

YEUNG, C. Y. and FIELD, E. (1969). Phenobarbitone therapy in neonatal hyperbilirubinaemia. *Lancet*, **2**, 135.

YOUNG, M. (1961). Blood pressure in the new-born baby. *Brit. med. Bull.*, **17**, 154.

ZEE, P. (1968). Lipid metabolism in the newborn. *Pediatrics*, **41**, 640.

4 Low Birth Weight

Definition

THE definition of a premature or immature infant as one with a birth weight of 2500 g. (5½ lb.) or less and/or a gestation period less than 37 completed weeks, which was proposed at W.H.O in 1948 (W.H.O 1948) and endorsed, as the international definition to be used by member countries, by the W.H.O Expert Group on Prematurity (1950), has now largely outlived its usefulness. The upper limit of 2500 g. was based mainly on the known birth weight distribution in white infants. It was anticipated then, and was demonstrated subsequently, that the definition is inappropriate in many areas. Even in more advanced countries a substantial minority of so-called prematures are low weight babies, born at or near term. In Britain about 7 per cent of live born infants are considered premature on a birth weight criterion but of these over one-third are born after 37 completed weeks of gestation. Nearly one-half of all prematures and over one-half of all surviving prematures have birth weights between 2,250 and 2,500 g. (5 and 5½ lb.). Few of these infants cause anxiety either in the immediate postnatal period or at later ages. In this country the majority of infants of 2,000 g. (4 lb. 6 oz.) or less require special postnatal care because of functional immaturity. At and below this birth weight level there is also a marked increase in stillbirth and neonatal death rates and in the proportion of surviving infants who appear subsequently to be handicapped in physical, mental and emotional development.

The W.H.O. Expert Committee (1961) has now recommended that the term 'low birth weight' should be used instead of 'premature' to describe infants included in the previous definition.

Factors Affecting Birth Weight and Gestation

Low birth weight and shortened gestation are related to social background, constitutional factors in the mother and fetus and circumstances arising during the course of the pregnancy.

Social factors. The association between low birth weight and low social class is well known, as is the influence of maternal height on birth weight (Baird, 1964). Although maternal height may be, in part, genetically determined, the frequently observed association between height and social circumstances suggests that small stature of mother is more often the result of poor nutrition during her own growing period in childhood. An Edinburgh study (Drillien, 1957) suggested that the social class into which a woman marries (*i.e.* that of her husband) has only a minor influence on her chance of having an infant of low birth weight compared with the social class in which she was born and brought up (*i.e.* that of her father).

The association of social class with birth weight becomes weaker as birth weight decreases, infants in the birth weight range 2,000–2,500 g. being the most likely to be born to mothers in the lower social classes (Drillien and Richmond, 1956; Drillien, 1964).

Maternal factors. The incidence of low birth weight varies with age, parity and marital status of the mother. For all parities the proportion of low weight infants as well as of perinatal losses is lowest for those born to mothers aged 20–34 years and for all maternal ages the incidence is highest in first births and lowest in second births (Walker, 1965). The incidence is also raised in the offspring of unmarried mothers. However, it is likely that the effect of these factors is related to associated social class differences as well as to variations in maternal physiology.

Smoking in the latter half of pregnancy is associated with a small but definite reduction in birth weight (amounting on average to about 170 g./6 oz.) and coincident upon this an increased fetal wastage, particularly in mothers who are, for other reasons, in groups of higher than average risk (Butler and Alberman, 1969).

Maternal reproductive capacity also appears to have an important bearing on the mother's liability to have an infant of low birth weight and shortened gestation period. This is particularly so when one is considering the smallest infants of birth weight 2,000 g. or less. Mothers of very small infants not only have difficulty in conceiving, with fewer conceptions for any given duration of marriage and long unwanted gaps after marriage and between conceptions, but also lose more of their other conceptions by abortion, stillbirth and neonatal death than do mothers in the general population (Wilson *et al.*, 1963; Drillien, 1967).

Fetal factors. Weight at birth will vary according to sex and whether the infant results from a single or multiple birth. It has been generally assumed that, for like birth weights, females are rather more mature than males at all gestational ages and twins are more mature than singletons. However, recent studies suggest that weight differences by sex develop mainly during the last 4 to 6 weeks of the normal 40 week gestation period and mean weights of singletons and twins are not much different until after 32 to 34 weeks' gestation (Lubchenco *et al.*, 1963; Butler and Alberman, 1969).

Infants with developmental malformations (Warkany *et al.*, 1961), chromosomal abnormalities and certain conditions known to be due to single gene defects (Schutt, 1965) are likely to be of low birth weight and frequently are markedly underweight for their gestational age.

Pregnancy factors. Low birth weight may be due to maternal complications during the course of or coincident with the pregnancy, as a result of premature delivery, whether spontaneous or induced, and/or because certain maternal complications appear to affect intra-uterine growth. Severe third-trimester complications such as toxaemia and antepartum haemorrhage or some chronic disease of the mother are present in less than one-third of pregnancies resulting in low birth weight infants (Baird, 1964). Pregnancy is least likely to be complicated when the low birth weight infant is born after 37 completed weeks of gestation. At birth weights of 2,000 g. or less, severe late pregnancy complications are present in about one-half of cases and in many of these labour will be induced or delivery effected by caesarean section because of the mother's condition. A substantial proportion of the infants born to mothers with toxaemia or chronic disease are not only of low birth weight but also underweight for gestation period. In the absence of late pregnancy complications many mothers of infants of 2,000 g. or less give a history of threatened abortion in the early weeks (Turnbull and Walker, 1956).

Small-for-dates Infants

In recent years there has been growing recognition of the importance of gestational age as well as of birth weight in classifying low weight infants. Some infants are small because of premature delivery, some because of retarded intra-uterine growth and others because of both these factors in combination. Aetiology, perinatal mortality, the risk of immediate postnatal complication and later progress differ in those who are prematurely delivered and appropriate weight for gestational age and those who are small-for-dates (*i.e.* of birth weight inappropriately low for gestational age).

The infant small for gestational age has been defined in several different ways. All definitions comprise those infants of lowest birth weight at a given gestational age, the criteria most commonly used being birth weights below the 10th percentile (Lubchenco *et al.*, 1963; Neligan, 1965), or below 2 standard deviations from the mean which is between the second and third percentiles (Gruenwald, 1963; McDonald, 1965).

Various descriptive labels have been attached to this condition, such as intra-uterine growth retardation, chronic fetal distress, pseudoprematurity or dysmaturity. These terms imply an aetiology which may or may not be implicated, for which reason the neutral term small-for-dates (or light-for-dates) is to be preferred.

The aetiology associated with inappropriately low weight for gestational age is multiple. Among maternal factors are young age, primiparity, short stature, low social class, toxaemia, and smoking. Retarded growth may be due to genetic factors, to adverse environmental influences in early fetal life, in which case congenital defects are likely to be present in addition to retarded growth, and to late pregnancy complications, among which toxaemia and/or essential hypertension appear to be the most important.

The conception of placental insufficiency leading to chronic fetal malnutrition has been invoked to account for the triad of maternal hypertension or toxaemia, pathological change or small weight of the placenta, and fetal growth retardation (Gruenwald, 1963). Placental insufficiency as indicated by falling maternal oestriol excretion is frequently associated with the clinical picture of the small-for-dates infant and low maternal oestriols may be considered an indication for induction or caesarean section (Frandsen and Stakemann, 1963).

In Britain gestational age can be estimated with reasonable accuracy in only

	24	25	26	27	28	29	30	31	32	33	34	35	36	37	38	39	40	41	42	43	44
	WEEKS GESTATION																				
OBSTETRICAL DATA																					
1 WKS FROM ONSET LNMP																					
2 FETAL MOVEMENT (16 WKS GEST)																					
3 FETAL HEART (1ST HEARD @ 20 WKS)																					
4 UTERINE GROWTH (SYMPHYSIS-FUNDUS)			25 CMS		26 CMS		28 CMS		30 CMS		31 CMS		32 CMS		33 CMS		32 CMS				
(1) PHYSICAL EXAMINATION - INFANT																					
1 VERNIX	APPEARS	COVERS BODY														DECREASES IN AMOUNT		NO VERNIX			
2 BREAST TISSUE	NONE										2 MM			4 MM		7 MM OR MORE					
3 NIPPLES									BARELY VISIBLE		WELL DEFINED, FLAT AREOLA					WELL DEFINED, RAISED AREOLA					
4 SOLE CREASES	NONE								1, ANTERIOR TRANSVERSE		2, ANTERIOR TRANSVERSE			ANTERIOR 2/3 SOLE		CREASES INVOLVING HEEL					
5 EAR CARTILAGE	PINNA SOFT, STAYS FOLDED										RETURNS SLOWLY FROM FOLDING			THIN CARTILAGE SPRINGS BACK		FIRM, REMAINS ERECT FROM HEAD					
6 EAR FORM	FLAT, SHAPELESS										BEGINNING INCURVING OF PERIPHERY			PARTIAL INCURVING, UPPER PINNA			WELL-DEFINED INCURVING, WHOLE OF UPPER PINNA				
7 GENITALIA - TESTES & SCROTUM	UNDESCENDED						TESTES HIGH IN CANAL, SMALL RUGAE INFERIORLY						TESTES LOWER, MORE RUGAE			TESTES DESCENDED IN PENDULOUS SCROTUM, RUGAE COMPLETE					
LABIA & CLITORIS	LABIA MAJORA WIDELY SEPARATED, PROMINENT CLITORIS												LABIA MAJORA NEARLY COVER LABIA MINORA			LABIA MINORA & CLITORIS COVERED					
8 HAIR (APPEARS ON HEAD @ 20 WKS)	EYEBROWS & LASHES, EYELIDS REOPEN						FINE, WOOLLY HAIR								HAIR SILKY, SINGLE STRANDS						
9 LANUGO (APPEARS @ 20 WKS)	LANUGO OVER ENTIRE BODY				VANISHES FROM FACE					SLIGHT LANUGO OVER SHOULDERS					NO LANUGO						
10 SKIN TEXTURE	THIN									SMOOTH, MEDIUM THICKNESS								DESQUAMATION			
11 SKIN COLOR & OPACITY	TRANSLUCENT, PLETHORIC. NUMEROUS VENULES (ABDOMEN)													PINK, FEW LARGE VESSELS OVERALL			PALE PINK, NO VESSELS SEEN				
12 SKULL FIRMNESS	SOFT TO 1 INCH FROM ANTERIOR FONTANELLE											SPRINGY AT EDGES OF FONTANELLE, CENTER FIRM			BONES HARD, SUTURES EASILY DISPLACED			BONES HARD, CANNOT BE DISPLACED			
(2) NEUROLOGIC EXAMINATION																					
1 POSTURE - RESTING	LATERAL DECUBITUS				HYPOTONIA		SLIGHT INCREASE IN TONE, LOWER EXTREMITY				FROG-LIKE		TOTAL FLEXION								
RECOIL							SLIGHT, LOWER EXTREMITIES				NONE UPPER EXT GOOD LOWER EXT		SLOW UPPER EXT			GOOD UPPER EXT					
2 TONE - HEEL TO EAR	NO RESISTANCE						SLIGHT RESISTANCE				DIFFICULT		ALMOST IM-POSSIBLE		IMPOSSIBLE						
SCARF MANEUVER	NO RESISTANCE										MIN RESISTANCE		FAIR RESISTANCE		DIFFICULT						
NECK EXTENSORS							SLIGHT				FAIR		GOOD								
NECK FLEXORS									MINIMAL						FAIR						
3 REFLEXES - MORO	BARELY APPARENT			COMPLETE, EXHAUSTIBLE				GOOD, COMPLETE			NO ABDUCTION				COMPLETE WITH ABDUCTION						
PUPILS TO LIGHT				REACT																	
GRASP	FEEBLE			FAIR				SOLID, INVOLVES ARMS						MAY PICK INFANT UP							
ROOTING	MINIMAL C̄ REINFORCEMENT			GOOD C̄ REINFORCEMENT				GOOD													
CROSSED EXTENSION	SLIGHT WITHDRAWAL						WITHDRAWAL				WITHDRAWAL & EXTENSION				WITHDRAWAL, EXTENSION & ABDUCTION						
AUTOMATIC WALK											MINIMAL				FAIR, TOES		GOOD, HEELS				
TRUNK ELEVATION											SLIGHT			GOOD							
GLABELLAR TAP							APPEARS					PRESENT									
HEAD TURNS TO LIGHT									APPEARS				PRESENT								
	WEEKS GESTATION																				
	24	25	26	27	28	29	30	31	32	33	34	35	36	37	38	39	40	41	42	43	44

FIG. 12. Guide to clinical estimation of gestational age.

(1) Farr *et al.*, 1966: Usher *et al.*, 1966.

(2) Robinson, 1966: Amiel-Tison, 1968.

about 60 to 80 per cent of pregnancies and in a much smaller proportion in under-developed countries, for which reason an assessment of maturity must frequently be made on clinical grounds.

Various criteria have been suggested for assessing maturity (Mitchell and Farr, 1965). These have been summarised in the Guide to Clinical Estimation of Gestational Age* used at the Newborn and Premature Center, University of Colorado Medical Center and reproduced in Fig. 12.

Radiological measurement of ossification centres is of little value as small-for-dates infants commonly show delay in appearance of these centres. There may also be retardation in growth of breast tissue in these infants.

A decrease in intra-uterine growth affects first the weight, then length and to a much smaller extent the head circumference. Thus, the percentile rankings for these measurements are discrepant in small-for-dates infants.

Some cases of gross interpair differences in size and nutritional status at birth of monochorionic twins may be due to placental anastomoses through which the one

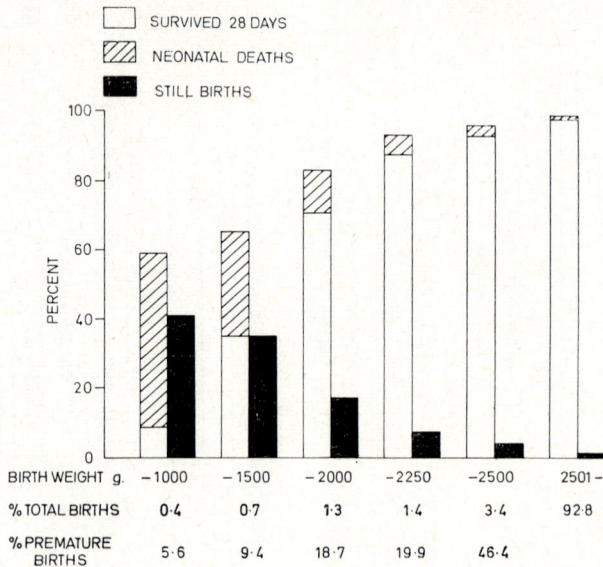

Fig. 13. Stillbirth and neonatal death rates by birth weight, based on all births in England and Wales, 1967.

twin continuously 'transfuses' the other (Benirschke, 1961). Placental anastomoses can be demonstrated frequently in monochorionic placentae but usually these produce no disturbance, both twins maintaining separate circulations.

Perinatal Mortality

Mortality by birth weight. The infant's chance of being born alive and of surviving the neonatal period is closely related to birth weight, as shown in Fig. 13

* Reproduced by permission of L. O. Lubchenco and F. C. Battaglia, Co-Directors of the Newborn and Premature Center and Lange Medical Publications, Los Altos, California.

which was constructed from data for all births in England and Wales in 1967 (Chief Medical Officer, Ministry of Health, 1968).

In the lowest birth weight group (1,000 g./2 lb. 3 oz. or less) over 40 per cent of infants were stillborn and of those live born, only 12 per cent survived for longer than 28 days, whereas among those in the birth weight range 2,001 to 2,500 g. (4 lb. 6 oz. to 5 lb. 8 oz.) 5 per cent were stillborn, and of those born alive, 96·5 per cent survived the neonatal period.

Improvements in survival rates in recent years are most marked for those in the lowest birth weight groups. In the 5 year period 1962–67 the survival rate of live-born infants of 1,500 g. or less increased from 34·4 per cent to 39·2 per cent, compared with an increase from 95·6 per cent to 96·5 per cent for those who were 2,001 to 2,500 g. at birth. Where intensive care units have been established, improvement is even more striking (Drillien, 1958; Walker, 1965).

Mortality by Sex. For all birth weights and gestation periods, perinatal mortality (stillbirth and neonatal death) is higher for males, with the exception of a small excess of losses in females of 1,001 to 1,500 g. (2 lb. 3 oz. to 3 lb. 4 oz.) born between 32 and 36 weeks' gestation and largely due to fatal malformations of the central nervous system. Apart from this group earlier gestations show the biggest preponderance of losses in males (Butler and Bonham, 1963).

Mortality by pathological findings in the infant and intra-uterine growth status. In nearly one-quarter of perinatal losses of low weight infants, fetal death occurs before the onset of labour and necropsy reveals no lesions other than those attributed to anoxia. These infants tend to be small for their gestational age and in some cases this associated with maternal toxaemia. One-fifth of all perinatal losses are due to fatal congenital malformations and again many of these infants fall into the small-for-dates category. Small-for-dates infants are also over-represented in deaths from massive pulmonary haemorrhage and pulmonary infection. On the contrary hyaline membranes and intraventricular haemorrhage are confined largely to perinatal losses of prematurely delivered infants of appropriate weight for gestational age (Butler and Bonham, 1963; Butler and Alberman, 1969).

Later Progress of Low Weight Infants

Morbidity. An increase in early illness, especially infective illness, is to be expected in children who were of low birth weight since they tend to come from poorer homes than heavier children.

A prospective study in Edinburgh of health and sickness during the first 5 years of life (Drillien, 1964) indicated that although the overall incidence of medical illness at all ages was higher in those who had been of low birth weight, after the age of 2 years differences in morbidity by birth weight appeared to be due to differing standards of maternal care and not to birth weight *per se*. In the first 2 years respiratory infections were common and the prevalence was between 20 and 30 per cent higher in boys of low birth weight than in girls of like weight from similar types of home.

As would be expected, all types of congenital malformations, both major and minor, are commonly associated with low birth weight. In particular the incidence of visual defects such as persisting squint and myopia increases steadily as birth weight decreases.

Physical growth. Since growth in childhood is related to the economic status of the home, any comparisons of physical stature and growth rates in children who were of different weight at birth must allow for the preponderance of fathers in the lower social classes in samples of low weight infants.

In general (Drillien, 1964), in the first 5 years weight increments are the same for children from similar homes whatever the birth weight, though there is a tendency for low weight infants to catch up to some extent in height, with the result that they tend to be not only of rather small stature but relatively underweight for their height at 5 years.

Children who were between 2,000 and 2,500 g. at birth and born after 37 completed weeks of gestation and those of very low birth weight (1,500 g. and under) are the most likely to be markedly undersized at 5 years. When standards of maternal care are taken into account more marked differences are found by birth weight; children of low birth weight and twins appear to suffer more from a poor environment (both as regards morbidity and growth) than heavier single children.

Behaviour. Many observers report an excess of behaviour problems in children who were of low birth weight (Lubchenco et al., 1963; Wortis et al., 1964; Drillien, 1964). The varieties of behaviour disturbance described by different authors cover a wide range from nail-biting, nightmares and masturbation to nervousness, overdependence and temper tantrums. No typical pattern of disturbed behaviour emerges from a study of the literature, except that most observers make mention of overactive, restless behaviour, particularly in those of very low birth weight.

A number of possible explanations come to mind to account for behaviour disturbance.

1. Since low birth weight is associated with poor socio-economic background, children who were of low birth weight are more likely to be subjected to stressful family situations.

2. Particularly in the first few months of life experiences of the very small infant will differ from those of normal weight infants. It is unlikely that he will be breast-fed. He may suffer total separation from the mother by being nursed in an incubator. He will be kept in the hospital nursery for an extended period after his mother has returned home. After his discharge from maternity hospital he is more likely to require later hospitalisation and suffer further separations, particularly as a result of his increased susceptibility to lower respiratory infections.

3. The mother's responses to the infant and her handling when she gets him home may be different from those of a mother whose infant has caused no anxiety postnatally. The mother of a very small infant may be tense and anxious and have feelings of inadequacy, possibly exacerbated by what she has seen of the paraphernalia accompanying current techniques of infant care in hospital. Feeding

and other difficulties of management may result in her obtaining little pleasure from her child in the early months.

4. There is the further possibility that behaviour disturbances may have an organic basis and may be due to brain damage resulting either from the low birth weight itself or from the commonly associated perinatal complications.

Prechtl (1960) reported finding an excess of behaviour problems at 2 to 3 years in normal weight children born following obstetric complications, particularly in those who had exhibited minor neurological abnormalities in the neonatal period. Drillien (1964) found a raised incidence of behaviour disturbance reported in school in all birth weight groups when there had been a history of complications of pregnancy and/or delivery, disturbed behaviour increasing with the severity of obstetric complications. Severe obstetric complications appeared to lower the resistance level to early familial stress, particularly in males, twins and those who were 2,040 g. (4½ lb.) or less at birth.

Mental development. A more important question than increased susceptibility to infection, possible inferiority in physique and increase in disturbed behaviour, is whether or not those who were of low birth weight are intellectually inferior to their larger-born contemporaries. A number of long-term follow-up studies since World War II have confirmed that children with birth weights of 2,000 to 2,500 g. do not show much increase in the incidence of severe handicap as compared with heavier children from similar homes, but below this weight there appears to be a steady increase in incidence of mental retardation and neurological and physical defects as birth weight decreases, and this cannot be accounted for solely by impoverished environment.

In one prospective study in Edinburgh (Drillien, 1968) of children born in 1953–60, about four-fifths of survivors with birth weights of 1,250 g. (2 lb. 12 oz.) or less, had moderate or severe handicaps at 7 years (in most cases necessitating education in special schools for the mentally or physically handicapped), as did nearly one-half of those between 1,250 and 1,500 g. (2 lb. 12 oz. and 3 lb. 4 oz.) and one-fifth of those between 1,500 and 2,000 g. (3 lb. 4 oz. and 4 lb. 6 oz.). Of the children considered to have moderate or severe handicaps, 40 per cent suffered from neurological defects, mainly cerebral diplegia, hemiplegia and epilepsy with or without mental retardation; 35 per cent exhibited mental retardation only; 18 per cent had major or multiple physical defects and 7 per cent dull intelligence and severe hyperkinetic behaviour disorders.

A current study of the later progress of low weight infants born in 1966–68 suggests that the incidence of severe handicap at school age is likely to be lower than in the earlier study, particularly in those of 1,500 g. or less, and that one-third rather than one-half of these very small infants may exhibit mental, neurological or physical defects at later ages.

Although it is now established that low birth weight is significantly associated with an increased incidence of various handicaps, two fundamental questions remain, to a large extent, unanswered. Firstly, what are the basic causes of the different handicaps affecting low weight infants; and, secondly, why do some infants suffer severe disability whilst others of like birth weight and similar obstetric history escape relatively unscathed?

Various defects as well as low birth weight and premature delivery may all be due to developmental anomalies. This is obviously so in a minority of low weight infants who have major or multiple congenital defects, which must have originated at an early stage of intra-uterine existence. However, most low weight infants who are subsequently found to have handicaps suffer from mental and neurological abnormalities which could have originated in early prenatal life, although the same clinical picture could have resulted from adverse influences in later pregnancy, during labour and delivery, in the early postnatal period or from some combination of adverse factors operating at different times.

The timing of the damage is of major importance, since if maternal complications or the premature delivery itself are the cause of later handicap, improvements in antenatal care of mothers and postnatal care of infants might be expected to improve the child's chance of later normality. On the other hand, if the infant is born prematurely because of developmental defect already present, such improvements might lead to the survival of an increasing number of defective children.

Factors affecting prognosis. A number of circumstances have been suggested as significant associations with an excess of mental and neurological defects in low weight infants.

Maternal and pregnancy factors. Women with a history of difficulty in conceiving and/or frequent abnormal outcome in their conceptions are more likely to give birth to infants of low birth weight; in addition the low weight infant born to a mother with this sort of history is more likely to suffer from significant handicap than the like weight infant born to a mother with no such history (Drillien, 1968).

Potentially hypoxia-producing complications of late pregnancy, such as severe toxaemia and chronic cardiac or renal disease, are associated with a higher incidence of both perinatal loss and later handicap, particularly in male infants.

Environmental factors. The infant born to parents of good intelligence from a good social background is less likely to exhibit handicap necessitating special education than the infant born to poor type parents of low intelligence. This applies particularly to the incidence of mental retardation alone without additional neurological or physical defects. However, it should be remembered that intellectual ability rated as low average or dull in a child whose parents and siblings are of superior intelligence may indicate as marked a degree of retardation and present the same domestic problems as a much lower level of ability necessitating education in special school in a child whose parents and siblings are themselves of low average intelligence.

Several recent long-term studies have demonstrated that, irrespective of the type of home, there is a steady scaling down in intellectual ability and educational performance as birth weight decreases, even when one excludes the most severely handicapped children who are ineducable (Wiener, 1968; Wiener *et al.*, 1968; Drillien, 1969).

Fetal factors. The incidence of definite disability increases with decreasing birth weight in both boys and girls, but at any given birth weight there is a significant excess of boys with handicaps (Heimer *et al.*, 1964; Bacola *et al.*, 1966; Drillien, 1967). The preponderance of females in samples of surviving infants of 2,000 g. or less appears to be due entirely to the increased chance of survival of females compared to males of similar birth weight. It is reasonable to suppose that the biological vulnerability of the male, which leads to a greater wastage in the early stages of gestation and an increased perinatal mortality rate, is likely also to lead to an increased risk of cerebral damage in surviving male infants of low birth weight.

The low weight infant with a congenital malformation, whether or not this is handicapping in itself, is more likely to present at later ages with mental and neurological defects than the like weight infant with no anomaly, suggesting that in many cases the total picture of mental, physical and neurological defect originated during the period or organogenesis in early pregnancy (Drillien, 1968).

The nutritional status of the low weight infant both pre- and post-natal may have a bearing on later intellectual performance. It has been known for many years that, in some mammalian species, lowering the mother's plane of nutrition towards the end of gestation can materially reduce the size of the newborn, and following nutritional set-back before birth some young animals not only fail to catch up in stature but also tend to lag further behind with increasing age (Dawes, 1968). It has also been demonstrated that the imprint of differential food intake during suckling persists in spite of unlimited food intake at later ages (McCance, 1962).

More recently the emphasis has shifted to brain rather than overall body growth and it has been shown that in some animals the brain may be permanently affected if nutritional restrictions are imposed at a time when it is undergoing its period of fastest growth (Dobbing, 1968). In the human the period of most rapid brain growth probably occurs during the last few months of normal gestation and to a lesser extent during the first few months of postnatal life, and the hypothesis has been put forward that malnutrition during this critical period may affect the physical composition of the brain in like manner.

The suggestion that small-for-dates infants may have a higher incidence of mental and neurological defects than like weight prematurely delivered infants is not yet substantiated. Studies carried out in Paris by Minkowski and his colleagues (Minkowski *et al.*, 1966) would seem to indicate that in the human, growth, structure and function of the brain are not noticeably affected by unfavourable gestational circumstances which may affect physical growth. These workers showed that brain growth and maturation of small-for-dates infants were appropriate for normal weight infants of like gestational age, as were neurological maturity and electroencephalographic findings.

Since there are differences in feeding behaviour and postnatal weight gain in infants of similar birth weight but different gestational age, it may be inappropriate to select weight for gestational age at birth as a measure of the adequacy of nutrition during what may be a critical period of brain development. It cannot be assumed that postnatal weight of the prematurely delivered infant will continue along the percentile curve appertaining at birth. An infant delivered at 30 weeks, whose weight for gestational age is on the 50th percentile, may by 34 weeks be well below the tenth percentile and continue at that level, weighing no more than the 37 week small-for dates infant when both have reached a post-conceptional age of 40 weeks.

There is some evidence that with immediate feeding of low weight infants with undiluted breast milk (Davies and Russell, 1968) or low electrolyte full strength cow's milk formulae, postnatal weight loss is reduced, hyperbilirubinaemia and hypoglycaemia are less often evident and later mental and neurological status is improved.

Postnatal factors. Infants of low birth weight, especially those who are prematurely delivered, are particularly liable to initial apnoea, later cyanotic attacks and severe respiratory distress. Initial apnoea does not seem to be associated with an increase in later handicap though there is an increase in those having cyanotic attacks some hours or days after satisfactory respiration has been established (Bacola *et al.*, 1966). However, in these cases one needs to consider whether damage resulted from anoxia or whether the apnoeic attacks themselves were evidence of pre-existing brain damage. The later status of infants who suffered from severe respiratory distress (which must produce marked and prolonged hypoxia) is not obviously different from that of infants of similar birth weight without respiratory distress.

Hyperbilirubinaemia is common in the low birth weight infant but there is not much evidence that the infant who has been subjected to indirect serum bilirubin levels of between 16 and 20 mg. per cent is at later disadvantage as compared with the baby of like birth weight without hyperbilirubinaemia. Higher levels are seldom seen at the present time as a rise above 20 mg. is usually considered an indication for exchange transfusion. There is some evidence that damage may be caused by lower levels in the case of very small infants with respiratory difficulties and acid base disturbances and there may be a case for earlier exchange transfusion in such circumstances (Stern and Denton, 1965).

Hypoglycaemia is also common in infants of low birth weight, particularly in those who are markedly underweight for their gestational age. The growth of the brain is less affected by intra-uterine malnutrition than any other part of the body, while the growth of the liver is considerably decreased. The tendency to hypoglycaemia is thought to be due to the metabolic needs of the relatively large brain exceeding the capacity of the small liver to produce sufficient glucose.

Cornblath *et al.* (1966) defined hypoglycaemia as sequential blood glucose values under 30 mg. per 100 ml. during the first 72 hours of life, under 40 mg. thereafter in the full-sized infant born at term and under 20 mg. in the infant of low birth weight after a $3\frac{1}{2}$ to $4\frac{1}{2}$ hours' fast. They reported an incidence of 5·7 per cent in low weight infants, and noted that among affected infants males predominated (2:1), and all were of low weight for gestational age and often the smaller members of twin pairs. Low weight infants who had been hypoglycaemic on these criteria were more likely to show mental retardation at ages 3 to 5 years and some abnormality on neurological evaluation than controls of like weight and sex. However, these workers draw attention to the fact that a part of the symptomatology and residual damage may be due to other causes, since low blood glucose levels may be associated with a variety of existing central nervous system abnormalities.

An attempt was made (Drillien, 1965) to assess the probable causes of the individual defects found in the one-third of a group of surviving children of birth weight 2,000 g. or less who exhibited moderate or severe handicaps at seven years. In one-half it seemed likely that the defect was developmental in origin (that is, had originated at an early stage of gestation) and that low birth weight and/or premature delivery was the result rather than the cause of the defect. Definite developmental anomalies were seen in some of these children. None of the mothers suffered from severe toxaemia or other chronic diseases likely to lead to fetal hypoxia, although a number had hydramnios, repeated threatened abortion and antepartum haemorrhage. The mothers frequently had a poor obstetric history of habitual abortion, perinatal losses and other abnormal offspring and/or were considered relatively infertile because of difficulty in conceiving. In one-quarter of the cases of handicap it seemed probable that the fetus had suffered cerebral damage as a result of intra-uterine hypoxia or malnutrition due to chronic disease of the mother or severe toxaemia. In a further one-quarter of cases the cause of handicap was uncertain. Most of these children had been less than 1,500 g. at birth and came from poor homes.

While the incidence of later handicaps due primarily to developmental abnormality cannot be affected by improvement in perinatal care, this is not to say that additional damage may not be caused by adverse factors during this period. The apparent decrease in significant handicap in very low weight infants in the past 10 years gives hope that the later status of potentially normal low weight infants may be improved by measures aimed at reducing hypoxia, pre- and post-natal malnutrition and biochemical disturbances.

C. M. DRILLIEN

References

AMIEL-TISON, C. (1968). Neurologic evaluation of the maturity of newborn infants. *Arch. Dis. Childh.*, **43**, 89.

BACOLA, E., BEHRLE, F. C., de SCHWEINITZ, L., MILLER, H. C. and MIRA, M. (1966). Perinatal and environmental factors in late neurogenic sequelae. *Amer. J. Dis. Child.*, **112**, 359.

BAIRD, D. (1964). The epidemiology of prematurity. *J. Pediat.*, **65**, 909.

BENIRSCHKE, K. (1961). Twin placenta in perinatal mortality. *N.Y.St.J. Med.*, **61**, 1499.

BUTLER, N. R. and ALBERMAN, E. D. (1969). *Perinatal Problems: The Second Report of the 1958 British Perinatal Mortality Survey.* Edinburgh: Livingstone.

—— and BONHAM, D. G. (1963). *Perinatal Mortality: The First Report of the 1958 British Perinatal Mortality Survey.* Edinburgh: Livingstone.

Chief Medical Officer of the Ministry of Health (1968). *Annual Report for 1967.* London: H.M.S.O.

CORNBLATH, M., JOASSIN, G., WEISSKOPF, B. and SWIATEK, K. R. (1966). Hypoglycemia in the newborn. *Pediat. Clin. N. Amer.*, **13**, 905.

DAVIES, P. A. and RUSSELL, H. (1968). Later progress of 100 infants weighing 1,000 g. to 2,000 g. at birth fed immediately with breast milk. *Develop. Med. Child Neurol.*, **10**, 725.

DAWES, G. S. (1968). *Foetal and Neonatal Physiology: A Comparative Study of the Changes at Birth*. Chicago: Year Book Medical Publishers, Inc.

DOBBING, J. (1968). Vulnerable periods in developing brain. In *Applied Neurochemistry*. Ed. A. N. Davison, and J. Dobbing, Oxford: Blackwell.

DRILLIEN, C. M. (1957). The social and economic factors affecting the incidence of premature birth. *J. Obstet. Gynaec. Brit. Emp.*, 64, 161.

—— (1958). Growth and development in a group of children of very low birth weight. *Arch. Dis. Childh.*, 33, 10.

—— (1964). *The Growth and Development of the Prematurely Born Infant*. Edinburgh: Livingstone.

—— (1965). Possible causes of handicap in babies of low birth weight. *J. Obstet. Gynaec. Brit. Cwlth.*, 72, 993.

—— (1967). The incidence of mental and physical handicaps in school age children of very low birth weight. *Pediatrics*, 39, 238.

—— (1968). Causes of handicap in the low weight infant. In Nutricia Symposium *Aspects of Praematurity and Dysmaturity*. Ed. J. H. P. Jonxis, H. K. A. Visser, J. A. Troelstra, Leiden: H. E. Stenfert Kroese N.V.

—— (1969). School disposal and performance for children of different birth weight born 1953–60. *Arch. Dis. Childh.*, 44, 562.

—— and RICHMOND, F. (1956). Prematurity in Edinburgh. *Arch. Dis. Childh.*, 31, 390.

FARR, V., MITCHELL, R. G., NELIGAN, G. A. and PARKIN, J. M. (1966). The definition of some external characteristics used in the assessment of gestational age in the newborn infant. *Develop. Med. Child Neurol.*, 8, 507.

FRANDSEN, V. A. and STAKEMANN, G. (1963). The clinical significance of oestriol estimations in late pregnancy. *Acta endocrinol.* (kbh.), 44, 183.

GRUENWALD, P. (1963). Chronic fetal distress and placental insufficiency. *Biol. Neonat.*, 5, 215.

HEIMER, C. B., CUTLER, R. and FREEDMAN, A. M. (1964). Neurological sequelae of premature birth. *Amer. J. Dis. Child.*, 108, 122.

LUBCHENCO, L. O., HANSMAN, C., DRESSLER, M. and BOYD, E. (1963). Intrauterine growth as estimated from liveborn birth-weight data at 24 to 42 weeks of gestation. *Pediatrics*, 32, 793.

MINKOWSKI, A., LARROCHE, J. C., VIGNAUD, J., DREYFUS-BRISAC, C. and SAINT-ANNE DARGASSIES, S. (1966). Development of the nervous system in early life. In *Human Development*. Ed. F. Falkner, Philadelphia: W. B. Saunders.

MITCHELL, R. G. and FARR, V. (1965). The meaning of maturity and the assessment of maturity at birth. In *Gestational Age, Size and Maturity*. Ed. M. Dawkins, and W. G. MacGregor, *Clinic in Developmental Medicine, No. 19*. London: Heinemann.

McCANCE, R. A. (1962). Food, growth and time. *Lancet*, 2, 621, 671.

McDONALD, A. D. (1965). Retarded foetal growth. In *Gestational Age, Size and Maturity*. Ed. M. Dawkins, and W. G. MacGregor, *Clinic in Developmental Medicine, No. 19*. London: Heinemann.

NELIGAN, G. A. (1965). A community study of the relationship between birth weight and gestational age. In *Gestational Age, Size and Maturity*. Ed. M. Dawkins, and W. G. MacGregor, *Clinic in Developmental Medicine, No. 19*. London: Heinemann.

PRECHTL, H. F. R. (1960). The long term value of the neurologic examination of the newborn infant. *Little Club Clinics in Developmental Medicine, No. 2*. Ed. M. Bax, R. MacKeith, London: Heinemann.

ROBINSON, R. J. (1966). Assessment of gestational age by neurological examination. *Arch. Dis. Childh.*, 41, 437.

SCHUTT, W. (1965). Foetal factors in intrauterine growth retardation. In *Gestational Age, Size and Maturity*. Ed. M. Dawkins, and W. G. MacGregor, *Clinic in Developmental Medicine, No. 19*. London: Heinemann.

STERN, L. and DENTON, R. L. (1965). Kernicterus in small premature infants. *Pediatrics*, 35, 484.

TURNBULL, E. and WALKER, J. (1956). The outcome of pregnancy complicated by threatened abortion. *J. Obstet. Gynaec. Brit. Emp.*, 63, 553.

USHER, R., McLEAN, F., SCOTT, K. E. (1966). *Judgment of Fetal Age : II.* Clinical significance of gestational age and an objective method for its assessment. *Pediat. Clin. N. Amer.*, 13, 835.

WALKER, J. (1965). Medical factors in the causation of prematurity and intrauterine growth retardation. In *Gestational Age, Size and Maturity.* Ed. M. Dawkins, and W. G. MacGregor, *Clinic in Developmental Medicine, No. 19.* London: Heinemann.

WARKANY, J., MONROE, B. B., SUTHERLAND, B. S. (1961). Intrauterine growth retardation. *Amer. J. Dis. Child.*, 102, 249.

WIENER, G. (1968). Scholastic achievement at age 12–13 of prematurely born infants. *J. spec. Educ.*, 2, 237.

—— RIDER, R. V., OPPEL, W. C., HARPER, P. A. (1968). Correlates of low birth weight. Psychological status at 8–10 years of age. *Pediat. Res.*, 2, 110.

WILSON, M. G., PARMELEE, A. H. Jr. and HUGGINS, M. H. (1963). Prenatal history of infants with birth weights of 1,500 g. or less. *Pediatrics*, 63, 1140.

World Health Organisation (1948–9) *Manual of the International Statistical Classification of Diseases, Injuries and Causes of Death.* Geneva: W.H.O.

—— (1950). Expert group on prematurity (final report.) *Wld. Hlth. Org. tech. Rep. Ser.* No. 27.

—— (1961). Public health aspects of low birth weight. Third report of expert committee on maternal and child health. *Wld. Hlth. Org. tech. Rep. Ser.* No. 217.

WORTIS, H., BRAINE, M., CUTLER, R. and FREEDMAN, A. M. (1964). Deviant behavior in 2½ year-old premature children. *Child Develop.*, 35, 871.

5   Nutrition and Feeding

ADEQUATE nutrition is a prime necessity for all living creatures and the young of most higher species are dependent on their parents for food. In man, the period of total dependence is relatively far longer than in other mammals and children are therefore especially liable to malnutrition. When food supplies are limited, it is infants and children who suffer first and most severely and the nutrition and feeding of the young constitute a major task for the health services in developing countries (Swaminathan, 1968). In countries where good quality food is plentiful and available to all, where standards of food processing and handling are high and where domestic hygiene is generally satisfactory, serious nutritional disorders affect only the exceptional few and are of comparatively little importance in ordinary clinical practice. Nevertheless, it must never be forgotten that malnutrition starts as soon as the supply of nutrients stops and that its florid manifestations appear very quickly when adverse conditions such as natural disasters, industrial depression or warfare disrupt food supplies or diminish the capacity of parents to provide for their children. Even in the most affluent society, hunger and starvation are always just around the corner.

Conditions of plenty are no guarantee of good nutrition, for children may be inadequately fed through ignorance of their needs or low standards of parental care. The food habits of minority religious or racial groups may be inappropriate to the circumstances in which they live and their children may develop nutritional disorders in consequence (Nutrition Society Symposium, 1967). Those responsible for the health of children must have a sound knowledge of nutritional principles if they are to advise and instruct mothers and others caring for young children and to recognise situations predisposing to malnutrition in time to take preventive action.

Improved nutrition has certainly been one, if not the sole, factor responsible for the acceleration of growth and maturation of children which has occurred in countries with a high standard of living during the present century (Wolff, 1955). It is probable, however, that the pendulum has swung too far in the direction of overnutrition amongst the most privileged population at a time when undernutrition is still a major problem for nearly half the world. The very early introduction of soft solids into the infant's diet and the high-pressure advertising of sweets, proprietary foods, drinks, ice-cream, vitamin preparations, etc., through all available mass media require much more critical evaluation in terms of child nutrition and health in adult life than they commonly receive (Forbes, 1957). Thus the largely unregulated fortification of infant foods with vitamin D during and after World War II produced the situation in which many toddlers were getting 4,000 units daily (ten times the recommended intake) and some showed symptoms of hyper-calcaemia as a result (Morgan *et al.*, 1956). The excessive use of refined sugar and sticky carbohydrates is not only a nutritional hazard but is also an important factor producing dental caries. Many infants in affluent countries are overweight and tend to remain so during childhood and into adult life. The adverse effects of life-long obesity are evident from the high mortality and morbidity rates for diabetes and cardiovascular disease in obese adults and the American Academy of Pediatrics (1967) has stressed the need for early treatment of obesity. Unfortunately, the results of attempting to reduce the weight of young children by dietary restriction are disappointing (Asher, 1968). Whilst the elimination of disease due to nutritional deficiency from infant and childhood communities is wholly desirable, it may reasonably be assumed that there is an optimum nutritional status which it is not advantageous to exceed.

The Digestive System

The digestive tract of the infant differs in several respects from that of the older child and its capacity is correspondingly limited.

APPETITE. It has been shown experimentally (Brobeck, 1957) that appetite is under the control of twin centres laterally placed in the hypothalamus and satiety, or inhibition of appetite, by similar centres situated medially. The appetite centres are activated by a variety of stimuli, *e.g.* hunger contractions of the stomach (see below), hypoglycaemia and possibly cold. When food is taken, the satiety centres are stimulated and appetite is inhibited, *i.e.* a sense of repletion is experienced. This alternating mechanism is well adjusted to the requirements of growth and activity, though it may be upset by psychological disturbances, physical disease or inability to satisfy the appetite. Thus unrelieved hunger or malnutrition will tend to inhibit appetite rather than increase it. Food intake is also influenced by the appearance, smell and taste of food. Consistent neglect of the sensation of repletion can raise the threshold at which this is experienced and so produce a vicious circle of over-eating, increased appetite and over-eating. Since the young infant is wholly dependent on the food offered, natural appetite can be disturbed by either under-feeding or compulsive feeding, or by lack of opportunity for selection.

THE MOUTH AND OESOPHAGUS. In early infancy, the absence of teeth precludes the chewing of solid food, while salivary digestion is negligible, though saliva is secreted from birth. Milk is normally obtained by sucking, which consists of suction to maintain the nipple far back in the infant's mouth and co-ordinated movements of the jaws on the areolar area behind the nipple, so expressing milk into the mouth. At the same time, milk is forced from the breast by the 'draught' and by these combined forces the infant obtains his feed. The reflex act of sucking is followed by swallowing, inhibition of respiration and closure of the larynx, in a patterned sequence of sucking, swallowing, breathing, controlled by a centre in the medulla. By the third day, oesophageal peristalsis is co-ordinated with swallowing, but in the first 12 hours after birth the oesophageal response is unco-ordinated (Gryboski, 1965).

THE STOMACH in early infancy lies with its long axis placed transversely and only gradually changes to reach the adult form and position at about 11 years of age. When it fills with food, there is tonic contraction of the fundus and waves of contraction are rapidly stimulated. These originate near the pylorus and subsequently at the cardiac end of the stomach, passing towards the pylorus. The findings in the newborn, however, are not consistent and Smith (1959) considers that there is unpredictable relaxation of the pylorus and 'massive, gentle, non-peristaltic movement' associated with emptying of the stomach. When the food is entirely fluid in early infancy, the stomach begins to empty rapidly, often within 5 minutes, but total emptying time is slower in infancy than in later life.

'Hunger contractions' occur when the stomach is empty and are frequent and intense in infancy. The interval between feeding and the next hunger period is variable but generally between 2 and 4 hours in the young infant. The recognition of the physiological basis, variability and intensity of hunger in the infant is essential for rational infant feeding. In older children the interval between taking food and the appearance of hunger contractions is longer. The influence of psychological factors on appetite is well known but it should also be remembered that for a healthy appetite to develop the stomach must be given a reasonable time to empty after a meal. Increased fat in the diet will tend to delay emptying and so reduce appetite, whereas a carbohydrate meal is quickly passed on. The osmotic pressure of the gastric contents also influences emptying and the stomach regulates this by secreting or absorbing water.

AIR-SWALLOWING is a normal procedure during feeding or crying in the infant. Air usually enters the stomach with the first inspiration and rapidly passes through the intestinal tract, reaching the colon within a few hours after birth. Some degree of air-swallowing always occurs during a feed and, if not excessive, the gas bubble rises to the fundus of the stomach and is eructated by the infant. This is facilitated by holding the baby upright at intervals during feeding and at the end. If the infant does not bring up his 'wind' in this way, the air tends to pass through the pylorus with the food and cause distension of the small bowel and consequent discomfort. Colic due to air-swallowing should be distinguished from a type of colic which may occur in healthy babies during the first 3 months and gives rise to prolonged screaming, usually in the evening. The cause of this 'three month colic' or 'evening colic' is unknown (Illingworth, 1959).

THE SMALL INTESTINE is variable in length, being about 300 cm. at birth and 450 cm. at one year. Movement in the small intestine in childhood is thought to be similar to that described in the adult but, as in the case of the stomach, the intestinal movement of the young child is much more susceptible to outside influences. Apart from the movement of the villi, three types of movement have been described—rhythmic segmentation, pendulum or swaying movements and 'travel-wave' or 'peristaltic rush'. The last of these is particularly readily excited in infants and young children, with the result that diarrhoea may follow such different stimuli as fright, infection or even the taking of food.

The digestion of fat is less effective during the first year than in later life. Digestion of starch by pancreatic amylase may also be deficient in the early months but the disaccharidase enzymes, which split maltose, lactose and sucrose into their constituent monosaccharides, are usually present from birth, though lactase may be inadequate in the infant born before term. Protein digestion is efficiently carried out by even the least mature newborn infant.

THE LARGE INTESTINE is relatively more capacious in the infant than in the adult. Digestion is virtually complete by the time the intestinal contents pass the ileo-colic sphincter and transport from caecum to rectum is very rapid. During this phase, water is absorbed so that the material is converted from a liquid to a solid consistency; absorption is less complete in the young infant, so that the stools remain semi-solid.

DEFAECATION. This is a reflex act which is not under voluntary control in early infancy, when it commonly occurs three or more times a day, though the frequency is variable. Not until the stools are becoming formed is sphincter control acquired, and since this is a gradual process, it is understandable that control is less perfect in young children than in adults.

When voluntary control is firmly established, most children adopt a rhythm of one bowel action a day at approximately the same hour, but either a more or less frequent rhythm is quite consistent with good health. 'Constipation' and 'diarrhoea' should be judged, not by the frequency of bowel actions (unless there is a sudden change in the child's usual pattern) so much as by the consistency of the stools.

STOOLS. At birth the intestine contains semi-fluid, viscid meconium, which is sterile and practically odourless. Its dark green colour is due to bile pigments and in their absence, as in biliary atresia, the meconium is light grey in colour. The material consists of mucopolysaccharides secreted into the intestinal lumen, digestive secretions and swallowed amniotic fluid and desquamated cells. Meconium is usually passed within a few hours of birth but passage may be delayed by a plug of inspissated meconium in the rectum. In the absence of pancreatic trypsin (as in cystic fibrosis), the meconium may have the consistency of putty and cause serious obstruction (meconium ileus).

From about the fourth day after birth, the material passed changes to the yellow semi-formed stool characteristic of the first few months. In the case of breast-fed babies, the stool is mustard-yellow and acid in reaction, and may be passed daily but often only once every second or third day. Artificially fed babies usually pass at least one stool a day, paler yellow in colour, more formed, and neutral or faintly alkaline. The infant's stool contains about 85 per cent of water, only very small amounts of protein and little or no sugar. The fat content is relatively high (approximately 35 to 40 per cent of the dried weight). The stools smell sour and lack the faecal odour of the stools in later life, which is due to the presence of indol and skatol and to the action of putrefactive bacteria in the large bowel. The presence of undigested curds is an indication that the food is passing too rapidly or that the cow's milk curd is proving too indigestible.

The stools become darker when mixed feeding is established and later become more formed, assuming the colour and odour of the adult stool during the second year of life.

INTESTINAL FLORA. Organisms rapidly appear in the meconium during the first 24 hours, due partly to invasion from below but principally to oral ingestion of organisms before food is taken. The upper part of the small intestine remains relatively free from organisms for a longer time in the breast-fed than in the artificially fed infant, possibly due to the higher gastric acidity in the former. There is also a striking difference between the character of the faecal flora of the breast-fed and that of the artificially fed infant, the difference in reaction of the stools being at least partly responsible. During the period of breast-feeding, the infant's stools are characterised by an almost pure growth of Lactobacillus bifidus, whereas on mixed feeding or cow's milk, there is a mixed flora. It has been suggested that this difference may have a bearing on the relative freedom from gastro-intestinal upsets observed in breast-fed babies.

Nutritional Requirements

CALORIES.* When it is considered that the infant may double, or more than double, his birth-weight in the first 5 months of life, it will be realised that his caloric requirements will be relatively much higher than those of an adult. They are normally supplied by approximately 110 cals. per kg. (50 per lb.) body-weight per day during the first 6 months and by 100 cals. per kg. (45 per lb.) during the second, as compared with the needs of a man weighing 70 kg. (154 lb.) on moderately active work who requires 3,000 calories, *i.e.* approximately 43 cals. per kg. (20 per lb.). Throughout childhood the caloric requirements remain high in order to supply the calls of both growth and energy expenditure. Individual variations are so wide, however, that the following recommended allowances (Department of Health and Social Security, 1969) can only be taken as an approximate guide in planning the feeding of large numbers: at 1 to 2 years, 1,200 cals.; at 2 to 3 years, 1,400 cals.; at 3 to 5 years, 1,600 cals.; at 5 to 7 years, 1,800 cals.; at 7 to 9 years, 2,100 cals.; and at 9 to 12 years, 2,300 cals. for girls and 2,500 for boys. It must be emphasised that these are only averages, and there will be great differences between children of the same age, determined by their sex, rate of growth, energy expenditure and metabolic activity. Moreover, the needs of the individual child will vary greatly from day to day and at different periods of the year. In the early teens, the requirements will be conditioned very largely by the age of occurrence of the pubertal spurt of growth. At 15 to 18 years, the calorie requirements have been estimated at 2,300 for girls and 3,000 for boys.

FLUID. The infant requires approximately 150 ml. of fluid per kg. (2½ fl. oz. per

* The large Calorie (kilocalorie) used in dietetics to express energy represents the amount of heat required to raise the temperature of 1 litre of water from 15° to 16°C and is a thousand times greater than the small calorie used in physics.

lb.) body weight per day; in older infants and children, average fluid requirements are proportionately less, but temperature and activity will cause great variation. Whilst thirst is usually a reliable guide, it is sometimes found that a child who is constipated, with dry hard stools, is suffering from excessive fluid absorption in the large bowel and that the condition can be relieved by a higher fluid intake.

PROTEIN supplies amino acids essential for growth and the replacement of tissue proteins which are constantly undergoing breakdown in the body. Whilst fat and carbohydrate, the main sources of energy, are to some extent interchangeable in metabolism, the essential amino acids cannot be formed from them and the food must therefore contain a sufficient quantity of suitable protein.

Ample supplies of fat and carbohydrate can spare protein, however, and the amount of protein required depends on this protein-sparing effect, on the quality of the protein, and on other factors such as its state of subdivision and the timing of feeds. The breast-fed infant is receiving protein of high quality and thrives on only about 2 g. of total protein per kg. per day (representing less than 10 per cent of total calories), whereas more than this will be needed when protein is of inferior nutritive value. The infant fed cow's milk may receive 3 g. of protein or more per kg. per day: it is not clear whether this is required because cow's milk protein is of lesser biological value or whether such an intake is unnecessarily high. The growing child is normally in a state of nitrogen retention and the younger the child the greater the retention relative to the body weight. Intake of protein above the needs of the infant leads to increased nitrogen retention but useful storage of protein probably does not occur (Holt and Snyderman, 1965). If sufficient milk is consumed to ensure an adequate intake of nitrogen, none of the essential amino acids will be deficient.

After the first year, the daily minimum requirement of high quality protein falls gradually to about 1·0 g. per kg., though the actual allowance should be higher than this, since daily allowances must not only supply the calculated minimum requirement but also allow a generous margin for individual variation. Recommendations by the Joint FAO/WHO Expert Group (1965) for requirements based on milk protein are as follows:

Age (months)	Protein requirement (g. per kg. per day)
0–3	2·3
3–6	1·8
6–9	1·5
9–12	1·2

In the diets of healthy children, it is found that protein usually represents at least 10 per cent of total calories, though this is probably more than double the minimum requirement of first-class protein. The inclusion of a half to one pint of milk daily in the diet of children, together with the amounts of meat, cheese, eggs or fish normally eaten, will provide an ample supply of first-class protein. In countries where animal protein is not normally included in the staple diet, it is

5

of much greater importance to ensure that the vegetable protein consumed is of high biological value. Most plant proteins are deficient in at least one of the essential amino acids but by a judicious mixture of various proteins the child's requirements can be adequately covered.

CARBOHYDRATE is the main source of glucose, which circulates in the blood to provide for energy requirements and is stored in the liver as glycogen. Owing to the rapid metabolism and variable activity in childhood, the calls for rapidly assimilable carbohydrate are higher than in the adult and the craving of children for sweet or starchy foods is physiological within limits, though liable to become excessive if over-indulged. Young children kept for several hours without carbohydrate may develop symptoms of hypoglycaemia and with longer deprivation ketosis may occur. Ketone bodies, the intermediary products of breakdown of fat, appear in the blood and urine when the liver is unable to cope with excessive demands for fat metabolism such as occur during carbohydrate starvation. Ketosis occurs most readily in early life, owing to the immaturity of the liver and to the high demands for available glucose which tend to cause too rapid depletion of liver glycogen.

Carbohydrate provides a ready source of calories, without requiring the kidneys to excrete an additional load of solute. A too exclusively carbohydrate diet, however, tends to produce fat rather than muscular development. The minimum carbohydrate requirements have been estimated as 3 g. per kg. per day for infants and 2·5 to 3 g. in the case of older children: the normal intake of the healthy child is considerably higher than this (10 to 14 g. for infants and 8 to 10 g. for older children). Although the carbohydrate present in milk is lactose, artificially fed infants are able to digest other sugars such as cane sugar and dextrimaltose, and the use of added lactose in artificial feeding is unnecessary.

FAT is, weight for weight, the most fruitful source of energy, supplying 9·0 calories per g. compared with 4·0 cals. per g. in the case of protein and carbohydrate. It is valuable as a stored reservoir of calories in the body and certain fats also supply fat-soluble nutrients such as vitamins A and D. Human milk and cow's milk both contain about 3·5 per cent of fat (the percentage varying considerably in different samples), yielding approximately half the total calories of a milk diet. Jersey and Guernsey milks having a higher fat content should be avoided in the artificial feeding of young infants. In general, it is found that a high fat intake is not well tolerated by many young children, being liable to result in ketosis and indigestion (probably related to the effect of fat in causing gastric and intestinal inertia).

INORGANIC ELEMENTS. The inorganic elements required in the diet are iron and iodine: calcium, sodium and potassium: phosphorus, sulphur and chlorine: and other elements in minute traces.

Iron is necessary for the formation of haemoglobin, muscle myoglobin and certain tissue enzymes. It must be supplied in the diet to provide for growth and to replace the small losses from the skin and in the excreta. The daily requirement is only about 1 mg. per day in childhood but a daily intake of at least 6 mg. is recommended to allow for individual variation and because only a proportion of food iron is absorbed. Additional iron may be required by girls after puberty and to replace any abnormal blood loss. There is usually no iron deficiency in healthy infants up to the age of 3 or 4 months but after this age it is important that iron-containing foods such as meat and green vegetables should be added to the diet. The iron content of both human and cow's milk is low and a breast-fed infant of 3 months may be getting less than 1 mg. of iron daily from the milk. Iron is often added to dried milk during manufacture so that artificially fed infants may obtain it from this source. Infants born before term will require early supplements of iron, since the total available iron in the body (mainly in the haemoglobin mass) is relatively small and is inadequate to meet the demands of the rapidly growing infant.

Calcium is necessary for growth of the skeletal system and for maintenance of the plasma calcium at the normal level of 9 to 11 mg. per 100 ml. in children (though the limits are rather wider in young infants). When there is gross deficiency of calcium in the diet or failure of absorption and utilisation due to lack of vitamin D, rickets and osteoporosis occur. The plasma calcium level is regulated by the actions of parathyroid hormone and thyrocalcitonin, which maintain an equilibrium between blood and bone calcium. When this mechanism breaks down and the plasma calcium falls below 6 mg. per 100 ml., tetany develops. It is difficult to state the optimum intake of calcium for, as the dietary content falls, absorption from the intestine becomes more efficient. The daily intake for children on adequate amounts of vitamin D should be at least 500 to 700 mg. daily, depending on age, and some have recommended that 1·0 g. should be allowed daily. Milk and cheese are rich sources of calcium and if the equivalent of at least one pint (568 ml.) of milk a day is included in the diet there is no danger of primary calcium deficiency.

Phosphorus is not only required for skeletal development but is also widely distributed in the tissue fluids and forms an essential constituent of phospholipids, phosphoproteins and nucleoproteins. The level of plasma inorganic phosphorus varies with season and age, being highest in infancy (up to 7 mg. per 100 ml.) and falling during childhood (4 to 6 mg. per 100 ml.). Phosphorus deficiency will not occur on a mixed diet containing milk, since it is present in most foods.

Iodine requirements in infancy are normally provided by milk and deficiency will only occur in breast-fed infants when the maternal diet is grossly deficient. In districts where there is little iodine in the soil and water, the deficiency can be remedied by the routine use of iodised table-salt (see endemic goitre, p. 537).

Copper, *cobalt*, *manganese and zinc* are constituents of certain enzymes and, though essential for metabolism, are present in animal tissues only in minute quantities. With the exception of copper (Cordano *et al.*, 1964), deficiencies of these trace elements are not known to occur in human infants.

Fluorine. Although it is doubtful whether fluorine is an essential constituent of human diet, it has been shown conclusively that populations dependent on water supplies containing less than 1 part per million of fluorine have an abnormally high rate of dental caries. In areas where the fluorine content of water is excessively high (*e.g.* 5 p.p.m.), dental fluorosis results in mottling of the enamel of the teeth, which are otherwise healthy. The raising of the fluorine content of low-fluorine water supplies to 1 p.p.m. has been abundantly justified as a harmless public health measure which is effective in lowering the incidence of dental caries. In spite of the considerable resistance which attempts at fluoridation of water have encountered, this is now becoming increasingly accepted as a desirable means of combating one of the major causes of dental ill-health in childhood.

Vitamin Requirements

There are still considerable gaps in our knowledge of the requirements of vitamins during infancy and childhood and recommended allowances are usually gross over-estimates based on inadequate evidence. They should be considered as estimates designed to cover minimum requirements, *i.e.* to prevent deficiency, and to allow a liberal safety margin. The Panel on Recommended Allowances of Nutrients of the Department of Health and Social Security (1969) define their recommended intakes as the amounts sufficient or more than sufficient for the nutritional needs of practically all healthy persons in a population. The daily allowances suggested for infants and children are as follows:

TABLE 3

Age years	Vitamin A µg retinol equivalents	Vitamin D i.u.	Thiamine mg.	Niacin mg.	Riboflavin mg.	Vitamin C mg.
0–1	450	400	0·3	5	0·4	15
1–2	300	400	0·5	7	0·6	20
2–3	300	400	0·6	8	0·7	20
3–5	300	400	0·6	9	0·8	20
5–7	300	100	0·7	10	0·9	20
7–9	400	100	0·8	11	1·0	20
9–12	575	100	0·9–1·0	13–14	1·2	25

VITAMIN A AND CAROTENOIDS. Vitamin A (Retinol) is necessary for the maintenance and growth of epithelium. It is obtained mainly from fats, especially fish liver oils, and there are substantial stores in the human liver. The carotenoid pigments found in green vegetables and carrots are pro-vitamins which are partly converted to vitamin A. Although the major manifestations of deficiency (xerophthalmia in infants and night-blindness with keratosis in children) are now comparatively seldom seen in Britain, their occurrence during periods of economic depression (Spence, 1931) is a reminder that an adequate intake must be assured. In parts of Asia, vitamin A deficiency is still an important cause of blindness and death in infancy. The recommended allowance of vitamin A and carotenoids is based on a mixed diet and is expressed in terms of retinol equivalents (1 µg. retinol equivalent is equal to 1 µg. of retinol (3·33 i.u.) or 6 µg. of β-carotene).

Vitamins A and D are usually given to infants in a single preparation. Prolonged and extreme overdosage with vitamin A produces changes in bones and skin and other abnormalities, whilst excess of carotene produces yellow staining of the tissues (Moore, 1965). In normal circumstances, however, there is evidently a very wide range of vitamin A intake which will protect against deficiency symptoms and which will not produce signs of overdosage.

VITAMIN B COMPLEX. The human requirements of a number of the components of the vitamin B complex, *e.g.* folic acid, biotin, pyridoxine (vitamin B_6), cobalamin (vitamin B_{12}) and pantothenic acid, are not accurately known and even in the case of thiamine (aneurin, vitamin B_1), riboflavin and nicotinic acid (niacin) the recommendations are to some extent empirical. Thiamine and riboflavin are widely distributed in natural foods, occurring in milk, meat, eggs, fish, green vegetables and fruits. Niacin also occurs in meat and wholemeal bread but to a lesser extent in milk and vegetables. Niacin deficiency is most likely to occur in populations where the staple diet is maize, and is otherwise very restricted. It is usually unnecessary to supplement a mixed diet in childhood with vitamin B complex and thiamine deficiency in infants (infantile beri-beri) is only likely to occur in the breast-fed infants of mothers whose diet is almost entirely limited to milled rice. Where it is thought desirable to supplement the diet with vitamin B complex, this can be done by including marmite or a yeast preparation.

VITAMIN C (ASCORBIC ACID). Vitamin C is essential for the formation of intercellular substances and for various other metabolic processes. The human infant, unlike the calf, cannot synthesise vitamin C, which must be supplied in the diet. Since human milk contains 4 to 7 mg. per 100 ml., unless the mother's diet is grossly deficient, the requirements of the breast-fed baby are normally supplied from this source. Cow's milk contains 2 mg. per 100 ml. or less, and artificially fed infants require additional vitamin C in the form of fruit juice or ascorbic acid (see Chapter 14).

Since vitamin C is thermolabile and destroyed by alkalis, preparations should not be boiled or have alkali added. The recommended allowances are usually exceeded, average intakes being 25 mg. by infants and 50 mg. in older children: there is no risk of over-dosage.

VITAMIN D promotes the absorption of calcium from the intestinal tract and contributes to the maintenance of plasma calcium levels. Deficiency causes nutritional rickets, which was formerly common in Britain but to-day is mainly a disease of large tropical cities (Mitchell, 1967). Vitamin D_3 (cholecalciferol) can be synthesised in the skin by the action of ultra-violet light but this is an unreliable source, since it depends on the amount of exposure to sunshine. In temperate climates, especially in winter, this is often very small and it may also be inadequate in crowded tropical cities, where traditional practices deny sunlight to the children. The secretion of vitamin D in human milk is correspondingly variable and breast-fed babies are unlikely to receive much from this source. Cow's milk contains little of the vitamin and it is therefore necessary to add vitamin D_2 (calciferol) to the diet of all milk-fed infants. In artificially fed infants, this is best achieved by adding the vitamin to dried or evaporated milk during manufacture but when the infant is breast-fed or when fresh cow's milk is used, a daily intake of fish liver oil or some other supplement by mouth must be assured. When mixed feeding is started and foods of animal origin, such as dairy products and eggs, are given, sufficient vitamin D may be obtained from these sources to prevent rickets. Because of the wide individual variation in response to the vitamin, however, it is advisable to continue supplementing the diets of all children, at least until the age of 2 years.

The recommended daily intake of vitamin D from all sources is 400 international units (10 μg. of cholecalciferol): many children receive more than this but a modest surplus is unlikely to produce signs of overdosage, though gross excess may precipitate hypercalcaemia in susceptible infants. At one time it was considered that infants of low birth weight required more vitamin D because of their rapid rate of postnatal growth but rickets appearing in such infants is generally due to calcium deficiency and cannot be corrected even by considerably larger doses of vitamin D. Thus 400 i.u. daily is sufficient for infants and children of all ages, including infants born before term, and this intake should be assured until the age of 5 years, after which the intake may be less since the contribution of sunlight is greater.

Natural cod-liver contains from 8,000 to 30,000 i.u. vitamin D per 100 g. edible portion and halibut-liver oil 20,000 to 100,000 i.u. Care must be taken to avoid overdosage if the latter is used and the idea that vitamins have a general tonic effect must be dispelled. Cod-liver oil compound (British Welfare Foods 1958 Standard) issued through child health centres is a preparation containing 10,000 i.u. vitamin D and 60,000 i.u. vitamin A per 100 g., the daily requirements being contained in one teaspoonful (5 ml.). More palatable syrups containing standard doses of vitamins A and D are now available. In the United Kingdom, dried milk contains not more than 90 to 100 i.u. of vitamin D per oz. of dried powder and infant cereals not more than 300 i.u. per dry oz. (10·6 i.u. per g.). The use of vitamin-fortified foods and supplements must be guided by calculation of the vitamin intake from all sources: in 1960 the great majority of British children received from 250 to 1,200 i.u. of vitamin D daily (Bransby *et al.*, 1964), but there is some evidence that intakes may have fallen more recently (Arneil, 1967).

VITAMIN K is an essential factor in the formation of prothrombin and other coagulation factors in the liver. It is obtained from plant foods and can be synthesised by bacterial action in the intestine. In the newly born infant, prothrombin activity in the blood is usually low but excessive hypoprothrombinaemia may result in haemorrhagic disease of the newborn. When due to vitamin K deficiency, the bleeding tendency can be corrected by administration of synthetic vitamin K_1 (phytomenadione) in a dosage of 1 to 2 mg. intramuscularly. Larger doses of vitamin K analogues are liable to cause haemolysis and kernicterus. Haemorrhage due to vitamin K deficiency is only liable to occur in older children in the presence of biliary obstruction or malabsorption of fats (since vitamin K, like vitamins A and D, is fat-soluble).

Infant Feeding

For successful infant feeding, the diet should be adequate in total calories, fluid content and bulk. The intake of essential constituents should suffice to cover the infant's current needs and enable him both to meet the stresses of daily life and to fulfil his genetic potential. The baby should be encouraged to establish a feeding regimen which will satisfy his hunger and keep him contented, and this in turn should lead to a healthy appetite throughout childhood. Digestion should be allowed to take place with the minimum of disturbance. Regular bowel action should be established and maintained without the use of laxatives.

In many parts of the world, these objectives can only be attained by natural feeding at the mother's breast because there is no satisfactory alternative but in our society they can be achieved either by breast-feeding or by artificial feeding with cow's milk. Great improvements in artificial feeding have made possible the steady decline in breast-feeding which has taken place in Britain, the United States and some other countries during recent years. Some of the reasons for this change are the greater employment of women outside the home, the dictates of fashion and the example of others, the limitations on social activities by breast-feeding and subtle pressures from relatives and the advertisers of infant foods. Lactation represents a considerable physiological stress and when to this are added the psychological and social strains of modern urban civilisation, it is not surprising that some mothers experience tiredness and minor ill-health during breast-feeding (Hytten *et al.*, 1958). In addition, there is the undoubted fact that many infants are underfed on the breast: the mother who does not know how much the baby is getting may become anxious, whereas with a bottle she can see exactly how much he takes and derives pleasure from watching the milk go in (Gunther, 1963).

Notwithstanding the attractions of artificial feeding, however, breast-feeding has advantages which make it desirable to encourage its practice generally, although the individual woman should be allowed and helped to feed her baby in the way she prefers. Human milk contains adequate quantities of the food elements necessary for good nutrition in the early months of life. It contains the types of protein and fat best suited to the human infant and forms a soft, easily digestible curd in his stomach. Provided that the supply of milk is sufficient, breast-fed infants thrive and few are overweight, in contrast to the artificially fed infant, who is often obese. Cow's milk provides the human infant with more protein and salts: while there is no proof that this is harmful, neither is there any good evidence that rapid gain in weight, high nitrogen retention and early maturation of tissues are beneficial, and many believe that they are not (Mac Keith, 1963). Even in good social circumstances, bottle-fed infants tend to have a greater incidence of minor ill-health than those on the breast (Mellander *et al.*, 1959: Hooper, 1965) and in poor socio-economic conditions, these differences may have serious implications. There are other possible advantages of breast feeding, such as the comfort of the infant in contact with the soft breast, the sense of achievement experienced by the mother who has breast-fed her infant successfully, and psychological benefits whose importance is difficult to estimate. The fact that sudden death in infancy occurs almost exclusively in artificially fed babies may also have relevance to infant feeding but its significance can not yet be assessed.

In conclusion, there is much to be said in favour of breast-feeding and many women derive pleasure and gain confidence from feeding their infants themselves, but artificial feeding can be just as satisfactory and the decision should be made by the mother herself without any coercion. This, of course, applies only to countries where standards of hygiene are good and there are adequate supplies of cow's milk. In many developing countries, the arguments for breast-feeding are much more cogent, since the mortality from infection and gastro-intestinal disturbances is so high among artificially fed infants.

Breast-feeding

LACTATION is usually established in from 3 days to a week after parturition. Before this time the breasts contain colostrum, a yellow secretion having considerable nutritive value and possibly some anti-infective properties also (Macy and Kelly, 1961). It has a relatively high protein content, containing less fat and carbohydrate than the later milk. The change from colostrum to milk secretion is not a sudden process taking place on a particular day, but gradual over several days or even weeks. Nevertheless, women whose lactation is adequate by the tenth day are more likely to breast-feed successfully than those whose lactation is inadequate at this time (Miller, 1952).

The supply of breast milk is partly dependent on demand and the most important stimulus to secretion is a vigorously hungry infant who empties the breast at each feed. When the infant is sucking feebly, emptying the breast manually or by pump at the end of the feeds will often increase the supply. The size of the breast is deceptive, a small firm breast often giving a greater milk yield than a large pendulous one. Elderly women are generally less successful in breast-feeding than younger women of similar parity and, in first lactations, capacity declines progressively as maternal age increases (Baird et al., 1958). Maternal physique, health and nutritional status exert a relatively small effect on lactation in comparison with age, parity and the functional capacity of the breast (Hytten and Thomson, 1961). Nevertheless, if lactation is not to be a drain upon the nutritional economy of the mother, energy and nutrients lost in the milk must be replaced. The mother's diet influences the composition of her milk (Gunther, 1968) and it should therefore be well-balanced, containing fresh vegetables, eggs and the equivalent of one and a half pints of milk per day in fresh milk or dairy produce. A liberal caloric intake should be assured, and the mother should drink water freely, but excessive fluid intake is to be avoided as it tends to impair lactation (Illingworth and Kilpatrick, 1953). Fresh air, adequate rest and a reasonable amount of exercise are most desirable: worry and fatigue are likely to affect the milk supply adversely.

PREPARATION FOR BREAST-FEEDING. During pregnancy, the mother should be told about the ways of feeding her baby and if she shows any desire to breast-feed, she should be given advice and encouraged to do so. This is particularly important during a first pregnancy, as successful breast-feeding of a first infant usually means that subsequent infants will also be breast-fed. Any psychological, physical or economic difficulties which can be overcome at this stage should be recognised early and not left until too late. If the mother does not wish to breast-feed, however, there must be no manifestation of disapproval which may make her feel guilty.

When a mother has decided to breast-feed, she will need advice concerning the preparation of her breasts. However, confidence in her ability to breast-feed must not be undermined by too much emphasis on detail, which may give her the impression that serious difficulties are anticipated. During the latter months of pregnancy, the breasts should be bathed at least once a day and carefully dried. This will tend to improve the circulation and render the nipples less tender and

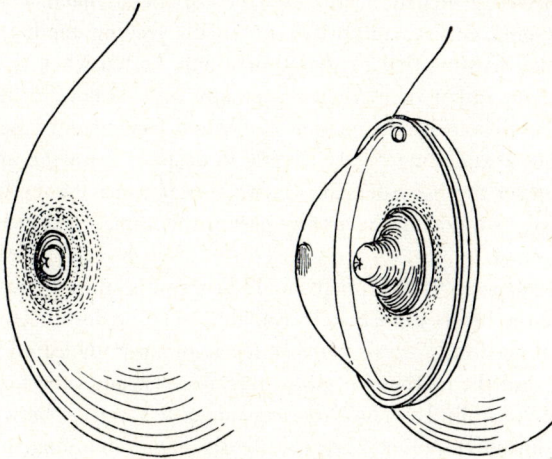

FIG. 14. Plastic shell applied over a
retracted nipple.

less liable to crack. The mother should be warned against clothing pressing tightly on the nipples and breasts. A properly fitting support should be worn, particularly by women with heavy breasts. If the nipples are found to be retracted, plastic shells (Fig. 14) should be worn under a firm support during the later months of pregnancy. The nipple protrudes through the opening in the shell and its attachments to deeper structures are gradually stretched. It is important that the breasts should be examined well before the end of pregnancy, as it is usually impossible to correct retraction after delivery. Scrubbing the nipples or attempts to harden them with alcohol are wholly undesirable, predisposing to cracks and infection. Some clinics use the methods of Waller (1946), who obtained excellent results by instructing pregnant women in massage of the breasts and expression of secretion during the later months of pregnancy: it was found that the subsequent free flow of milk was thus more readily established, with a significant diminution of breast engorgement, and that 83 per cent of the instructed mothers successfully breast-fed their infants as compared with 42 per cent of a control group.

TECHNIQUE OF FEEDING. Depending on the condition of the mother, the baby should be put to the breast two or three times during the 24 hours after delivery. He will only obtain small amounts of colostrum during a few minutes' sucking but lactation will be stimulated and the sucking reflex reinforced. Mother and baby will have the opportunity of adapting to one another before suckling begins in earnest.

In establishing the subsequent regimen, it is essential to bear in mind that it is intended primarily for the benefit of the baby, secondarily for the benefit of the mother, and only thirdly and lastly for the convenience of the nurse. Among primitive peoples, the baby is usually put to the breast when he cries and, since hunger is the strongest emotion in the young infant, an irregular feeding regimen is established, based primarily on the demands of the stomach. During the first half of the present century, authorities on infant feeding tended to go to the opposite extreme, insisting that the baby must only be fed when they thought he ought to be hungry rather than when he actually was. This rigid 'feeding by the clock' did nothing to increase the incidence of breast feeding and indeed frequently led to the mother abandoning breast-feeding in despair. With the present fashion of feeding whenever the baby demands it, we appear to have gone full-circle, but at least this has the support of the greater part of the human race, who breast-feed as a matter of course.

For practical purposes, the regimen should be a compromise between the baby's demand to have the breast immediately available when he desires food or comfort, his physiological need of intervals between feeds for sleep, digestion and emptying of the stomach, and the mother's need for rest, exercise and time for the secretion of a fresh supply of milk. In view of the considerable variation between infants in the speed of stomach emptying, the need for sleep and emotional and personality characteristics, it is only reasonable that the regimen should be flexible, especially in early infancy.

In the newborn period, it is most desirable that the baby should be with the mother as much of the time as practicable. In the case of babies born in hospital, 'rooming-in' with the mother should be the normal procedure. If the baby is deposited in a nursery and only brought to the mother at certain arbitrary 'feeding times', the mother is likely to return home without having had a real opportunity of getting to know her baby, or recognising whether he is crying because he is hungry, or wet, or cold, or troubled with wind, or requires to have his position changed. This is a common cause of anxiety in the mother and may result in breast-feeding being abandoned immediately on return home from hospital. Where an early discharge scheme is operated, a very short period in hospital (48 hours) is preferable to several days from the point of view of establishing breast-feeding, since there can then be continuity of advice from the time lactation starts. This depends, of course, on close liaison between hospital and domiciliary services but experience shows that a well-organised scheme has no adverse effect on breast-feeding (Arthurton and Bamford, 1967).

For the first 10 days, the baby should be put to the breast when he is hungry, which is likely to be about 8 times in the 24 hours. Except at night (when it is found that some newborn babies can sleep for 6 hours without distress), the infant should not go more than 4 hours without being fed. It is exceptional for infants born at term to require feeding more than 8 times in the 24 hours after the first 10 days. When the mother resumes household work, her time and other commitments will have to be considered as well as the baby, and the feeding schedule gradually regularised. This does not mean, however, that if the infant wakes ravenously hungry at 5·15 a.m. he must be left screaming until his feed is due at 6 a.m. This certainly does no good to the baby and is extremely distressing to the mother, whose milk supply may be affected in consequence.

In the course of the first few weeks it will usually be found that the number of times the baby sleeps for 4 hours between feeds gradually increases and that he can thus slide into a 4-hourly feeding programme rather than be forced into it. The times usually adopted are 6 a.m., 10 a.m., 2 p.m., 6 p.m., 10 p.m., and 2 a.m. if necessary. Some infants require feeding more frequently and others establish an irregular pattern, so that the ultimate result must often be a compromise between infant's demands and mother's convenience. No hard-and-fast rule can be given as to when the night feed can be omitted, though it is obviously a great advantage to the mother (not to mention the father) when she can get 6 or more hours undisturbed sleep. If the infant does not require a 2 a.m. feed, the 10 p.m. feed can often be given between 11 p.m. and midnight, thus allowing the mother to go out for an evening without having to rush home early to feed the baby. Later, this late feed can often be omitted if the baby is thriving, but it should be continued when weight gain is not satisfactory.

The right breast should be given first at one feed and the left breast at the next, in order to ensure that both are equally stimulated. It is usually best for the baby to suck at both breasts at each feed even when feeding 7 or 8 times in the day. The total time of nursing at each feed should not exceed 20 minutes, as a normally sucking infant will have obtained the greater part of his feed in less than half this time. Often when the infant is put to one breast the 'draught' or 'let-down' reflex causes milk to spurt from both breasts: if the draught is exceptionally strong, quantities of milk may be ejected at high pressure resulting in choking and refusal to feed by the infant. When an abundant milk supply flows copiously in this way, the use of only one breast at each feed or shortening the time on each breast may help to reduce the supply to manageable proportions.

While feeding, the mother should be comfortably seated and she will usually prefer a low chair with her feet so placed that the arm holding the baby can be rested on her thigh. If possible, the mother should rest for a short while before each feed, since an atmosphere of anxiety or hurry will inevitably react on both the infant and the supply of milk. The infant should be held in the crook of the mother's elbow, with the head slightly raised (Fig. 15). It is not uncommon to see infants fed in a horizontal position, which makes it difficult for the infant to swallow and is liable to result in regurgitation into the nasopharynx. There must be a clear airway to allow the infant to breathe comfortably while sucking. If there is any nasal obstruction, the nose should be gently cleaned with cotton wool and care should be taken that a pendulous breast is supported off the baby's face with the mother's free hand. During and at the end of feeding, the infant should be held erect until he brings up his 'wind' (see p. 106).

COMPOSITION OF BREAST MILK. Milk secreted by different women varies in composition depending on inherent differences, environmental factors such as

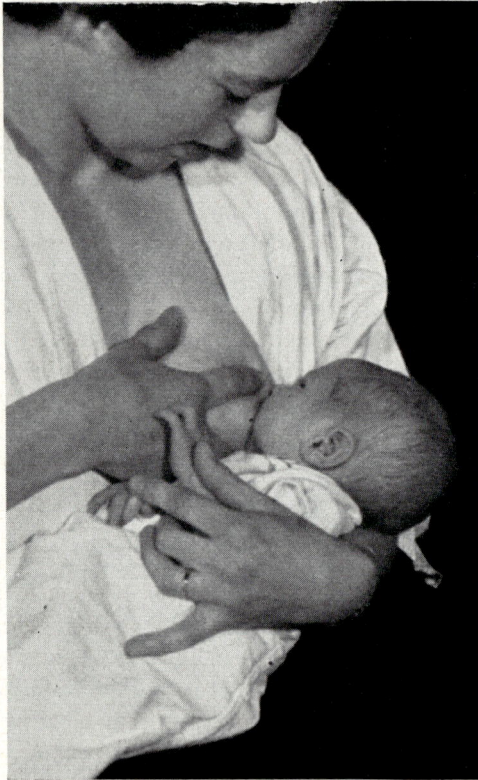

FIG. 15. Breast-feeding. The infant is held with
the head slightly raised and the breast is
supported by the mother's hand to allow
the infant a clear airway.

exposure to sunshine, and the diet consumed. Samples of human milk from the same woman also vary considerably, depending on which breast they are taken from, the time of day and whether they represent the first or the last part of the feed, the milk at the end of a feed having a higher content of fat than the 'fore-milk'. The composition of individual samples will therefore not be representative and a full 24 hours' collection must be pooled for analysis. Average values for the percentage composition of human milk are shown in Table 4.

The protein consists of lactalbumin and caseinogen, which are present in the proportions of 0·75 and 0·50 per cent respectively. The fat content is the most variable factor (other than total volume) and the carbohydrate content the least. Human milk has a caloric value of approximately 70 calories per 100 ml. (20 cal./fl. oz.) and the average infant's caloric requirements will therefore be supplied by 150 ml. per kg. body weight per day (2½ fl. oz./lb.), which will also satisfy his needs for fluid. In practice, it is found that many large active babies take considerably more than this amount.

Except in rare cases of intolerance to milk, it is seldom that the quality of the mother's milk is unsuitable for her infant, though babies are frequently weaned on this supposition, especially as breast milk has a thin watery appearance when compared with cow's milk. In cases of feeding difficulty, the fault is much more likely to lie in the quantity of milk or the technique of feeding. Occasionally it is found that a woman who is on a grossly deficient diet is secreting milk which has a deficient vitamin content: here the remedy lies in correction of the maternal diet. Iron-deficiency anaemia in the mother should also be treated, though normally the iron content of the milk is not increased by increased maternal intake.

Most substances ingested during lactation will appear in the milk, often only as minute traces but sometimes in larger quantities, the concentration depending on the dose taken by the mother. A few drugs, such as thiouracil, are concentrated by the mammary gland and appear in greater amounts in the milk than in the maternal blood. In many cases, the presence of drugs in breast milk will be quite harmless to the infant but some may affect him, when either the drug must be withdrawn or breast-feeding stopped.

Some laxatives may be secreted in the milk and affect the infant's bowels: senna in ordinary dosage can safely be given to the nursing mother, however. Heavy smoking may result in the appearance of appreciable quantities of nicotine and excessive consumption of alchohol in the appearance of alcohol in the milk. Moderate consumption of alcohol will not affect the infant. Penicillin, streptomycin, tetracycline and other antibiotics, chemotherapeutic agents such as sulphonamides and isoniazid, and some sedative drugs are secreted, but usually not in amounts that will affect the baby. However, adverse effects from some anticonvulsant drugs such as bromides and phenytoin have been reported. A full list of drugs secreted in human milk has been published by Knowles (1965). It should be noted that the greater use of antibiotics and other drugs for dairy cattle has increased the risk of such substances being found in cow's milk as well.

COMPLEMENTARY AND SUPPLEMENTARY FEEDS. A complementary feed is an artificial feed given immediately after a breast-feed when the breast milk supply is inadequate for the infant's requirement. A supplementary feed is an artificial feed completely replacing one of the breast feeds. Complementary feeding should be looked on as a temporary measure designed to tide over a period of deficient lactation: by complementing the feeds, it is possible to maintain the milk supply by regular stimulation of the breasts and at the same time to satisfy the infant: the complement is reduced as the breast milk increases in amount. It is essential to give the complement after the infant has been put to the breast, not before, otherwise he will not suck vigorously on the breast.

Supplementary feeds are given when the mother's health or occupation necessitates the omission of one or more breast-feeds. Thus a working mother may be able to breast-feed at night and in the morning but not at mid-day, while one who has to be free in the evening may wish to breast-feed during the rest of the day.

Difficulties in Breast-feeding

Most of the difficulties are encountered during the first 2 or 3 weeks and early weaning is unlikely to become necessary if breast-feeding has been satisfactorily established in that time. Careful antenatal preparation and close supervision by experienced staff during the puerperium are the principal determinants of success, since many of the problems can be solved by relatively simple measures. Apart from the recognisable difficulties, lactation may sometimes fail for no apparent reason. Possibly there are genetic factors which make breast-feeding less universally practicable amongst civilised and urban peoples than in primitive communities, where successful breast-feeding is essential for the survival of the infant. In these circumstances, it is understandable that, by natural selection, profuse lactation becomes virtually a racial characteristic, whereas in societies in which the majority of artificially fed infants will survive, there is not nearly the same likelihood of poor-lactating strains dying out. In Britain and North America, these may now form a substantial proportion of the population, so that some women have a greater potential for lactation than others.

The commonest difficulty encountered during the puerperium is *breast engorgement*. In minor degrees, the breast feels heavy and uncomfortable and may be appreciably harder than normal on palpation. Manual expression of milk and support of the breast will usually relieve the engorgement until the infant is able to empty the breast effectively. In more severe degrees, the breast becomes oedematous and the flow of milk obstructed. Here the breast must be rested and the engorgement relieved by the administration of stilboestrol (1 to 5 mg.). The infant should only be returned to the breast when oedema has subsided and there is a free flow of milk again. If there is any evidence of *mastitis*, with flushing of the breast, pain and fever, an antibiotic should be given promptly.

Sore or cracked nipples cause great discomfort and may be due to the infant's continued sucking on an engorged breast. In some women, however, the skin appears to be exceptionally fragile. From the start of feeding, the nipples should be kept scrupulously clean, being carefully dried and covered with gauze after each feed. The infant should not be allowed to suck on a sore nipple but should be taken off the affected breast until the lesion has healed. Sore nipples should be treated with cetrimide cream for a few days. *Breast abscess* is liable to arise from a cracked nipple or from neglected mastitis. The infant must be taken off the affected breast until the abscess has been treated and healed: it may be possible to continue breast-feeding subsequently but often the mother prefers not to do so. Nipples that are too large or too small for the infant to suck comfortably, or that are severely retracted or inverted, will in some cases make breast-feeding impossible, though with perseverance and temporary manual expression of milk the infant may some-times learn to feed satisfactorily.

Apart from disorders of the breast or nipple, the principal difficulties that arise in breast-feeding are (1) underfeeding, (2) inability of the infant to suck, (3) unwillingness of the infant to suck ('breast shyness'), (4) over-anxiety or fear on the part of the mother, and (5) interference on the part of relatives.

Under-feeding is usually due to an inadequate supply of breast milk. Commonly the reduction in milk supply is only transient due to resumption of household duties and anxiety, increased by the unhappy crying of the infant. Unfortunately, breast-feeding is all too often abandoned completely owing to such temporary decrease in the quantity of milk. The underfed infant fails to gain weight, goes ravenously to the breast and still appears hungry and restless at the end of the feed. In prolonged under-feeding, the infant becomes apathetic and appetite is diminished rather than increased. When under-feeding is suspected and examination of the infant reveals no other abnormality, a small complementary feed of unsweetened milk may be offered after each feed. The infant will then be satisfied, gain weight and cease his restless crying. As the mother's confidence is restored, her milk supply increases again and, in favourable cases, the complementary feeds are refused after 2 or 3 weeks and full breast-feeding can continue. Occasionally it may be necessary to demonstrate the inadequacy of the breast-feeds, either to convince the mother or to settle any diagnostic doubt. This is accomplished by test-weighing, in which the infant is weighed before and after feeding, the difference in weight representing the weight of the milk consumed. It is not necessary to undress the baby, as it is only the difference in weights that is significant: a napkin wetted during the feed should not be changed until the baby has been re-weighed. Since the amount of milk varies considerably at different feeds, usually being greatest in the early morning and least in the afternoon, the amount taken during at least three feeds should be averaged in order to obtain an estimate of the daily intake. Test-weighing should seldom be resorted to, since it is generally unnecessary and may engender an undesirably obsessive approach to breast-feeding.

When the milk supply remains inadequate despite careful supervision and the infant is failing to thrive on complementary feeding, breast-feeding should be abandoned. No hard and fast rule can be laid down as to how long to persist in attempts to establish satisfactory lactation but even when the mother is eager to go on, there is little point in continuing if she is supplying less than half of the infant's requirements.

Inability of the infant to suck may be due to low birth weight, cerebral damage or maldevelopment, feebleness due to disease, or abnormality of the lips and mouth. In the case of an infant who has previously sucked well, the mouth should be carefully examined for local lesions, of which thrush is the most common. The 'sucking blisters' often seen on the lips of young infants do not cause any disability. It is extremely rare for shortness of the fraenum ('tongue-tie') to cause difficulty in sucking, and the practice of cutting the fraenum in young infants is wholly unnecessary. It should be remembered that the tip of the tongue grows forward as the infant develops and what may appear to be 'tongue-tie' is usually a perfectly normal state in early infancy.

Breast-shyness. The infant who is both hungry and able to suck but refuses the breast presents a problem requiring patience and ingenuity for its solution. Painful local lesions of the mouth must of course be excluded. It will sometimes be found that the infant has a blocked airway or that the nipple is too large or too small for his mouth. In other cases the trouble is due to difficulty in initiating the flow of milk, and here moistening of the nipple with milk may encourage vigorous sucking. The possibility of the draught being too forceful and copious is referred to above. Temporary sedation with chloral hydrate will sometimes prove effective in overcoming breast-shyness for which no cause can be found.

Over-anxiety or fear can usually be relieved by sympathetic supervision and it is most important that the mother should gain confidence in handling and feeding her baby during the lying-in period. Sometimes difficulty may arise from unexpressed repugnance to the idea of breast-feeding, to dislike of an unwanted baby or to the realisation that breast-feeding will interfere with other activities. Such causes of reluctance to feed should have been fully discussed before the baby was born but occasionally a mother who wanted, and fully intended, to feed her infant herself changes her mind when it comes to the reality of breast-feeding. Tactful advice may help her to overcome her reluctance but she should not be persuaded to breast-feed against her will. In these cases, and when the mother has decided not to breast-feed from the beginning, lactation may be suppressed by the administration of oestrogens. This must be done very carefully when the mother is over 35 or predisposed to thromboembolism, because the hormonal suppression of lactation may increase the risk of deep venous thrombosis (B.M.J. 1968).

Interference by relatives, who are often well-meaning but misguided, is a frequent cause of failure of breast-feeding. Some grandmothers are actively jealous of their daughter's breast-feeding and possessing the baby and, though the motivation may not come into consciousness, they are only too eager to get the baby off the breast and take over the management of the bottle feeding. It is also sometimes found that the father dislikes the intimacy of the mother-child breast-feeding relationship and is glad to see it broken.

CONSTIPATION AND DIARRHOEA. There is considerable variation in the frequency with which healthy infants pass stools. In the breast-fed infant, 2 or even 3 days may elapse between each bowel movement, although on artificial feeding at least one stool is usually passed daily. If the stools are of normal consistency for age and are passed without difficulty, the fact that they are infrequent does not justify the diagnosis of constipation nor is it an indication for medication. When the stool is harder than normal and causes discomfort on defaecation or shows streaks of blood on the outside, the anus should be carefully examined for the presence of a local lesion and if necessary a rectal examination performed. Simple constipation can usually be overcome by increasing the fluid intake or giving a simple natural laxative such as one or two teaspoonfuls of stewed prune juice. In more obstinate cases, milk of magnesia or senna is generally effective: stronger laxatives are inadvisable if they can be avoided. The aim in both infants and older children is to establish a natural and regular bowel action and not to rely on purgatives.

The diagnosis of diarrhoea should only be made when stools are abnormally fluid and not if they are merely small and frequent. The passage of small dark 'hunger stools' is an indication of underfeeding. Diarrhoea is usually due to infection though it may be a manifestation of intolerance of a constituent of the diet. Rarely in very hot weather it may be due to over-feeding, which may occur if no fluid other than milk is offered to relieve thirst.

CONTRA-INDICATIONS TO BREAST-FEEDING are very few. Maternal diseases such as advanced cardiac or renal disease, malignant disease, psychiatric disorders or pulmonary tuberculosis will usually constitute contra-indications, though each case must be judged on its merits. Breast-feeding should always cease if the mother becomes pregnant again during lactation. In the case of active tuberculosis, segregation of the infant from birth until the mother's condition is inactive, coupled with B.C.G. vaccination, is the logical procedure. Maternal diabetes is not necessarily a contra-indication, since the diabetic mother whose condition is controlled with insulin can successfully breast-feed without ill effect. The secretion of drugs in the milk, *e.g.* when the mother is epileptic or is on anti-thyroid treatment, is considered above. In a few predisposed women, breast-feeding may cause or increase jaundice in the infant, since the milk contains a steroid (pregnane-3 (α), 20(β)-diol) which inhibits the activity of glucuronyl transferase in the infant's liver (Gartner and Arias, 1966). This should not be considered a contra-indication to breast-feeding, but, if the serum bilirubin approaches dangerous levels (20 mg. per 100 ml.), breast-feeding should be stopped for a few days and can then be safely resumed.

Artificial Feeding

Choice of Milk

If a mother does not wish to feed her infant on the breast or is unable to do so, the alternative is artificial feeding, which in Britain is nearly always based on the use of cow's milk. The digestive system of the human infant is better adapted to human milk than to cow's milk and so some modification of the latter is advisable. If the average composition of human and cow's milk is compared, it is seen that human milk has a higher carbohydrate and a lower mineral content and that the total and relative proportions of the milk-proteins are different (see Table 4). It must be remembered, however, that there is wide variation in the composition of different samples of both human and cow's milk.

Unmodified cow's milk forms a larger and tougher curd than human milk and the buffering action is three times as great. In fact, the percentage of fat and the caloric value are the only two factors which correspond closely on average analysis and both of these are variable in individual samples. Although the total amount of fat is approximately the same, the fat of cow's milk differs from that of human milk and is not so well absorbed by the young infant, having a lower content of un-saturated fatty acids. It has been suggested that the best ratio of unsaturated to saturated fatty acids and the best distribution of chain lengths of saturated fatty acids for each species is provided by its own particular milk (Widdowson, 1965).

Cow's milk can be modified to make it more suitable for infant feeding in a variety of ways, *e.g.* dilution, boiling, evaporation, drying, or the addition of

TABLE 4

	Human milk	Cow's milk
Caloric value (per fl. oz.)	20	18–20
(per 100 ml.)	70	70
Carbohydrate (lactose) per cent	7	4·75
Fat	3·5–4	3·5–4
Total protein	1·25	3·4
Lactalbumin	0·75	0·4
Caseinogen	0·5	3·0
Total minerals	0·2	0·73

sodium citrate or lactic acid, and all these methods have been employed. Fresh cow's milk, boiled and diluted with water, is still used in this country but it has important disadvantages. It has a low content of vitamins and iron. It is bulky to store, requires refrigeration if kept for more than a short time and constitutes a good culture medium for bacteria. Sugar must be added, since dilution reduces the lactose content too low. Digestive disturbances are more common in infants fed on fresh cow's milk. This is therefore not a good method of feeding infants, except possibly when domestic standards are very high and the mother is fully alive to the need for additions of vitamins and iron to the diet.

Dried and Evaporated (Condensed) Milks

The use of either dried or evaporated (condensed) milk has to a large extent replaced the use of fresh milk in infant feeding in Britain, since 'processed' milk from which a proportion of the water has been removed by heat has certain practical advantages as regards sterility, storage and preparation. The cow's milk curd is rendered less tough and more readily digestible by the processing and in practice this has lessened the need to give dilute feeds, so reducing the incidence of underfeeding. Additions of vitamins and iron can be made during the process of manufacture, thus ensuring that all infants receive these essential nutrients, regardless of the quality of maternal care. One possible disadvantage of these milks is that the mineral content of the reconstituted milk is unaltered by the process of drying or evaporating. When given at full strength to infants in the first week or two of life, there is a risk that the high phosphate content will cause elevated levels of blood phosphorus and low levels of calcium which may precipitate tetany (Oppé and Redstone, 1968). This is only likely to occur in a minority of infants but the risk must be borne in mind, especially in feeding infants born before term. There may be a case for reducing the mineral contents of these milks but this is unlikely to be done on a large scale without more accurate assessment of the practical importance of these effects.

Dried milk powder is prepared commercially either by roller-drying or by spray-drying. In the former process, liquid milk (either whole, skimmed or partially skimmed) is run over heated rollers, and the powder formed is scraped off. In spray drying, a fine jet of liquid milk is forced under high pressure into an enclosed tower where the droplets of milk meet a moving current of hot air, the dried particles falling to the bottom. In both processes, burnt particles are removed before packing. Dried and evaporated milks used for infant feeding are fortified with vitamin D before heating, and many proprietary brands contain additional iron, vitamin A and vitamin C

Evaporated milk is prepared by reducing the water-content of liquid milk by boiling in a vacuum of 28 to 29 in. mercury, the milk at this pressure boiling at a temperature of between 102° and 130°F. Unsweetened evaporated milk is run out when sufficiently concentrated, cooled, homogenised and subsequently sealed in tins and sterilised (the Food and Drugs Act, 1959, requires minimum standards of 31 per cent total solids, inclusive of 9 per cent butterfat). The average percentage composition of some dried and evaporated milks is shown in Table 5.

TABLE 5

Percentage Composition of Types of Dried and Evaporated Milks
(These are examples, and there are small variations between different
proprietary brands)

	Dried milk		Evaporated milk
	Full cream	Half cream	
Fat	27·5	16·5	9·1
Protein	24·5	30·3	8·6
Lactose	38·0	43·8	12·5
Ash or mineral matter	6·0	6·9	1·8
Water	4·0	2·5	68·0

Types of Dried Milk

A great many proprietary brands are on the market, and the manufacturer's literature must be consulted for the exact individual compositions, which are controlled under the Food and Drugs Act, 1959. The majority to these dried milks are manufactured so that 1 drachm by weight of powder made up to 1 fl. oz. with water will form 1 fl. oz. of reconstituted milk or 'modified milk mixture' having the caloric value of whole milk. Since the specific gravity of the various brands varies, a measure which contains 1 drachm by weight is usually provided by the manufacturers.

The popularity of proprietary dried milks is due to their being designed so that, when reconstituted as directed, they provide a feed for infants of different ages, with little or no further modification. They mix easily with water and most have vitamins and iron added. National Dried Milk is satisfactory for infant feeding if properly used, though it is not quite so easy to mix with water and the fat tends to separate after mixing. Some paediatricians believe that it produces more irritating stools than the commonly used proprietary brands. The following are the more important types of dried milk available:

Full Cream dried milk. When reconstituted, this represents whole cow's milk and, since the toughness of the curd is modified by the drying process, is suitable without further modification for feeding normal infants. It can be used suitably diluted from birth, though some prefer to use a half cream milk in the first few weeks (see below).

Partly skimmed dried milk ($\frac{3}{4}$, $\frac{1}{2}$ or $\frac{1}{4}$ cream) is modified by the drying and removal of a proportion of the cream, with consequent increase in the proportions of protein and carbohydrate. The tin must be labelled 'should not be used for babies except under medical advice'. These modified dried milks are useful when it is desired to give an infant milk of low fat content, *e.g.* following diarrhoea.

Skimmed dried milk has too low a caloric value for routine use in infant feeding and the tin must be labelled 'unfit for babies'. It may be valuable for short periods during recovery from a digestive upset or when there is failure of fat absorption.

'Humanised' dried milks. In these, the percentage composition of the dried milk is so modified that when the milk is reconstituted by addition of the appropriate amount of water, it has the approximate composition of breast-milk. Thus the percentage of carbohydrate is raised and an adjustment effected in the relative proportions of caseinogen and lactalbumin. These milks are suitable for infants without further modification but are unnecessarily expensive for routine use.

In addition to the above types, a large number of modified and synthetic milks are available for feeding infants in special circumstances, *e.g.* intolerance or allergy to certain constituents of milk.

Types of Evaporated Milk

As in the case of dried milk, there are a number of proprietary brands of evaporated milk available for infant feeding which only require the addition of the appropriate amount of water, and sugar as required.

Full cream unsweetened evaporated milk is cow's milk which has been heated to reduce the volume to between one-half and one-third of that of the original milk. When reconstituted by adding the appropriate amount of water, it can be used in the same way as whole cow's milk, the toughness of the curd being modified as in dried milk. The concentrated evaporated milk has 50 calories per fl. oz. and 1 part to 3 parts of water thus has 12·5 calories per fl. oz. (raised to 17·5 cals./fl. oz. by the addition of 1 drachm of sugar to 3 fl. oz.). This mixture with its low fat-content (2·3 per cent) is suitable for very young infants but after the first few weeks a stronger mixture is necessary, *e.g.* 1 part of concentrate to 2 parts of water; this has 17 cals./fl. oz., which is raised to 20 by adding 1 drachm of sugar to 4 fl. oz. of mixture.

Skimmed unsweetened evaporated milk is similarly processed after the removal of fat and must be sold as 'unfit for babies'. The same observations apply to its use as to skimmed dried milk.

Sweetened condensed milk is unsuitable for the routine feeding of healthy infants owing to its high carbohydrate and low protein content. It may be useful in the feeding of feeble immature infants, when it is desired to give a high calorie, easily assimilated feed over a short period. If used over a long period it is likely to result in a fat, flabby infant with low resistance to infection.

Feeding with dried milk. This is now the most popular form of artificial feeding in this country. In recent years, the practice has increased of feeding all healthy infants born at term with full cream dried milk from the start of milk feeding, diluting it suitably during the first week or two, but thereafter giving it at fully reconstituted strength ('full-strength'). While many babies thrive on this regimen, a small proportion develop abdominal discomfort, excessive wind and slow weight gain, which are attributed to fat intolerance because a change to half cream milk usually results in prompt improvement. Depending on their views of the frequency and seriousness of these disturbances, paediatricians may recommend that half cream milk be given to all infants for the first few weeks, thereafter changing to full cream milk, or that all infants be given full cream milk from the start and that only infants who exhibit signs of intolerance be changed to half cream milk. The protagonists of the latter view maintain that early feeding with half cream milk complicates infant feeding unnecessarily and may lead to many infants being unsatisfied. On the other hand, there is evidence that cow's milk fat may interfere with calcium absorption in early infancy (Southgate *et al.*, 1969) and the incidence of fat intolerance is considered by some to be high. More information is needed before a firm recommendation can be made: it is the author's preference to use half cream milk routinely for the first few weeks, changing to full cream milk if the infant is thriving and appears hungry and nearly always by the end of 4 weeks.

The healthy newborn infant should be offered boiled water, which may be sweetened with glucose, for the first feed and if this is taken well he may then be given half-strength dried milk, gradually strengthening the feed over the next few days. After the first week the infant should be offered as much full-strength feed as required to satisfy him. Many proprietary dried milks have sugar already added but when this has not been done, one to two teaspoonfuls of cane sugar should be added to each feed, the amount depending on the volume of the feed. The complex calculations formerly undertaken to determine the precise feed to be given are no longer considered necessary, since the infant's appetite, weight gain and general well-being are the best guides. It may occasionally be useful, however, to determine whether a particular baby is receiving at least the theoretical requirement of an average infant of his age and birth weight. This is done by calculating the expected body weight on the basis of birth weight plus 30 g. (one ounce) per day of postnatal life, omitting the first 10 days. This formula is valid until 3 months of age and thereafter 500 g. (approx. one lb.) are added for each additional month of age. Once the expected weight has been worked out, the total fluid needs are based on the average daily requirement of 150 ml. per kg. (2½ fl. oz./lb.). Thus, an infant weighing 3,000 g. at birth and aged 50 days has an expected weight of 4,200 g. and a daily fluid requirement of approximately 630 ml.: a five-months-old infant of birth weight 4,000 g. has an expected weight of 7,400 g. and a daily fluid requirement of 1,110 ml. When the daily fluid requirement has been estimated in this way, it can be divided by the number of feeds to establish the amount of each feed.

It must be emphasised that the value of this simple rule-of-thumb method is solely to calculate the theoretical average requirement to serve as a yardstick to the infant's actual intake and not to dictate what he 'should' have. In hot weather it is advisable to offer additional water to drink between feeds since thirst may tempt the baby to take more milk than he needs. If there is a tendency to loose stools, the added sugar should be reduced in quantity.

Technique of Artificial Feeding

Many of the principles applicable to breast-feeding are equally important in artificial feeding, the differences relating mainly to the use of the feeding bottle and teat. It must be remembered that the risk of infection is greater in artificially fed infants than in those who are breast-fed and scrupulous care of equipment and attention to detail are essential.

Bottles and teats may be sterilised by heat or by antiseptics, the latter method being preferable in the home because of its ease, reliability and low cost. In the sodium hypochlorite (Milton) method, the bottle and teat are thoroughly cleansed after use and then immersed in hypochlorite solution, which must be made up freshly every day. When the next feed is due, the bottle is removed from the solution, drained and filled with the milk mixture without further rinsing. In the boiling method, the cleansed bottle and teat are placed in a pan a quarter full of water, the lid is put on and the water boiled vigorously for at least 5 minutes, thereafter being allowed to cool until the equipment can be remo ed by hand. In large hospitals, the technique of terminal sterilisation is often used, the bottle being filled with mixture, the teat and a cover applied, and the whole heated to 100°C. for 25 minutes at normal pressure, cooled rapidly and transferred to a refrigerator until required. Other hospitals use the hypochlorite method: some manufacturers are now producing sterilised feeds in disposable bottles, the use of which avoids the need for milk preparation rooms and staff but creates its own problems of storage and disposal.

The upright glass feeding bottle is commonly used in this country, although plastic bottles are becoming more popular. The narrow-necked bottle is gradually giving way to the wide-necked bottle, which is easier to clean and fill (Fig. 16). The teat should be of a size and consistency such that the baby can take it well back into the mouth and suck vigorously on it. The hole should be just large enough for him to obtain the feed quickly and easily but not so large that it pours out and chokes him. Teats with different sizes of hole can be bought: a small hole can be enlarged by inserting a hot needle. As air has to pass into the bottle through the teat to prevent the formation of a vacuum, the teat should be removed from time to time from the baby's mouth during the feed.

The feed is generally warmed to approximately body temperature before it is given to the infant, though experience in some hospitals suggests that a cold feed

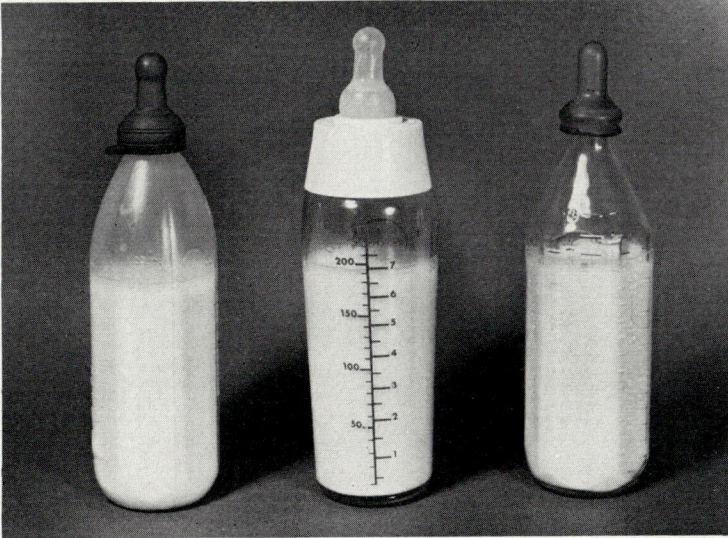

FIG. 16. Different types of feeding bottle. Narrow-necked plastic, wide-necked glass and narrow-necked glass (left to right).

is just as acceptable. The infant should be held in a comfortable position as for breast-feeding and should never be fed lying on his back. The practice of leaving a baby to feed himself from the bottle lying beside him or hanging from a string is to be condemned, as milk is liable to enter the Eustachian tubes and excessive air may be swallowed.

VITAMIN SUPPLEMENTS. Although breast-fed infants are less likely to suffer from vitamin deficiencies than artificially fed infants, an adequate intake of vitamins C and D should be assured by giving orange juice or rose hip syrup and a vitamin D preparation from the age of one month. The infant fed on fresh cow's milk runs a considerable risk of vitamin deficiency and must have adequate vitamin supplements from one month until the end of the second year. By that time he should be receiving sufficient vitamins from his food, provided that he is on a full mixed diet with plenty of fruit and vegetables. The fortification of modern dried and evaporated milks with vitamins and iron has made supplements less necessary for infants fed on these preparations but unless it is quite certain that the milk is fortified and that the intake is adequate, it is wise to insist on supplementary vitamins for these infants as well, care being taken that the intake from all sources, especially of vitamin D, is not excessive.

WEANING. The infant is weaned from his mother's milk by gradual introduction of other types of food. Most infants can digest a variety of foods from an early age, and there is therefore no lower age limit to weaning but it is generally unnecessary

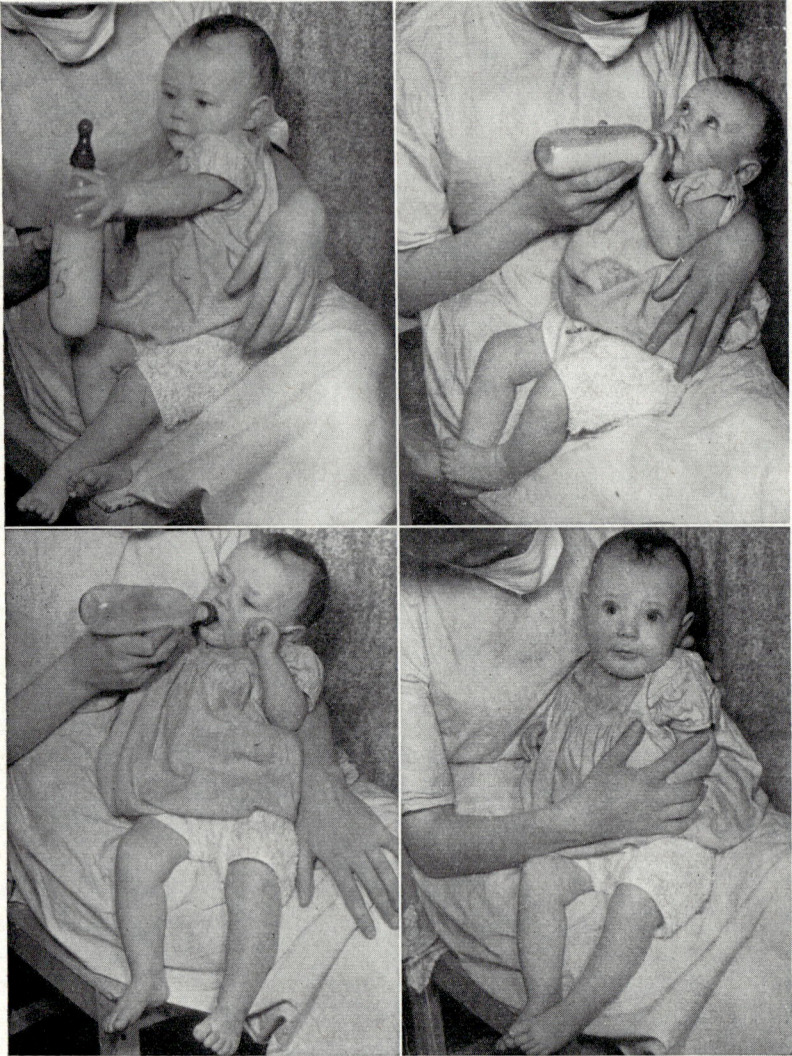

FIG. 17. Feeding behaviour of a six-month-old infant. (*a*) Recognises bottle and grasps it with both hands: (*b*) recognises nurse: (*c*) begins to lose interest as feed nears completion and no longer holds bottle: (*d*) eructates wind at end of feed.

to start before 4 months of age. Since mixed feeding provides a rich source of iron, it is desirable to introduce these foods by 5 or 6 months at the latest; an additional advantage of this policy is that the infant becomes accustomed early to feeding from a spoon and later difficulties are avoided.

The kind of food chosen to start weaning is not of great importance but it is customary to introduce a cereal food first, giving a small amount with a spoon before one of the feeds, usually the 10 a.m. feed. Once the infant has become used to the taste the amount can be increased each day and after a week or two a different food may be introduced before the 6 p.m. feed. Thereafter additions are made at the 2 p.m. feed and the quantity and variety of food gradually increased. Pre-cooked cereals are favoured by many mothers to start with, since they only require to be mixed into a little milk to the right consistency for feeding. Egg yolk, finely divided meat and vegetables, mashed potato and coarser cereals can follow. Many foods suitable for infants are now supplied in tins, which most mothers find more convenient than home-prepared foods. The reaction to a new taste is often refusal and the baby should be offered a variety of foods with a chance of indulging preferences rather than being forced to eat them.

The length of time that breast-feeding should be continued will depend to some extent on the health of the mother, on the adequacy of her lactation and on her own wishes: while some mothers breast-feed satisfactorily until the infant is 9 months old, few wish to continue after that age. A practical policy is to omit one breast-feed each week during the sixth or seventh month, until the baby is off the breast early in the seventh or eighth month. When cow's milk is introduced into the diet, it is advisable to use fortified dried milk. This need not be given from a bottle but can be offered in a cup, since most infants can drink readily from a cup by the age of 4 months or earlier. After the age of one year, it may be more convenient to give the baby fresh cow's milk, which should be pasteurised or boiled, but in that case vitamin supplements should be given as well.

The infant who is artificially fed can be accustomed to mixed feeding in the same way as the breast-fed infant. It has become fashionable to introduce cereals from the age of 2 or 3 months or even younger, but this is only necessary for those few infants who are not satisfied by full feeds of milk (*e.g.* 1,200 ml. of full-strength dried milk per day). The majority of infants will be contented and thrive on milk until 4 or 5 months, and earlier introduction of solids merely adds to the mother's work without corresponding benefit.

From the age of about 5 months, the infant may be given a hard rusk to chew on, though little will be actually eaten until the teeth have erupted.

Diet for Older Children

Studies on self-selected diets during the toddler period, in which older infants were allowed to eat freely from a large selection of foods, showed not only that they throve on what they chose but that they selected diets that were adequate in quantity and practically optimal in composition (Davis, 1928). The appetite factor is all-important and if the child develops healthy feeding habits when he is young, he will amply cover his requirements from the average family diet when he is older. In the case of children from the poorest homes, the factor most likely to be deficient is first-class protein, since meat and cheese are expensive items, and the diet will tend to contain too high a proportion of starch. The general provision of milk and meals in schools has gone a long way to remedy these defects, though previous failure to establish good feeding habits and appetite may defeat the intention. Thus Le Gros Clarke (1942, 1943) carried out investigations on the child's reaction to school meals and found that, when no persuasion was exerted, green vegetables were refused by over 50 per cent of girls aged 5 to 10, and by 44 per cent of girls aged 10 to 13: the percentage of boys in the same age groups was significantly lower. In underdeveloped countries, and amongst immigrant communities in this country, food habits and cultural or religious taboos on available foods may prove an important contributory factor in malnutrition (Burgess and Dean, 1962).

Milk is particularly valuable during childhood and adolescence, since it not only provides first-class protein but is also a rich source of calcium. Children up to 5 years of age should have a pint (600 ml.) of milk daily: after this age less may be taken if other first-class protein and calcium-containing foods are included in the diet, but even then at least half a pint should be taken as long as the child is growing. When younger children are unwilling to drink enough milk, the consumption of animal protein should be increased by giving cheese, lean bacon or mince according to preference.

During the weaning period, vegetables and other foods should be sieved, but subsequently a reasonable amount of roughage in the diet is useful in maintaining regular bowel action. If there is a tendency to constipation, increased fluid intake, regular exercise and an increase in green vegetables and fruit in the diet will usually achieve the desired result.

As a general rule, the diet of older children will inevitably fall into line with the diet of the adults with whom they live, varying from country to country and from household to household. Many children are very conservative, being happy to eat the same few well-liked foods and turning up their noses at anything unfamiliar. Variety is as important as good cooking in establishing sound feeding habits and educating the palate, however, and the mother and school should endeavour to avoid monotony by varying the diet and occasionally introducing something entirely new.

R. G. MITCHELL

References

American Academy of Pediatrics. Committee on Nutrition (1967). Obesity in childhood. *Pediatrics*, 40, 455.

ARNEIL, G. C. (1967). *Dietary Study of 4,365 Scottish Infants—1965*. Scottish Home and Health Department.

ARTHURTON, M. W. and BAMFORD, F. N. (1967). Paediatric aspects of the early discharge of maternity patients. *Brit. med. J.*, 3, 517.

ASHER, P. (1966). Fat babies and fat children. *Arch. Dis. Childh.*, 41, 672.

BAIRD, D., HYTTEN, F. E. and THOMSON, A. M. (1958). Age and human reproduction. *J. Obst. Gyn. Brit. Emp.*, 65, 865.

BRANSBY, E. R. BERRY, W. T. C. and TAYLOR, D. M. (1964). Study of the vitamin D intakes of infants in 1960. *Brit. med. J.*, 1, 1661.

British Medical Journal (1968). Thrombosis and inhibition of lactation. *Brit. med. J.*, 4, 1.

BROBECK, J. R. (1957). Neural control of hunger, appetite and satiety. *Yale J. Biol.*, **29**, 565.

BURGESS, A. and DEAN, R. F. A. (Ed.) (1962). *Malnutrition and Food Habits*. London: Tavistock.

CORDANO, A., BAERTL, J. M. and GRAHAM, G. G. (1964). Copper deficiency in infancy. *Pediatrics*, **34**, 324.

DAVIS, C. M. (1928). Self-selection of diet by newly weaned infants. *Amer. J. Dis. Child.*, **36**, 651.

Department of Health and Social Security (1969). Recommended intakes of nutrients for the United Kingdom. *Rep. Publ. Hlth Med. Subj.*, *No. 120*. London: H.M.S.O.

FORBES, G. B. (1957). Over-nutrition of the child: blessing or curse? *Nutrit. Rev.*, **15**, 193.

GARTNER, L. M. and ARIAS, I. M. (1966). Studies of prolonged neonatal jaundice in the breast-fed infant. *J. Pediat.*, **68**, 54.

GRYBOSKI, J. D. (1965). The swallowing mechanism of the neonate. *Pediatrics*, **35**, 445.

GUNTHER, M. (1963). The comparative merits of breast and bottle feeding. *Proc. Nutr. Soc.*, **22**, 134.

—— (1968). Diet and milk secretion in women. *Proc. Nutr. Soc.*, **27**, 77.

HOLT, L. E. and SNYDERMAN, S. E. (1965). Protein and amino acid requirements of infants and children. *Nutr. Abst. Rev.*, **35**, 1.

HOOPER, P. D. (1965). Infant feeding and its relationship to weight gain and illness. *Practitioner*, **194**, 391.

HYTTEN, F. E. and THOMSON, A. M. (1961). Nutrition of the lactating woman. In *Milk: the Mammary Gland and its Secretion*. Ed. S. K. Kon, and A. T. Cowie. New York: Academic Press.

—— YORSTON, J. and THOMSON, A. M. (1958). Difficulties associated with breast feeding. *Brit. med. J.*, **1**, 310.

ILLINGWORTH, R. S. (1959). Evening colic in infants. *Lancet*, **2**, 1119.

—— and KILPATRICK, B. (1953). Lactation and fluid intake. *Lancet*, **2**, 1175.

Joint FAO/WHO Expert Group Report on Protein Requirements (1965). FAO Nutrition Meetings Report, Series No. 37: WHO Technical Report, Series No. 301.

KNOWLES, J. A. (1965). Excretion of drugs in milk—a review. *J. Pediat.*, **66**, 1068.

LE GROS CLARKE, F. (1942). *The School Child and School Canteen*.

—— (1943). *The School Child's Taste in Vegetables*. (Both publ. Herts. County Council).

MAC KEITH, R. C. (1963). Is a big baby healthy? *Proc. Nutr. Soc.*, **22**, 128.

MACY, I. G. and KELLY, H. J. (1961). Human milk and cow's milk. In *Milk: the Mammary Gland and its Secretion*. Ed. S. K. Kon and A. T. Cowie. New York: Academic Press.

MELLANDER, O., VAHLQUIST, B., MELLBIN, T. (1959). Breast feeding and artificial feeding. *Acta paed. Scand.*, **48**, Suppl. 116.

MILLER, R. A. (1952). Factors influencing lactation. *Arch. Dis. Childh.*, **27**, 187.

MITCHELL, R. G. (1967). Modern views on rickets and hypercalcaemia. *World Rev. Nutr. Diet.*, **8**, 207.

MOORE, T. (1965). Vitamin A deficiency and excess. *Proc. Nutr. Soc.*, **24**, 129.

MORGAN, H. G., MITCHELL, R. G., STOWERS, J. M. and THOMSON, J. (1956). Metabolic studies in two infants with idiopathic hypercalcaemia. *Lancet*, **1**, 925.

Nutr. Soc. Symposium (1967). Food habits and nutritional status of minority groups in the United Kingdom. *Proc. Nutr. Soc.*, **26**, 191.

OPPÉ, T. E. and REDSTONE, D. (1968). Calcium and phosphorus levels in healthy newborn infants given various types of milk. *Lancet*, **1**, 1045.

SMITH, C. A. (1959). *The Physiology of the Newborn Infant*. 3rd edit. Springfield: Thomas.

SOUTHGATE, D. A. T., WIDDOWSON, E. M., SMITS, B. J., COOKE, W. T., WALKER, C. H. M. and MATHERS, N. P. (1969). Absorption and excretion of calcium and fat by young infants. *Lancet*, **1**, 487.

SPENCE, J. C. (1931). Nutritional xerophthalmia and night blindness. *Arch. Dis. Childh.*, 6, 17.

SWAMINATHAN, M. (1968). The nutrition and feeding of infants and pre-school children in the developing countries. *World Rev. Nutr. Diet.*, 9, 85.

WALLER, H. (1946). The early failure of breast feeding. *Arch. Dis. Childh.*, 21, 1.

WIDDOWSON, E. M. (1965). Absorption and excretion of fat, nitrogen and minerals from "filled" milks by babies one week old. *Lancet*, 2, 1099.

WOLFF, O. H. (1955). Obesity in childhood: a study of the birth weight, the height, and the onset of puberty. *Quart. J. Med.*, 24, 109.

6 Postnatal Growth

Growth and Development

ALTHOUGH growth and development are closely related and both continue from the moment of conception to the point at which adulthood is reached, they are essentially two different processes. *Growth* implies increase in size, typically coupled with

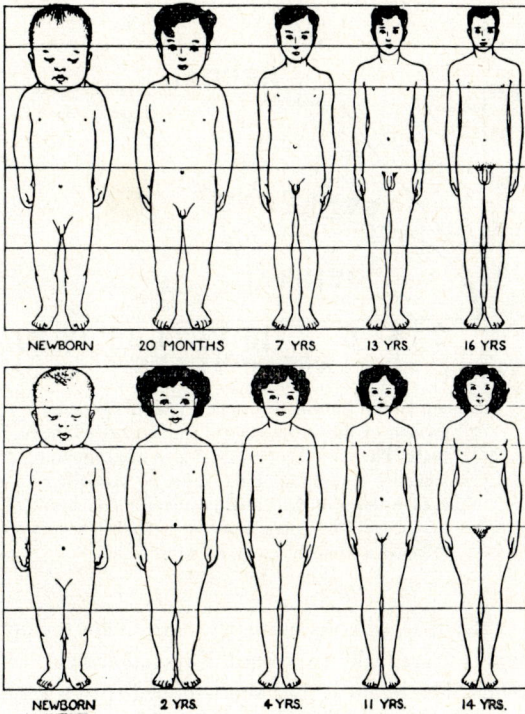

FIG. 18. Diagram showing relative proportions of the body from birth to adolescence.

cell-division and enlargement of protoplasmic and skeletal structure, whereas *development* represents increasing maturation of tissue, organs, or of the whole individual until full maturity of structure and function is attained. As a general rule the more mature organ or individual will be larger than the less mature, but this is

137

not necessarily the case. The thymus, for example, is actually smaller in the adult than in later childhood.

There are wide differences between the rates of growth of different organs and tissues at different stages of development. This is reflected in the changing proportions of the body during infancy, childhood and adolescence (Fig. 18). In the newborn infant the head represents approximately one-quarter of the total crown-heel length and the legs (heel to perineum) approximately three-eighths. In the adolescent, the head represents one-seventh and the legs approximately one-half. The

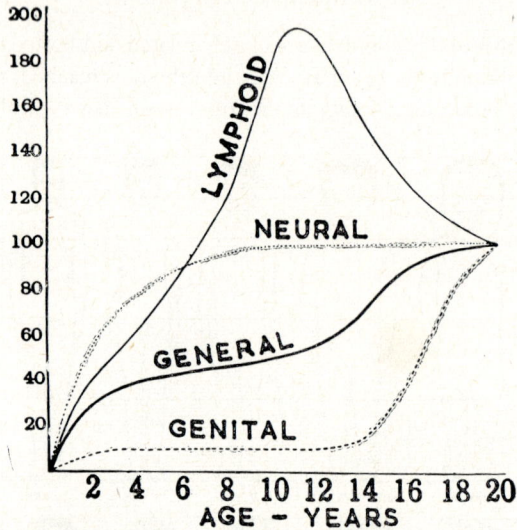

FIG. 19. Graph showing the major types of postnatal growth of the various parts and organs of the body. The several curves are drawn to a common scale by computing their value at successive ages in terms of their total postnatal increments (to 20 years). (After Scammon, R. E., 1930. 'The Measurement of Man'. Minnesota).

same figure shows also that, whereas in the newborn infant the umbilicus lies well below the mid-point, it gradually rises until in the adolescent it lies considerably above the mid-point. The infant is thus short-limbed with a relatively large head and thick trunk, compared with the adolescent.

PATTERN OF GROWTH. Scammon (1930) described four distinct types of growth, characteristic of different organs or tissues, which proceed concurrently. These are illustrated in Fig. 19, where each is shown diagrammatically as the percentage increment from birth (0) to maturity (100) in each year of age. The general type (heavy unbroken line) is the pattern followed by the body as a whole and by most of its external dimensions with the exception of the head and neck. The respiratory and digestive organs, the kidneys, spleen, musculature, aorta, blood-volume, etc.

conform approximately to this pattern, which shows rapid increment during infancy, a slowing-down during childhood, a further rapid increment with the approach of puberty and adolescence, and subsequent deceleration. The genital type (broken line), which is characteristic of the testis, ovary, epididymis, uterine tube, prostate, prostatic urethra and seminal vesicles, shows minimal increment during infancy and childhood followed by rapid growth with onset of puberty. In striking contrast to this, the neural type of growth, shown by a dotted line and representing the brain, meninges, optic apparatus and most head dimensions, is characterised by extremely rapid increment during the first 4 years, reaching nearly 60 per cent of the total at 2 years and nearly 90 per cent at 6 years. Subsequent growth from 6 to 20 years is

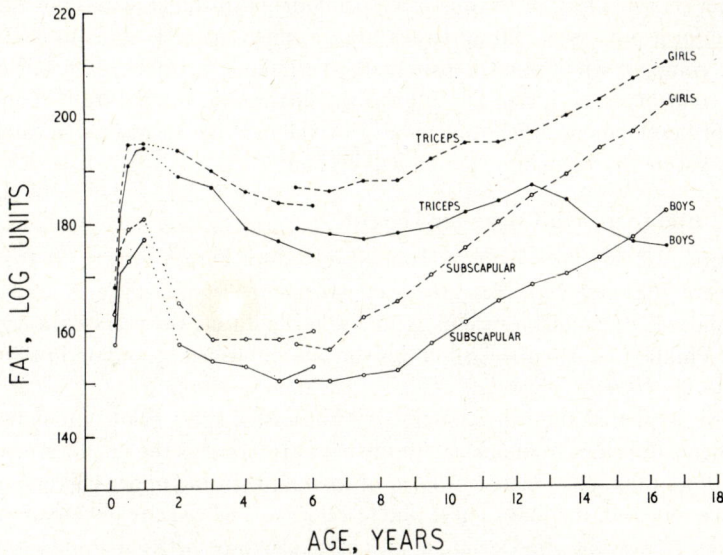

FIG. 20. Amount of subcutaneous fat on the back of the arm (triceps) and on the chest (subscapular) from birth to age 16. Distance curves; measurements by skinfold calipers, reported as logarithms of readings less 1·8 mm. (From Tanner, 1962).

minimal, representing only 10 per cent of the total increment from birth to maturity, though development (particularly of the cortex) continues more actively than over-all growth. The lymphoid type of growth (light unbroken line), which characterises the thymus and lymph-nodes, is again radically different from the other three types, since it reaches a maximum greatly in excess of the final increment at 10 to 12 years, and there is subsequently an absolute and relative decrease in lymphoid and thymic tissue during the succeeding 8 years.

A further growth-pattern may be added, that of the body fat, illustrated in Fig. 20. The amount of subcutaneous fat may be measured at certain sites by picking up a fold of skin and fat between thumb and forefinger, and measuring its thickness with a special, constant-pressure caliper. Figure 20 shows the curves for fat over the triceps and under the angle of the scapula, for healthy girls and boys.

The amount of fat increases from birth to about 9 months (in the average child; the peak may be reached as early as 6 months or as late as 12 or 15 months). The amount of fat then decreases until age 6 to 8 years, when it begins to increase once more. At adolescence limb fat in boys decreases (see triceps Fig. 20); the body fat shows a temporary slowing down of gain, but no actual loss in the average boy. In girls at adolescence there is a slight halting of the limb fat gain, but no loss; the trunk fat shows only a steady rise till adulthood.

Whilst it will be realised that diagrammatic representations of these growth patterns are no more than general approximations, and that growth increments of many of the organs cannot be accurately measured by longitudinal methods during life, they serve to illustrate the important point that postnatal growth is not a simple and uniform process of getting larger from birth to maturity. It is in contrast a highly complex symposium of patterns and rhythms, to which each organ and tissue contributes its quota. The adult is the final result, but the child at any one stage of development differs not only in overall size but in qualitative make-up from what he has been and what he will become.

The Human Growth Curve for Height

Figure 21 shows the most famous of all records of human growth. It concerns the height of a single boy, measured every six months from birth to 18 years. This is the oldest longitudinal record in existence, made during the years 1759–1777 by Count Philibert de Montbeillard on his son and published by Buffon in a supplement to the *Histoire Naturelle*.

Above is plotted the height attained at successive ages; below are shown the increments in height from one age to the next expressed as the rate of growth per year. If we think of growth as a form of motion, then the upper curve is one of distance travelled, the lower curve one of velocity. The velocity or rate of growth naturally reflects the child's state at any particular time better than does the distance achieved, which depends largely on how much the child has grown in all the preceding years. The blood and tissue concentrations of those substances whose amounts change with age are thus more likely to run parallel to the velocity than to the distance curve. In some circumstances, indeed, it is the acceleration rather than the velocity curve which best reflects physiological events; it is probable, for example, that the great increase in secretion of the endocrine glands at adolescence is manifested most clearly in acceleration of growth.

Figure 21 shows that in general the velocity of growth decreases from birth (and actually from as early as the fourth month of fetal life), but that this decrease is interrupted shortly before the end of the growth period. At this time, from 13 to 15 years in this particular boy, there is a marked acceleration of growth, called the adolescent growth spurt. From birth until age 4 or 5 the rate of growth in height declines rapidly, and the the decline, or deceleration, gets gradually less so that in some children the velocity is practically constant from 5 or 6 up to the beginning of the adolescent spurt. A slight increase in velocity is sometimes said to occur between about 6 and 8 years, providing a second wave on the general velocity curve.

Although Fig. 21 seems to show its presence, examination of many other individual records from age 3 to 13 fails to reveal it in the great majority; if it occurs at all, it is only in a minority of children.

As the points of Fig. 21 show, growth is in general a very regular process. The more carefully measurements are taken, with precautions, for example, to minimize the decrease in height that occurs during the day for postural reasons, the more regular does the succession of points in the graph become. Figure 22 shows the

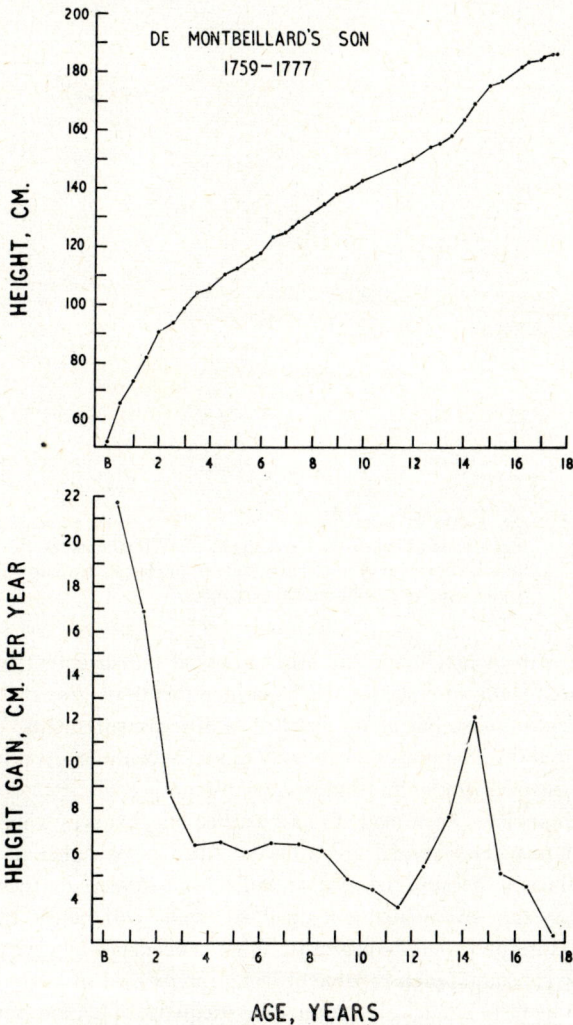

DE MONTBEILLARD'S SON
1759—1777

HEIGHT, CM.

HEIGHT GAIN, CM. PER YEAR

AGE, YEARS

FIG. 21. Growth in height of de Montbeillard's son from birth to 18 years, 1759–77. Above: distance curve, height attained at each age. Below: velocity curve, increments in height from year to year (data from Scammon, 1927, Amer. J. phys. Anthropol.).

fit of a smooth mathematical curve to a series of measurements taken on a child by the same observer every 6 months from age $3\frac{1}{2}$ to 10. None of the points deviates from the line by an amount more than measuring error. This is generally true, although in some children regular seasonal variations (discussed later) super-impose an added 6-month rhythm about the curve. There is no evidence for

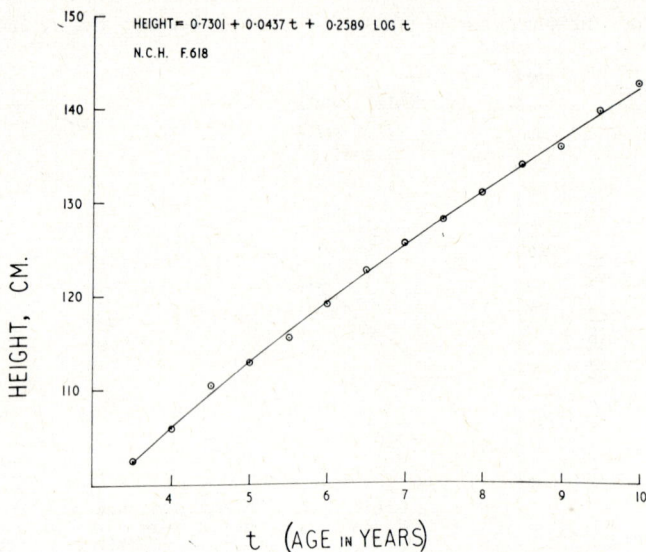

FIG. 22. Curve of form $y = a + bt + c$ log. t fitted to stature measurements taken on a girl by R. H. Whitehouse every 6 months from age $3\frac{1}{2}$ to 10 years (data from Harpenden Growth Study—see Israelsohn in Tanner, 1960).

'stages' of growth in height (or any other physical measurement) except for the spurt associated with adolescence. Perhaps increments of growth at the cellular level are discontinuous; but at the level of bodily measurements, even of single bones measured by X-rays, we can only discern complete continuity, with a velocity that changes gradually from one age to another.

Many attempts have been made to find mathematical curves which fit, and thus summarise, human and animal growth data. Most have ended in disillusion or fantasy; disillusion because fresh data failed to conform to them, or fantasy because the system eventually contained so many parameters that it became impossible to interpret them biologically. What is needed is a curve or curves with relatively few constants, each capable of being interpreted in a biologically mean-ingful way. The fit to empirical data must be adequate, of course, within the limits of measuring error. Part of the difficulty arises because the measurements usually taken are themselves biologically complex. Stature, for example, consists of leg length and trunk length and head height, all of which have rather different growth curves. Even with such relatively homogeneous measurements as humerus length or calf-muscle width, it is not clear what purely biological assumptions should be made as the basis for the form of the curve. The assumption that cells are continuously dividing leads to a different formulation from the assumption that cells are adding constant amounts of non-dividing material, or amounts of material at rates varying from one age period to another.

But fitting a curve to the individual values is the only way of extracting the maximum information about an individual's growth from the measurement data. This conclusion becomes increasingly inescapable when the effect of environmental circumstances on growth rate (e.g. illness on height growth) is investigated, or when two different measurements are being compared for the consistency of each as the child grows up. The individual's consistency can only be measured by deviations from his own growth curve. A change of rank order of two individuals from one age to another in a measurement may represent not inconsistency but consistently differing rates of change, one individual having a small velocity in the measurement, and the other individual a larger one.

More than one curve is needed to fit the postnatal age range. It seems that two curves may suffice, at least for many measurements such as height and weight. A curve of the form shown in Fig. 22 appears to fit well from a few months after birth to the beginning of adolescence. The adolescent spurt is fitted well by the Gompertz curve, a skew S-shaped exponential, which expresses the assumption that in equal small intervals of time the organism loses equal proportions of its remaining power to grow.

Types of Growth Data

The curves just discussed have to be fitted to data on single individuals. Yearly averages derived from different children each measured once only do not, in general, give the same curve. Thus the distinction between the two sorts of investigation is very important. The method of study using the same child at each age is called longitudinal; that using different children at each age is called cross-sectional. In a cross-sectional study each child is measured once only and all the children at age 10, for example, are different from those at age 9. A study may be longitudinal over any number of years; there are short-term longitudinal studies extending from age 3 to 5, for instance, and full birth-to-maturity longitudinal studies in which the children may be examined once, twice, or even more times every year from birth until 20 or over.

In practice it is always impossible to measure exactly the same group of children every year for a prolonged period; inevitably some children leave the study and others, if that is desired, join it. A study in which this happens is called a mixed longitudinal study and special statistical techniques are needed to get the maximum information out of its data. One particular type of mixed study is that in which a number of relatively short-term longitudinal groups are interlocked; here we may have groups of 0 to 6, 5 to 11, 10 to 16, and 15 to 20 to cover the whole age range. Problems arise at the 'joins' unless the sampling has been remarkably good, but the whole age range is covered for estimates of mean yearly velocity in the research time of 5 years.

Both cross-sectional and longitudinal studies have their uses, but they do not give the same information and cannot be dealt with in the same way. Cross-sectional surveys are obviously cheaper and more quickly done, and can include far larger numbers of children. They tell us a good deal about the distance curve of growth and it is essential to have them as part-basis for constructing standards for height and weight and other measurements in a given community (see below). Periodic cross-sectional surveys are valuable in assessing the nutritional progress of a country or a socio-economic group and the health of the child population as a whole. But they have one great drawback: they can never reveal individual differences in rate of growth or in the timing of particular phases such as the adolescent growth spurt. It is these individual rate differences which chiefly throw light on the genetical control of growth and on the correlation of growth with psychological development, educational achievement, and social behaviour. Longitudinal studies are laborious and time consuming; they demand great perseverance on the part of those who make them and those who take part in them; and they demand very high technical standards, since in the calculation of a growth increment from one occasion to the next, two errors of measurement occur. They are the indispensable base, however, on which the diagnosis and treatment of disorders of growth rest, for the clinical approach is a longitudinal one, and each child treated with human growth hormone or an anabolic steroid represents an attempt to alter an individual pattern of growth velocity.

Cross-sectional data can in some important respects be misleading. Figure 23 illustrates the effect on 'average' figures produced by the individual differences in the age at which the adolescent spurt begins. Figure 23A shows a series of individual velocity curves from 10 to 18 years, each individual starting his spurt at a different age. The average of these curves, obtained simply by treating the values cross-sectionally and adding them up at age 10, 11, 12, etc., and dividing by 5, is shown by the dashed line. This line in no way characterises the 'average' velocity curve; on the contrary, it is a travesty of it. It smoothes out the adolescent spurt, spreading it along the time axis. It does not take account of the 'phase-differences' between the individual curves. Figure 23B shows the same individual curves, but arranged so that their peak velocities coincide; the average curve then characterises the group in a proper manner. In passing from Fig. 23A to 23B the time-scale has been altered so that in Fig. 23B the curves are plotted not against chronological age but against a measure which arranges the children according to how far they have travelled along their course of development; in other words, they are arranged according to their true developmental or physiological growth status.

Averages computed from cross-sectional data inevitably produce velocity curves of this flattened, distorted type; and, equally, distance curves show the distortion by not rising sufficiently rapidly at adolescence. Until recently all the published height and weight standards used in hospitals and schools incorporated this distortion. However, it is possible to construct curves whose fiftieth percentile

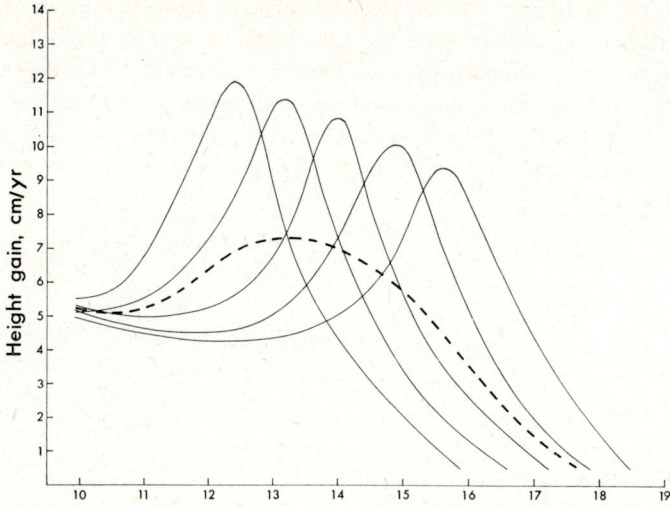

FIG. 23A

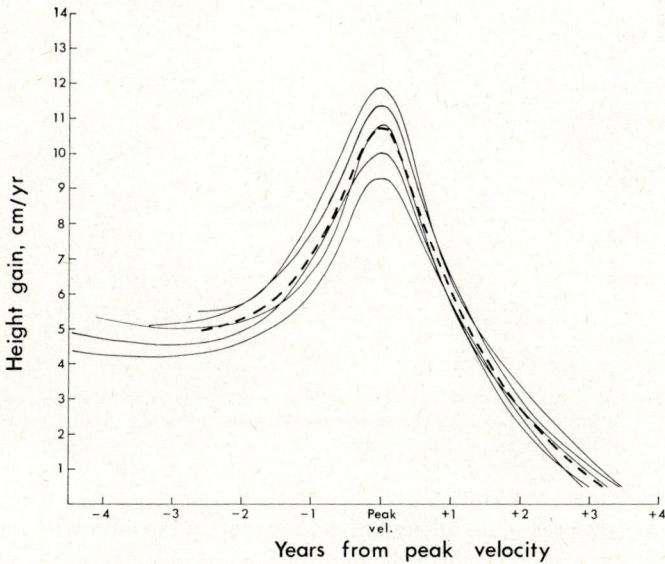

Years from peak velocity

FIG. 23B

FIG. 23. The relation between individual and mean velocities during the
adolescent spurt. (A) The individual height velocity curves of 5
boys of the Harpenden Growth Study (solid lines), with the mean
curve (dashed line) constructed by averaging their values at each
age. (B) The same curves all plotted according to their peak
height velocity (from Tanner, Whitehouse and Takaishi, 1966).

represents the actual growth of a typical individual by taking the shape of the curve from individual longitudinal data, and the absolute values for the beginning and end from large cross-sectional surveys (Tanner, Whitehouse and Takaishi, 1966). Figures 24 and 25 show height-attained and height-velocity curves for the 'typical' boy and girl in Britain in 1965, determined in this way. By 'typical' is meant that boy or girl who has the mean birth length, grows always at the mean

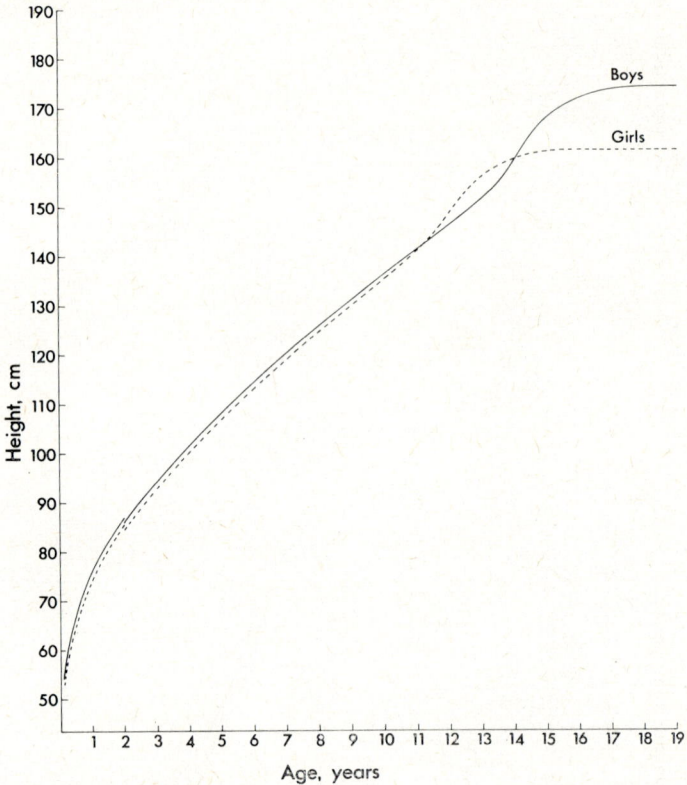

FIG. 24. Typical individual height-attained curves for boys and girls (supine length to the age of 2 years). Integrated curves of Fig. 25 (from Tanner, Whitehouse and Takaishi, 1966).

velocity, has the peak of the adolescent growth spurt at the mean age, and, finally, reaches the mean adult height at the mean age of cessation of growth. There is of course a certain danger in showing such a smooth, average curve, for measurements on a single individual are naturally less regular, however expert the measurer. Practically no individual follows the fiftieth percentile curve of Fig. 24 and 25; but most have the same shaped curve. However, some individuals, mostly late-maturing boys, seem to have a slight dip in the velocity curve just before the adolescent spurt starts. These are such a small minority that they were ignored when the typical-individual curves were constructed, but they may be important when we have to consider what is the normal prepuberal velocity for a boy who is a very late maturer.

Boys' and Girls' Height Curves

Figures 24 and 25 show the height curves from birth to maturity. Up to age 2 the child is measured lying down on his back. This measurement is called supine length, and averages about 1 cm. more than the measurement of standing height taken in the same child. The supine length-stature difference causes the break in the line in Fig. 24 at age 2. Figure 24 shows the typical girl as slightly shorter than

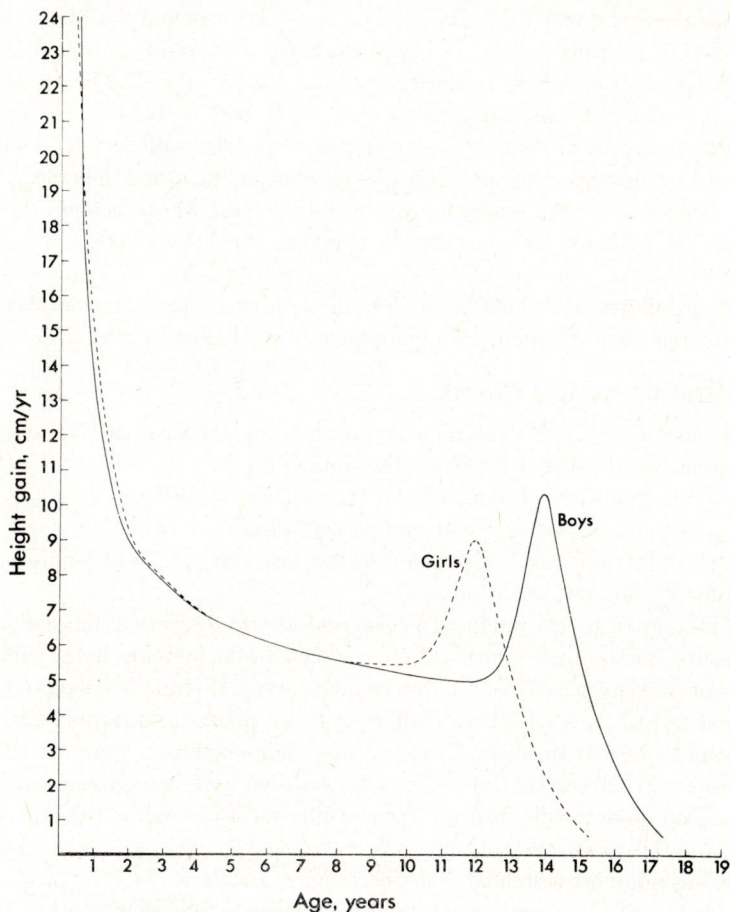

FIG. 25. Typical individual velocity curves for supine length or height of boys and girls. These curves represent the velocity of the typical boy and girl at any given instant—for construction, see text (from Tanner, Whitehouse and Takaishi, 1966).

the typical boy at all ages until adolescence. She becomes taller shortly after age 11·0 because her adolescent spurt takes place 2 years earlier than the boy's. At age 14·0 she is surpassed again in height by the typical boy, whose adolescent spurt has now started. In the same way, the typical girl weighs a little less than the boy at birth, equals him at age 8, becomes heavier at age 9 or 10, and remains so till about age 14½.

The velocity curves given in Fig. 25 show these processes more clearly. At birth the typical boy is growing very slightly faster than the typical girl, but the velocities become equal at about 7 months and then the girl grows faster to 4 years. From then till adolescence no difference in velocity can be detected. The sex difference is best thought of, perhaps, in terms of acceleration, the boy decelerating harder than the girl over the first 4 years (see also Deming, 1957; Deming and Washburn, 1963). In Britain in 1965 the typical girl begins the adolescent height spurt at about age 10·5 and reaches peak height velocity at approximately 12·0. The boy begins his spurt and reaches his peak just 2 years later. The boys' peak is higher than the girls', averaging in our data 10·3 ± 0·2 cm./year compared with the girls' 9·0 ± 0·2 cm./year (as 'instantaneous' peaks, i.e., peaks obtained by fitting smoothed curves to the observations; the velocities over that whole year which includes the peak moment are naturally less, averaging 9·5 cm./year for boys and 8·4 cm./year for girls).

Girls are always in advance of boys (i.e., closer to their final mature status), even at birth; this very important sex dimorphism is considered in more detail below.

Standards for Normal Growth

The doctor or nurse examining or treating a child suspected of abnormal growth has usually one of three questions in mind.

(1) Is the child's *size* (height, weight, etc.) within normal limits for his age, sex, population, socio-economic group, and parents' sizes?

(2) Has this child's *rate of growth* over the past year, say, been within normal limits for his age, sex, etc.?

(3) Has my treatment produced a *change in the rate of growth* of this child?

The first question arises when the child is seen for the first time in the clinic, the school or perhaps in a public health screening survey. It requires standards of size attained at each age, which we shall refer to as 'distance standards'. Charts of height and weight attained at each age exist for children of many countries but they have to be revised each decade or so, since children have been getting larger and growing up more rapidly in many parts of the world during the last 50 years or more, and this process is still going on (see below).

The second, more searching, question requires standards for *velocity* or rate of growth. The third question really requires standards for acceleration or rate of change of growth velocity, but none are available at present. However, just as in the past abnormality of velocity could be detected, though not properly quantified, from distance plots, so unusual accelerations can be detected from the velocity charts given here.

Charts of height attained, height velocity, weight attained, and weight velocity for girls and boys from birth to maturity are given in Figs 26 to 29. (The detailed values will be found in Tanner, Whitehouse and Takaishi, 1966 and the charts are available commercially from Creaseys of Hertford, Herts, both in this form and in a

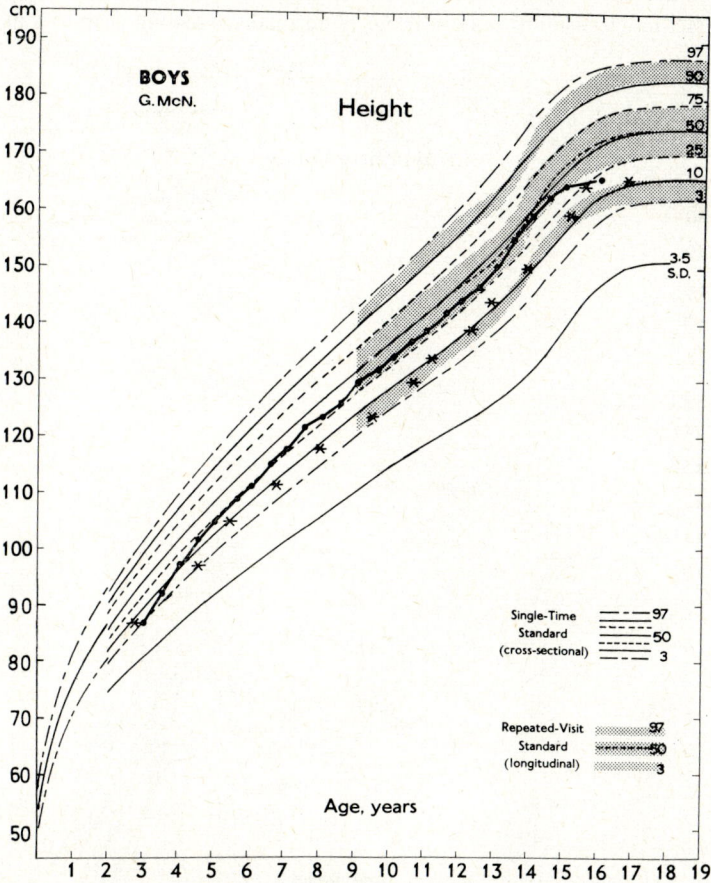

FIG. 26 A. Standard chart of height attained for boys (from Tanner, Whitehouse and Takaishi, 1966), with normal boy, followed longitudinally, plotted. Stars represent height plotted against skeletal age instead of chronological age (note skeletal age is in advance of chronological age after age 4).

form from birth to 5 only, giving a magnification of this section.) Each standard is given in terms of percentiles, so that the interpretation of a child's position is direct. If a child is at the 3rd percentile this means that 3 per cent of British children are less tall, or are growing less fast (if a velocity standard) than he is; if at the 50th then 50 per cent of children are smaller, if at the 97th then 97 per cent of children are smaller. In growth-disordered children who are much below the 3rd percentile it is convenient to use a multiple of the standard deviation for height at the given age to express how far down the chart the child is; for example he may be 3·5 S.D. below the mean. The S.D's. at each age are tabulated in the reference cited; the 3·5 S.D. line however has been put in on the height charts.

Age on the charts is given in terms of decimals, or tenths of a year, not in months. It is in fact much easier to work in terms of decimal age than in years and months,

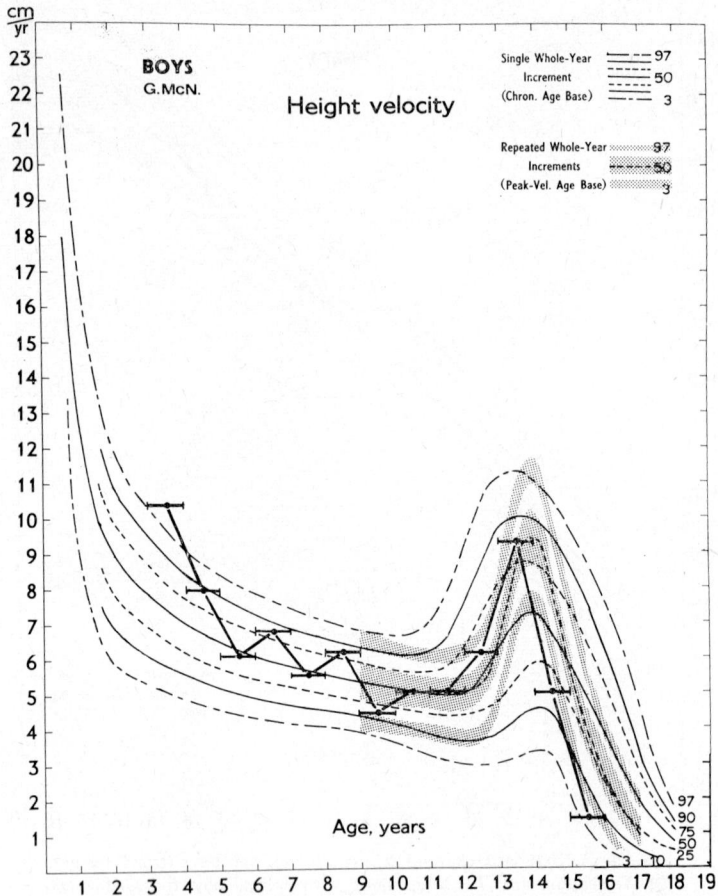

FIG. 26 B. Standard height velocity chart for boys with yearly velocities of boy of FIG. 26 A plotted.

and practically imperative to do so when calculating velocities. Table 6 gives the conversion and is used as follows:

(1) Record the date of examination as a five figure number, the first two figures being the year (e.g. '69) and the next three the decimal of the year corresponding to the date, i.e. January 1st 1969 is 69·000, February 1st 1969, 69·085, etc. An examination carried out on January 7th 1969 is recorded as 69·016. Calendars can be premarked.

TABLE 6

TABLE OF DECIMALS OF YEAR

	1 JAN.	2 FEB.	3 MAR.	4 APR.	5 MAY	6 JUNE	7 JULY	8 AUG.	9 SEPT.	10 OCT.	11 NOV.	12 DEC.
1	000	085	162	247	329	414	496	581	666	748	833	915
2	003	088	164	249	332	416	499	584	668	751	836	918
3	005	090	167	252	334	419	501	586	671	753	838	921
4	008	093	170	255	337	422	504	589	674	756	841	923
5	011	096	173	258	340	425	507	592	677	759	844	926
6	014	099	175	260	342	427	510	595	679	762	847	929
7	016	101	178	263	345	430	512	597	682	764	849	932
8	019	104	181	266	348	433	515	600	685	767	852	934
9	022	107	184	268	351	436	518	603	688	770	855	937
10	025	110	186	271	353	438	521	605	690	773	858	940
11	027	112	189	274	356	441	523	608	693	775	860	942
12	030	115	192	277	359	444	526	611	696	778	863	945
13	033	118	195	279	362	447	529	614	699	781	866	948
14	036	121	197	282	364	449	532	616	701	784	868	951
15	038	123	200	285	367	452	534	619	704	786	871	953
16	041	126	203	288	370	455	537	622	707	789	874	956
17	044	129	205	290	373	458	540	625	710	792	877	959
18	047	132	208	293	375	460	542	627	712	795	879	962
19	049	134	211	296	378	463	545	630	715	797	882	964
20	052	137	214	299	381	466	548	633	718	800	885	967
21	055	140	216	301	384	468	551	636	721	803	888	970
22	058	142	219	304	386	471	553	638	723	805	890	973
23	060	'45	222	307	389	474	556	641	726	808	893	975
24	063	148	225	310	392	477	559	644	729	811	896	978
25	066	151	227	312	395	479	562	647	731	814	899	981
26	068	153	230	315	397	482	564	649	734	816	901	984
27	071	156	233	318	400	485	567	652	737	819	904	986
28	074	159	236	321	403	488	570	655	740	822	907	989
29	077		238	323	405	490	573	658	742	825	910	992
30	079		241	326	408	493	575	660	745	827	912	995
31	082		244		411		578	663		830		997
	JAN. 1	FEB. 2	MAR. 3	APR. 4	MAY 5	JUNE 6	JULY 7	AUG. 8	SEPT. 9	OCT. 10	NOV. 11	DEC. 12

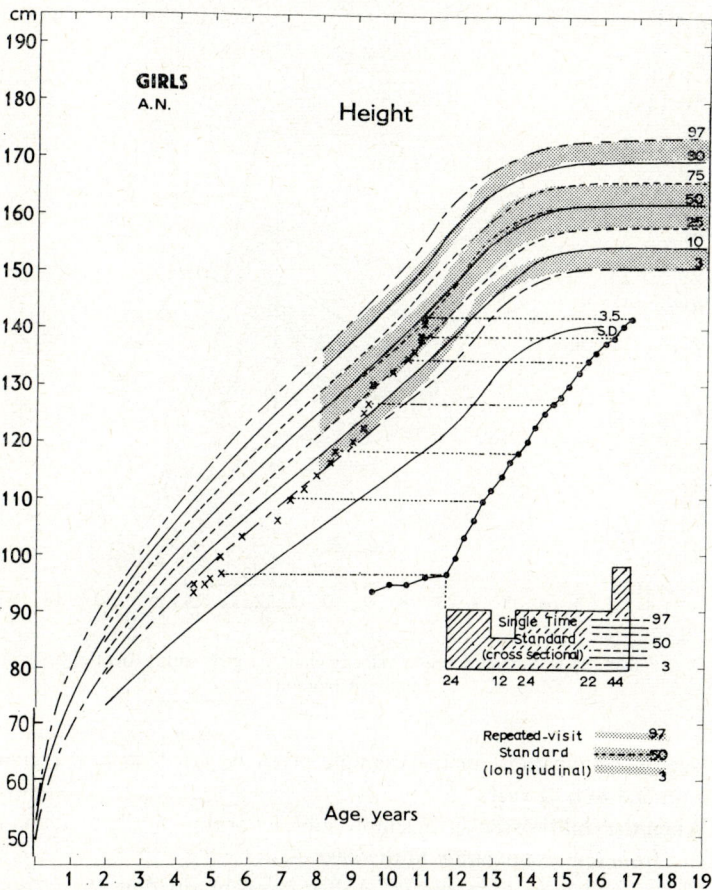

FIG. 27 A. Standard chart of height attained for girls (from Tanner, Whitehouse and Takaishi, 1966), with patient with growth hormone deficiency, treated with human growth hormone, plotted. Note 'catch-up' (dose indicated by shading in IU/week).

(2) Immediately underneath write the date of birth of the child, also in the decimal system. Thus a boy born on June 23rd 1959 has the birth date 59·474.

(3) Subtract date (2) from date (1) in a normal arithmetic manner. The answer

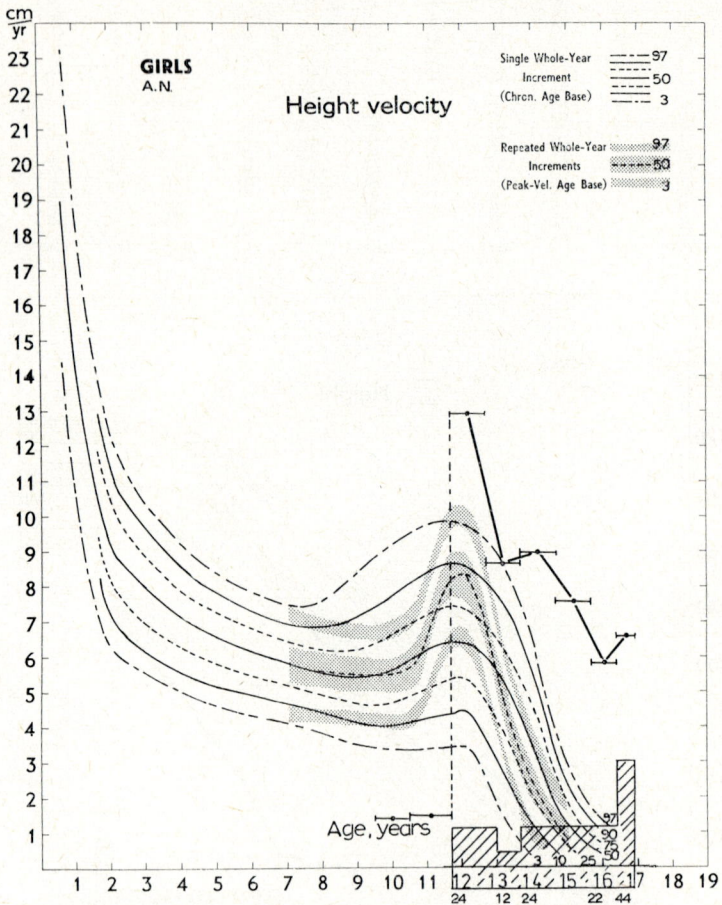

FIG. 27 B. Standard height velocity chart for girls with patient of
FIG. 27 A plotted.

is the age at examination; in the example given 69·016 less 59·474 giving age 9·542, rounded to 9·54 years.

(4) When the child is seen again simply subtract arithmetically to obtain the age increment from one examination to the next.

(5) The growth velocity in cm./yr. is then given by dividing the increment of height in cm. by the age increment in years. This may necessitate a pocket slide rule, but no other equipment is necessary and the velocity is accurately calculated.

In the charts the percentile lines marked with numerals are cross-sectional type standards, and the dotted line with the shaded areas starting at age 8 in girls and 10 in boys are longitudinal-type standards. On the first occasion that a child is seen, his plot in the distance standards should be interpreted on the cross-sectional lines; but when he is followed as he grows then the interpretation should be made

Name   Date of Birth   Reg. No.

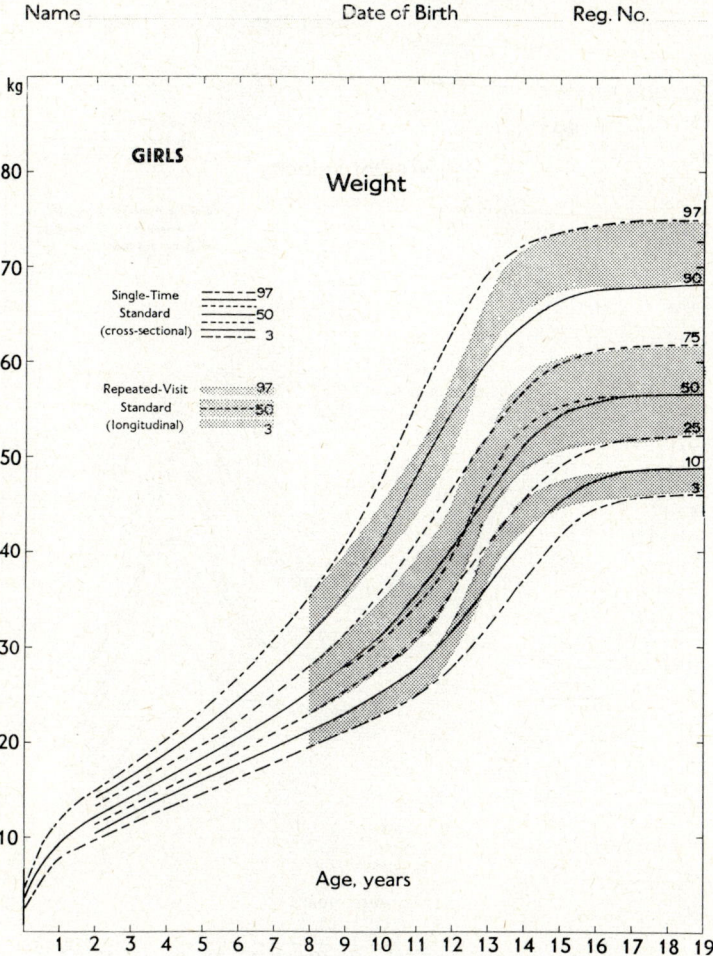

FIG. 28 A. Standard chart of weight attained for boys (from Tanner, Whitehouse and Takaishi, 1966).

at adolescence on the longitudinal type curves. Similarly when only a single increment is available for a child then the velocity should be interpreted on the cross-sectional lines. When a series of velocities are available, then the interpretation is made on the longitudinal lines.

In following clinical cases it is often useful to plot height against bone age (estimated as described below) as well as against chronological age. In Fig. 26 the height and height velocity of a healthy boy are plotted (though he was probably growth-retarded when first seen which explains his unusually high velocity in the first year). In general a child tends to follow a given height percentile throughout the whole growing period, and ends up as an adult at this same percentile. Hence

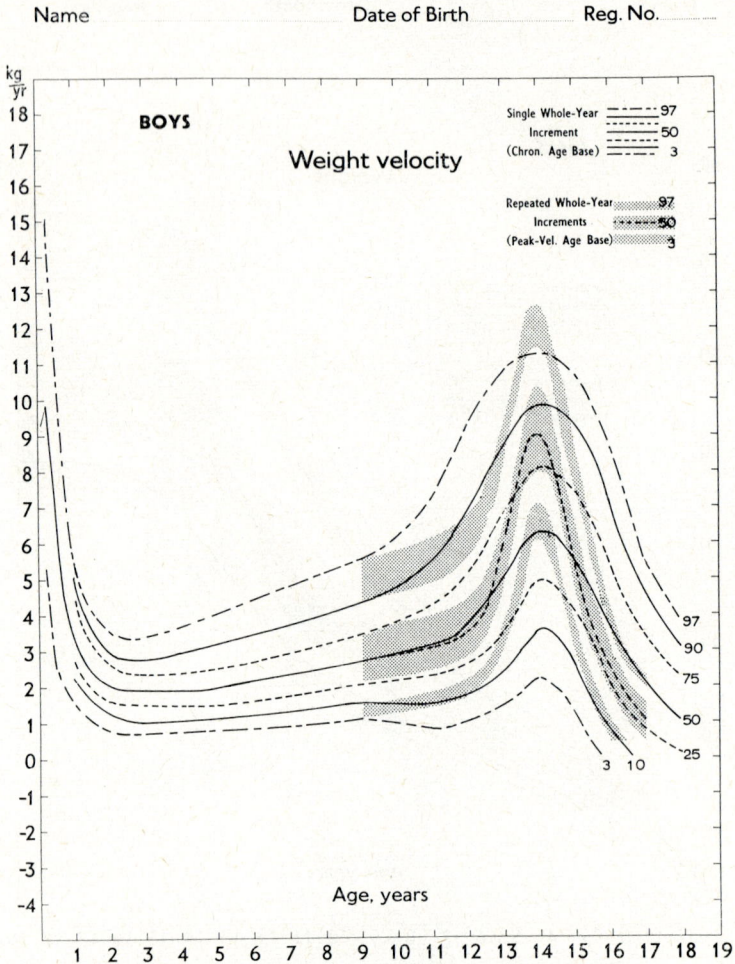

FIG. 28 B. Standard chart of weight velocity for boys.

one can make a reasonable guess at the expected adult height when a number of points are available for plotting. But if the child is a slow maturer, as signified by a delayed bone age, then his final height will be nearer his height for bone age than his height for chronological age. (The child in Fig. 26 is a fast maturer, but exemplifies well this rule.) Practical experience seems to indicate that the best estimate is one which lies about midway between the two predictions. Some children however do change their percentile position as a result of a specially large or small adolescent spurt. The amount of the spurt is to a considerable degree independent of the amount of growth before (see Chapter 7).

The method of plotting velocity is shown in Figs. 26B and 27B. The velocity,

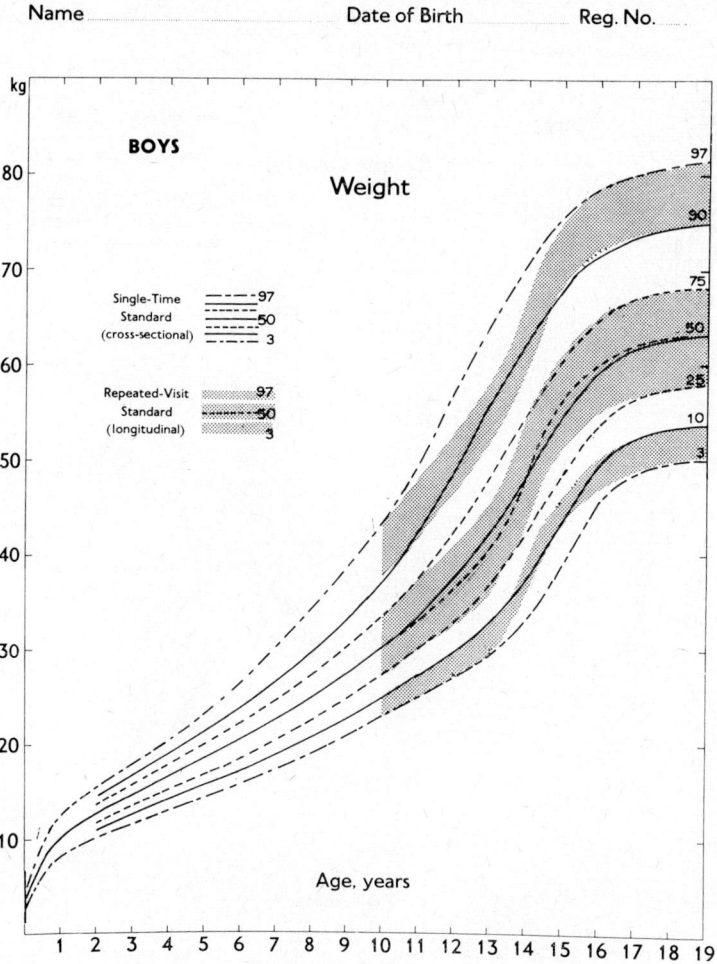

FIG. 29 A. Standard chart of weight attained for girls (from Tanner, Whitehouse and Takaishi, 1966).

calculated in cm./yr., is plotted at the mid-point of the interval from one examination to the next, with the length of this interval indicated by the solid line with vertical ends on it. (The interpretation depends somewhat on how long this interval has been; hence it is important to display it.) When treatment occurs it is perhaps visually better not to join the velocity plots before and during it (since the line would look as if it started to rise before the treatment began) but to draw a line vertically upwards at the moment treatment began (or ended) as in Fig. 27B. These velocity standards are appropriate only for interpretation of a whole year's growth, or a longer period. For shorter periods the variation is greater; thus if one plots a six-monthly velocity (multiplied by 2 to correct it to cm./yr.) then the limits

Name _____   Date of Birth _____   Reg. No. _____

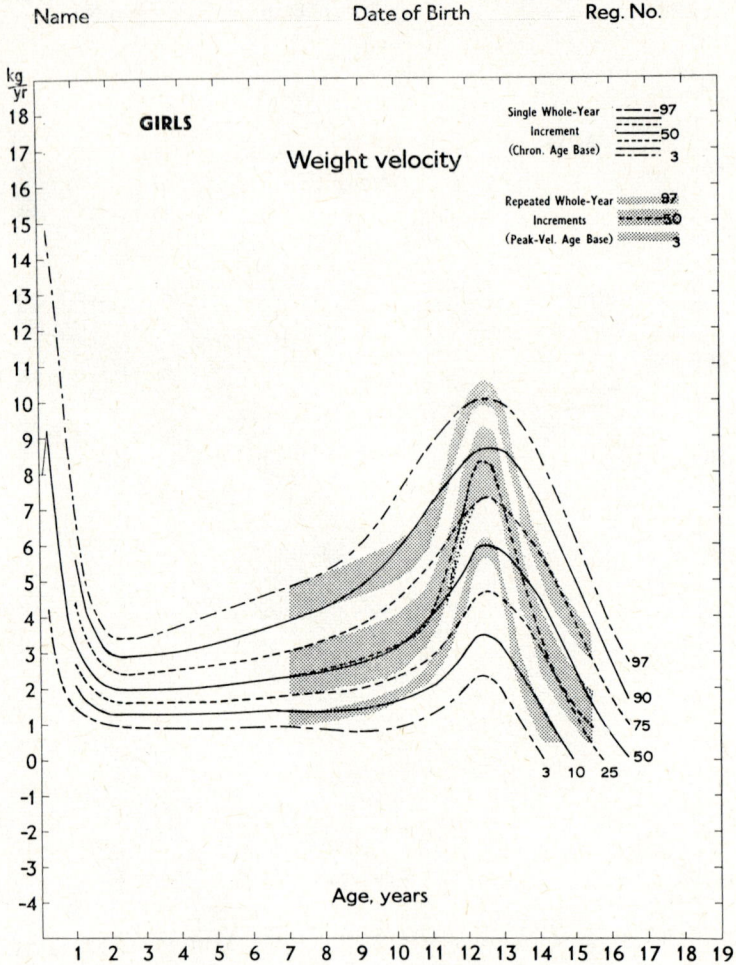

FIG. 29 B. Standard chart of weight velocity for girls.

of normality should be wider, and a child at or below the third centile might be perfectly normal (see Tanner, Whitehouse and Takaishi, 1966). Velocity plots have to be regarded a little differently from distance ones. Even a healthy child will not stay on the same velocity percentile throughout growth unless he is close to the fiftieth. A child who grew consistently along the third velocity percentile would end up a dwarf; indeed this is what children with gonadal dysgenesis typically do.

Conversely a child consistently at the ninetieth would soon come to be abnormally large.

It is obvious enough that the girl illustrated in Fig. 27 responded to the administration of human growth hormone by a great acceleration in growth. But sometimes it is by no means so clear whether or not a treatment has altered growth rate. Though no standards for acceleration are yet available, our empirical data enable us to say that from age 3 to the beginning of puberty a difference of over 2 cm./yr. between two successive years' velocities (that is, an acceleration from year 1 to year 2 of over 2 cm./yr./yr.) is very unusual in healthy children. This figure may therefore serve as a guide to a significant effect of treatment.

When assessing whether a child is within normal limits for height for age it is really desirable to compare him with standards drawn from the same region and the same socio-economic group, but this is not at present practicable. Regional differences are in fact quite small in Britain; social class differences are larger (see below). More important than these variables however is height of the parents and other near relatives. A child who is a little below the third percentile and has parents at the third and twentieth is probably perfectly normal, whereas one of the same size with parents at the seventieth and ninetieth certainly needs careful investigation. A visual impression may be obtained by plotting the parents' heights in the child's chart, at the 19-year-old level. Since the average difference in stature between British men and women is approximately 13 cm. or 5 inches, this amount is added to the mother's height before her position is plotted on the boy's chart, or subtracted from the father's height when his position has to be plotted on the girl's chart. A more accurate allowance for parents' height can be made in the light of the correlation coefficients between parents and children at successive ages. In principle a correction can be calculated, the application of which places the child at a new percentile, with parental height now allowed for. Publication of these corrections may be expected in the course of the next year or two.

Anthropometric Techniques

Besides height and weight, measurements of sitting height (giving leg length by subtraction from height), shoulder and hip width (biacromial and bi-iliac diameters), circumferences of arm, calf and head and skinfold measurements of subcutaneous fat are often useful in assessing the growth of a child. Span has been used in the past to give an indication of arm length, but has little to recommend it; it is hard to take accurately and combines both arm length and chest breadth. Standards are available, however, as also for sitting height, in Provis and Ellis (1955). Endocrinologists have often used pubes-vertex (upper segment) and pubes-heel (lower segment) as measures of trunk and legs but the measuring errors are larger and no good standards exist; sitting height and stature are preferable.

Standards for sitting height plotted against stature are given for boys and girls in Fig. 30. A plot is shown of a normal child (Fig. 30A) and of one with achondroplasia (Fig. 30B). Deviations from the normal range are rare, even in a growth disorder clinic. The standards show the way in which sitting height increases more than leg length at adolescence: up till then the curve of sitting height on stature is more or less linear, but at adolescence it turns quite sharply upward. The adolescent spurt in stature is mostly in trunk length.

As we are required to assess the velocity of growth, accuracy of measurement of

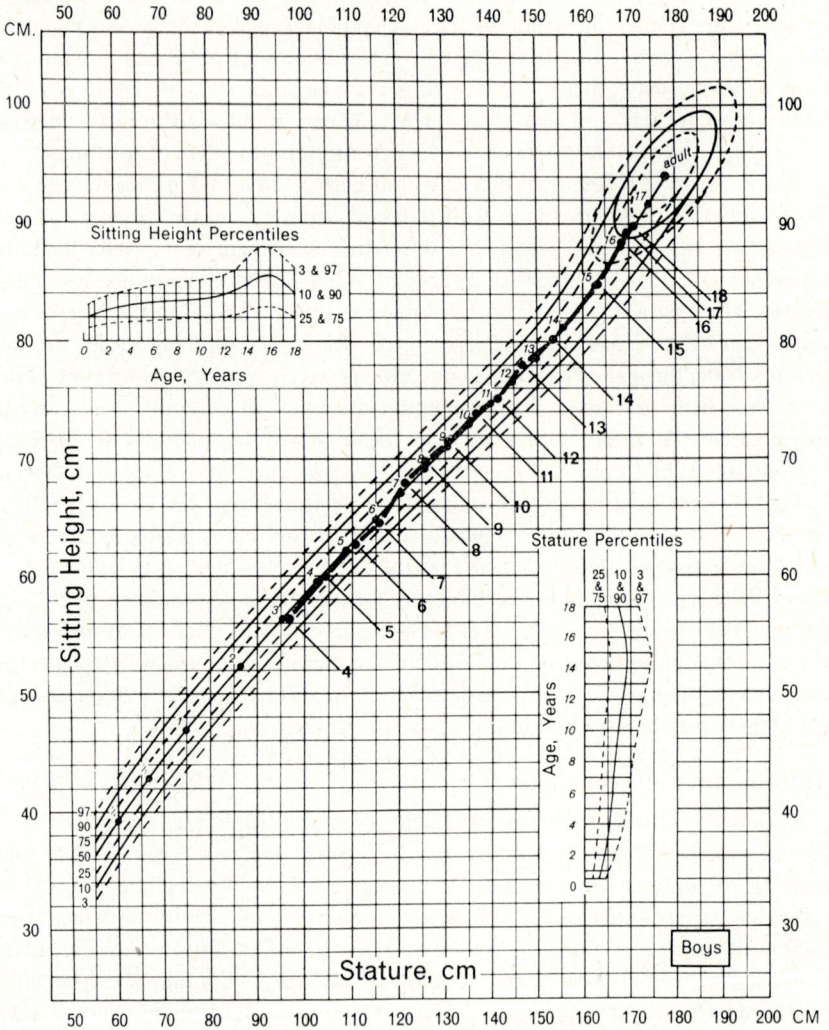

Fig. 30 A. Standard chart of sitting height for stature (boys), with healthy boy's progress plotted (Tanner and Whitehouse, unpublished).

stature and other dimensions is essential. Stature and supine length are both very reliable measurements if taken with proper technique. Two observers should differ by 4 mm. or less on 95 per cent of occasions. But this accuracy can only be achieved if constant care is exercised. Untrained or casual personnel, who fail to position the child properly, may quite well differ by 1·5 cm. in their measurements. Two summating errors of this magnitude can turn a three monthly velocity of 12·0 cm./yr., which represents a good response to human growth hormone, say,

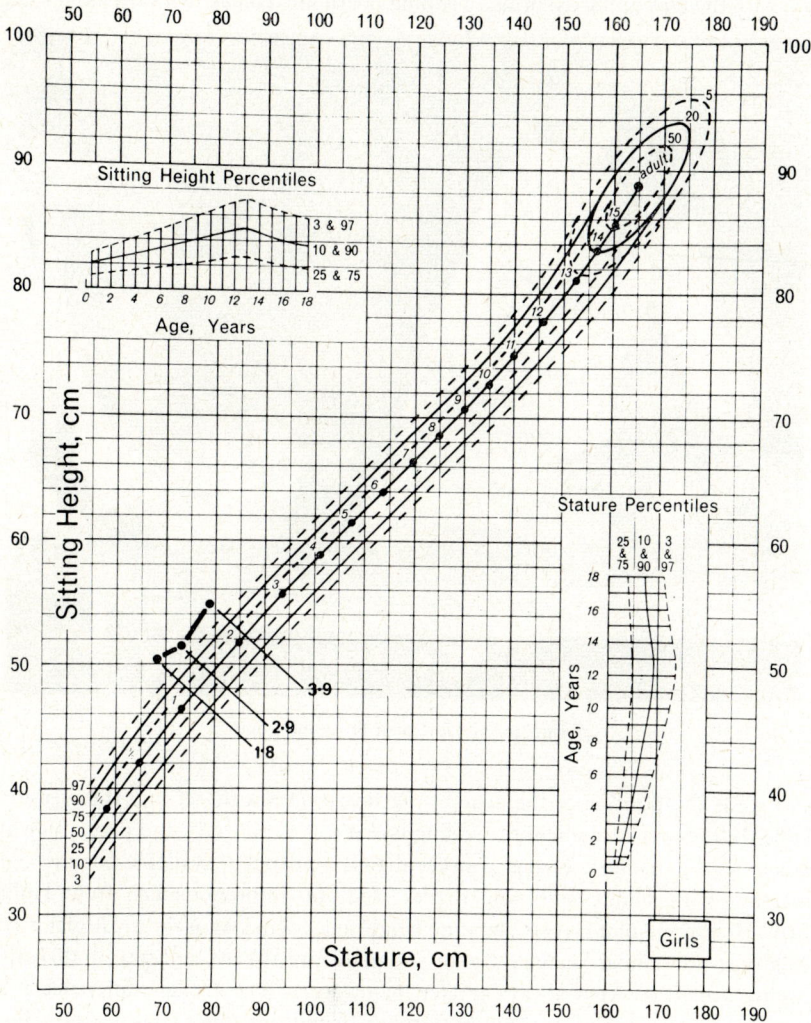

FIG. 30 B. Standard chart of sitting height for stature (girls), with achondroplasiac plotted.

into 2·0 cm./yr., a hypopituitary rate. Thus measurements should never be left to the haphazard attention of whichever nurse or doctor happens to be in the clinic that day; in any paediatric endocrinology clinic there should be one or two nurses, technicians or radiographers specially trained in simple anthropometry.

The methods for measuring supine length and stature are illustrated in Figs 31 and 32. Supine length is taken with the child lying on a flat surface on his back. One observer holds the head in contact with a board at the top of the table, and another straightens the legs, turns the feet to right angles with the leg (that is to say, with the toes upwards) brings a sliding board into contact with the child's heels

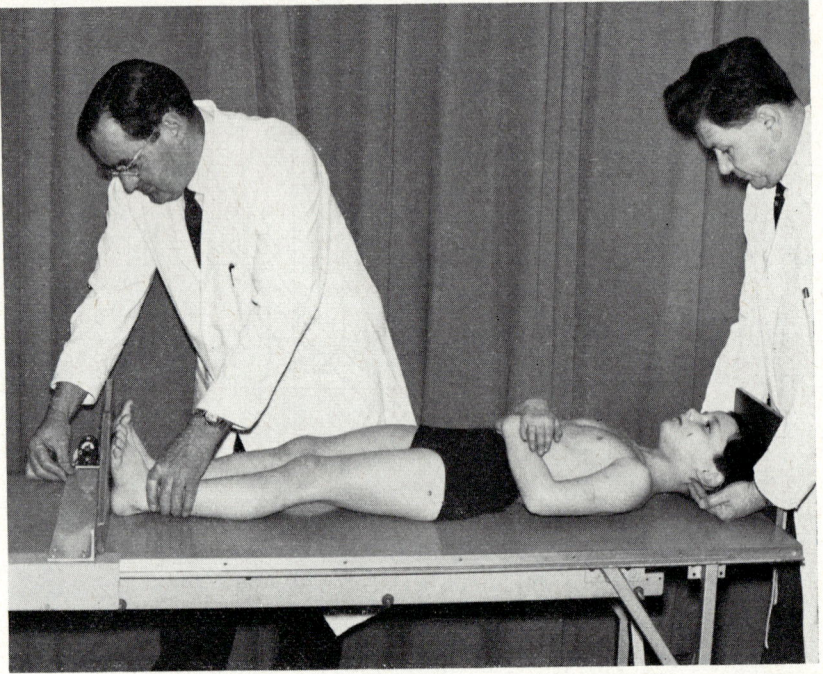

FIG. 31. Measurement of supine length.

and reads the position of the edge of the board on a scale set into the measuring table. In the best equipment the sliding board moves on a rack and pinion to which a counter is attached, giving a direct digital read-out. (Available commercially, together with stadiometers and digital read-out anthropometers, from Holtain Ltd.) By the age of 2·0 years standing height may be taken in the great majority of children; the standards above are for supine length till 2·0, and stature thereafter. Supine length is nearly always greater than stature. The average difference at age 2 to 5 is a little under 1 cm., but unfortunately children differ considerably, due to their posture. Thus in passing from one measurement to the other a difference of from zero to 2·5 cm. may occur. At ages between 2 and 3 years inclusive, both measurements should be taken.

Stature is measured without shoes, the child standing with his heels and back in contact with an upright surface. His head is held so that he looks straight forward with the lower borders of his eye sockets in the same horizontal plane as his external auditory meati (*i.e.* the head *not* tipped with nose upwards). A movable head piece, with digital read-out in modern equipment, or a triangular block, is slid down until it touches the child's head. During the measurement the child should be told to take a breath, relax the shoulders and stretch up to be as tall as possible, and the observer aids this by applying gentle upward pressure under the mastoid processes. Care must be taken (usually by a second observer when dealing with small children) to prevent the heels coming off the ground. The stretching

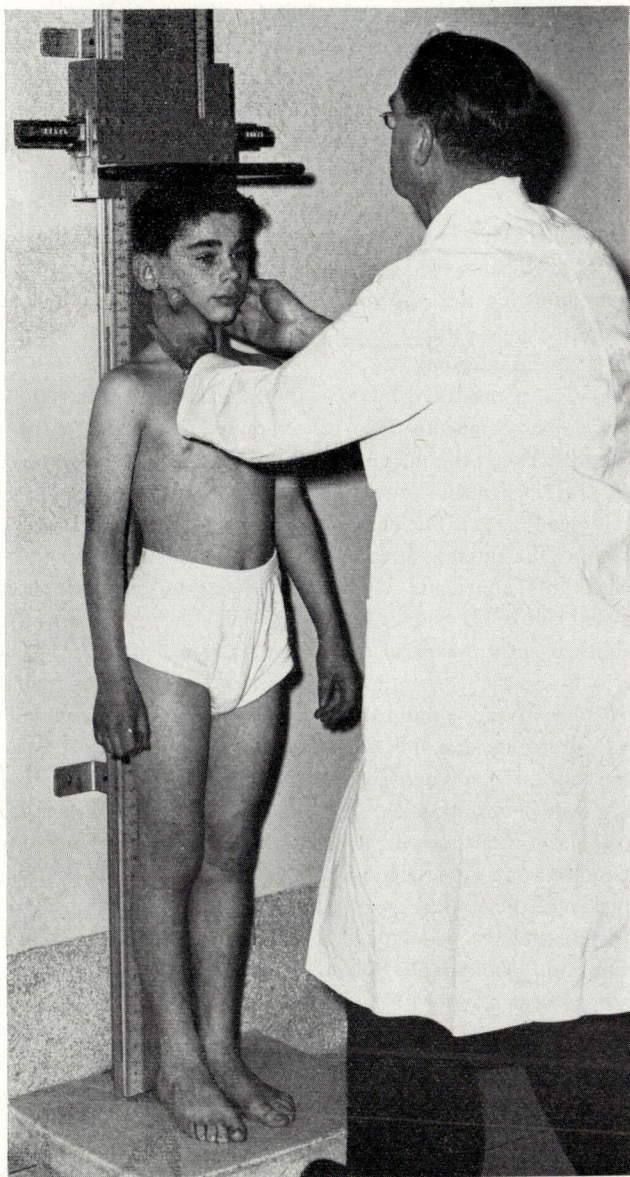

FIG. 32. Measurement of stature.

minimises the variation in height which occurs from morning to evening, which can otherwise be as much as 2 cm. Stature and supine length should be recorded to the last completed mm.

Weight is easier to measure than stature but much less useful, since it consists of a conglomerate of all the tissues, which, as we have seen, do not all have the same growth curves. Thus if a child is putting on weight, this may be because of muscular and skeletal growth or fat growth only. Failure to gain weight, or actual loss of weight in an older child, may signify nothing except a better attention to diet and exercise, whereas failure to gain height or muscle would call for an immediate investigation. Some children and adults who are 'over-weight' by the traditional weight-for-height tables are simply athletes with heavy muscles. If one wants to assess how fat a child is, the best thing is to measure the amount of subcutaneous fat directly.

Weight should be taken in the nude or with the child wearing only a standard gown or pair of light pants the weight of which is known and can be allowed for (preferably by adjusting the zero of the machine). The standards are for nude weight. A beam balance without loose weights should be used, and it should be regularly checked and adjusted.

Subcutaneous fat is measured by the skinfold technique. At certain sites in the body the skin and subcutaneous tissue can be pulled up away from the underlying muscle in a fold between the measurer's thumb and forefinger. Special constant-pressure calipers (Harpenden skinfold calipers) are then applied to the fold and the reading taken (see Fig. 33). The most reliable sites are over the triceps, under the scapula and above the anterior superior iliac spine; standards for the first two have been published by Tanner and Whitehouse (1962) and an example is given in Fig. 34. The left side of the body is used for all one-sided measurements, following a long-established anthropological convention. The exact location of the sites to pick up the folds and the technique of measurement are very important if comparison is to be made with the skinfold standard; the error between observers is greater for these measurements than for the other body measurements discussed here. Before embarking on skinfold measurements the anthropometrist should seek a brief training from someone skilled in the technique. Not all babies and children give a valid skinfold measurement; some are so fat that a true double fold cannot be properly pulled away from the muscle. When this is so, the measurement should be abandoned since the reading is spurious.

Further details of how to take all the measurements cited here are given in Falkner (1960) and photographs showing the technique are in Tanner (1964). Sitting height is best taken with an anthropometer, the child stretching to his maximum, aided by gentle pressure from the observer; crown-rump is measured instead up till age 2. Head circumference may be required in infancy for special diagnostic purposes. It is taken with a metal or plastic tape (linen tapes stretch): Standards will be found in Westrupp and Barber (1956).

In reporting growth data confusion still arises between means referring to children all aged, say, exactly 6·0, children aged 6·0 to 6·99, and children aged

5·5 to 6·49. The best terminology is to label the means of these age groups 6·0, 6+ and 6± respectively.

Charts exist in which limits of expected weight for height at a given age are displayed, or log weight for height. Tables of ratios such as weight/height, or

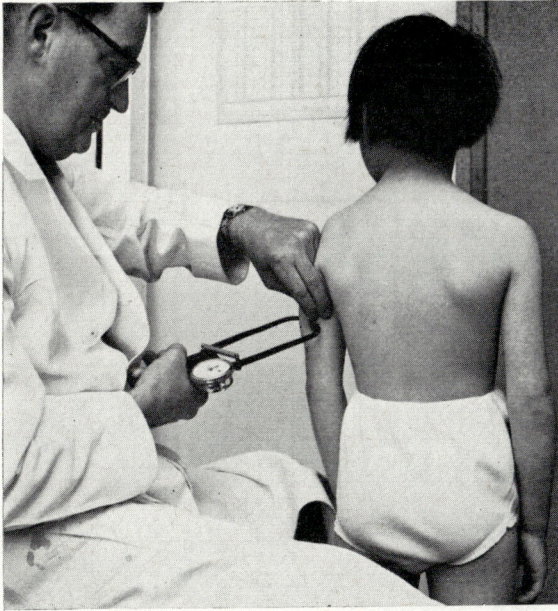

FIG. 33. Measurement of triceps skinfold.

$\sqrt[3]{\text{Wt.}}/\text{Ht.}$ have also been reported. In general it suffices, however, to consider the percentile positions of the child for height and for weight separately; any discrepancy between the two is then obvious. The next step is to look at the percentiles for skinfolds to see if the child is very fat or thin. Some guide to the amount of muscle may be found in considering arm circumference less the triceps skinfold.

Growth during Infancy

In the returns of the Registrar-General 'infancy' refers to the first year of life; in the school system 'infants' is a term characterising children aged 5 to 7 years; and in legal parlance 'infancy' extends from birth till age 18. From the point of view of growth and development the first year after birth constitutes a somewhat special period, as does the second year also, though to a lesser extent. Growth is most rapid during this time, though steadily decelerating, and the correlations of length and weight from one age to the next are lower than subsequently, indicating that more children are changing position relative to each other. Recognition of pathologically small children in child health clinics during this period of life would result in better treatment of growth hormone failure and other conditions, now usually only recognised at school entry. Recognition must depend on length measurements as well as weight however. Changes in body composition are also more marked than later, body water decreasing and protein concentration increasing. After the initial

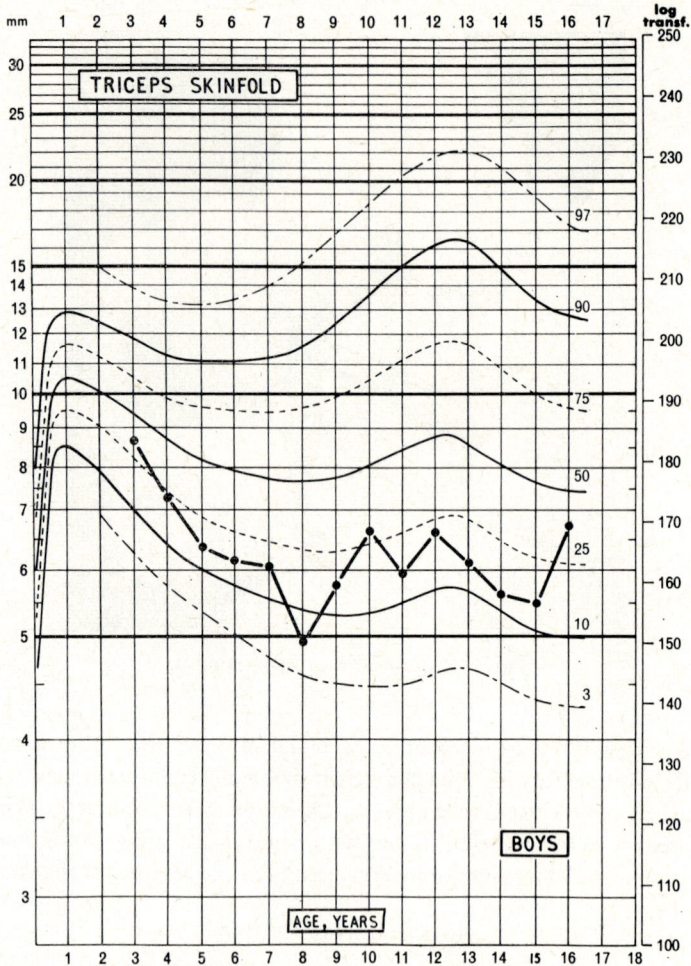

FIG. 34. Standards for triceps skinfold for boys (from Tanner and Whitehouse, 1962), with normal boy plotted.

loss in the newborn period the infant gains on average 4·5 kg. (10 lb.) during the first six months. There is a small negative correlation between birth weight and weight gain in the first 6 months, and also between birth length and gain in length (Tanner, 1963). Thus on average small babies tend to catch up the others, and large babies to slow down. (The idea that an infant should double or treble his birth weight by particular ages is misleading.) During the second 6 months the gain averages about 2·5 kg. (5½ lb.).

Supine length at birth (singletons at term) averages about 51 cm. in males and 50 cm. in females (or 20 in. and 19½ in.). The range is approximately 4 cm. either side of this. The average gain in length for boys is about 8 cm. in the first 3 months, 6 cm. in the second 3 months, and 9·5 cm. during the subsequent 6 months.

THE HEAD. At birth, 6 fontanelles are normally present, the large anterior and small occipital fontanelles lying in the midline and the small paired fontanelles (the sphenoidal and mastoid) lying in relation to the antero-inferior and postero-inferior angles of the parietal bone respectively. They represent sheets of membrane (persisting parts of the membranous skeleton). Of these the anterior fontanelle is of principal interest clinically, since its size, tension, and time of closure may be modified by disease. Thus increased intracranial pressure in infancy will be recognisable by bulging or tension of the fontanelle, and when acting over a long period will increase the size and shape of the bony aperture; rickets and cretinism will delay closure. Even in health, however, there is wide individual variation in the age at which the fontanelle is no longer clinically patent. Aisenson (1950) in a series of 1,677 New York infants found that the age of closure varied from 4 to 26 months and that the mean age of closure was 13·5 months. In infants included in the Oxford Child Health Survey, however, Acheson and Jefferson (1954) found that the mean age of clinical closure was slightly later, viz. 16·3 months (boys) and 18·8 months (girls). Mean age of radiological closure was 17·9 and 19·7 months respectively.

Circumference of the head increases extremely rapidly during infancy, the increase reflecting the general growth of nervous tissue shown in Fig. 19. The average circumference at birth of 34·6 cm. (13½ in.) increases by approximately 5 cm. (2 in.) during the first 3 months and by a further 3·2 cm. (1¼ in.) during the second 3 months; at 12 months the mean circumference is 46·6 cm. (18·3 in.) and during the second year a further increase of 2·5 cm. (1 in.) occurs. Measurements of girls are on the average slightly less than those of boys at all ages, the difference being about 1 cm. (½ in.) from 6 months to 2 years of age (Meredith, 1946).

The Pre-school Period

From the age of 2 to 5 years, growth proceeds more slowly than during infancy with an average annual increment of approximately 2 to 2·25 kg. (4½ to 5 lb.) in weight and a slightly decelerating increase in height (approximately 9 cm. (3½ in.) between 2 and 3 years of age, and 6 cm. (2½ in.) between 4 and 5 years). The increase in height, however, coupled with the loss of subcutaneous fat, is often sufficient to give the child a thinner appearance and to cause parental concern unless it is pointed out that it is normal for the rounded contours of infancy to be gradually replaced by the more linear ones of childhood during this phase of development. Although the pre-school child is less vulnerable than the infant, he is exposed to a wider range of risks, particularly infections, and growth may be affected by adverse environmental conditions during this period.

Childhood and Adolescence

During the early school period (5 years to onset of puberty) the child shows a slight increase of annual weight increment and a slightly falling height increment. The growth of lymphoid tissue at this time often results in the tonsils being regarded as abnormally large when they are in fact following their course of physiological development.

At puberty a spurt in growth and a change in body composition occurs, as detailed in the next chapter.

Developmental Age: Fast and Slow Tempo of Growth

The chronological age of a child described in terms of time-since-birth is used as a yardstick in defining his date of entry and exit from the educational system, his capacity to undertake employment, his liability to military service, and his capacity to assume civil responsibility including marriage. Yet if a hundred boys, of, say, exactly 14 years of age are grouped together, it will be immediately obvious that there are enormous differences between them, not only with regard to size but also in respect of development as evidenced by musculature, pitch of voice, and development of body hair. If a group of a hundred girls of the same age is added, the developmental differences become even more striking. At the lower end of the scale one may well have a boy who would be mistaken for a child of 10 or 11, and at the other end a girl who would pass for a mature woman. Although the differences are most obvious in the early teens, owing to the widely varying age of onset of puberty and the appearance of secondary sexual characters, they are also recognisable in large groups of infants or children in any one age group. As early as 1908, Crampton put forward the view that 'physiological age' or developmental age, as distinct from chronological age, was a fundamental concept in studying children. Boas named this difference between individuals in rate of development '*tempo of growth*' (see Tanner, 1959). Some play out their childhood slowly, and come late to puberty; others travel 'allegro' and enter puberty early. The differences of age at puberty are illustrated in Fig. 45 in the next chapter.

There are numerous possible measures of developmental age that are applicable throughout part or all of the period of growth. They range from the number of erupted teeth to the percentage of water in muscle cells. The various developmental 'age' scales do not necessarily coincide, and each has its particular use. The most generally useful, however, is skeletal maturity or bone age.

SKELETAL MATURITY. Skeletal maturity is a measure of how far the bones of an area have progressed toward maturity, not in size but in shape and in their relative positions one to another, as seen in a radiograph. The sequence of changes of shape through which each of the bone centres and epiphyses passes is the same in all individuals. Skeletal maturity is judged both from the number of centres present and from the stage of development of each.

In principle any or all parts of the skeleton could be used to give an assessment of skeletal maturity, but in practice the hand and wrist form the most convenient area and the one generally used. The hand is an area where a large number of bones and epiphyses develop, and a radiograph of it is easily made without exposing the remainder of the body to measurable doses of radiation. It itself requires only a very small dose of X-rays (Garn, Helmrich, Flaherty, and Silverman, 1967). This is of the order of 4 millirads, a figure which should be compared with the amount received from unavoidable everyday background radiation, which is 100 millirads per year at sea level rising to 300 millirads at 2,000 metres. There is no evidence that 4 millirads does any harm whatever; indeed it would be surprising if it did, since it represents the dose obtained unavoidably by every child who spends a week on holiday in the mountains.

For the radiograph the left hand is used, placed flat on an X-ray cassette with the palm down and the tube positioned 30 inches above the knuckle of the middle finger. The skeletal maturity assessment is made by comparing the given radiograph with a set of standards. There are two ways in which this may be done. In the older 'atlas' method, the radiograph is matched successively with the standard Greulich–Pyle (1959) plates representing ages 5·0, 6·0, and so on. The age of the standard with which the radiograph most nearly coincides is recorded as the skeletal 'age', interpolation between standards being made if it is thought to be justifiable. In the more recently developed 'maturity points' method (see Acheson, 1966) a series of standard stages is given for each individual bone, independent of age, and each bone of the radiograph is assigned a score corresponding to the stage it has reached. The scores are mathematically weighted to produce the best overall estimate of total maturity. The scores for the individual bones are added; thus the whole hand radiograph scores a total of so many weighted maturity points. This score is then compared with the range of scores of a standard group of children of the same age and a percentile status is assigned, just as it would be for height. A skeletal age may also be assigned, this being simply the age at which the given score lies at the fiftieth percentile. This method is somewhat finer in gradation and easier to use than the atlas method, although it is slightly more time-consuming. The standards are those of Tanner, Whitehouse and Healy (1962), and it must be remembered that they are based on a large random sample of Scottish urban and rural children, who are 6 to 9 months less advanced than the North American well-off middle-class children on whom the Greulich–Pyle method was standardised. Thus the two methods do not lead to the same result in terms of bone age, unless a correction is made.

In the Greulich–Pyle standard, boys and girls have a different series of plates, since the girls are more advanced. The Tanner–Whitehouse stages for each individual bone are common to both sexes, and the sequence of appearance and development of one bone relative to another in the hand is also closely similar. Hence in this method only one set of standards is used. The skeletal maturity score at any given chronological age is simply higher for girls than for boys (Fig. 35).

Skeletal maturity provides a true common scale of development, which measures such as 'height age', sometimes used by paediatricians, and indeed IQ, fail to do.

This is because every healthy individual reaches the same skeletal maturity eventually. The skeletal score represents a 'per cent of maturity attained'; thus a low score for age can be unequivocally taken to signify retardation in the true sense of delay in

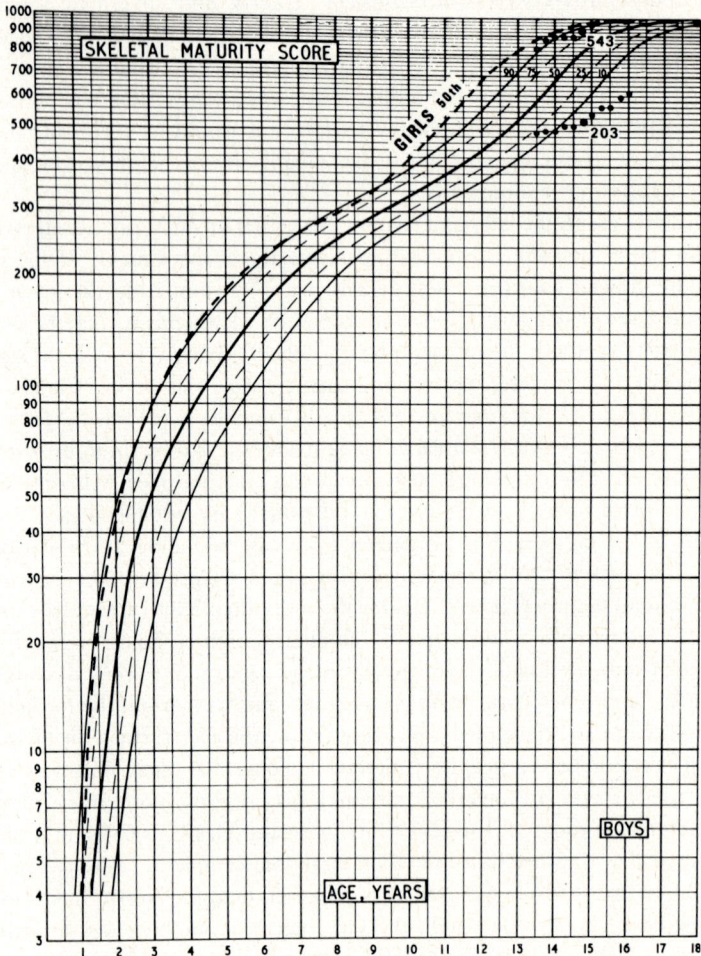

FIG. 35. Tanner-Whitehouse skeletal maturity standards for boys. Dashed line shows the 50th percentile for girls. The dots show skeletal maturity scores from 13½ onwards of the early- and late-maturing boys represented in Fig. 45 at age 14.75. The larger dots represent the age illustrated in Fig. 45 (from Tanner, 1969).

skeletal maturing. Final adult height or final IQ, on the other hand, varies from individual to individual. For this reason height age and mental age are more closely related to final height and final IQ than to advancement/retardation. Hence height ages cannot be validly compared from one individual to another as a measure of maturity status.

Standards are available for skeletal development of the pelvis and knee and ankle, besides the hand and wrist. Indeed, at ages under 1 year the knee and ankle provide better estimates of maturity than the hand, and in work upon infants and newborns the stages described by Vincent and Hugon (1962) should be used with locally derived norms.

DENTAL MATURITY. Dental maturity can be obtained by counting the number of teeth erupted and relating this to standard figures in much the same way as skeletal maturity. The deciduous dentition erupts from about 6 months to 2 years of age

TABLE 7

Deciduous dentition		Date of eruption
Central incisors	upper lower	8th month
Lateral incisors	upper lower	10th month
First molars		12th month
Canines		18th month
Second molars		24th month

TABLE 8

Permanent dentition		Date of eruption
First molars	lower	6th year
	upper	6th–7th year
Central incisors	lower	6th–7th year
	upper	6th–7th year
Lateral incisors	lower	7th–8th year
	upper	8th–9th year
First pre-molars	upper	10th year
Canines	lower	10th–11th year
First pre-molars	lower	11th year
Second pre-molars	upper	10th–12th year
Canines	upper	11th–12th year
Second pre-molars	lower	11th–12th year
Second molars		12th year
Third molars		17th–25th year

and can be used during this period. The permanent or second dentition provides a measure from about 6 to 13 years. From 2 to 6 and from 13 on little information is obtainable from the teeth by simple counting, but stages of calcification of teeth as seen in jaw radiographs can be used in just the same way as calcification in the bones of the hand and wrist. The average ages of eruption of deciduous and permanent teeth are given in Tables 7 and 8.

RELATIONS BETWEEN DIFFERENT MEASURES OF MATURITY. Skeletal maturity is closely related to the age at which adolescence occurs, that is, to maturity measured by secondary sex character development. Thus the range of chronological age within which menarche may normally fall is about 10 to $16\frac{1}{2}$ years, but the corresponding range of skeletal age is only 12 to $14\frac{1}{2}$.

Furthermore, children tend to be consistently advanced or retarded in maturity during their whole growth period, or at any rate after about age 3. Thus girls with an early menarche are skeletally advanced not only at the age at which menarche takes place, but at previous ages too. The correlation between menarcheal age and skeletal age at menarche itself is about 0·85, and between menarcheal age and skeletal age at chronological age 5 or 6 is about 0·55. The correlation becomes less the further back in growth one goes.

Dental maturity partly shares in this general skeletal and bodily maturation. At all ages from 6 to 13 children who are advanced skeletally have on average more erupted teeth than those who are skeletally retarded. Likewise those who have an early adolescence on average erupt their teeth early (see also Garn, Lewis and Kerewsky, 1965a). Girls on average have more erupted teeth than boys of the same age.

But this relationship is not a very close one. Quantitatively it is the relative independence of teeth and general skeletal development which should be emphasised. This is not surprising, in that the teeth are part of the head of the organism, and as we have already seen, the head is advanced over the rest of the body and for this reason its growth curve and growth control differ somewhat from the general growth curve.

Evidently there is some general factor of bodily maturity throughout growth, creating a tendency for a child to be advanced or retarded as a whole; in his skeletal ossification, in the percentage attained of his eventual size, in his permanent dentition, doubtless in his physiological reactions, and possibly in his intelligence test results also. But not too much should be made of this general factor. It should be especially noted how very limited is the loading, so to speak, of brain growth in it. There is little justification in the facts of physical growth and development for the concept of 'organismic age' in which almost wholly disparate measures of developmental maturity are lumped together.

Set under this general tendency are groups of more limited maturities, which vary independently of it and of each other. The teeth constitute two of these limited areas (primary and secondary dentition being largely independent of each other); the ossification centres another; the brain at least one more. Some of the mechanisms behind these relations can be dimly seen. In children who lack adequate thyroid gland secretion, for example, tooth eruption, skeletal development, and brain organisation are all retarded; whereas in children with precocious puberty, whether due to a brain disorder or a disease of the adrenal gland, there is advancement of skeletal and genital maturity without any corresponding effect upon the teeth or, as far as we can tell, upon the progression of organisation of the brain.

SEX DIFFERENCES IN DEVELOPMENTAL AGE. Girls are on average ahead of boys in skeletal maturity from birth till adulthood, and in dental maturity also during the whole of the permanent dentition eruption (though not, curiously, in primary dentition). It would seem therefore that the sex difference lies in the general maturity factor (as well as in various more detailed factors). Girls are usually ahead of boys in motor development also and in certain forms of aptitude tests.

The skeletal age difference begins during fetal life, the male retradation being due, probably indirectly, to the action of genes on the Y-chromosome. Children with the abnormal chromosome constitution XXY (Klinefelter's syndrome) have a skeletal maturity indistinguishable from the normal XY male, and children with the chromosome constitution XO (Turner's syndrome) have skeletal maturities approximating to the normal female XX, at least until puberty. The male retardation may be established as early as the differentiation of testis or ovary, or, more probably, it may be caused by the secretion by the fetal gonads or adrenals of sex-specific hormones. At birth boys are about four weeks behind girls in skeletal age, and from then till adulthood they remain about 80 per cent of the skeletal age of girls of the same chronological age. The percentage difference in dental age is not so great, boys being about 95 per cent of the dental age of girls.

The sex difference is not precisely the same for all bones, nor for all teeth. There is a sex-bone and sex-tooth interaction. Thus in girls the canines erupt on average 11 months earlier than in boys, whereas the first molars erupt only two months earlier. Similar effects are seen in skeletal ossification, particularly in knee and elbow (Garn, Rohmann, and Blumenthal, 1966).

The sex difference in skeletal maturity is not confined to man but occurs in chimpanzees, gorillas, and rhesus monkeys, and in rats also.

DEVELOPMENTAL AGE AND THE PREDICTION OF ADULT HEIGHT. The age at which growth ceases is related much more closely to the age at which adolescence occurs than to chronological age. After the age of 9 the amount of growth left to occur, and hence final adult stature, can be predicted better by reference to skeletal age than to chronological age. This can sometimes be of practical educational or social importance. For example, girls usually enter the Royal Ballet School at 9 or 10 years old, and thereafter they undergo a very rigorous and specialised training and are vocationally oriented to becoming dancers. But the exigencies of the corps de ballet require that the dancers shall all be within certain rather narrow height limits. If a girl grows up to be too short or too tall her career may be over. We cannot as yet control the extent to which children grow—and perhaps we should not when we can—but we can at least warn on entry those whose chances of ending between the required height limits are statistically rather small. The prediction of adult height requires knowledge of chronological age, bone age, and present height. We use either the Greulich–Pyle atlas for bone age and then the Bayley–Pinneau (1952) tables, or the Tanner–Whitehouse skeletal maturity and an associated multiple regression equation. The accuracy is such that 90 per cent of predictions from age 9 on lie within $\pm 1\frac{1}{2}$ inches of true final height. This is rather better than predictions based on height of parents.

Local, Hormonal, Genetic and Environmental Factors Controlling Growth

Local Factors

Vascular abnormalities operative during the growth period are liable to increase or diminish growth of the affected part. Thus binding the feet of Chinese girls resulted in abnormally small feet, whereas the increased blood supply to a limb with an arteriovenous aneurysm may cause overgrowth of the limb (Fig. 36). The

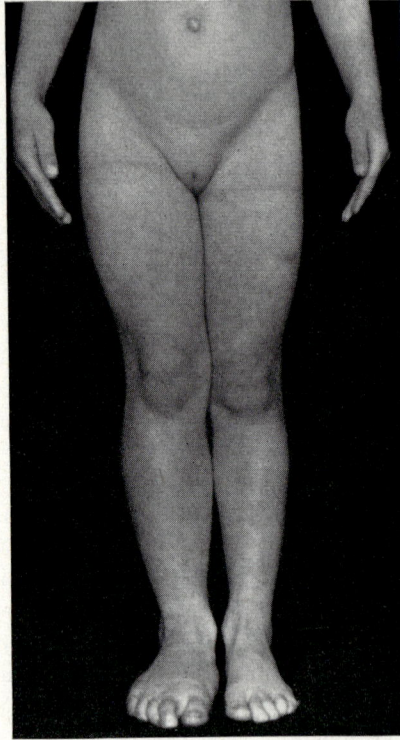

FIG. 36. Overgrowth of the right lower extremity due to arterio-venous aneurysm.

mechanism of this latter effect is not understood; it may well be that the increased pressure of blood in some way causes increase in size of cells, perhaps by effects on membrane permeability. Local hydrodynamic factors are known to affect growth of mouse fetuses (Healy, McLaren, and Michie, 1960). A certain percentage of children with low birth weight and subsequent short stature have one side (or part of a side) of the body noticeably larger than the other (Silver's syndrome, see Tanner and Ham, 1969); whether this is due to hydrodynamic factors operating in utero is not known, nor whether cell size or cell number is affected.

If the nerve supply to a part is defective, for example following poliomyelitis, the part affected—for example a leg—may grow less than the symmetrical part. Again the mechanism is not understood.

Transverse lines of increased density occur at the ends of the long bones in many children. They may follow a general infection; but may also appear apparently unrelated to any disease. Most disappear as growth proceeds. The exact way in which they are formed is still not clear (see Marshall, 1968).

Endocrine Factors

The endocrine glands are of great importance in the control of growth and development, being one of the chief agents for translating the instructions of the genes into the reality of the adult form, at the pace and with the result permitted by the available environment.

The hormones particularly concerned in growth are thyroxine from the thyroid gland, cortisol and adrenal androgens from the cortex of the adrenal gland, testosterone from the Leydig cells of the testes, oestrogens from the ovary, insulin from the islets of Langerhans in the pancreas and growth hormone from the pituitary gland. The pituitary in addition produces thyroid-stimulating hormone (TSH), adrenocorticotrophic hormone (ACTH), and at least two gonadotrophic hormones.

THYROID HORMONE begins to be secreted by the fetal pituitary around the fifteenth to twentieth week probably under the stimulus of fetal TSH. It affects protein synthesis in the brain of the fetus and young child and is necessary for the brain's normal development. In its absence nerve cell bodies, dendrites and axons are reduced in size, and the number of connections between dendrites is decreased. These changes are irreversible if they persist for very long. During childhood, so far as growth is concerned the action of thyroid hormone is permissive and not controlling. In hypothyroidism, growth in size and skeletal, dental and intellectual maturity are all delayed. The rate of secretion appears to drop gradually during the first 2 years after birth and then remains practically constant till adolescence.

GROWTH HORMONE. The most important hormone controlling growth from birth till adolescence is pituitary growth hormone or somatotrophin. This is a polypeptide which has a greater degree of species (or really order) specificity than other pituitary hormones. Consequently only human or monkey growth hormone has a growth-stimulating effect in man. It seems that growth hormone is not secreted continuously, but in response to a variety of stimuli, chiefly a drop in blood sugar and a rise in blood alpha-amino-acids. Exercise and emotion are also associated with increases in blood hormone level. The fetus probably secretes greater amounts of growth hormone than the child. Nothing is yet known about variation in secretion rates with age in childhood, or whether the level rises at adolescence and is part cause of the adolescent growth spurt. It used to be said that secretion started at 2 to 3 years only, but this is now known to be wrong; children who lack the ability to secrete growth hormone usually grow slowly and are small from birth onwards. An example of the growth of a girl lacking the hormone is shown in Fig. 27 above,

7

together with her response to administration of exogenous hormone. Her thyroid and adrenal functions were normal.

Growth hormone causes the incorporation of amino-acids into tissues to form new protein. In experimental animals it specifically causes growth in muscle and other non-fatty tissue; control animals fed the same amount and not given the hormone put on more fat and less protein. The same is almost certainly true in man.

ADRENAL GLANDS. The amount of cortisol and mineralo-corticoids secreted increases during childhood in proportion to the increase in body size, but no more. The role of cortisol in normal growth is not known; at normally encountered levels it may have little effect. But excessive amounts of cortisol or allied substances (cortisone, prednisone, etc.), either secreted in response to chronic stress or given by a paediatrician for intractable asthma or other disease, have a powerful growth-retarding effect. This is manifested by small size and delayed bone age, and cannot be counteracted by growth hormone. Amounts of steroid equivalent to 15 mg. cortisone a day are sufficient to have this effect in the pre-school and school child.

The androgenic hormones secreted by the adrenal are chiefly dehydroepiandrosterone and its sulphate and 11 β-hydroxyandrosterone; in peripheral blood androsterone sulphate is also found. These substances are secreted during all childhood in most children (see Tanner and Gupta, 1968) but only in small quantities before puberty. Their function before puberty is obscure. Their role at puberty is discussed in the next chapter.

It is possible that differences between individuals in tempo of growth are wholly or partly due to small differences in habitual hormonal balance, but our techniques at present are not sufficiently sensitive to be able to detect these.

Most endocrine glands secrete their hormones in response to the stimulus of an activating hormone from the pituitary gland. Thus thyroxine is secreted in response to pituitary thyroid-stimulating hormone, cortisol in response to adrenocorticotrophic hormone, and so on. The pituitary hormones are themselves secreted in response to the arrival of specific releaser substances originating in nearby areas of the brain, chiefly the median eminence of the hypothalamus. The releaser substances, in turn, are secreted or switched off in response to certain defined stimuli, in some cases a drop or rise in the level of the hormone in the blood, sensed by specialised cells also in the hypothalamus. Thus a feedback circuit is established: sensor-releaser-pituitary hormone-peripheral hormone-sensor. Outside influences can play on the circuit, particularly at the junctions peripheral hormone-sensor, and sensor-releaser. Thus nervous impulses from other parts of the brain may alter the threshold of the sensor. The way puberty is believed to be initiated provides an example. Before puberty the sensor for oestrogen is set so it responds by discontinuing the release of FSH when blood oestrogen is still at a very low level. Then impulses arrive which diminish the sensitivity of the sensor so that now it only responds to a high level of oestrogen. In consequence FSH is not switched off, blood oestrogen rises, and development of the breasts and uterus occurs. Influences from outside the organism affect endocrine function as a rule by this type of action. It is believed, for example, that severe psychological stress may cause dwarfism in certain children by switching off their secretion of growth hormone. This may be either by affecting the sensor or by raising the threshold at which the neural growth hormone releaser is secreted.

Some hormones are released usually or sometimes without the full circuit being involved. There is good evidence that a rise in the level of blood thyroxine is sensed directly at the pituitary level, switching off the secretion of TSH immediately, rather than at the level of the hypothalamus.

Regulation of Growth; Canalisation and Catch-up

It is thought that the processes of growth are self-stabilising, or, to take another analogy, 'target-seeking'. Children, no less than rockets, have their trajectories, governed by the control systems of their genetical constitution and powered by energy absorbed from the natural environment. Deflect the child from his growth trajectory by acute malnutrition or illness, and a restoring force develops so that as soon as the missing food is supplied or the illness terminated the child catches up toward his original curve. When he gets there, he slows down again to adjust his path onto the old trajectory once more.

The property of returning to the original growth curve after being pushed off trajectory has been called canalisation by Waddington (1957). The unusually large velocity occurring during this process has been named 'catch-up' by Prader, Tanner and von Harnack (1963). An example is given in Fig. 27 above; a similar catch-up occurs when, for example, a state of malnutrition is corrected or a cortisol-producing tumour is removed. The velocity during a period of catch-up may reach three or more times the average velocity for the chronological age. The allied term 'compensatory growth' is normally used to refer to growth of organs or parts rather than to the whole animal and describes a different phenomenon. Thus when one kidney is removed the other undergoes compensatory growth or hypertrophy; when a limb of an amphibian is removed, it, or something similar, may grow again and this also may be called compensatory growth (see Goss, 1964).

The mechanism of canalisation is at present very little understood. Females are better canalised than males, in respect of most characters, in man and all other mammals that have been investigated. Thus girls slow their growth less in response to malnutrition or disease than boys (see Tanner, 1962, p. 127).

The earlier and the more prolonged the stress, the more difficult it is for regulation to be fully effective in restoring the pre-stress situation. Rats may be malnourished from birth till 21 days by being placed in an over-numerous litter so that the mother's milk is insufficient. At weaning (21 days postbirth) they are smaller than well-fed rats. If after weaning they are allowed unlimited access to food, they do show a catch-up, but it is insufficient to bring them up to the size of the well-fed rats; they remain small throughout their lives (Widdowson and McCance, 1960). If, in contrast, rats are malnourished from 21 days to 77 days and then fed without restriction, a complete catch-up in weight occurs by 133 days in females and a very nearly complete one in males (Widdowson, Mavor, and McCance, 1964). It must be remembered that the rat is born very early compared with the human, and the human equivalent to the rat suckling-period starvation is starvation *in utero*.

The evidence leads us to suppose that it is both the duration of the malnutrition and the magnitude of the normal rate of growth at the time the malnutrition is applied that determine whether a full catch-up is possible. If true, this means that the critical factor is the amount of unsatisfied growth potential accumulated. A possible mechanism for growth regulation has been elaborated elsewhere (Tanner, 1963).

Heterochrony and Dysharmonic Development

The multitude of chemical reactions going on during differentiation and growth demands the greatest precision in linkage. Thus for normal acuity of vision to occur the growth of the lens of the eye has to be harmonised closely with the growth in depth of the eye-ball, so that the point of focus of the light rays lies exactly on the retina. It is small wonder that the success of this co-ordination varies, and most people are just a little farsighted or nearsighted.

The regulative forces harmonising the velocity of growth of one part with that of another do not always succeed, even in arriving within an acceptable area around the target. If the original genetic forces begin by being too unbalanced, as in trisomy, normal development cannot occur.

Variation in the speed of development of different structures and functions (heterochronisms) underlie many individual differences in bodily structure. Examples are the longer arms and legs relative to trunk in men as opposed to women, or in black as opposed to white races. It is an open question to what extent similar heterochronisms may explain differences in personality structure. Some psychological abnormalities or culturally excessive deviations from the average (analogous with an inconvenient degree of nearsightedness) may arise from insufficient harmonisation of the speeds at which different structures and functions develop. This could occur either for genetical reasons, the child carrying, by chance, a relatively dysharmonic set of genes, or for environmental reasons, the development of one area of the personality having been speeded up by external forces, perhaps early in childhood, while another was relatively retarded.

Sensitive or Critical Periods

The much-discussed critical periods are extreme examples of this linking of differential growth events. By 'critical period' is meant a certain stage of limited duration during which a particular influence, from another area of the developing organism, or from the environment, evokes a particular response. The response may be beneficial, indeed perhaps essential to normal development, or it may be pathological. The term 'sensitive period' is now displacing the term critical period. This describes the usual situation more accurately, since usually these periods consist of a number of hours, days or weeks during the beginning and end parts of which the organism is slightly sensitive to the specific influence, with a period of maximum sensitivity in the middle. It is not as a rule an all-or-none phenomenon.

An example of a sensitive period is the first to twelfth weeks of pregnancy during which a fetus is at risk from the presence of rubella virus in the mother. Another, normally occurring, example is in the differentiation of the brain in the rat into male or female type. During the first 5 days after birth the male rat's testes secrete testosterone or an allied hormone which causes the brain to be irrevocably differentiated as male. Experiments show that giving testosterone either before or after this limited period does not cause the effect; if testosterone secretion is prevented during these 5 days, then the brain differentiates, again irreversibly, as female (see Harris and Levine, 1965).

Interaction of Heredity and Environment in Controlling Growth

Rate of growth at any age is the outcome of the interaction of genetical and environmental factors. The genetical control of rate seems to be independent of the genetical control of final size and, to a large extent, of shape; and environmentally produced changes in rate do not necessarily produce any alteration in final physique. Size and shape are themselves to a large extent affected separately by genetical and environmental influences.

Final size and shape also reflect the continuous interaction of hereditary and environmental forces. It is a long way from the possession of a certain set of genes to the acquisition of a height of 6 feet or the development of the menarche at age 12·5. Furthermore, it is a truism in modern genetics that this interaction may be nonadditive. This means that bettering the nutrition by a fixed amount will not in principle produce an increase of 10 per cent, say, in the height of all persons but only in persons of certain 'susceptible' genotypes. It is therefore impossible to specify in general the relative importance of heredity and environment in contributing to the variance of a particular trait. The nearer optimal the environment, the more the genes have a chance to show their hand, it is true; but this is a general statement only and undoubtedly many subtle and specific interactions occur.

Hereditary factors are, however, clearly of immense importance in the control of growth. The fundamental plan is laid down very early. An immature limb-bud removed from a fetal or newborn mouse and implanted under the skin of an adult mouse of the same inbred strain will continue to develop until it closely resembles an adult bone. Furthermore, the cartilage scaffolding of the bone, removed at a stage preceding actual bone formation, will do the same (Felts, 1959). The structure of the adult bone, in all its essentials, is implicit in the cartilage model of months before. The later action of the bone's environment, represented by the muscles pulling on it and the joints connecting it to other bones, seems limited to the making of finishing touches.

Genetics of Growth

The genetical control of rate of growth is manifested most simply in the inheritance of age at menarche. Identical twin sisters growing up together under average West European economic conditions reach menarche an average of 2 months apart (see Tanner, 1962). Nonidentical twin sisters, with the same proportion of identical genes as ordinary sisters, reach menarche on average about 10 months apart. The sister–sister and mother–daughter correlation coefficients for menarcheal age are both about 0·4, which is only slightly below the same correlations for height. Thus a high proportion of the variability of age at menarche in populations living under European conditions is due to genetical causes. The inheritance is probably transmitted as much by the father as the mother, and is due not to a single gene, but to many genes, each of small effect.

This genetical control evidently operates throughout the whole process of growth, for the conclusions regarding age at menarche apply also to skeletal maturity at all

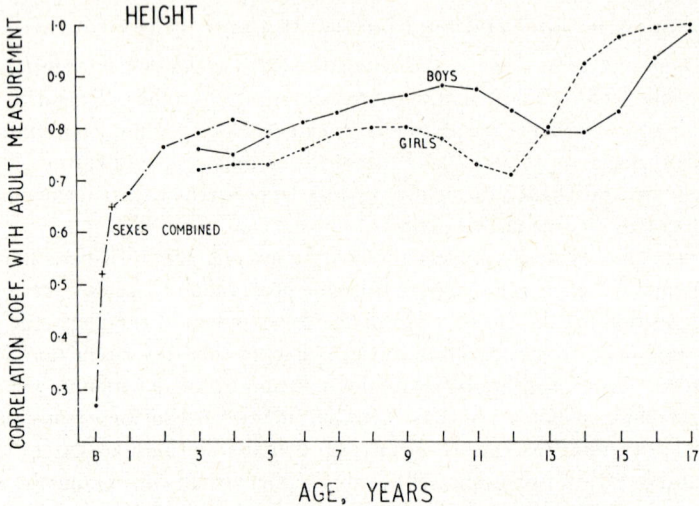

Fig. 37. Correlations between adult height and heights of the same individuals as children (from Tanner, 1962).

ages, and to the eruption of the teeth, both in age and in sequence (Garn, Lewis and Kerewsky, 1965a; Garn, Lewis and Polachek, 1960).

Not all genes are active at birth. Some are not switched on till later and some can express themselves only in the physiological surroundings provided by the later years of growth. The effects of the latter are said to be 'age-limited'.

This is the probable explanation of the curve described by the correlations between measurements of a child at successive ages and his measurements as an adult, which have been obtained in long-term longitudinal studies. The curves for height are illustrated in Fig. 37. The correlation of length at birth with adult height is very low, since birth weight reflects uterine conditions and not fetal genotype. The child's genes increasingly make themselves felt and the correlation rises steeply during the first 3 years. After this a small, steady rise occurs till adolescence; at this time the correlation for height drops, simply because some children are early and others late developers. If skeletal age is used instead of chronological age the correlation continues to rise gradually.

The correlation coefficients between the height of the parent and the height of the child at successive ages from birth describe very similar curves. The correlation when the child is born is about 0·25 and it then rises to reach a plateau by the time the child is about 3.

Race and Ecological Conditions

There are racial differences in rate and pattern of growth, leading to the racial differences seen in adult body build. Some of these are clearly genetically controlled, whereas others depend perhaps on climatic differences and certainly on nutritional ones (see Tanner, 1966a, for review).

We must suppose that in each of the major populations of the world the growth of its members was gradually adjusted, by means of selection, to the environmental conditions in which they evolved. We should be able to see the remnants of this process in modern populations—the remnants only, because relatively recent migrations have much altered the distributions of peoples, so that many no longer live in the areas in which they evolved. There is, in fact, a quite close positive relation between the linearity of peoples, as judged by their adult weight for height, and the average annual temperature of where they live (Roberts, 1953; Schreider, 1957).

Negroes are ahead of white races in skeletal ossification at birth. This probably reflects an inherited difference in hormone secretion during the late fetal period, for negroes' permanent teeth also erupt earlier, and the basis of these is laid down *in utero*, though later than the primary teeth, whose eruption differs less between the races. The negro child maintains his advancement (which is paralleled by advancement in motor development) for about 2 or 3 years if living in good economic circumstances. After this the African child comes to equal, or more usually to fall behind, the European in maturity. This may be a natural occurrence, the mean velocity curves of the two races having different shapes, just as do the velocity curves of males and females in both races. Or it may reflect simply the better nutrition of the European.

Season of the Year

In most European and American data a well-marked seasonal effect on velocity of growth can be seen. Growth in height is fastest in the spring and growth in weight fastest in the autumn. The average velocity of height in the March to May quarter may be almost twice that in the September to October quarter. Children differ surprisingly, however, both in the time of year at which they grow fastest, and in the degree to which they show the seasonal trend at all.

Nutrition

Malnutrition delays growth, as is shown from the effects of famine associated with war. In Fig. 38 the heights of children in Stuttgart, Germany, are plotted at each year of age from 1911 to 1953. There is a uniform increase at all ages from 1920 to 1940 (see discussion of secular trend following), but in the later years of both world wars the height drops as the food intake of the children becomes restricted.

Children subjected to an episode of acute starvation recover more or less completely by virtue of their regulative powers, provided the adverse conditions are not

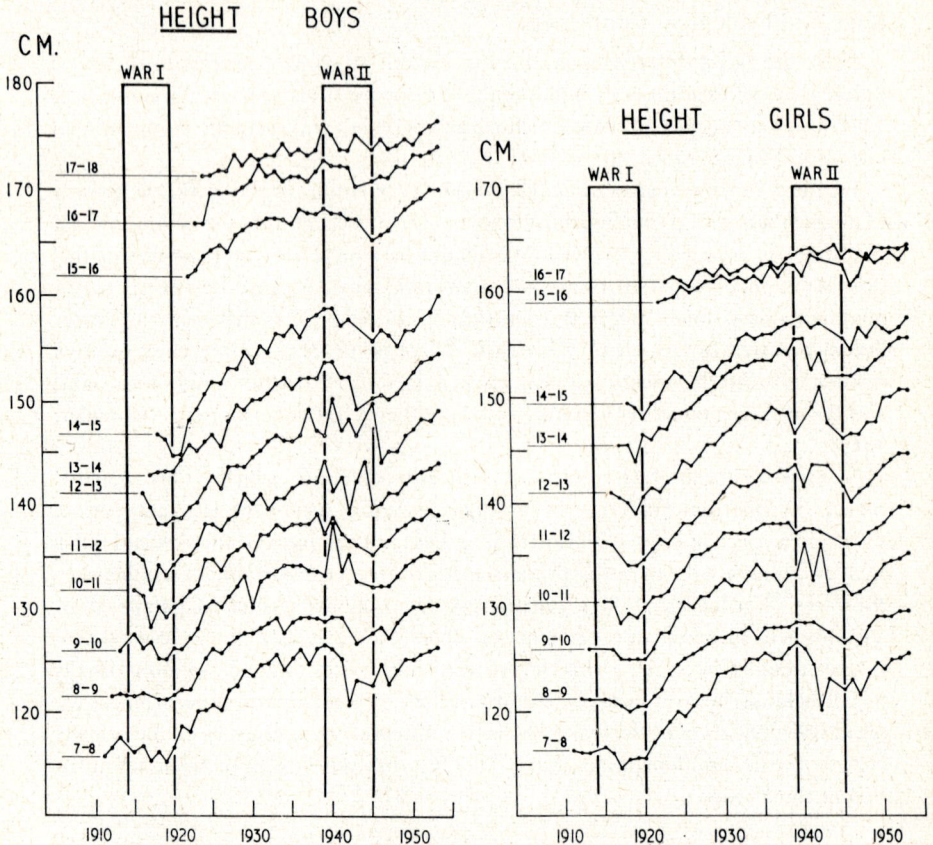

FIG. 38. Effect of malnutrition on growth in height. Heights of Stuttgart schoolchildren (7–8 to 14–15 Volkschule; 15–16 upwards, Oberschule) from 1911 to 1953. Lines connect points for children of same age and express secular trend and effect of war conditions (data from Howe and Schiller, 1952, and personal communication. From Tanner, 1962).

too severe and do not last too long. Chronic malnutrition is another affair. Most members of some populations, and some members of all populations, grow to be smaller adults than they should, because of chronic undernourishment during all or most of their childhood.

Disease

Minor and relatively short illnesses such as measles, influenza, antibiotic-treated middle ear infection, or even pneumonia cause no discernible retardation of growth rate in the great majority of well-nourished children (Tanner, 1962; Meredith and Knott, 1962). In children with a less adequate diet they may cause some disturbance, thought this has not been securely established. Often children with continuous colds, ear disease, sore throats, and skin infections are on average smaller than others, but inquiry reveals that they come from economically depressed and socially disorganised homes where proper meals are unknown and cleanliness too much trouble. The small size is more likely to be due to malnutrition than to the effects of the continued minor disease (Miller, Court, Walton and Knox, 1960).

Major diseases which take the child to a hospital for a month or more or keep him in bed at home for several months may cause considerable slowing down of growth, followed by a catch-up when the disease is cured. The mechanism of the retardation probably varies from one disease to another; in some an increased secretion of cortisol may be the cause.

Acheson (1966) thinks that even a relatively mild disease or subnutrition will cause the formation of new cartilage to slow down while permitting the turning of cartilage into bone to continue. Such an imbalance would result in a reduced final height. While this probably occurs in severe disorders, there is little evidence that it occurs in mild diseases or temporary undernutrition.

Psychological Disturbance

Really severe psychological stress seems capable of retarding growth. In a famous experiment, Widdowson (1951) studied (as she thought) the effects of increased rations on orphanage children living on the poor diet available in Germany in 1948. What she succeeded in showing was that the presence of a sadistic house-sister inhibited the children's growth, even in the face of adequate caloric intake.

Socio-economic Class: Number of Children in Family

Children from different socio-economic levels differ in average body size at all ages, the upper groups being larger (Tanner, 1962; Graffar and Corbier, 1966). In most studies socio-economic status has been defined according to father's occupation, though in recent years it is becoming clear that in many countries this does not distinguish people's living standards or style of living as well as formerly.

The difference in height between children of the professional and managerial classes and those of unskilled labourers in Britain is currently about 2·5 cm. (1 in.) at 3 years rising to 5 cm. (nearly 2 in.) at adolescence. In weight the difference is less, since the lower socio-economic class children have a greater weight for height, due to greater relative breadth of bone and muscles.

Part of the socio-economic height difference is due to earlier maturation of the well-off, though some is due to their being larger as adults. There is also the difference in height and weight of the child according to his number of siblings, his growth being slower the more siblings he has at home. The difference disappears when adulthood is reached (for full discussion see Tanner, 1966c).

The causes of the socio-economic differential are multiple and complex. Differences in nutrition are certainly important, and all the habits of regular meals, sleep, exercise, and general organisation that distinguish, from this point of view, a good home from a bad one. The growth differences are more related to home conditions than to the economic conditions of the families, and home conditions reflect to a considerable degree the intelligence and personality of the parents. It is perhaps therefore not altogether surprising that more intelligent children are at all ages taller than less intelligent children of the same occupational background. This association probably represents a complex mixture of environmental and genetical effects, the one reinforcing the other. There is evidence that the height differential between social classes in the adult population is kept in existence by a system of social mobility which for some reason produces an average movement of tall persons upward and short persons downward (Schreider, 1964; Tanner, 1966c).

Secular Trend

During the last hundred years there has been a striking tendency for children to become progressively larger at all ages (Tanner, 1966b). This is known as the 'secular trend'. The magnitude of the trend in Europe and America is such that it

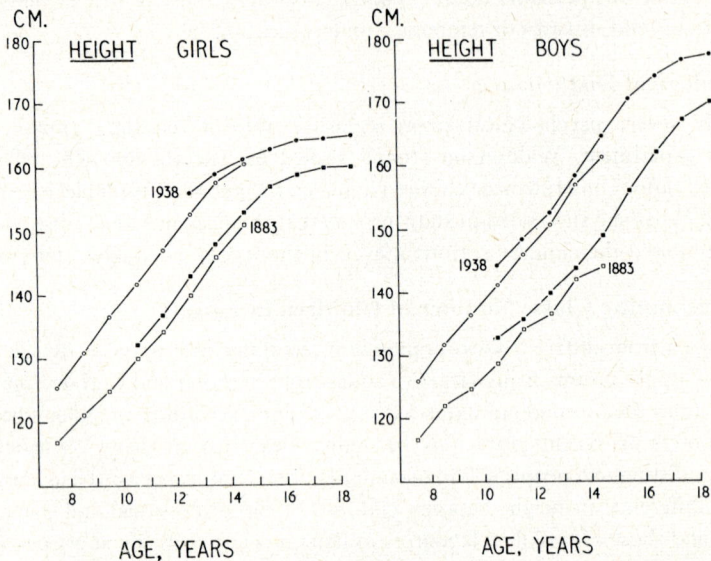

FIG. 39. Secular trend in increase of height. Height of Swedish girls and boys measured in 1883 and 1938–9. Elementary schools age 7–14, secondary schools 10–18. Distance curves, cross-sectional (data from Broman, Dahlberg and Lichtenstein, 1942. From Tanner, 1962).

dwarfs the differences between socio-economic classes. In Fig. 39 are plotted the heights of Swedish boys and girls measured in 1883 and 1938. The difference amounts to about 1½ years of growth. At the age when growth ceases, as shown by the 18-year-old girls in the figure, the secular trend is less than in childhood, but it still exists.

The data from Europe and America agree well: from about 1900, or a little earlier, to the present, children in average economic circumstances have increased in height at age 5 to 7 by about 1 to 2 cm. each decade, and at 10 to 14 by 2 to 3 cm. each decade. Pre-school data show that the trend starts directly after birth and may, indeed, be relatively greater from age 2 to 5 than subsequently. The trend started, at least in Britain, a considerable time ago, because Roberts, a factory physician, writing in 1876 said that 'a factory child of the present day at the age of

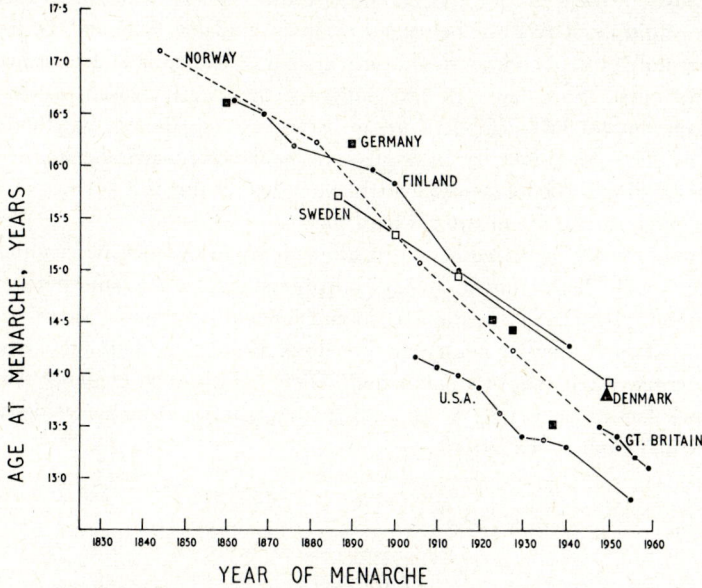

Fig. 40. Secular trend in age at menarche 1830–1960 (from Tanner, 1962, where sources given).

nine years weighs as much as one of 10 years did in 1833 . . . . each age has gained one year in forty years'. The trend in Europe is still continuing at the time of writing (1969) but there is some evidence to show that in the United States the best-off sections of the population are now growing up at something approaching the fastest possible speed.

During the same period there has been an upward trend in adult height, but to a considerably lower degree. One of the difficulties is that in earlier times final height was not reached till 25 years or later, whereas now it is reached at 18 or 19. Data do exist, however, which enable us to compare fully grown men at different periods. They lead to the conclusion that in Western Europe men increased in adult height little if at all from 1760 to 1830, about 0·3 cm. per decade from 1830 to 1880, and about 0·6 cm. per decade from 1880 to 1960. The trend is apparently still continuing in Europe.

Most of the trend toward greater size in children reflects a more rapid maturation; only a minor part reflects a greater ultimate size. The trend toward earlier maturing is best shown in the statistics on age at menarche. A selection of the best data is illustrated in Fig. 40 (the sources are detailed in Tanner, 1966*b*). The trend is about 4 months per decade since 1850 in average sections of Western European populations. Well-off persons show a trend of about half this magnitude, having never been so retarded in menarche as the worse-off. Details on average age of menarche of various populations and the methods for collecting these statistics will be found in Tanner (1966*b*).

The causes of the trend (or acceleration of growth as it is sometimes called) are probably multiple. Certainly better nutrition is a major one, and perhaps in particular more protein and calories in early infancy. A lessening of disease may also have contributed. Some authors have supposed that the increased psychosexual stimulation consequent on modern urban living has contributed, but there is no positive evidence for this. Girls in single-sex schools have menarche at exactly the same age as girls in coeducational schools, but whether this is a fair test of differences in psychosexual stimulation is hard to say.

The trend toward increased height in adults does not necessarily have the same causes. Probably better nutrition has contributed to it also, but there may in addition be a genetical explanation. If some degree of dominance occurs in genes increasing stature, then increased outbreeding, producing more heterozygotes, would increase the height of a population. There is increasing evidence that such dominance does in fact occur. As for outbreeding, that has been increasing steadily since the invention of the bicycle.

J. M. TANNER

References

ACHESON, R. M. (1954). A method of assessing skeletal maturity from radiographs. *J. Anat.*, 88, 498.

—— (1966). Maturation of the skeleton. In *Human Development*. Ed. F. Falkner. Philadelphia: Saunders.

—— and JEFFERSON, E. (1954). Some observations on closure of anterior fontanelle. *Arch. Dis. Childh.*, 29, 196.

AISENSON, M. R. (1950). Closing of anterior fontanelle. *Pediatrics*, 6, 223.

BAILEY, N. (1946). Tables for predicting adult height from skeletal age and present height. *J. Pediat.*, 28, 46.

BALDWIN, B. T. (1921). *Physical Growth of Children from Birth to Maturity*. Iowa City: Univ. Iowa Press.

BAYLEY, N. and PINNEAU, S. R. (1952). Tables for predicting adult height from skeletal age: revised for use with the Greulich-Pyle hand standards. *J. Pediat.*, 40, 423.

CLARK, W. E. LE GROS and MEDAWAR, P. B. (1945). (Ed.) *Essays on Growth and Form*. London: Oxford.

CLEMENTS, E. M. B. (1953). Changes in the mean stature and weight of British children over the past seventy years. *Brit. Med. J.*, 2, 897.

—— (1954). The age of children when growth in stature ceases. *Arch. Dis. Childh.*, 29, 147.

CRAMPTON, C. R. (1908). Physiological age—a fundamental principle. *Amer. phys. educ. Rev.* 13, nos. 3, 4, 5, 6 (also *Child Devel.*, 1944, 15, 3).

DEMING, J. (1957) Application of the Gompertz curve to the observed pattern of growth in length of 48 individual boys and girls during the adolescent cycle of growth. *Hum. Biol.*, **29**, 83.

—— and WASHBURN, A. H. (1963). Application of the Jenss curve to the observed pattern of growth during the first eight years of life in forty boys and forty girls. *Hum. Biol.*, **35**, 484.

ELLIS, R. W. B. (1946). Height and weight in relation to onset of puberty in boys. *Arch. Dis. Childh.*, **20**, 97.

—— (1948). Puberty growth of boys. *Ibid.*, **23**, 17.

FALKNER, F. (1960) (Ed.) Child development: an international method of study. *Ann. Paediat. Suppl.*, **72**, 237.

—— (1966) (Ed.) *Human Development*. Philadelphia: Saunders.

FELTS, W. J. L. (1959). Transplantation studies of factors in skeletal organogenesis. I. The subcutaneously implanted immature long-bone of the rat and mouse. *Am. J. phys. Anthrop.* N.S., **17**, 201.

GARN, S. M. HELMRICH, R. H., FLAHERTY, K. M. and SILVERMAN, F. N. (1967). Skin dosages in radiation-sparing techniques for the laboratory and field. *Am. J. phys. Anthrop.*, **26**, 101.

—— LEWIS, A. B. and KEREWSKY, R. S. (1965a). Genetic, nutritional and malnutritional correlates of dental development. *J. dent. Res.*, **44**, 228.

—— —— —— (1965b). X-linked inheritance of tooth size. *J. dent. Res.*, **44**, 439.

—— —— and POLACHECK, D. L. (1960). Sibling similarities in dental development. *J. dent. Res.*, **39**, 170.

—— ROHMANN, C. G. and BLUMENTHAL, T. (1966). Ossification sequence polymorphism and sexual dimorphism in skeletal development. *Am. J. phys. Anthrop.*, **24**, 101.

GOSS, R. J. (1964). *Adaptive Growth*. London: Logos.

GRAFFAR, M. and CORBIER, J. (1966). Contribution à l'étude de l'influence socio-économique sur la croissance et le développement de l'enfant. *Courrier*, **16**, 1.

GRUELICH, W. W. and PYLE, S. I. (1959). *Radiographic Atlas of Skeletal development of the Hand and Wrist*. 2nd ed. Stanford: Stanford Univ. Press.

HARRIS, H. A. (1933). *Bone Growth in Health and Disease*. London: Oxf. Univ. Press.

HARRIS, G. W. and LEVINE, S. (1965). Sexual differentiation of the brain and its experimental control. *J. Physiol.*, **181**, 379.

HEALY, M. J. R., McLAREN, A. and MICHIE, D. (1960). Foetal growth in the mouse. *Proc. Roy. Soc. B.*, **153**, 367.

MARSHALL, W. A. (1968). Problems in relating the presence of transverse lines in the radius to the occurrence of disease. *Sym. Soc. Study Hum. Biol.*, **8**, 245.

MEREDITH, H. V. (1946). Physical growth from birth to two years: II. Head circumference. *Child Develop.*, **17**, 1.

—— and KNOTT, V. B. (1962). Illness history and physical growth. III. Comparative anatomic status and rate of change for school children in different long-term health categories. *Am. J. Dis. Child.*, **103**, 146.

MERMINOD, A. and Internat. Childr. Center Paris (1962). (Ed.) The growth of the normal child during the first three years of life. *Modern Problems in Paediatrics VII*. New York: Karger.

MILLER, F. J. W., COURT, S. D. M., WALTON, W. S. and KNOX, E. G. (1960). *Growing up in Newcastle-upon-Tyne: A Continuing Study of Health and Illness in Young Children Within their Families*. London: Oxf. Univ. Press.

PATON, R. G. and GARDNER, L. I. (1963). *Growth Failure in Maternal Deprivation*. Springfield: Thomas.

PRADER, A., TANNER, J. M. and VON HARNACK, G. A. (1963). Catch-up growth following illness or starvation. *J. Pediat.*, **62**, 646.

Provis, H. S. and Ellis, R. W. B. (1955). An anthropometric study of Edinburgh school-children: Part I. Methods, data and assessment of maturity. *Arch. Dis. Childh.*, **30**, 328.

Rix, R. E. (1956). Development and care of the teeth, in *Child Health and Development*. Ed. R. W. B. Ellis. 2nd ed. London: Churchill.

Roberts, D. F. (1953). Body weight, race and climate. *Am. J. phys. Anthrop.* N.S. **11**, 533.

Scammon, R. E. (1930). The measurement of the body in childhood. In *The Measurement of Man*. University of Minnesota.

Schreider, E. (1957). Gradients écologiques, régulation thermique et différenciation humaine. *Biotypologie*, **18**, 168.

—— (1964). Récherches sur la stratification sociale des caractères biologiques. *Biotypologie*, **25**, 105.

Shuttleworth, F. K. (1938). Sexual maturation and the skeletal growth of girls age six to nineteen. *Monogr. Soc. Res. Child Dev.*, **3**, No. 1.

Simmons, K. (1944). The brush foundation study of child growth and development. II. Physical growth and development. *Monogr. Soc. Res. Child Devel.*, **10**, No. 1.

—— and Greulich, W. W. (1943). Menarcheal age. *J. Pediat.*, **22**, 518.

Stuart, H. C. (1946). Normal growth and development during adolescence. *New Eng. med. J.*, **234**, 666, 693, 732.

Tanner, J. M. (1951). Notes on the reporting of growth data. *Hum. Biol.*, **23**, 93.

—— (1952). The assessment of growth and development in children. *Arch. Dis. Childh.*, **27**, 10.

—— (1959). Boas' contributions to knowledge of growth and form. In *The Anthropology of Franz Boas*. Ed. W. Goldschmidt. Mem. Amer. Anthropol. Assoc. No. 89.

—— (1960). (Ed.) *Human Growth*. London: Pergamon Press.

—— (1962). *Growth at Adolescence*. 2nd ed. Oxford: Blackwell.

—— (1963). The regulation of human growth. *Child Dev.*, **34**, 817.

—— (1964). *The Physique of the Olympic Athlete*. London: Allen and Unwin.

—— (1966a). Growth and physique in different populations of mankind. In *The Biology of Human Adaptability*. Ed. P. T. Baker and J. S. Weiner. Oxford: Clarendon.

—— (1966b). The secular trend towards earlier physical maturation. *T. Soc. Geneesk.*, **44**, 524.

—— (1966c). Galtonian eugenics and the study of growth. The relation of body size, intelligence test score, and social circumstances in children and adults. *Eugen. Rev.*, **58**, 122.

—— (1969). Growth and endocrinology of the adolescent. In *Endocrine and Genetic Diseases of Childhood*. Ed. L. Gardner. Philadelphia: Saunders.

—— and Gupta, D. (1968). A longitudinal study of the excretion of individual steroids in children from 8 to 12 years. *J. Endocr.*, **41**, 139.

—— and Ham, T. (1969). Low-birth-weight dwarfism with asymmetry (Silver's syndrome): treatment with human growth hormone. *Arch. Dis. Childh.*, **44**, 231.

—— and Whitehouse, R. H. (1962). Standards for subcutaneous fat in British children. Percentiles for thickness of skinfolds over triceps and below scapulae. *Brit. Med. J.*, **1**, 187.

—— —— and Healy, M. J. R. (1962). A new system for estimating skeletal maturity from the hand and wrist, with standards derived from a study of 2,600 healthy British children. Paris: Centre Internationale de l'Enfance.

—— —— —— and Takaishi, H. (1966). Standards from birth to maturity for height, weight, height velocity and weight velocity: British children. *Arch. Dis. Childh.*, **41**, 454, 613.

Todd, T. W. (1933). Growth and development of the child. *White House Conference on Child Health*. New York.

VICKERS, V. S. and STUART, H. C. (1943). Anthropometry in the pediatrician's office. *J. Pediat.*, **22**, 155.

VINCENT, M. and HUGON, J. (1962). L'insuffisance pondérale du prématuré Africain au point de vue de la santé publique. *Bull. Wld. Hlth. Org.*, **26**, 143.

VOGT, E. C. and VICKERS, V. S. (1938). Osseous growth and development. *Radiology*, **31**, 441.

WADDINGTON, C. H. (1958). *The Strategy of the Genes. A Discussion of some aspects of Theoretical Biology*. London: Allen and Unwin.

WATSON, E. H. and LOWREY, G. H. (1962). *Growth and Development of Children*. 4th ed. Chicago: Year Book med. publ.

WEIR, J. B. DE V. (1952). The assessment of growth of schoolchildren with special reference to secular changes. *Brit. J. Nutrit.*, **6**, 19.

WESTROPP, C. K. and BARBER, C. R. (1956). Growth of the skull in young children. *J. Neurol. Neurosurg. Psychiat.*, **19**, 52.

WIDDOWSON, E. M. (1951). Mental contentment and physical growth. *Lancet*, **1**, 1316.

——, MAVOR, W. O. and McCANCE, R. A. (1964). The effect of undernutrition and rehabilitation on the development of the reproductive organs in rats. *J. Endocr.*, **29**, 119.

—— and McCANCE, R. A. (1960). Some effects of accelerating growth. I. General somatic development. *Proc. R. Soc. B.*, **152**, 188.

7 Puberty and Adolescence

THE term puberty is used in the medical and legal literature to describe several slightly different phases of sexual maturation lying between childhood and adulthood, *e.g.* the point in time at which procreation becomes possible, or the period leading up to or following this point. The term 'non-pubescent' is applied to children showing no evidence of secondary sexual characters or genital maturity; 'pubescent' to those in whom secondary sexual characters and early genital development are appearing. The term 'adolescent' was used by Ellis and others to refer to girls who had passed menarche (the first menstruation) but not yet reached maturity, and to boys in a roughly similar stage. However this usage seems more likely to confuse than clarify, especially as psychologists have now begun to use adolescence as referring specifically to psycho-social changes. In this chapter the terms puberty and adolescence are used quite interchangeably. At adolescence the transition from one phase of development to the next is not an abrupt one, since even the menarche (which is most readily determined in point of time) is not necessarily coincident with ovulation, and the time-relationship between the appearance of the various indices of sexual development is to a considerable extent variable. Although the physical and emotional changes which occur during the process of sexual maturation follow each other with a rapidity which is only comparable to the speed of development of the infant during the first 2 years of life, sexual maturation represents a transition period lasting 3 or more years, and involving physical and emotional problems peculiar to itself.

Manifestations of Sexual Maturation

This period is characterised by five closely interrelated features:

1. The adolescent spurt of growth (see Chapter 6), which commonly begins early in the process of maturation, reaches a maximum shortly before menarche in girls and subsequently decelerates rapidly until adult stature is reached. Rapid increase in weight often continues after deceleration in height has begun, and the period of maximum weight-gain is not necessarily coincident with that of height. There is a change in body composition, particularly in boys, fat being lost and muscle greatly increased.

2. The appearance of secondary sexual characters.

3. Rapid growth and development of the gonads and genitalia.

4. A general readjustment of endocrine balance resulting in the establishment of menstruation and ovulation in girls and of spermatogenesis in boys.

5. Emotional development and personality changes, which may be manifested by a variety of behaviour difficulties, frustration and self-consciousness before adult poise is attained.

Although some children are more fortunate than others in passing easily from childhood to adult life, the transition is often one of difficulty and embarrassment, and should always call for sympathetic handling. The rapidity of growth tends to make the adolescent awkward and ungainly; the boy may be dismayed by his large hands and feet, his acne and breaking voice, and the girl by transient obesity, or by her breast development and problems of menstruation. Both sexes usually experience an increase of appetite coincident with their maximum growth; minor digestive disturbances, probably related to the rise in gastric acidity which occurs during puberty, and symptoms suggestive of mild hypoglycaemia are common. Vasovagal instability, manifested by blushing, tachycardia, or even fainting attacks, is much more frequent at this time than during childhood.

The Adolescent Growth Spurt: Physical and Physiological Changes

At puberty, a very considerable change in growth rate occurs. For a year or more the velocity of growth approximately doubles: a boy is likely to be growing at a rate he last experienced at about age 2. During the year which includes the moment of peak height velocity a boy usually grows between 7 and 12 cm. and a girl between 6 and 11 cm. The average age at which the peak occurs varies more from one population to another than does the magnitude of the peak, depending on environmental and perhaps genetic factors. In moderately well-off children in West Europe the peak is reached on average at about 14·0 in boys and 12·0 in girls; in the United States it is reached about 6 months earlier in the corresponding socio-economic group.

Practically all skeletal and muscular dimensions take part in the spurt, though not to an equal degree. Most of the spurt in height is due to acceleration of trunk length rather than length of legs. There is a fairly regular order in which the dimensions accelerate; leg length as a rule reaches its peak first, followed by the body breadths, with shoulder width last. Thus a boy stops growing out of his trousers (at least in length) a year before he stops growing out of his jackets. The earliest structures to reach their adult status are the head, hands, and feet. At adolescence, children, particularly girls, sometimes complain of having large hands and feet. They can be reassured that by the time they are fully grown their hands and feet will be a little smaller in proportion to their arms and legs, and considerably smaller in proportion to their trunk.

The marked increase in muscle size in boys at adolescence leads to an increase in strength, illustrated in Fig. 41. Before adolescence boys and girls are similar in strength for a given body size and shape; after, boys are much stronger, probably due to developing more force per gm. of muscle as well as absolutely larger muscles. They also develop larger hearts and lungs relative to their size, a higher systolic blood pressure, a lower resting heart rate, a greater capacity for carrying oxygen in the blood, and a greater power for neutralising the chemical products of muscular exercise such as lactic acid (see Tanner, 1962). In short, the male becomes at adolescence more adapted for the tasks of hunting, fighting, and manipulating all sorts of heavy objects, as is necessary in some forms of food-gathering.

The increase in haemoglobin, associated with a parallel increase in the number

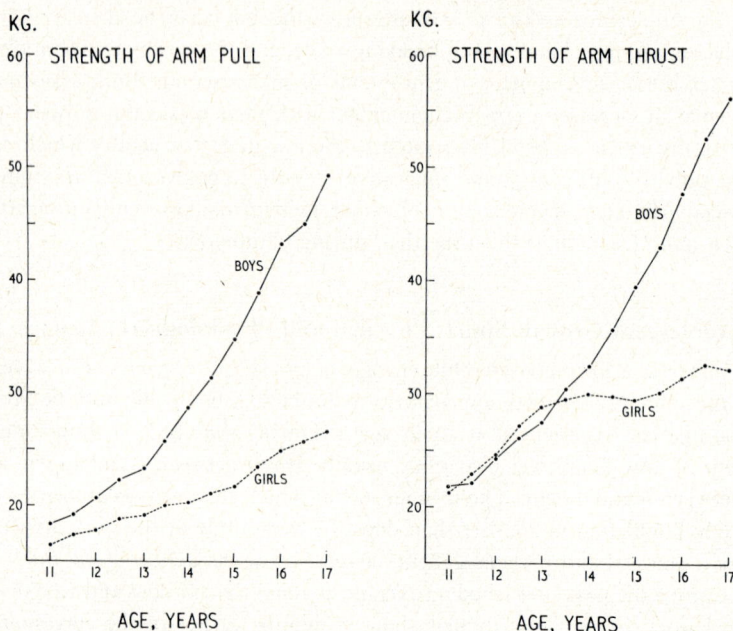

FIG. 41. Strength of arm pull and arm thrust from age 11 to 17 years. Mixed longitudinal data: 65-93 boys and 66-93 girls in each age group (data from Jones, 1949. From Tanner, 1962).

of red blood cells, is illustrated in Fig. 42 drawn from the data of Young (1963). The haemoglobin concentration is plotted in relation to the development of secondary sex characters instead of chronological age to obviate the spread due to early and late maturing. Girls lack the rise in red cells and haemoglobin, which is brought about by the action of testosterone.

It is as a direct result of these anatomical and physiological changes that athletic ability increases so much in boys at adolescence. The popular notion of a boy 'outgrowing his strength' at this time has little scientific support. It is true that the peak velocity of strength is reached a year or so later than that of height, so that a short period may exist when the adolescent, having completed his skeletal and probably also muscular growth, still does not have the strength of a young adult of the same body size and shape. But this is a temporary phase; considered absolutely, power, athletic skill, and physical endurance all increase progressively and rapidly throughout adolescence. It is certainly not true that the changes accompanying adolescence enfeeble, even temporarily. If the adolescent becomes weak and easily exhausted it is for psychological reasons and not physiological ones.

Development of Reproductive System

Whilst the order of appearance of secondary sexual characters is not exactly the same in all children, there is a general pattern for either sex to which most conform.

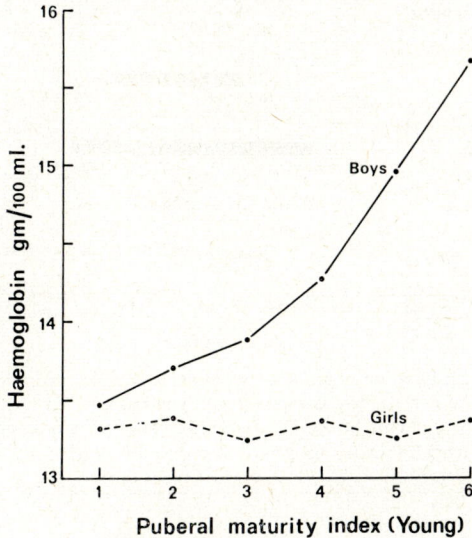

FIG. 42. Blood haemoglobin level in girls and boys according to stage of puberty. Cross-sectional data from Young, 1963 (from Tanner, 1962).

It is, for instance, very exceptional for axillary hair to appear before pubic hair, though this may occur. The speed with which one character follows another, however, varies greatly in different individuals and, although secondary sexual characters will ultimately accentuate the differences between the two sexes, transient characters of the opposite sex are often seen during pubescence. Thus, whilst breast-development is essentially a female character, a slight degree of gynaecomastia is frequently seen in boys. Deposition of fat over the hips and shoulders may also give pubescent boys a pseudofeminine contour which is lost during later adolescence.

Boys

The sequence of events in boys and girls is shown diagrammatically in Figs. 43 and 44. The solid areas in Fig. 43 marked *penis* and *testis* represent the period of accelerated growth of these organs, and the horizontal lines and the rating numbers marked *pubic hair* stand for its advent and development. The sequence and timings given represent in each case an average value for British boys. To give an idea of the individual departures from the average, figures for the range of ages at which the spurts for height, penis growth, and testis growth begin and

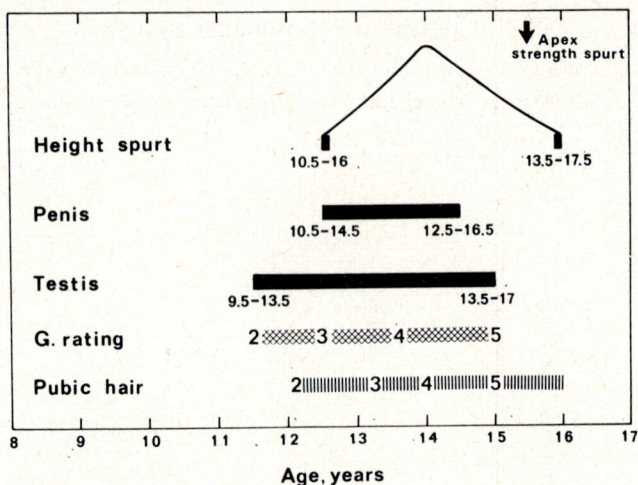

FIG. 43. Diagram of sequence of events at adolescence in boys. An average boy is represented. The range of ages within which some of the events charted may begin and end is given by the figures placed directly below them.

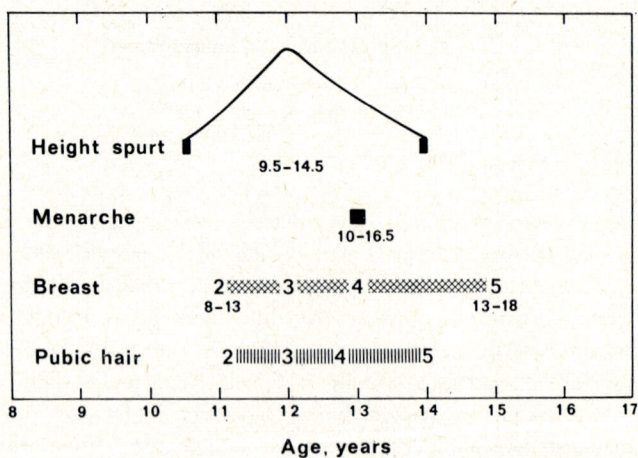

FIG. 44. Diagram of sequence of events at adolescence in girls. An average girl is represented. The range of ages within which some of the events charted may occur is given by the figures placed directly below them.

end are inserted under the first and last point of the curves or bars. The acceleration of penis growth, for example, begins on average at about age 12½, but sometimes as early as 10½ and sometimes as late as 14. The completion of penis development usually occurs at about age $14\frac{1}{2}$ but in some boys at $12\frac{1}{2}$ and others at $16\frac{1}{2}$. There are a few boys, it will be noticed, who do not begin their spurts in height or penis development until the earliest maturers have entirely completed theirs. At age 13 and 14 there is an enormous variability among any group of boys, who range all the way from practically complete maturity to absolute pre-adolescence. This is illustrated in Fig. 45. The psychological and social importance of this is very great.

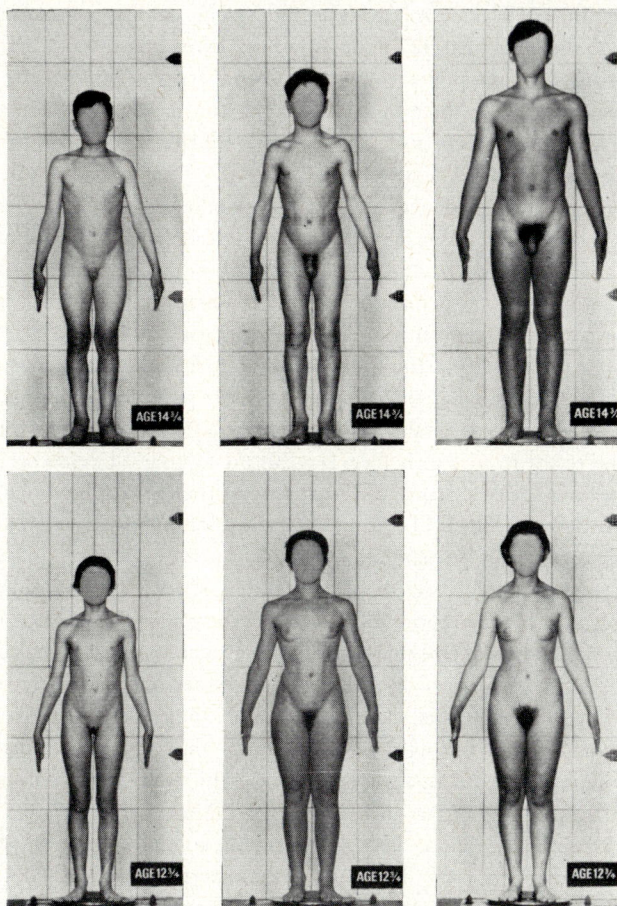

FIG. 45. Differing degrees of adolescence at the same chronological age. Upper row, 3 boys all aged 14·75 years. Lower row, 3 girls all aged 12·75 years (from Tanner, 1969).

Boys who are advanced in development are likely to dominate their contemporaries in athletic achievement and sexual interest alike. Conversely the late developer is the one who all too often loses out in the rough and tumble of the adolescent world; and he may begin to wonder whether he will ever develop his body properly or be as well endowed sexually as those others he has seen developing around him. A very important part of the educationist's and the doctor's task at this time is to provide information about growth and its variability to pre-adolescents and adolescents and to give sympathetic support and reassurance to those who need it (Tanner, 1958).

The earliest change in boys is usually the appearance of non-pigmented 'vellus' or fine hair at the root of the penis. This is followed by the stages of pubic hair development illustrated in Fig. 48. The moustache, at first consisting of short sparse hairs at the outer margin of the upper lip, extending towards the mid-line, usually appears at about pubic hair stage 4, and axillary hair usually begins at about this stage also. The spread of the face hair to the sides and lower border of the chin is a late development and seldom occurs till after stage 5 has been reached in both genital and pubic hair development.

The first unequivocal evidence of genital development may synchronise with the appearance of pigmented pubic hair, or may precede or follow it by a short interval. Both penis and testes show singularly little alteration throughout childhood; with the onset of pubescence the penis increases in both length and girth due to development of the corpus spongiosum and the corpora cavernosa, and the glans also enlarges in size. The body of the testis enlarges in relation to the epididymis and softens, the onset of testicular enlargement normally preceding penile growth. The stages through which the genitalia pass are shown in Fig. 47, below. An increase in weight of the testes from 2 g. before 11 years to 17 g. at 18 years occurs during sexual maturation (Stuart, 1946), and the body of the testis approximately trebles its length in the same time. The volume of the testes increases from about 2 ml. to 25 ml. on average; a good estimate of testicular size can be made in the clinic by comparison with a standard set of plastic models, known as the Prader orchidometer. The growth of the prepuce follows that of the glans. There is very commonly an increased production of smegma beneath it, necessitating scrupulous cleanliness. The scrotum becomes more pendulous and wider distally than proximally. Either the left or right testis may enlarge first, though the left testis is more commonly smaller than the right. The prostate, which has also remained small throughout childhood, enlarges rapidly during the later pubescent period, and becomes easily palpable on rectal examination. There are no reliable data as to when mature spermatogenesis occurs in relation to the clinical signs of sexual maturation. It may reasonably be assumed that spermatogenesis is not an 'all-or-none' process, but that the profuse production of mature spermatozoa is the end of a gradual process of maturation.

GYNAECOMASTIA. The nipples normally enlarge slightly during pubescence and the areolae become pigmented. In those boys in whom this stage of development is associated with transient fat deposition of feminine distribution, a considerable degree of subcutaneous fat may appear in the breast region and simulate breast development. Apart from this, however, a true gynaecomastia or development of mammary tissue, attached to the nipple and palpable as a firm nodule, occurs in a considerable number of pubescent boys. It may be unilateral or bilateral. In some cases, particularly when there is no excess of subcutaneous fat around the nipple, the breast-enlargement is closely similar to that first seen in pubescent girls. Whilst obvious pubescent gynaecomastia is likely to prove embarrassing and may cause some slight discomfort, it will commonly disappear spontaneously during later adolescence (usually within 18 months of its appearance).

VOICE. The 'broken voice' is a characteristic change observed in the adolescent boy. The change in pitch is due to the rapid growth of the larynx and lengthening of the vocal cords. During the period of 'breaking', the pitch is variable and the true adult pitch associated with full growth of the larynx may not be established until late adolescence. In addition to change in pitch, there is also a change in quality or timbre which distinguishes the voice (particularly the vowel sounds) of both male and female adults from that of children. This is dependent on the enlargement of the resonating spaces above the larynx, due to the rapid growth of the mouth, nose and maxilla which occurs during adolescence.

SKIN. The sebaceous and apocrine sweat glands, particularly of the axillae and genital and anal regions, develop rapidly during puberty and give rise to a characteristic odour; the changes occur in both sexes but are more marked in the male. Enlargement of the pores at the root of the nose and the appearance of comedones and acne, whilst liable to occur in either sex, are considerably commoner in adolescent boys than girls, since the underlying skin changes are the result of androgenic activity (Ellis, 1946). A roughening of the skin in certain areas (particularly over the outer aspects of the thighs and upper arms), associated with a mild degree of follicular keratosis, may be seen in both sexes during adolescence, but again is commoner in boys than girls.

Girls

The sequence of events in girls is shown in Fig. 44. The appearance of the 'breast bud' (stage 2 in breast development) is as a rule the first sign of puberty in girls, though the appearance of pubic hair sometimes precedes it. The uterus and vagina develop simultaneously with the breast. As in boys, there is a large variation in the age at which the various events occur. Menarche, the first menstrual period, is a late event in the sequence. It occurs almost invariably after the peak of the height spurt has been passed. Most frequently it coincides closely with the point of maximum deceleration (Tanner, 1969). On average girls grow about 6 cm. more after menarche, although gains of up to twice this amount may occur. The gain is practically independent of whether menarche occurs early or late.

The breast stages are illustrated in Fig. 49, and pubic hair stages in Fig. 48. Axillary hair appears usually at about the time of menarche. Details of individual variation of the course of puberty in girls will be found in Marshall and Tanner (1969) and are illustrated in Fig. 46.

Clinical evidence of genital development is shown by gradual enlargement of the labia majora and minora and the clitoris during pubescence, associated with fat deposition over the mons. Bartholin's glands become active. Rapid growth of the uterus occurs at the same time, though it does not assume adult proportions until late. The ovaries nearly double their weight during adolescence. The onset of menstruation is in some cases preceded by one or more periods of abdominal discomfort without bleeding. Menstruation may at first be irregular with scanty or excessive flow and irregular intervals between the periods. Dysmenorrhoea may occur. It is sometimes many months before a regular menstrual cycle is established.

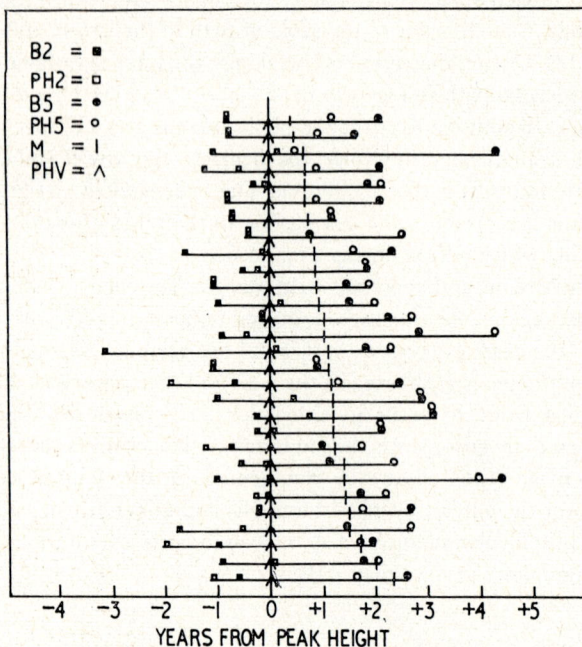

FIG. 46. Intervals between different events of puberty in a series of 29 girls. Girls are aligned by peak height velocity (from Tanner, 1969).

Although menarche will in some cases correspond with the first ovulation, it is not infrequent for a number of anovulatory cycles (which may extend over 1 to 3 years) to follow menarche. This is borne out by the observation that a period of 'adolescent sterility' commonly occurs amongst populations where marriage at or before menarche is the general rule. Although the onset of menstruation is often thought to be synonymous with capacity to procreate, this is not necessarily the case. Menarche is associated with changes in the vaginal mucosa, the cells maturing and increasing in glycogen content.

The diagrams of Figs. 43 and 44 must not be allowed to obscure the fact that children vary a good deal in the relative closeness with which the various events of puberty are linked together. At one extreme we may find a girl who has not yet menstruated, though she has reached adult breast and pubic hair ratings and is already 2 years past her peak height velocity; at the other we may find a girl who has passed all the stages of puberty within the space of 2 years. The means and ranges of the ages at which the various events occur are plotted for girls in Fig.

50; it can be seen that at ages between 12·0 and 14·0 girls may be found in any stage of puberty from complete pre-adolescence (not yet B2 or PH2) to complete maturity of appearance (B5 and PH5). The variability between individuals is equally marked in boys. The average boy takes about 2 years to pass from genital stage 2 to stage 4, but exceptional boys may take as long as 5 years. In both sexes the acceleration in skeletal development and the development of genitalia and breasts are rather closely linked. The growth of pubic hair is a little less closely bound up with skeletal and reproductive events.

The basis for some children having loose and some tight linkages between pubertal events is not known. Probably the linkage reflects the degree of integration of various processes in the hypothalamus and the pituitary gland, for breast growth is controlled by one group of hormones, pubic hair growth by another, and the height spurt probably by a third.

Clinical Maturity Grading

Since sexual maturation is closely related to growth and physical performance (Espenschade, 1940; Ellis 1948b; Jones, 1949), medical records should include

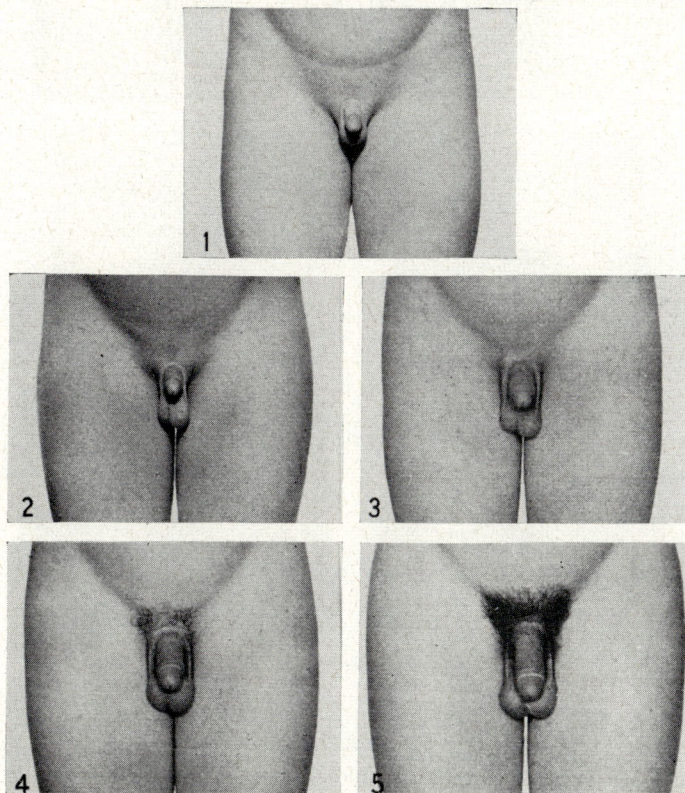

FIG. 47. Standards for genital maturity ratings in boys
(from Tanner, 1962).

some assessment of the stage of maturity reached at the time of examination. Genitalia in boys, pubic hair in both sexes, and breasts in girls may be rated using the stages illustrated in Figs. 47, 48 and 49.

The description of the genitalia stages are as follows (Tanner, 1962, 1969). In

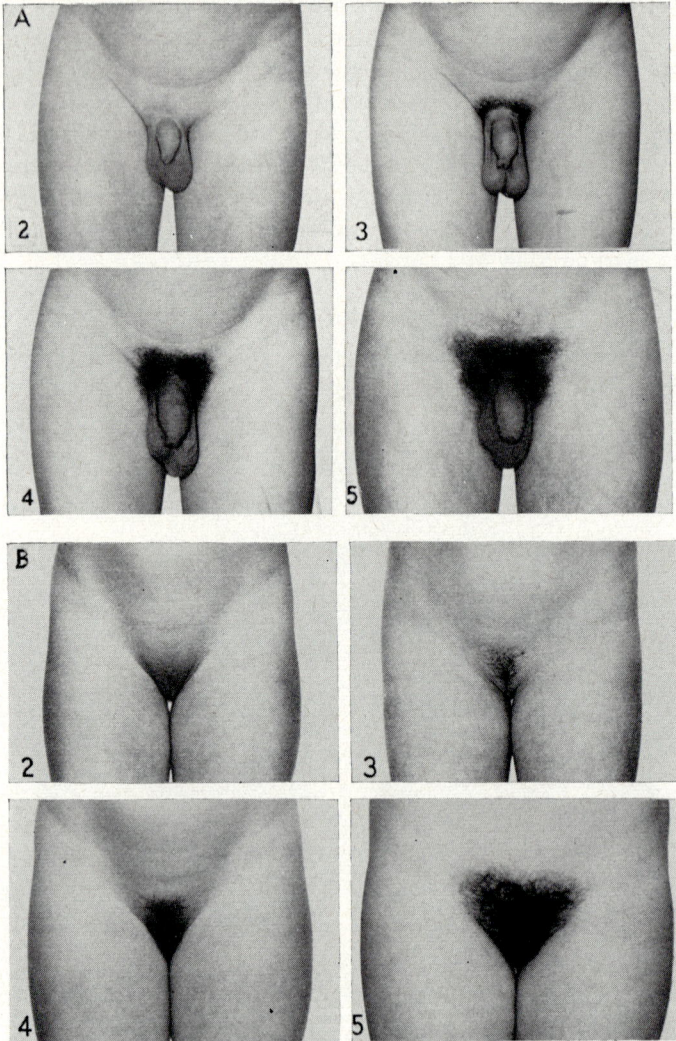

FIG. 48. Standards for pubic hair ratings in (A) boys and
(B) girls (from Tanner, 1969).

clinical studies, as distinct from school medical examinations, the size of the testes should also be recorded using the orchidometer.

STAGE 1. Preadolescent; Testes, scrotum and penis are about the same size and shape as in early childhood.

Stage 2. Scrotum and testes are slightly enlarged. The skin of the scrotum is reddened and changed in texture. There is little or no enlargement of the penis at this stage.

Stage 3. Penis is slightly enlarged, at first mainly in length. Testes and scrotum are further enlarged than in stage 2.

Stage 4. Penis is further enlarged, with growth in breadth and development of glans. Testes and scrotum are further enlarged than in stage 3; scrotal skin is darker than in earlier stages.

Stage 5. Genitalia are adult in size and shape.

The size of the testes can be measured if necessary, or more conveniently assessed by palpation in comparison with a string of plastic models of testicular shape (the

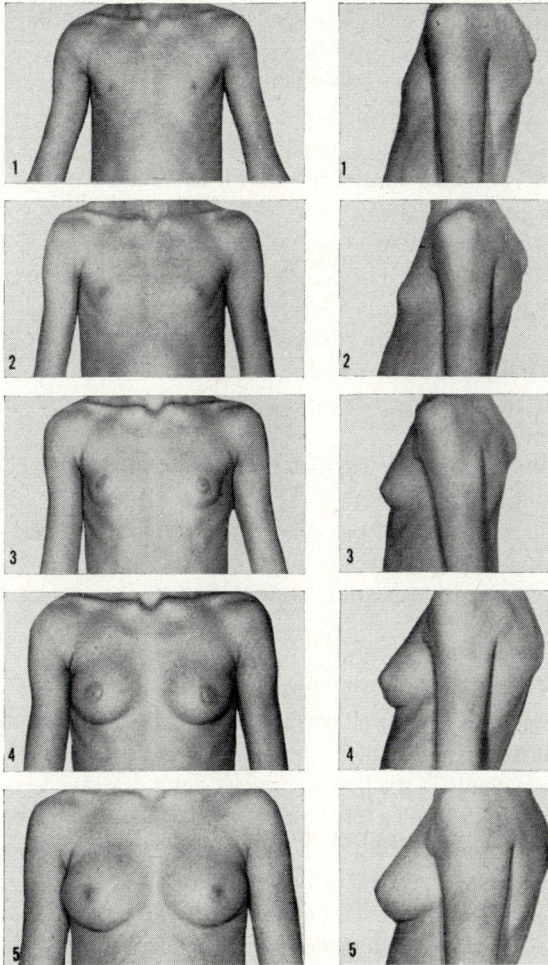

Fig. 49. Standards for breast development ratings
(from Tanner, 1969).

Prader Orchidometer). The models are marked according to their volumes in cubic centimetres; sizes 1 and 2 correspond to stage 1 in genital development; 3, 4 and 5 to stage 2; 6, 8 and 10 to stage 3; 12, 15 and 20 to stage 4; and 25 and 30 (depending on individual variations) to the adult stage 5.

The pubic hair stages, illustrated in Fig. 48 for boys and girls, are as follows.

STAGE 1. Preadolescent. The vellus over the pubes is not further developed than that over the abdominal wall, *i.e.* no pubic hair.

STAGE 2. There is sparse growth of long, slightly pigmented downy hair, straight, or slightly curled, chiefly at the base of the penis or along the labia.

STAGE 3. The hair is considerably darker, coarser and more curled. It spreads sparsely over the junction of the pubes.

STAGE 4. Hair is now adult in type, but the area covered is still considerably smaller than in the adult. There is no spread to the medial surface of the thighs.

STAGE 5. The hair is adult in quantity and type with distribution of the horizontal (or classically 'feminine') pattern. Spread is to the medial surface of the thighs but not up the linea alba or elsewhere above the base of the inverse triangle (spread up the linea alba occurs late and is rated stage 6).

The breast development stages (Reynolds and Wines, 1948), illustrated in Fig. 49, are as follows:

STAGE 1. Preadolescent. There is elevation of the papilla only.

STAGE 2. Breast bud stage. There is elevation of the breast and the papilla as a small mound. Areolar diameter is enlarged over stage 1.

STAGE 3. Breast and areola are both enlarged and elevated more than in stage 2, but with no separation of their contours.

STAGE 4. The areola and papilla form a secondary mound projecting above the contour of the breast.

STAGE 5. Mature stage. The papilla only projects, with the areola recessed to the general contour of the breasts.

The stage 4 development of the areolar mound does not ever occur in some girls; in probably a quarter it is absent and in a further quarter slight. Furthermore, when it does occur, it may persist well into adulthood. Thus stages 4 and 5 are not distinct in all girls.

The Development of Sex Dimorphism

The differential effects on the growth of bone, muscle, and fat at puberty increase considerably the difference in body composition between the sexes. Boys have a greater increase not only in the length of bones but in the thickness of cortex, and girls have a smaller loss of fat. The most striking dimorphism however are the man's greater stature and breadth of shoulders and the woman's wider hips. These are produced chiefly by the changes and timing of puberty but it is important to remember that sex dimorphisms do not only arise at that time. Many appear much earlier. Some, like the external genital difference itself, develop during fetal life. Others develop continuously throughout the whole growth period by a sustained differential growth rate. An example of this is the greater relative length and breadth of the forearm in the male when compared with whole arm length or whole body length (see Tanner, 1962; Hiernaux, 1968 for further discussion).

Part of the sex difference in pelvis shape antedates puberty. Girls at birth already have a wider pelvic outlet. Thus the adaptation for child-bearing is present from a very early age. The changes at puberty are concerned more with widening the

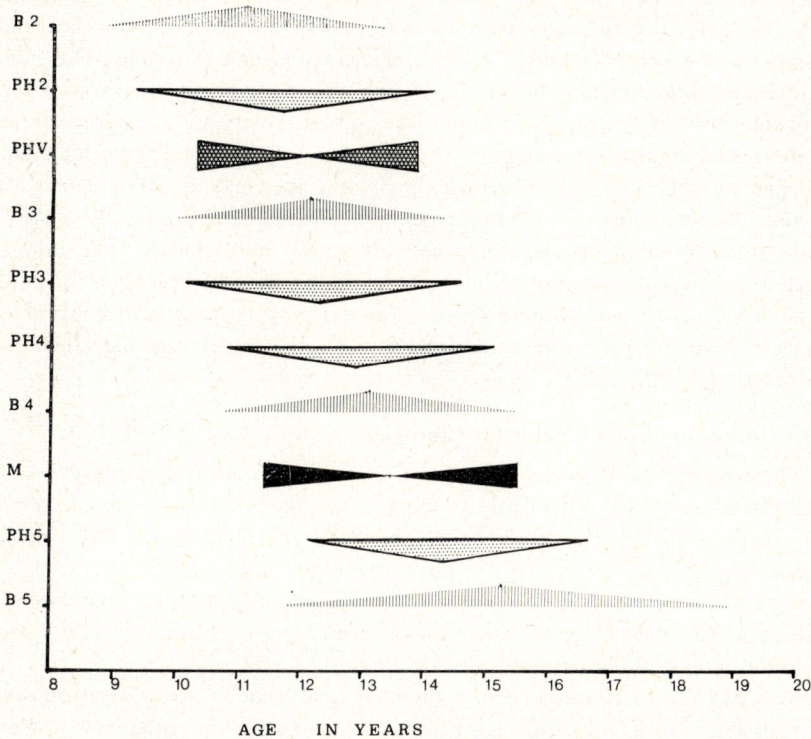

FIG. 50. Age on reaching each stage of puberty. The centre of each symbol represents the mean and the length of the symbol is equivalent to two standard deviations on either side of the mean (from Marshall and Tanner, 1969).

pelvic inlet and broadening the much more noticeable hips. It seems likely that these changes are more important in attracting the male's attention than in dealing with its ultimate product.

These sex-differentiated morphological characters arising at puberty—to which we can add the corresponding physiological and perhaps psychological ones as well—are secondary sex characters in the straightforward sense that they are caused by sex hormone or sex-differential hormone secretion and serve reproductive activity. The penis is directly concerned in copulation, the mammary gland in lactation. The wide shoulders and muscular power of the male, together with the canine teeth and brow ridges in man's ancestors, developed probably for driving away other males and ensuring peace from other animals, an adaptation which soon becomes social. A number of traits persist, perhaps through another mechanism known to ethologists as ritualisation. In the course of evolution a morphological character or a piece of behaviour may lose its original function and becoming further elaborated, complicated, or simplified, may serve as a sign stimulus to other members of the same species, releasing behaviour that is in some way advantageous to the spread or survival of the species. It requires little insight into human erotics to suppose that the shoulders, the hips and buttocks, and the breasts (at least in a number of widespread cultures) serve as releasers of mating behaviour. The pubic hair (about whose function the text-books have always preserved a cautious silence) probably survives as a ritualised stimulus for sexual activity, developed by simplification from the hair remaining in the inguinal and axillary regions for the infant to cling to when still transported, as in present apes and monkeys, under the mother's body. Similar considerations may apply to axillary hair, which is associated with special apocrine glands which themselves only develop at puberty and are related histologically to scant glands in other mammals. The beard, on the other hand, may still be more frightening to other males than enticing to females. At least ritual use in past communities suggests this is the case; but perhaps there are two sorts of beard.

The Endocrinology of Pubertal Changes

The events of puberty take place under hormonal control. As yet, however, our understanding of what is evidently a complex series of events, each with a feedback on others, is incomplete (see Donovan and Werff ten Bosch, 1965 and Tanner, 1969).

GONADOTROPHINS. The first event in the sequence of puberty, immediately preceding the morphological changes, is believed to be an increase in secretion of gonadotrophins by the pituitary.

Both FSH and LH are present in the blood and urine of prepubertal children though at a considerably lower level than at adolescence. The rising level of FSH causes the tubules of the testis and the follicles of the ovary to develop, and the rising level of LH causes the Leydig cells to enlarge and to secrete testosterone.

OESTROGEN. There is a low and relatively constant excretion of oestrogen by both boys and girls from age 3 to 7, after which a gradual rise takes place in both sexes until adolescence, when in girls excretion increases sharply and becomes cyclic. Cycles are established at about the time when breast buds appear. Oestrogens are responsible for the growth of the breasts, uterus and vagina. In boys a rise in oestrogen excretion occurs at a point between the beginning of stages G3, PH3 and G4, PH4. Probably this is responsible for the gynaecomastia seen in some boys.

TESTICULAR ANDROGENS. A small amount of testosterone is present in the blood of prepubertal boys and girls, but at puberty in boys a very large increase occurs, probably under the stimulus of LH from the pituitary.

ADRENOCORTICAL HORMONES. Two out of the three major groups of adrenocortical hormones circulate in the blood at relatively unchanged levels from birth on: these are cortisol and aldosterone. The excretion of cortisol metabolites increases in keeping with the increase of body size, but it has no particular spurt beyond this at adolescence.

The secretion of adrenal androgenic hormones, on the other hand, increases greatly at puberty, in both boys and girls. Before puberty very little dehydro-epiandrosterone (DHA) or DHA sulphate can be demonstrated in blood or urine. The androgen metabolites in the urine, that is the 17-oxosteroids, increase sharply at about the time the height spurt begins. This occurs in both sexes, but in boys the 17-oxosteroids reach a level about one and a half times that in girls (Fig. 51).

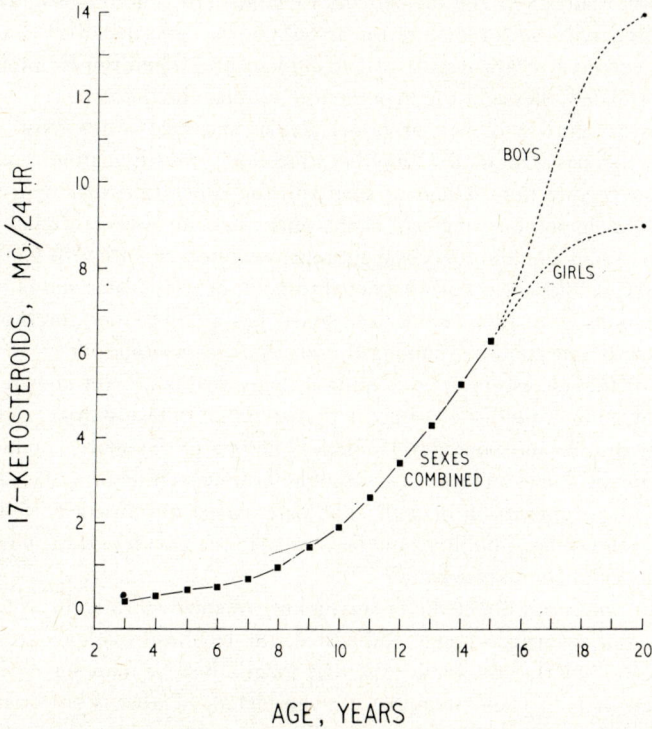

FIG. 51. Excretion of neural 17-ketosteroids from age 3 to 20 years (from Tanner, 1962: data for age 3 to 15 from Talbot *et al.*, 1943; extrapolation to age 20 based additionally on Hamburger, 1948, and Sprechler, 1951).

The sex difference is probably entirely due to the fact that testosterone is also partly metabolised to 17-oxosteroids so that the boys' levels include both adrenal and testicular androgen metabolites. It seems likely that the adrenal contribution is fairly similar in both sexes.

The cause of the increase in androgen secretion is far from clear. ACTH cannot be responsible, for it always causes a much greater increase in corticoid than in androgen secretion, yet the corticoids rise only slightly at puberty. Either some still unknown pituitary hormone is concerned ('adrenarche hormone') or else something modifies the response of the adrenal to ACTH at this time (see Tanner, 1962). This adrenal component of adolescence is sometimes referred to as 'adrenarche'.

The adrenal androgens are clearly important in bringing about some of the changes of puberty, particularly in girls, in whom they cause growth of the pubic and axillary hair. Occasionally children are seen in whom pubic and sometimes axillary hair develops very early, before the occurrence of other signs of sexual maturity. The patients are mostly girls and a high proportion have brain damage. Bone maturation is advanced and the patients are large. The condition is known as 'premature adrenarche' or 'premature pubarche' and is associated with levels of 17-oxosteroid excretion characteristic of late adolescence. The disorder probably represents an isolated release of the hypothetical 'adrenarche hormone'.

The differential growth of hair at pubes, axilla, and face seems most easily explicable on the basis of locally different thresholds to stimulation, coupled perhaps with a predilection of hair at each site for either testicular or adrenal hormone. On this hypothesis, the skin of the pubes has the lowest threshold and responds to the small amount of adrenal androgen secreted by both girls and boys early in puberty. Axillary hair has a higher threshold, develops later and is somewhat more responsive to testosterone; the beard has a still higher threshold to adrenal androgens and a more pronounced preference for testosterone.

The cause of the adolescent growth spurt in body size is not yet known. The excess of the male over the female spurt is probably due to testosterone, as is the excess of male muscle and bone development. The rest of the spurt, common to both sexes, must be due to an increase in growth hormone section or to the adrenal androgens or to a combination of both. The part played by growth hormone at adolescence is not yet clear, but it should become so in the next few years, now that methods for its estimation are reliable.

Much is still uncertain about the endocrinology of adolescence. The synergies of hormone action are exceedingly complicated, the technical methods are complex and costly, and the absolutely essential longitudinal studies on hormonal production have not yet been attempted. Further details of what is known in this field can be found elsewhere (Tanner, 1969; Tanner and Gupta, 1968).

The Initiation of Puberty

The manner in which puberty is initiated has a general importance for the clarification of developmental mechanisms. Certain children develop all the changes of puberty, up to and including spermatogenesis and ovulation, at a very early age, either as the result of a brain lesion or as an isolated developmental, sometimes genetic, defect. The youngest mother on record was such a case, and gave birth to a full-term healthy infant by caesarean section at the age of 5 years 8 months. The existence of precocious puberty and the results of accidental ingestion by small children of male or female sex hormones indicate that breasts, uterus and penis will respond to hormonal stimulation long before puberty.

Evidently an increased end-organ sensitivity plays little or no part in pubertal events.

The signal to start the sequence of events is given by the brain, not the pituitary. Just as the brain holds the information on sex, so it holds information on maturity. The pituitary of a newborn rat successfully grafted in place of an adult pituitary begins at once to function in an adult fashion, and does not have to wait till its normal age of maturation has been reached (Harris and Jacobsohn, 1952). It is the hypothalamus, not the pituitary, which has to mature before puberty begins.

Maturation, however, does not come out of the blue and at least in rats a little more is known about this mechanism. In these animals small amounts of sex hormones circulate from the time of birth and these appear to inhibit the prepubertal hypothalamus from producing gonadotrophin releasers. At puberty it is supposed that the hypothalamic cells become less sensitive to sex hormone. The small amount of sex hormones circulating then fails to inhibit the hypothalamus, gonadotrophins are released, and the level of sex hormone rises until the same feedback circuit is re-established, but now at a higher level of gonadotrophins and sex hormones. The sex hormones are now high enough to stimulate the growth of secondary sex characters and support mating behaviour (Donovan and Van der Werff ten Bosch, 1965).

Age at Puberty: Delayed Puberty

The factors controlling the age at which puberty begins have been discussed in the previous chapter, and the approximate average ages and ranges of the various stages are displayed in Figs. 43 and 44. Further details may be found in Marshall and Tanner (1969). At present the average age of menarche in British girls is approximately 13·0 years, and the range which covers 95 per cent of normal girls stretches from 11·0 to 15·0. Some girls with a delayed tempo of growth have menarche considerably later, although the sequence of events remains quite normal (for examples see Tanner, 1969). The cause of the slow tempo is not known.

The same occurs in boys and frequently leads to requests for medical advice. If a boy shows no signs of beginning puberty by his sixteenth birthday it is usually advisable for him to seek specialist opinion. The administration of testosterone for a limited period in cases where the bone age is very delayed causes an increase in growth rate, without premature closure of the epiphyses, and may have very beneficial psychological effects because of this action. It should always be accompanied, however, by studies of the rate of progression of bone age.

Care of the Adolescent

The structure of modern society provides greater problems for adolescents than for members of most other age groups and despite the increasing attention given to adolescence by teachers and employers, many of these problems remain largely unsolved. In a primitive community, the undertaking of adult work and responsibilities including marriage, together with the attendant adult privileges and outlets, is likely to be governed primarily by physical development and capacity. In civilised

society, the long period of apprenticeship necessary for most types of adult occupation and remuneration, the taboos on sexual outlet, and the over-riding emphasis
on chronological age rather than on development and maturation, give many
adolescents a sense of frustration which contributes to defiance of authority and
conflict with society unless their energies and interests can be directed into channels
which are socially desirable.

Since pubescence is essentially a period of sexual maturation, parents and other
adults must realise that sexual interests during this transition period are very
active and may even be as urgent as at any later period of the life span. Although
a more realistic attitude to sex is nowadays common, many adults (usually as a
direct result of their own early upbringing) still adopt a shamed or repressive
attitude to any sexual interest shown by the infant or child, and have already
transferred a sense of guilt and subterfuge before adolescence is reached. In such
cases it is clearly difficult or impossible for the adolescent to ask adult advice when
this is most needed, even supposing that the adults available are competent to give it
objectively. In the school environment, which is primarily concerned with academic
education or training, the adolescent often receives far less guidance in the field of
human relationships than his or her apprenticeship for adulthood requires.

It should also be realised that sexual impulse in the adolescent frequently takes
some time to be clearly canalised towards the opposite sex. During pubescence,
the child is likely to have an increasing interest in his or her own body, aroused
not only by the endocrine changes which are taking place but by the appearance of
secondary sexual changes and genital development. In some cases this is followed
by a transient attraction to members of the same sex. This may be regarded more
calmly if it is remembered that both boys and girls are producing hormones typical
of the opposite sex, and that as adolescence progresses, androgens will become
dominant in the male and oestrogens in the female. Admittedly a small proportion
of both sexes become emotionally arrested at this stage of development, but this
does not affect the fact that the great majority of those who pass through it, reach
the adult heterosexual phase which normally follows.

The adult attitude to masturbation, which according to Kinsey has been
practised by over 90 per cent of boys by the age of 17, must be carefully adjusted to
the individual concerned. It is now generally recognised that the only physical
effect that the practice is likely to have is that of the mildest temporary fatigue, but
that if it is accompanied by a profound sense of guilt, this latter may be emotionally
damaging. If a child is already suffering from a sense of guilt, only harm can be
achieved by adding to it. Masturbation is an experience which has been shared by
almost all adolescent boys and most adolescent girls, and is a perfectly normal
stage in sexual development, subsequently outgrown. For those in whom it creates
little or no guilt-feeling or anxiety, it is a phase which is left behind when adult
behaviour is established. In the exceptional case where obsessional masturbation
is accompanied by other evidence of profound emotional upset, it should be regarded
as a symptom, and the underlying disturbance investigated.

The hygiene of adolescence should be established or taught before puberty. The development of the apocrine sweat glands and the onset of menstruation make regular bathing during adolescence even more necessary than during childhood, but the principles of body-cleanliness should have been learnt much earlier and only require re-emphasis at this time. (Similarly sex education should not represent an emotional high-dive to be taken for the first time at puberty, but simply an amplification of existing knowledge of body function and structure built up gradually from early childhood). Girls should be forewarned of the onset of menstruation, and taught the use and disposal of sanitary towels. The advisability of girls taking part in organised games during menstruation must be decided for each individual. If physical exercise at this time can be carried out without discomfort or excessive fatigue, there is no contraindication to it or necessity to regard menstruation as a period of invalidism. However, many girls do in fact suffer considerable disturbance, at least during the first months or years after menarche, and in these cases their regimen should be modified accordingly. It should be emphasised to them that these disabilities will probably cease as the adult cycle is fully established.

J. M. TANNER

References

BRYAN, A. H. and GREENBERG, B. G. (1952). Methodology in the study of physical measurements of school children: Part II. Sexual maturation. *Hum. Biol.*, **24**, 117.

DONOVAN, B. T. and VAN DER WERFF TEN BOSCH, J. J. (1965). *Physiology of Puberty.* London: Arnold.

ELLIS, R. W. B. (1946). Height and weight in relation to onset of puberty in boys. *Arch. Dis. Childh.*, **21**, 181.

—— (1948a). Puberty growth of boys. *Arch. Dis. Childh.*, **23**, 17.

—— (1948b). Growth and physical performance of children in relation to maturity. *Proc. Roy. Soc. Med.*, **41**, 343.

—— (1950). Age of puberty in the tropics. *Brit. med. J.* **1**, 85.

ESPENSCHADE, A. (1940). Motor performance in adolescence. *Monog. Soc. Res. Child. Devel.*, **5**, No. 1.

GREULICH, W. W., DORFMAN, R. I., CATCHPOLE, H. R., SOLOMON, C. I. and CULOTTA, C. S. (1942). Somatic and endocrine studies of puberal and adolescent boys. *Monog. Soc. Res.*, **7**, No. 3.

HARRIS, G. W. and JACOBSOHN, D. (1952). Functional grafts of the anterior pituitary gland. *Proc. R. Soc.*, **139**, 263.

HIERNAUX, J. (1968). Shape differentiation of ethnic groups and of sexes through growth. *Hum. Biol.*, **40**, 44.

HOGBEN, H., WATERHOUSE, J. A. H. and HOGBEN, L. (1948). Studies on puberty, Part I. *Brit. J. Soc. Med.*, **2**, 29.

JONES, H. E. (1949). *Motor Performance and Growth.* Berkeley: Univ. Calif. Press.

MARSHALL, W. A. and TANNER, J. M. (1969). Variation in the pattern of pubertal changes in girls. *Arch. Dis. Childh.*, **44**, 291.

MONTAGU, M. F. A. (1946). *Adolescent Sterility.* Springfield: Thomas.

PROVIS, H. S. and ELLIS, R. W. B. (1955). An anthropometric study of Edinburgh school children: Part I. Methods and data with assessment of maturity. *Arch. Dis. Childh.*, **30**, 328.

REYNOLDS, E. L. and WINES, J. V. (1948). Individual differences in physical changes associated with adolescence in girls. *Amer. J. Dis. Child.*, **75**, 329.

—— —— (1951). Physical changes associated with adolescence in boys. *Amer. J. Dis. Child.*, **82**, 529.

RUNDLE, A. T. and SYLVESTER, P. E. (1962). Measurement of testicular volume. *Arch. Dis. Childh.*, **37**, 514.

SCHONFELD, W. A. (1943). Primary and secondary sexual characteristics: study of their development in males from birth through maturity with biometric study of penis and testes. *Amer. J. Dis. Child.*, **65**, 435.

SHUTTLEWORTH, F. K. (1937). Sexual maturation and the physical growth of girls aged six to nineteen. *Monog. Soc. Res. Child. Devel.*, **2**, No. 5.

SIMMONS, K. and GREULICH, W. W. (1943). Menarcheal age and the height, weight and skeletal age of girls age 7 to 17 years. *J. Pediat.*, **22**, 518.

STOLZ, H. R. and STOLZ, L. M. (1951). *Somatic Development of Adolescent Boys*. New York: Macmillan.

STONE, C. P. and BARKER, R. G. (1937). On the relationship between menarcheal age and certain measurements of physique in girls of the ages of 9 to 16 years. *Hum. Biol.*, **91**, 1.

STUART, H. C. (1946). Normal growth and development during adolescence. *New Eng. J. Med.*, **234**, 666, 693 and 732.

TANNER, J. M. (1958). Physical maturing and behaviour at adolescence. (*The Convocation Lecture of the National Children's Home*). London: National Children's Home.

—— (1962). *Growth at Adolescence*. 2nd ed. Oxford: Blackwell.

—— (1969). Growth and Endocrinology of the Adolescent. In *Endocrine and Genetic Diseases of Childhood*. Ed. L. Gardner. Philadelphia and London: Saunders.

—— and GUPTA, D. (1968). A longitudinal study of the excretion of individual steroids in children from 8 to 12 years old. *J. Endocr.*, **41**, 139.

—— WHITEHOUSE, R. H. and TAKAISHI, M. (1966). Standards from birth to maturity for height, weight, height velocity and weight velocity: British children. *Arch. Dis. Childh.*, **41**, 454, 613.

YOUNG, H. B. (1963). Ageing and adolescence. *Dev. Med. Child Neurol.*, **5**, 451.

8　The Development of Behaviour

THE study of behaviour development requires the observation, analysis and interpretation of the series of changes which enable a helpless newborn infant to become an independent adult. It is concerned with the nature of these changes, the order in which they occur and the ages at which they may be found. In addition investigators are interested in the intrinsic and environmental circumstances which appear to accelerate or retard them.

Behaviour development depends upon the maturation of the nervous system but is also influenced by a complex interplay between intrinsic and environmental factors which affect the child. The genetic make-up of the individual and his early intra- and extra-uterine experience will affect his physical, intellectual, and emotional growth and this in turn will determine whether he reacts favourably or unfavourably to later changes in his environment. These changes themselves are likely to have further effects on physical and behavioural development. The complexity of the interweaving of intrinsic and extrinsic factors through generations has been well illustrated by studies of children born to impoverished and ignorant parents. They tend to be undersized, intellectually retarded, handicapped in speech and uneducated as compared to the offspring of parents with more money and education (Birch, 1968). Since disease in childhood affects a developing organism it is liable to have far-reaching effects on the later maturation of physical growth and behaviour. For example, serious starvation in infancy may be followed by permanent stunting of growth. Impairment of hearing as a result of meningitis or otitis media may cause secondary retardation of speech development and impair the child's ability to make social contact with other children and adults at a later stage.

Normal behaviour development depends upon normal maturation in the nervous system and any disease of the brain is likely to have immediate and long-term effects upon the child's behaviour, but even then environmental influences have a part to play. It is impossible, for example, to teach a child to talk until a certain degree of neurological maturation has been achieved or to teach a child to walk until the neurological substrate required for the development of walking is present. On the other hand children who have limited opportunities for close human contact in infancy may be slow to speak though the neurological apparatus necessary for the development of spoken language is present.

Neligan and Prudham (1969) studied the norms for the developmental milestones of sitting, walking unsupported, using single words and using sentences in a large representative population of children in the City of Newcastle upon Tyne. They found that there was a closer correlation between the ages at which children passed the two motor milestones and the ages at which they passed the two linguistic milestones than there was between either of the motor milestones and linguistic milestones. They found that girls and first born children showed significant advancement in using sentences compared to other groups and that children in social classes III, IV and V showed significant precocity in walking. They made the not entirely unexpected observation that mothers' memories about milestones become progressively less accurate as their children grew older.

Children later excluded from normal school because of mental defect, cerebral palsy or deafness had shown previously significant delay in passing the milestones

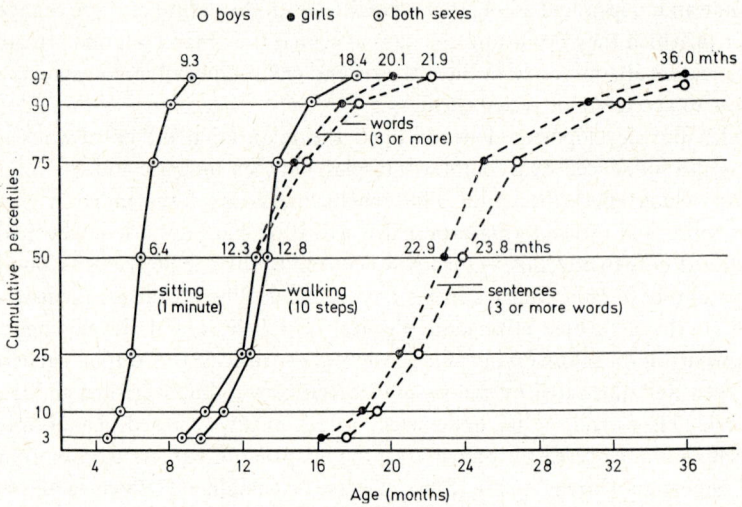

FIG. 52. Cumulative percentile curves for four standard developmental milestones.

of sitting and walking unsupported and using sentences. They were not so consistently retarded in using single words (Neligan and Prudham, 1969 *a* and *b*).

Even when behaviour development is slowed by adverse environmental conditions it is usual for the same sequence of maturation to be preserved; the child sits before he stands and stands before he walks. He babbles before he says his first words and says single words before he talks in phrases and sentences. There is truth in the old adage 'you cannot teach a child to run before he walks'.

Though there is regularity in the order in which particular 'milestones' of behaviour are reached by healthy children, there is a great variation in the ages at which they are achieved; some healthy children, for example, may say their first intelligible words by the age of 10 months yet be unable to walk without support until the age of 16 or 17 months, whereas others quite as healthy may walk unsupported by the age of 12 months but fail to say intelligible words until the age of 2 years or more (Fig. 52).

Attempts to relate behavioural changes to neurophysiological or neuropathological phenomena have not been very successful to date. It is apparent, for example, that many nerve tracts in the brains and the spinal cords of infants function very similarly to those in adults even before they are myelinated (Luria, 1966; Ellingson, 1964). Similarly attempts to relate electroencephalographic phenomena to the development of normal behaviour are still rather crude and elementary though progress has been made (Dreyfus-Brisac, 1964). The fact that developmental changes in behaviour cannot be related directly to neuroanatomical and neurophysiological findings means that higher nervous activities must be discussed using psychological rather than neurological or neuropathological terms (D'Ajuriaguerra and Hécaen, 1949).

Developmental Diagnosis

Developmental diagnosis consists of comparing the various achievements of the child under study with those of a representative group of children from the same community. For the purposes of systematic description it is convenient to consider arbitrarily defined categories of behaviour separately. Gesell (1940), for example, made separate assessments of motor, linguistic, adaptive and social behaviour. The categories of motor, linguistic and social behaviour are self-explanatory. By adaptive behaviour is meant that type of behaviour which is shown when the child is set to solve problems. These may be problems of everyday life, such as those encountered when he tries to feed himself using a spoon or to undress and dress, or they may be those presented to him when formal tests are given.

Inevitably there is some overlap in the categories described. The later social milestones of development, for example, depend upon there being normal linguistic development. Many items of adaptive behaviour depend upon there being normal motor function, but many of them also depend upon the child's concept of himself and of his environment. A baby of 6 months, for example, who is perfectly able physically to reach for an object which has been covered by a cloth, will not search for it because he has not developed the concept of 'object constancy' which is necessary before he can realise that the fact that something has disappeared from sight does not mean that it has 'gone'. Similarly many older children who have the manipulative ability to do up small buttons or tie their shoe-laces cannot do so because they are unable to conceptualise the process of tying knots. Many such items of adaptive behaviour are dependent upon the development of the ability to carry out what Piaget calls 'mental operations' which he defines as 'internalised reversible actions' (Piaget, 1950). Experiments by Piaget and his pupils have done much to enlarge our knowledge of the ages at which particular 'internalised reversible actions' can be demonstrated, but it has been pointed out by many workers that it is very difficult to assess the 'awareness' of a young infant from his responses to stimuli. For example, the fact that a fetus in utero will react by moving to the sound of a loud motor horn merely means that the fetus reacts to a loud noise and that the peripheral pathways for hearing are intact; it does not mean that the fetus is 'aware' of the sound at any conscious level.

Developmental diagnosis is of great clinical value, for it does help to identify categories of behaviour in which the child is defective. For example, a toddler of 18 months who was unable to sit without support or reach for objects but whose linguistic, adaptive and social performance was otherwise normal would be considered to show specific retardation of motor development. A child able to run and jump at the age of 2 years who could feed himself, and was able to take his socks and shoes off and make social relationships with his parents, but who had no words of spoken language, would be considered to have relatively normal adaptive and social behaviour but to show specific retardation of linguistic development. This could be due to impaired hearing or to poorly understood hereditary factors which cause specific retardation of speech development. By using the techniques of developmental diagnosis it is possible to suspect mental retardation in many children who are still too young for formal tests of intelligence. Most children who suffer from severe mental subnormality show global retardation of behaviour development though the retardation of motor development is usually less marked than that of linguistic, adaptive and social behaviour and in a minority of mentally handicapped patients motor development may be normal. Diagnosis of lesser degrees of mental subnormality must be made with caution and it may not be possible to make it until the child is 3 years of age or more, by which time standardised formal tests of intelligence can be employed. As children grow older assessment of behaviour development becomes in many ways easier and long range prediction of future development can be achieved with increasing accuracy (Illingworth, 1967; Ingram, 1969, and see also Chapter 9).

The Newborn Infant

The newborn baby makes reflex responses to auditory, gustatory and tactile stimuli but deliberate purposeful responses are lacking. He is completely dependent upon his parents for food, care and protection, but he is not inactive. His responses to environmental stimuli merit study for it is only in the newborn period that the reflex activities mediated through the spinal cord and brain stem which are later inhibited and submerged in patterns of voluntary movement can be examined adequately.

Motor Activities of the Newborn

The resting posture of the mature newborn is usually one of semi-flexion of the trunk and limbs, a modification of the fetal position of generalised flexion, though babies born by the breech with extended legs may keep their lower limbs in this position for some weeks after delivery. Because of their semi-flexed posture newborn babies tend to lie mostly on their sides when at rest or sleeping (Fig. 53). In babies born before term the resting posture is one of more marked flexion of the trunk and all four limbs.

The newborn baby has very little control of posture. When placed in the supine position his head falls back, but he should be able to maintain his head in a semi-extended position when he is held prone, something that the premature

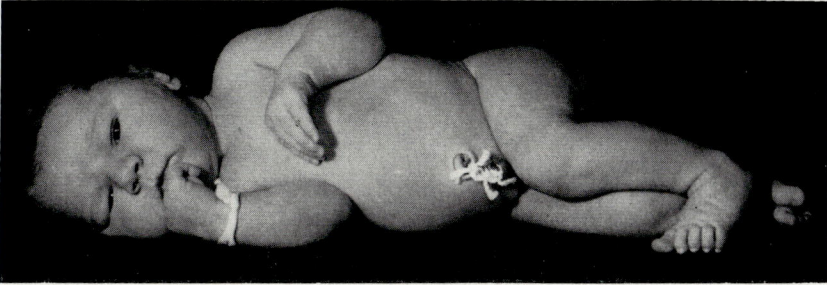

FIG. 53. The characteristic posture of the newborn baby is one of semiflexion of the neck, trunk and limbs. The hands are usually closed and the thumbs grasped in the palms. The posture is similar to that of the fetus in the womb.

infant is commonly unable to achieve (Fig. 54). In contrast to the rather free movements of the head which occur when the baby's position is changed, the postures of the upper limbs remain relatively constant.

In most babies the tonus of the flexor muscle groups is greater than that of the anti-gravity muscles for the first 6 to 8 weeks of life. Muscle tone varies greatly in

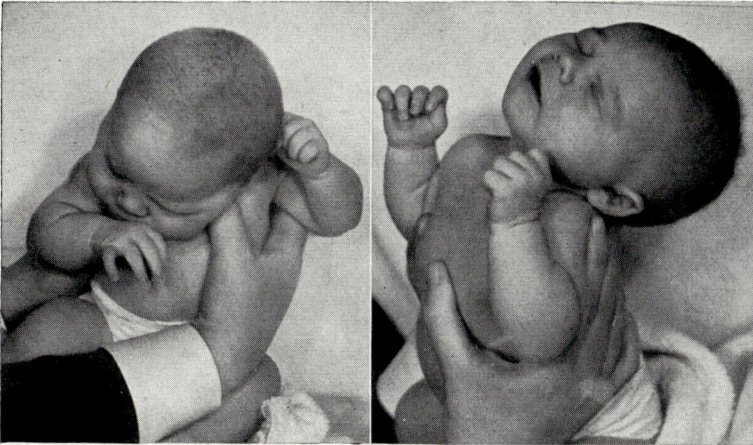

FIG. 54. Newborn infant aged 24 hours, showing inability to hold up head in erect position.

different babies and from time to time in the individual child. It tends to be increased when the baby is hungry or crying and relatively diminished when he is satisfied and comfortable.

Spontaneous movements appear random and purposeless in the newborn and

the limbs tend to move all in one piece from the proximal joints without coordin-
ated movements in the distal parts. Movements of the upper limbs commonly
result in the hands being placed in the mouth; sucking of the thumb and scratching
of the face occur within a few hours of birth and have even been observed in utero.
When the lower limbs are moved spontaneously, reciprocal pedalling or 'bicycling'
activity is often seen. Mass movements affecting the trunk and all four limbs, as in
yawning or stretching, are characteristic in the newborn period. Many of these
involuntary subcortically controlled movement patterns are strikingly similar to
those exhibited by lower forms of animal life and by decerebrate mammals.
Swimming and crawling movements resembling those found in amphibia and
reptiles may be demonstrated in the newborn. They become progressively inhibited
by higher nervous centres after the first 2 or 3 weeks of postnatal life, but may
persist for much longer periods in patients with severe developmental abnormalities
or birth damage of the brain (McGraw, 1943). There are dangers, however, in
interpreting too closely the sequential stages of early human development in terms
of behaviour development of lower animal forms (Carmichael, 1954).

Reflexes in the Newborn

A number of well defined reflexes should be present in the newborn infant and
their absence usually indicates abnormality of the nervous system or serious
systemic disease. It is important to remember, however, that the ease with which
particular reflexes may be elicited depends greatly upon the physiological state of
the infant. For example, the feeding reflexes are greatly enhanced by hunger and
depressed if the baby is satisfied, while the Moro reflex may be difficult to elicit in
some babies if they are too drowsy and in others if they are crying. Prechtl and
Beintema (1964) describe five states which should be recorded when any baby is
subjected to neurological examination. These are as follows:

STATE 1: eyes closed, regular respiration, no movements.
STATE 2: eyes closed, irregular respiration, no gross movements.
STATE 3: eyes open, no gross movements.
STATE 4: eyes open, gross movements, no crying.
STATE 5: eyes open or closed, crying.

Clearly in State 1 the baby is likely to be much less responsive to stimuli than in
State 3 or 4, whereas in 5 there is so much body movement and fluctuation in
muscle tone that neurological examination is likely to be unrewarding.

A number of feeding reflexes have been described in the newborn. They are all
subcortically mediated and are the most constantly present of the infantile reflexes.
The rooting or search reflex is the name given to the reflex orientation of the head
towards the touch stimulus in the peri-oral region. Two patterns of response have
been described by Prechtl (1958). In the first there is a repetitive side-to-side
movement of the head away from and towards the stimulus, the range of oscillation
of the head gradually diminishing until the stimulus is approximated to the mouth.
This response is characteristically found in prematurely born babies but it is present
in a proportion of mature babies for a week or two after birth. The second response,

which supersedes side-to-side head turning, is often present from birth in mature babies, and is called the 'directed head turning reflex'; this consists of a single, well directed, purposeful-looking movement of the head, which results in the infant's mouth being placed in contact with the touch stimulus.

What is often termed the 'sucking reflex' really comprises two reflexes; the lip reflex or lip phenomenon or 'l'épreuve des points cardinaux' (André-Thomas *et al.*, 1960) and the sucking reflex proper. The lip reflex can most easily be elicited by a gentle stroking stimulus in the peri-oral region moving towards the mouth

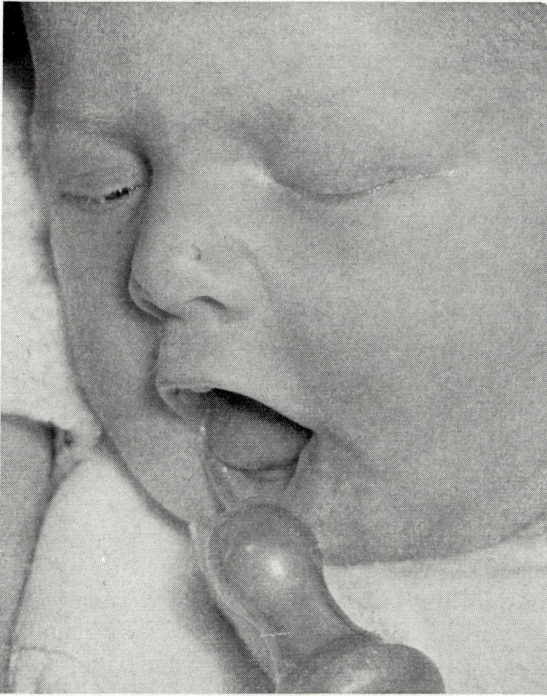

FIG. 55. The lip reflex in the newborn.

The response consists of mouth opening and a movement of the parted lips towards the stimulus so that the mouth is often open towards one side rather than in the mid-line. As the mouth opens the tongue usually protrudes at least as far forward as the lips and is curved so as to be concave superiorly, forming a trough into which the nipple or teat stimulus is taken and brought into the mouth. As the tongue and nipple are pulled into the mouth the infant closes the lips and often swallows (Fig. 55).

The actual sucking reflex consists of a reflex sucking movement elicited by a touch stimulus applied to the infant's lips, the front of his tongue, his gums or his hard palate.

The swallowing reflex is the name given to the swallowing movement which occurs when fluid or food is placed in contact with the walls or the back of the pharynx, on the back of the tongue, the epiglottis or the soft palate. In practice, the easiest way to elicit the swallowing reflex is to cause the infant to suck, for sucking will draw saliva towards the back of the mouth and usually this in turn produces swallowing. When successful feeding routines have been initiated the rooting, lip, sucking and swallowing reflexes are integrated closely one with the other. The movement of head rotation towards the nipple, mouth opening, tongue protrusion and retraction with the nipple on it with mouth closure, sucking and swallowing occurs so rapidly and so smoothly that where one reflex ends and the next begins may be difficult to determine. Feeding reflexes become less easily elicited in most babies after the age of 5 or 6 months, but the time at which they actually disappear is extremely variable. They may be elicited in many drowsy children aged 3 or 4 years (Ingram, 1962).

The Moro reflex may be elicited by changing the position of the head relative to the trunk. The child may be dropped in space so that his head is jerked gently backwards or an abrupt stimulus may be given by the examiner banging his hands onto the mattress beside the baby's head. It is believed that the Moro response depends upon proprioceptive impulses from the neck and not, as used to be believed, from the vestibular apparatus (Paine *et al.*, 1964). The response consists of a momentary flexion of the head, trunk and limbs so rapid that it can only be appreciated in slowed down cinematographic film and then a rather abrupt extension and abduction of the arms and legs. These movements are followed by slower flexion of the limbs and trunk so that the semi-flexion position of infancy is again assumed (Fig. 56). The reflex is very constantly present in healthy mature and premature babies. It is most easily elicited in the first 4 to 6 weeks of life, but is usually present in infants under the age of 3 months though after this time it becomes progressively difficult to elicit. It is almost invariably absent by the time the child can sit even momentarily without support. If there is lower or upper neurone damage affecting the limbs on one side the reflex will be asymmetrical even in early infancy. Severe retardation of motor development due to failure of the maturation of higher inhibitory functions in the cerebral cortex often results in persistence of the Moro reflex. However, brain damage acquired after the disappearance of the Moro reflex rarely, if ever, results in its reappearance.

The symmetrical tonic neck reflex is evoked by extension or flexion of the neck. When the child is in the prone position kneeling, extension of the head produces an increase of anti-gravity tonus in the limbs. When the head is flexed the limbs show a decrease in antigravity tone.

In the erect position the effect of flexion and extension of the head is somewhat different in the newborn baby. In this position extension of the head tends to cause flexion and adduction of the shoulders, flexion of the elbows and pronation of the forearms and an increase of anti-gravity tone in the lower limbs. In normal babies the symmetrical neck reflex becomes progressively difficult to elicit and identify after the age of 4 or 5 months, but in children with severe cerebral palsy it may be easily elicited throughout life.

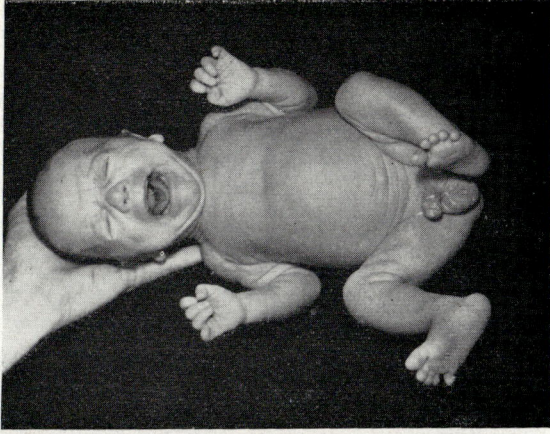

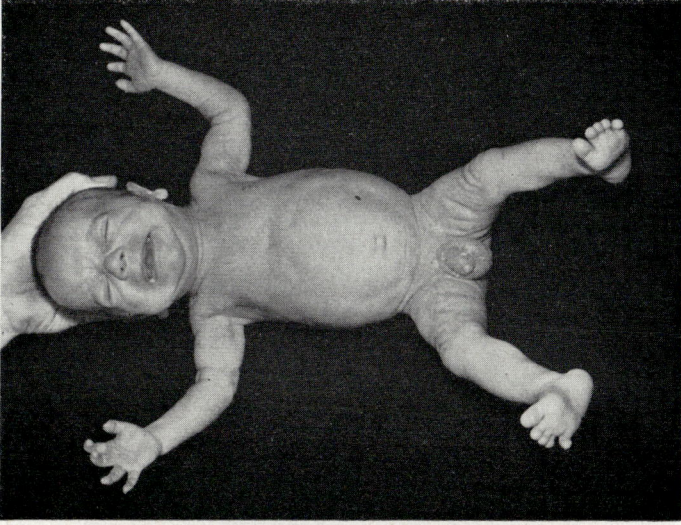

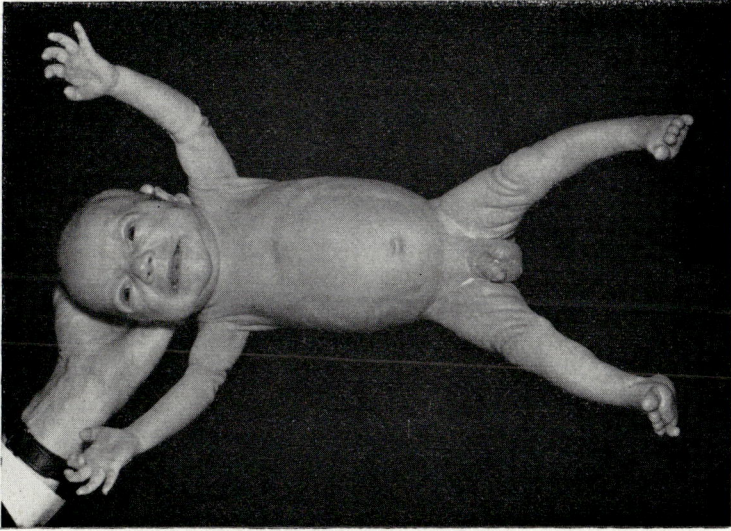

Fig. 56. Moro reflex, showing extension and abduction of limbs, followed by flexion and abduction.

(a)

(b)

(c)

The asymmetrical tonic neck reflex consists of the response of the limbs to rotation of the head. The reflex is best elicited when the child lying in the supine position himself spontaneously turns his head in one or other direction. The response consists of extension of the limbs on the side to which the head is turned and flexion of the contralateral limbs, so that 'a fencing position' is assumed (Fig. 57). The reflex is brisk in babies born after about 28 weeks' gestation, but declines in activity after about 36 weeks' gestation so that in many term infants the reflex may be quite difficult to demonstrate. Thereafter, however, it again

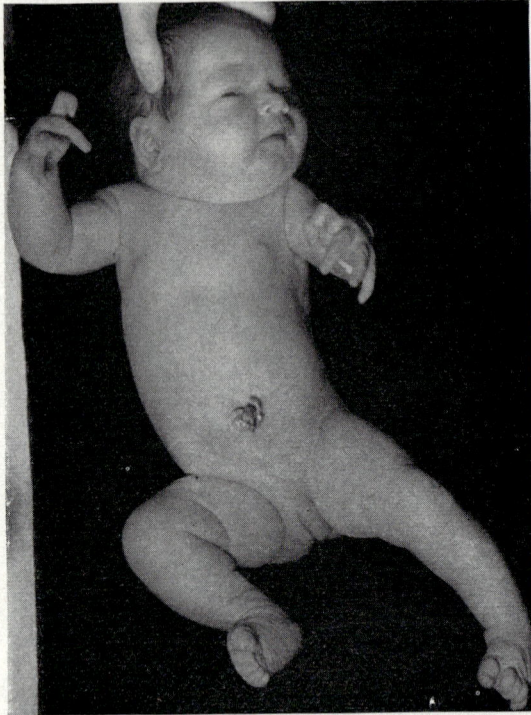

FIG. 57. Asymmetrical tonic neck reflex showing extension of limbs on side towards which head is turned, with flexion of contra-lateral limbs.

becomes easier to elicit and at the age of between 1 and 3 months *post partum* can be elicited quite readily. The persistence of an obligatory asymmetrical neck reflex after the age of 5 months should be viewed with concern for it may be one of the first signs of extra-pyramidal (choreoathetoid) cerebral palsy (Paine *et al.*, 1964).

The placing response is elicited by bringing an object into contact with the dorsum of the foot or the anterior aspect of the tibia. The foot is then raised in a stepping movement (Fig. 58). By reflex walking is understood the reciprocal placing response that may be elicited in newborn babies if they are placed with their feet on a flat surface and are tilted alternately sideways and slightly forwards.

Reciprocal placing movements in which there is a high stepping gait may then be elicited. The reflex is present in almost all newborn babies and is particularly brisk in prematures. It declines progressively from the age of 4 to 6 weeks and it is

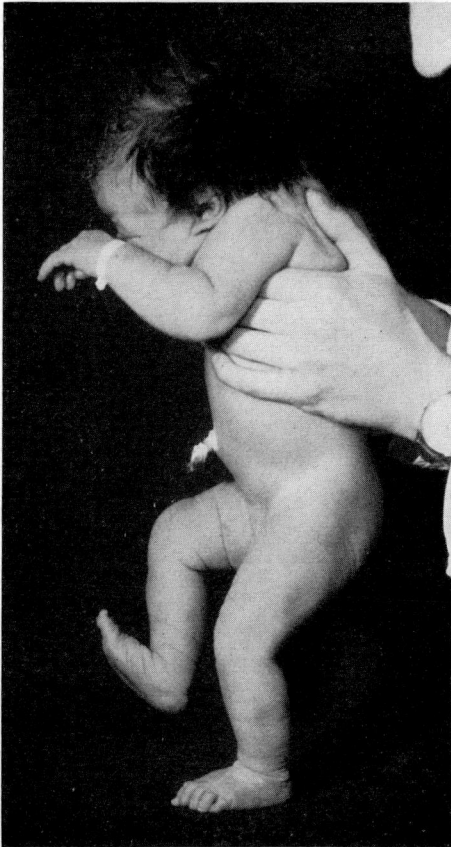

FIG. 58. Reflex stepping by newborn infant.

unusual to be able to elicit reciprocal walking after the age of about 3 months in normal babies.

Grasp reflexes in the hands and feet are easily elicited in the majority of mature newborn babies if a touch stimulus is moved distally along the palm or the sole (Fig. 59). The reflexes become less easy to elicit in the majority of babies at the age of 2 months, but there is considerable variation in the time of their disappearance. A marked asymmetry in the ease with which the grasp reflexes are obtained on the two sides may indicate the presence of hemiplegia.

The trunk incurvation response is elicited by exerting pressure medially beside the spine between the lower ribs and the pelvis. The response consists of a reflex incurvation of the trunk so that the spine is made concave on the side of the stimulus.

This reflex can nearly always be elicited in the newborn and it commonly persists until the baby is 2 or 3 months old (Fig. 60). Tendon jerks are much more variable in the newborn infant than they are in adults and their briskness depends to a

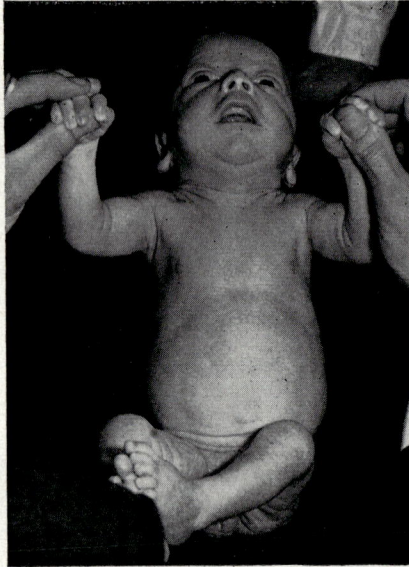

FIG. 59. The grasp reflexes are present at birth in both hands and feet. The most reliable stimulus is a touch of moderate pressure moving distally in the palm of the hand.

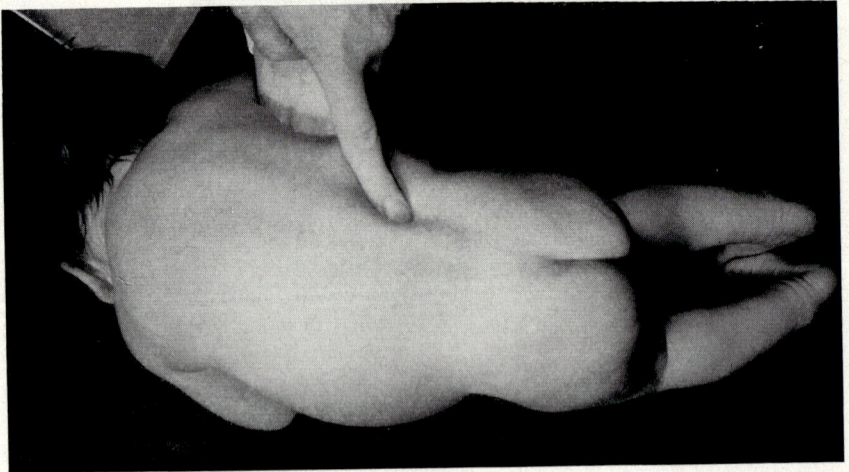

FIG. 60. The trunk incurvation response. Firm pressure in the newborn infant's loin causes the trunk to curve concavely on the side of the stimulus.

considerable extent upon the alertness or 'state' of the infant (Prechtl and Beintema, 1964). Thus they vary considerably from baby to baby and in individual babies from time to time. Biceps, supinator and knee jerks can usually be elicited easily but ankle and triceps jerks are often quite difficult to obtain. The plantar response

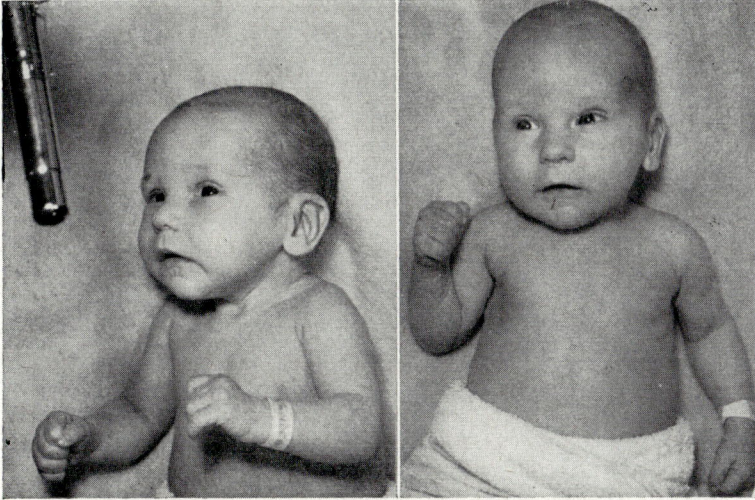

FIG. 61. Infant aged 4 weeks following a bright object with the eyes.

is extensor in the majority of newborn babies, but is flexor in a significant minority (Brain and Wilkinson, 1959).

The abdominal reflex is present in the newborn infant, but the response is much more diffuse and generalised than in the adult.

The vestibular apparatus can be shown to be active in the newborn baby, for if he is held in the examiner's hands and rotated the eyes move first in the direction of rotation and then in the opposite direction when rotation ceases and there is nystagmus. Vestibular reflexes become progressively important in maintaining the posture of the baby's head after the age of 2 or 3 weeks.

The newborn infant reacts to a bright light by blinking or screwing up the eyes, but in suitable conditions it can be demonstrated that even in the first week of life children can recognise contrasting shapes and if a striped rotating drum is placed within their field of vision saccadic movements of the eyes will result (Fantz, 1967). As they grow older the visual fixation of babies becomes more accurate (Fig. 61).

Motor Development in the First Two Years of Life

It is convenient to consider motor development in two ways. Firstly the positive 'milestones' of development should be noted. The ages at which achievements such as sitting without support or reaching for objects using the thumb and forefinger occur are examples of positive milestones. Secondly motor development may be

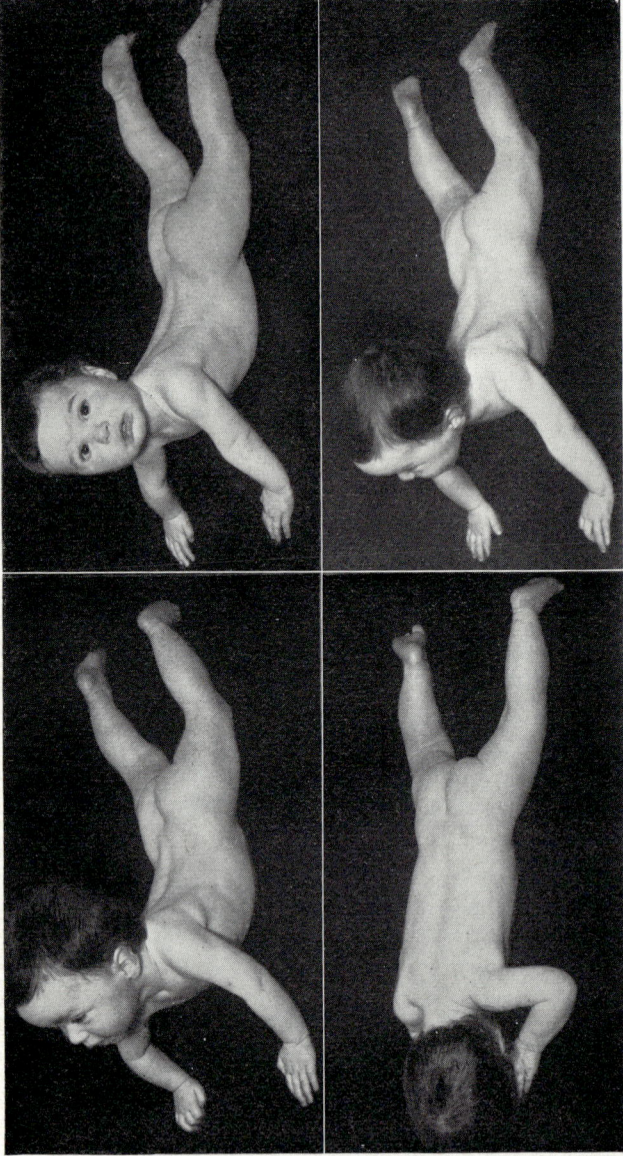

FIG. 62. By the age of 16 weeks the baby can support his upper trunk for a limited period when prone and can move head and eyes in a co-ordinated fashion.

measured to some extent by negative motor milestones. By negative motor milestones are understood the ages at which reflexes characteristic of the newborn disappear. For example, a child age 7 months showing brisk Moro, stepping and

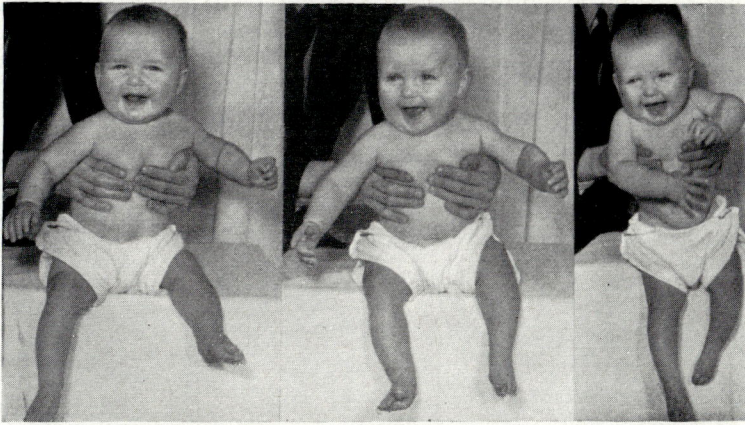

FIG. 63. By the age of 4 to 5 months supported sitting is possible and is much enjoyed.

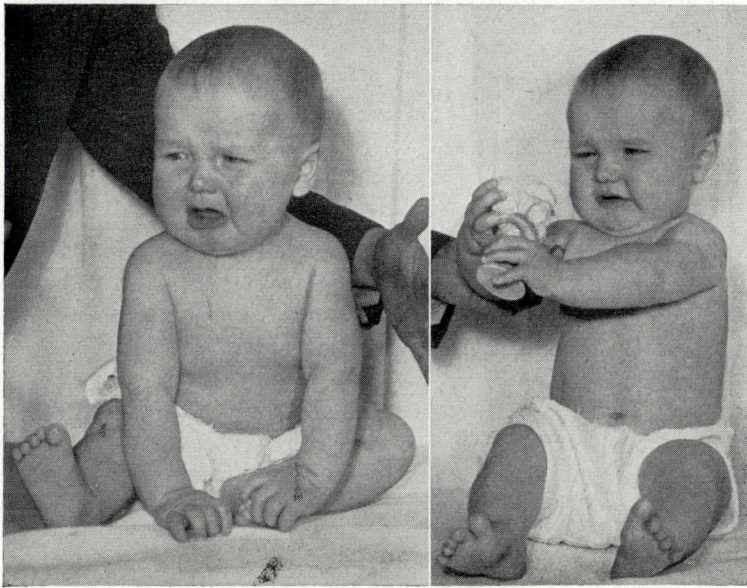

FIG. 64. Infant aged 6½ months. Can sit momentarily with support of arms but not without: grasps object with both hands.

grasp reflexes would be considered to be retarded, for by this age these reflexes should have been inhibited by the action of higher nervous centres.

Though they are necessarily inter-related, it is convenient for the purposes of

description to consider separately the development of postural control and manipulative skills.

As emphasised by Gesell (1940), it is universal that voluntary control of posture
proceeds in a cephalo-caudal direction so that the child acquires control of the
position of his head before he can maintain the position of his upper trunk and
can control his upper trunk before he is able to balance sitting unsupported or
standing.

Increasing control of posture is achieved by the integration of the tonic neck
activity typical of the neonate with the higher level vestibular and retinal reflexes

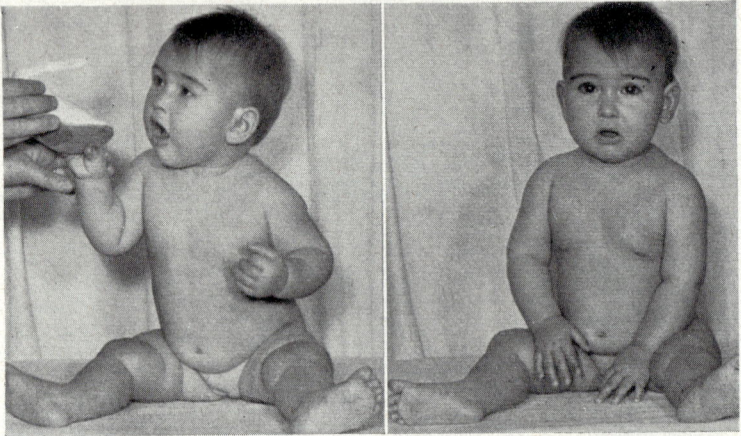

FIG. 65. Infant aged 8 months. Sits confidently without support; grasps
with one hand but shows flexion of contralateral limb while doing so.

and their subsequent inhibition by cortical centres which allow the child to alter
his posture voluntarily without losing balance. By the age of 4 weeks he can turn
his head from side to side when prone and support his head briefly when held in
the erect position. By the age of 6 weeks he is usually able to follow bright objects
moving near him by movements of the head and neck as well as of the eyes. Control
of the upper trunk which allows unsupported sitting is achieved usually between
5 and 7 months. Control of the lower trunk is achieved between the ages of 7 and 9
months and being able to balance in the standing position first supported and then
unsupported is achieved by most babies between the ages of 12 and 15 months
(Fig. 62, 63, 64, 68, 69). By the age of 7 or 8 months the baby 'helps' to pull
himself from the supine to the sitting position (Fig. 67).

There are, however, great variations in the ages at which these positive milestones of motor development are reached and also in their pattern. For example,
some children crawl on their bellies and pull themselves along with their arms
from the age of 5 or 6 months (Fig. 70); others crawl on their hands and knees
from the age of 8 or 9 months (Fig. 71); and some bottom-crawl in the squatting
position from the age of 9 or 10 months and may not walk if they are adept at this

until the age of 20 months or more. These variations, however, do not affect the general rule of the cephalo-caudal development of postural control.

The secondary effects of the child's progressively improving control of posture should not be neglected, for inevitably what he can see and learn about his environment is vastly increased when he can attain the sitting position and see

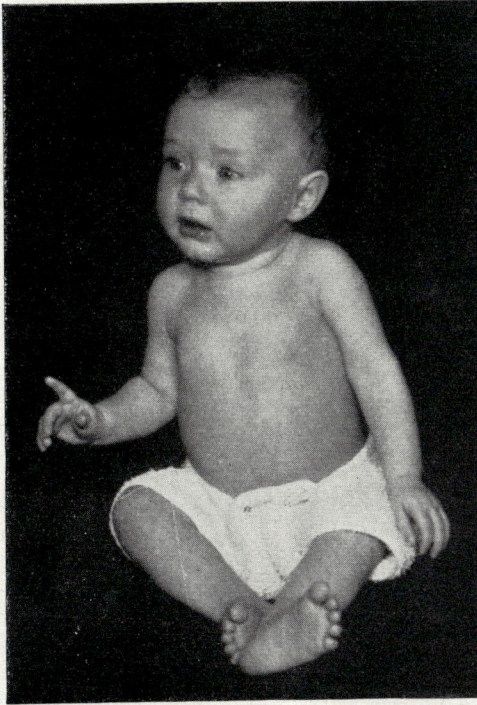

FIG. 66. Infant aged 10 months. Independent use of right hand without flexion of contralateral limb.

things at eye level instead of having to look up at them all the time. Moreover, as postural control improves so the living platform to which the limbs are attached becomes steadier and increasingly precise movements of the hands are possible. The child usually reaches for objects two-handed at the age of about sixteen weeks, but it is usually two or three weeks after this before he achieves useful grasping and is able to place objects in his mouth with precision (Fig. 72). From the age of between 24 and 28 weeks the baby may reach for objects one-handed with his fingers somewhat separated and opposed to the palm; quite marked associated movements of the contralateral upper limbs are usually present when he does so. As he grows older the child tends to use the thumb to a greater extent, opposing it to begin with to the ulnar border of the hand and as he grows older progressively

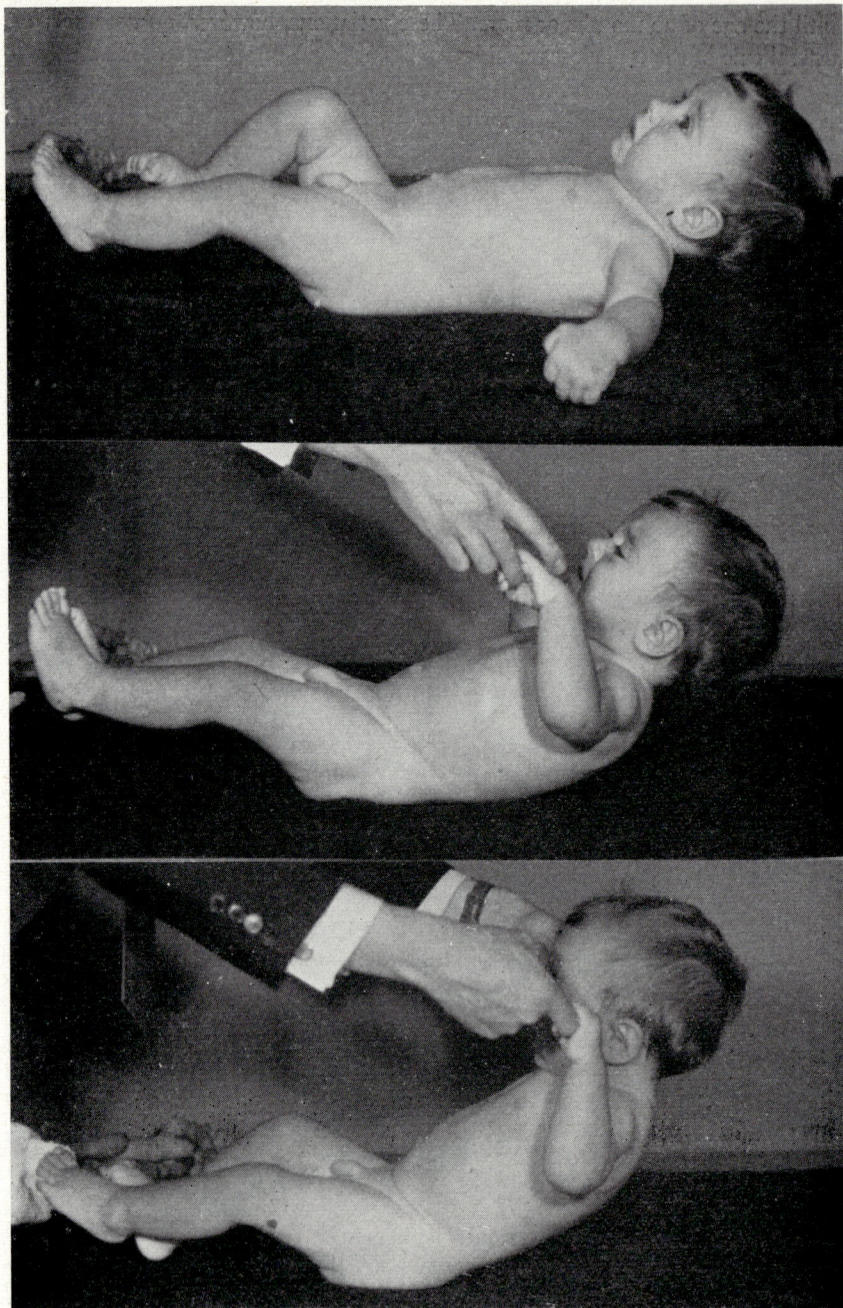

FIG. 67. Infant aged 8 months, showing characteristic use of arms to help to pull himself from supine to sitting position.

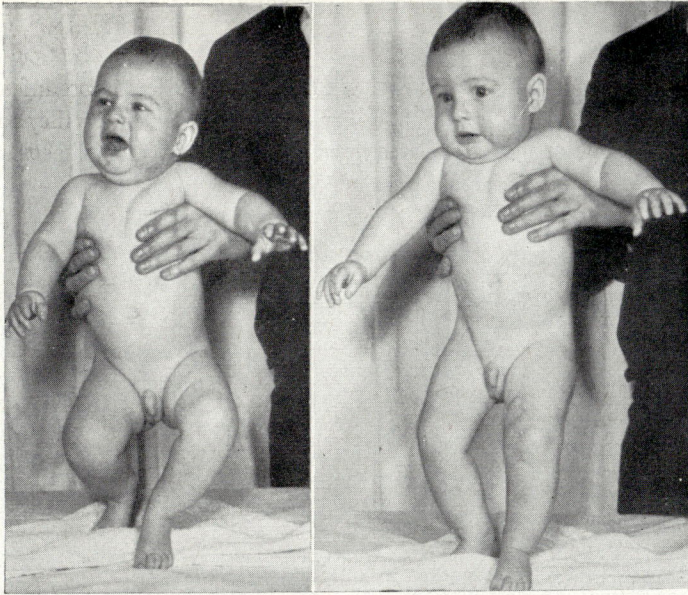

FIG. 68. Infant aged 5 months. Momentarily takes a little weight on lower limbs when held.

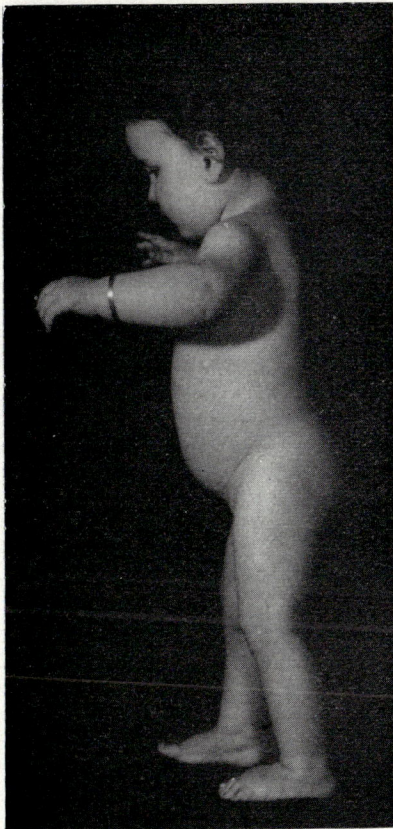

FIG. 69. Infant aged 11 months. Early unsteady steps, using elevated upper limbs to help balance.

to the radial side of the hand. Well before the age of a year, most infants have achieved a pincer grip using the thumb and first finger and when they reach for an object they do not show associated involuntary movements of the contralateral upper limb as at an earlier age (Gesell and Amatruda, 1947).

Preference in the use of hand, eye and foot develops gradually in childhood.

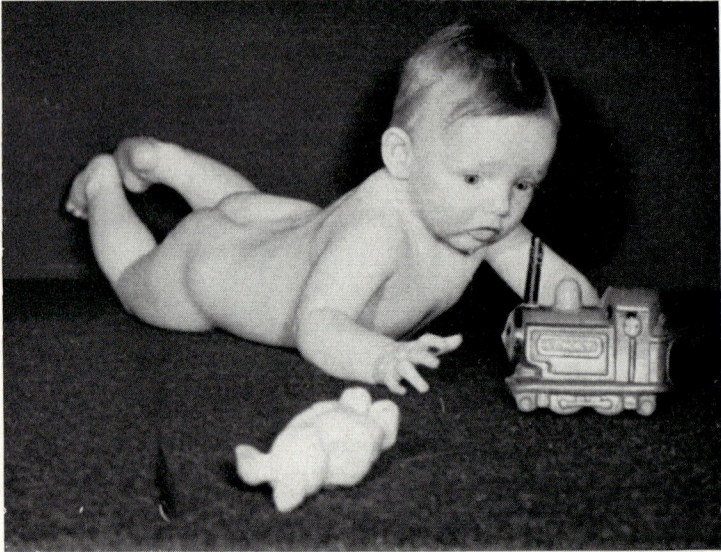

FIG. 70. Crawling on the abdomen is achieved by most babies between the ages of 7 and 9 months, but the extent to which crawling is used as a means of progression is extremely variable.

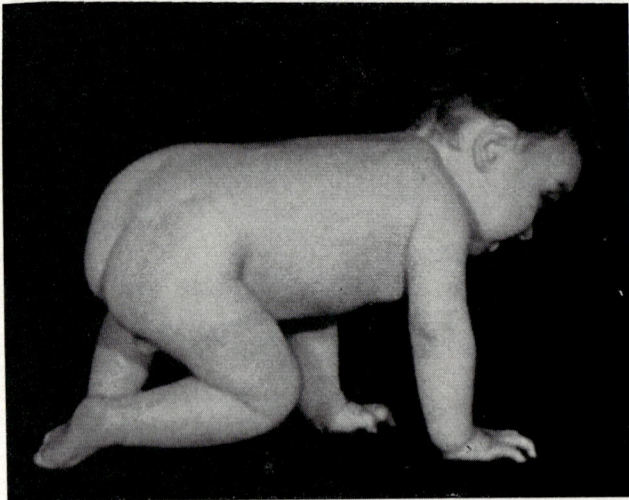

FIG. 71. By the age of 10 months crawling is usually on hands and knees and the limbs are used reciprocally.

There is no doubt that hereditary factors are important in determining lateral preference, but sinistrality does not appear to be inherited according to Mendelian rules. Environmental factors are of obvious importance. Right-handed parents, for

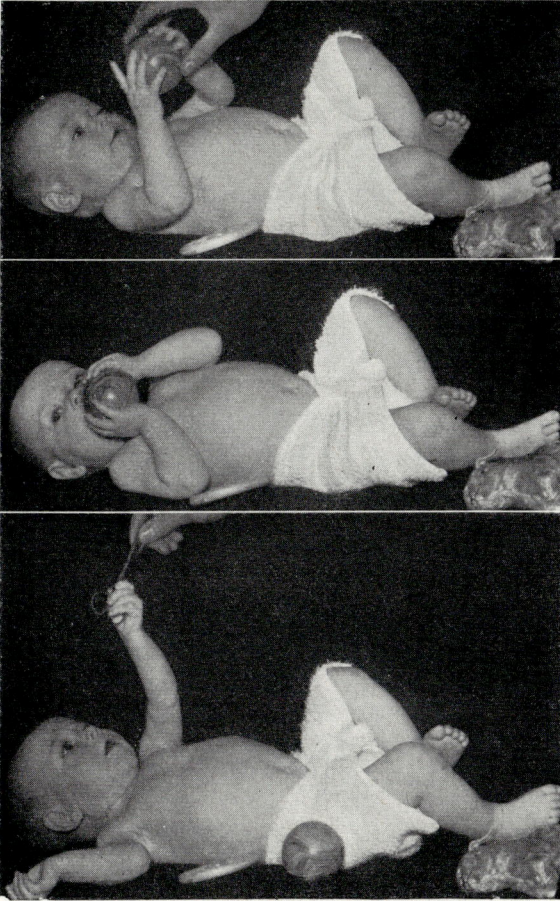

FIG. 72. Infant aged 6 months. From 4 to 5 months onward, he begins to reach for objects using all the fingers as a unit and usually with both hands operating similarly. He explores the things he picks up by putting them to his mouth and bites as well as sucks them.

example, usually encourage their babies to use their right hands for spoon feeding or for taking a cup. Various patterns in developing preference for one hand or another may be recognised. Some babies appear to be 'lateralised' from early infancy, whereas others may show little or no preference for one or the other hand for months or even years. Changes in apparent handedness are not uncommon in the first 2 years of life (Fig. 65).

With the development of voluntary control of motor activity, there are changes in muscle tone, in reflex activity and in posture at rest. Reflexes characteristic of the newborn baby, for example the stepping reflex and the Moro reflex, become inhibited as higher nervous centres develop, but some new reflexes appear. For example, as the activity of the asymmetrical tonic neck reflex declines, the 'parachute reflex' or 'falling reflex of Magnus' becomes manifest. This reflex is elicited by

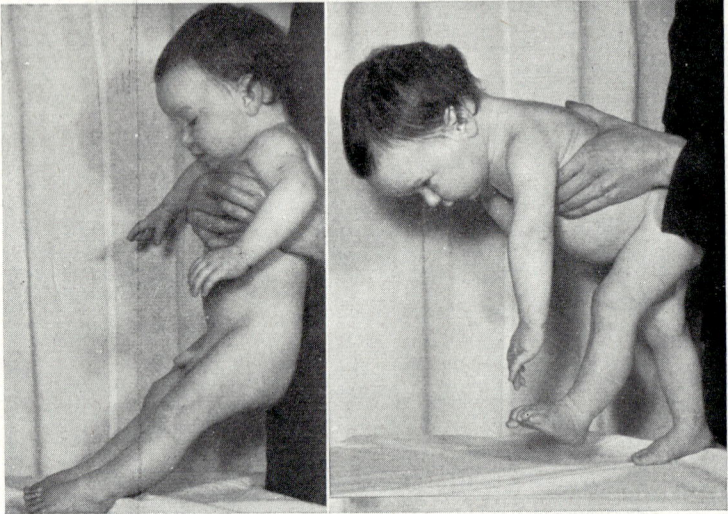

FIG. 73. Falling reflex of Magnus. When the infant is tilted forward quickly there is a reflex stepping movement forwards and the extended upper limb is placed anteriorly as though to break a fall.

holding the child in the erect position and abruptly tilting him forward. From between the ages of 7 and 9 months it is usual for normal babies to throw their upper limbs forward with the elbows extended as if to break their fall (Fig. 73). Neonatal reflexes which persist for a time are gradually integrated with these later appearing reflexes and are in turn controlled and to some extent submerged as voluntary control of movements and posture develops.

Thus whilst 'motor ages' may be assessed on the basis of the child's milestones of positive motor development, they may be assessed also, in a sense negatively, by studying the reflexes which are still present and which should have been lost. A study of infantile reflexes is not only crucial to determining stages of motor development, but may also be of value in detecting disease of the nervous system at an early stage. For example, a child aged 10 months with a congenital hemiplegia is likely to extend his unaffected upper limb in the parachute reflex, but fail to extend his paretic arm (Fiorentino, 1963).

As the child's voluntary control of motor activities becomes more complete there occur changes in resting posture and in the postures assumed when he is placed in different positions. The resting position of the newborn child is one of semi-flexion of the trunk and limbs; even when placed in the erect position with his feet on a flat surface so that the positive supporting reaction is provoked the lower limbs maintain a position of some flexion at the hips and knees. But the period during which the child prefers postures of flexion or semi-flexion, the so-called first flexor stage of infancy, is limited and is succeeded gradually between the ages of 8 and 12 weeks by a stage in which extensor postures of the trunk and limbs become apparent. This stage is usually at its peak when the infant is aged between 14 and 18 weeks. In this stage when placed in the erect position the baby takes more weight on his lower limbs and may be able to take all his own weight with minimal support to the hands. This 'reflex standing' is achieved by bringing into play the crossed extensor reflexes, the symmetrical neck reflex and the vestibular reflexes all of which tend to increase anti-gravity tone.

As the vestibular, symmetrical neck and crossed extensor responses gradually become inhibited, so reflex standing ceases to occur, and instead of demonstrating extensor postures of the trunk and limbs at rest the child's postures again become more flexed (Ingram, 1959; Bobath, 1966). It is at this stage, commonly at the age of 5 to 8 months, that first supported sitting and then unsupported sitting become possible—indeed unsupported sitting may be regarded as the major achievement of the second flexor stage. This stage in turn merges gradually into the second extensor phase between 9 and 12 months. This stage is characterised by the child beginning to assume the erect position, first pulling himself up by 'climbing' furniture or people and then gradually attaining spontaneous standing and walking (Fig. 69). Because of the predominance of voluntary activity by this age, postural reflexes are more difficult to elicit and less definite; but the study of muscle tone, tendon jerks and plantar responses similar to that used by neurologists concerned with adults, becomes of increasing clinical importance.

Some space has been devoted to a description of motor development in infancy since, for the first 10 or 12 months of life, it is on positive and negative motor milestones that the clinician has to rely for his assessment of the child's development. Yet motor milestones may be normal or nearly normal in a significant minority of children who later show signs of mental handicap. It is important, therefore, to avoid reassuring parents about the later intelligence of their infants because motor development appears to have been normal. Towards the end of the first year milestones of linguistic, adaptive and social behaviour become progressively more testable and important in developmental diagnosis.

Speech Development in Childhood

In the last 40 or 50 years speech development has attracted much research because of the clues it gives about the development of higher nervous activities—for example, the growth of concepts of time, person and direction (Ingram, 1969). Verbal behaviour of children under the age of about 2 years gives less information about the child's 'inner language' and his ability to conceptualise than it does at later ages.

It is possible to subdivide the study of speech development in a number of ways. A division by time into pre-linguistic utterances to one year, one word statements by the age of 2 years, two word phrases by the age of 3 years, and three or more word sentences by the age of 4, according to Gesell, is one such chronological subdivision (Gesell, 1925). It has the great virtue of simplicity but does not describe all the different ways in which a child's spoken language develops during the first 3 years of life. A more meaningful if more complex classification is by the aspects of levels of language which are being studied. This involves distinction between phonological, syntactical and semantic aspects of language. By phonology is understood the study of the articulation of the language and its sound systems. Syntax includes the study of grammatical performance on and in words (usually beginnings and endings of words in English) or morphology and the composition of sentences (or meaningful units) in terms of word order and grammatical relationships. Semantics covers the relationship of the language to cognitive activity. In addition it is necessary to take account of the growth of the child's comprehension of the spoken language to which he is exposed.

Pre-Verbal Speech Development

The first cry of the newborn characteristically consists of 'a' or 'e' or 'ae' sounds, usually nasalised: occasionally 'u' is the sound first uttered. Even in the newborn period the cry has an expressive quality, for it has been shown that experienced observers can distinguish between the recorded cries of babies in pain, healthy babies and babies with brain damage (Partanen et al., 1967; Wasz-Hockert et al., 1968). Within weeks consonants are added. Following Darwin (1877), Lewis (1951) distinguishes between sounds uttered in states of discomfort, especially hunger 'u', 'h', 'l', 'ng', 'm' and 'n', and those uttered in states of comfort such as 'g', 'k' and 'r' which are sounds commonly associated with burping and belching. They are typically produced in states of pleasure (Lewis, 1963).

The repertoire of sounds increases rapidly and by the age of 3 months most babies are making repetitive sounds for periods of a few minutes at a time especially after feeds. These utterances are usually repetitive chains of sounds such as 'mamamama', 'nananana' or 'nenenene'. Their utterance seems to be a form of vocal play and their purpose to please the child himself rather than a form of purposeful expression. It is worth noting nevertheless that babble contains sounds characteristically uttered in states of discomfort as well as those produced in states of comfort. It is rather characteristic of the third and fourth months of life that the child exploits his power to alter pitch and volume so that growls and shrieks are emitted apparently 'just for fun' (Lewis, 1951). By the age of 5 months all the sounds likely to be used in later spoken language will probably have been uttered 'accidentally' during babbling.

Even during the pre-verbal stage speech development will be influenced by the environment and particularly by the adults who regularly care for the child, though the influence of the environment has been minimised by some recent authors (Lenneberg, 1966). Babies commonly respond by crying to the sound of another baby crying even in the newborn period and by the second month of life may smile or turn their heads in the direction of a human voice. By the age of 4 months and perhaps even earlier the infant distinguishes between friendly and unfriendly intonational patterns. Friendly approaches will often be answered by vocalisation and are effective in evoking the child's own familiar babbling sounds (Gregoire, 1937).

It is difficult to say when the child begins to imitate what he hears, but certainly by the age of 6 or 7 months intonational patterns and rhythms are being copied and soon afterwards the first rudimentary attempts to imitate word sounds appear. It is probably at this stage that environmental influences play an important part in influencing the choice of the sounds which are produced. Parents, by approving of the child uttering particular sounds such as 'ma', 'da', encourage the repetition of constant sound sequences to refer to particular people or objects or situations. By the age of about a year the child is likely to produce 'words' appropriately even though these may be incorrectly pronounced and all the word sounds may not be uttered (Weir, 1962). Some authors regard the stage of babbling as crucial to the development of later spoken language (Weir, 1962; Lewis, 1951). Others have considered that the development of spoken language proceeds relatively independently of the preceding babbling phase (Jacobsen and Halle, 1956).

To begin with the child's spontaneous utterances consist of only two or three vowels and a limited number of consonants, most commonly 'p', 'b', 'm', 'w', 'f', 'v', 't', 'd' and 'n'. These are used more frequently at the beginnings of words than at the ends. Gradually, however, the number of consonants increases and the child begins to use them more successfully in the medial and final positions in words. 'Th', 'r', 'sh' and 's' sounds tend to be acquired last and they and clusters of consonants may be omitted or substituted by other phonemes even after the age of 4 years, especially when these are terminal or medial in position. Consonant blends such as 'hw', 'lfth' and 'tl' were found by Templin (1957) to be omitted or substituted by more than 25 per cent of her subjects age 8 years.

It is necessary to distinguish between passive vocabulary which consists of the words which the child understands, and active vocabulary which consists of the words he uses in spoken language. Passive vocabulary is usually considerably larger than active vocabulary. The extent of passive vocabulary can be measured using a number of tests; one of the best and most popular of which is the Peabody Word Recognition Test (Peabody, 1959) which has been standardised for English children by Brimer and Dunn (1963). The number of words in the child's passive and active vocabularies will depend to a large extent on the spoken language to which he has been exposed, to the socio-economic circumstances of his family, the education of his parents and his own intelligence. In most studies girls are found to have a slightly larger active vocabulary than boys, but at least two studies have suggested that boys have a larger passive or recognition vocabulary than girls. It has been estimated that the average two-year-old has a mean speaking vocabulary of 272 words, while by the age of 7 the subjects studied by Templin (1957) had a mean estimated vocabulary of about 20,000 words with a standard deviation of about 10,000—some indication of the great differences in the size of the vocabularies in different children. Most authors have found that there is a rapid increase in the number of words a child uses between the ages of 12 and 15 months, some slowing in the rate of the acquisition of vocabulary in the next 3 months and then a period of rapid vocabulary growth from the age of about 18 months.

The actual naming of objects and events marks a major development in the child's cognitive development. Naming involves classifying and a growing vocabulary implies growth in the child's powers of classification. Many examples of this growing classificatory ability can be found in the older anecdotal accounts of the development of child language (Stern and Stern, 1928). A word like 'dada' for example may be first used to apply to all men and then gradually comes to be applied to the child's father, or 'moo-cow' may initially be the name given to all four-footed animals before the child has learnt to identify by name cows, horses, dogs, pigs, etc. When he does utter a word the child does not necessarily mean exactly the same as an adult would mean if he used it. For example, when the child says 'uppy' it usually means that he wishes to be picked up. This does not mean, however, that the child associates the word 'uppy' with the antonym down or 'downy' or indeed realises that the state of being 'down' is necessarily the converse of being 'up'. The understanding of the meanings of words probably develops very gradually but the importance of the increasing mastery of spoken language shown by young children is of immense importance to cognitive development, as has been emphasised by Luria (1961).

Between the ages of 18 and 24 months words are first combined into phrases and shortly afterwards simple sentences appear. Initially these are usually of a simple subject—predicate structure, the predicate often consisting of another noun, as in 'Mummy egg' for 'Mummy has got an egg' or a verb as in 'all gone'.

It is not very rewarding to analyse utterances of this stage according to traditional grammatical rules, yet it is clear that the child has consistent grammatical rules of his own and tends to treat nouns in one way and verbs in another. Nonsense words treated as nouns by an adult will be treated as nouns even in a different context by the child and verbs will be treated as verbs (Brown, 1964). Generally nouns and verbs appear before adjectives and adverbs, and these in turn are mastered before prepositions, pronouns and conjunctions. Imperative and negative forms are mastered relatively early. On the other hand the correct use of personal pronouns and prepositions which require a sense of temporal or spatial relationships and conjunctions which often require a sense of causality are acquired comparatively late. Piaget has pointed out that until the child has a real concept of cause and effect he is unlikely to be able to describe coherently sequences of events which depend upon each other (Piaget, 1932). As the child's ability to conceptualise increases, so does the complexity of his grammar. Various arbitrary measures of his linguistic sophistication have been devised mostly based on analysis of 50 consecutive utterances elicited in certain standard situations (Templin, 1957). These include the mean number of words in utterances, the number of words contained in the longest utterance, the complexity of the utterance as measured by its grammatical completeness, the numbers of subordinate clauses and the use of particular parts of speech, especially prepositions. It has been shown in most studies that firstborn children score more highly than later-born children and that children of upper social class have higher scores than children of lower social class. Intelligent children have higher scores than unintelligent children.

It has long been recognised that children from culturally deprived backgrounds, especially those living in institutions, show slower speech development than children from emotionally healthy, middle-class homes (Templin, 1957). They have smaller vocabularies, use shorter sentences of simpler grammatical form, and use fewer past and future tenses and fewer subordinate clauses. More recently significant qualitative differences have been described. Bernstein (1965) contrasts the 'elaborated code' used by middle-class children to communicate ideas with the 'restricted code' used by children from culturally deprived backgrounds which allows much more limited interpersonal communication. The work of Labov (1966) and Cazden (1968) has demonstrated the very important determining effects of social environment on the developing spoken language of young children. Cultural deprivation is likely to have particularly profound effects upon the speech development of children who already have intrinsic handicaps such as mental deficiency or hearing impairment.

One of the major difficulties in studying the developing speech of children has been the lack of sophisticated measures of attainment. It is to be hoped that advances in general linguistics will allow for the future construction of tests of grammatical sophistication (Bellugi and Brown, 1964). Tests of articulatory development are already becoming available (Renfrew, 1964; Templin, 1957; Ingram *et al.*, 1970).

Adaptive Behaviour

Gesell (1940) suggests that adaptive behaviour may be described as 'a convenient category for those various adjustments, perceptual, orientational, manual and verbal, which reflect the child's capacity to initiate new experiences and to profit by past experience'.

As the child matures he becomes progressively able to adapt to new situations and to solve for himself problems which he meets in everyday life and in test situations. When he contrives means of dealing successfully with these situations, he may be said to 'adapt' to them. In a sense many of the everyday activities which the normal child learns to carry out for himself are tests of 'adaptation'; using a spoon efficiently, drinking from a cup, learning to take his own shoes and socks off, undressing and dressing, and toileting, may be regarded as forms of adaptive behaviour (Fig. 74). An observant mother carefully questioned about her child's practical abilities in the home setting can often give information which allows a reasonably accurate measure of adaptive behaviour development to be made. Gesell and Amatruda (1947) give norms for these everyday adaptive skills. For example, the child may be expected to be capable of taking some part in feeding himself by 18 months, by 21 months he should handle a cup well, and by 3 years he should be feeding himself quite efficiently (Fig. 74). He may begin to co-operate in the process of putting his clothes on as early as 12 months but not till 24 months will he normally be able to put on simple garments unaided. At the age of 3 years he should be able to put on his shoes and to undo buttons if they are easily accessible.

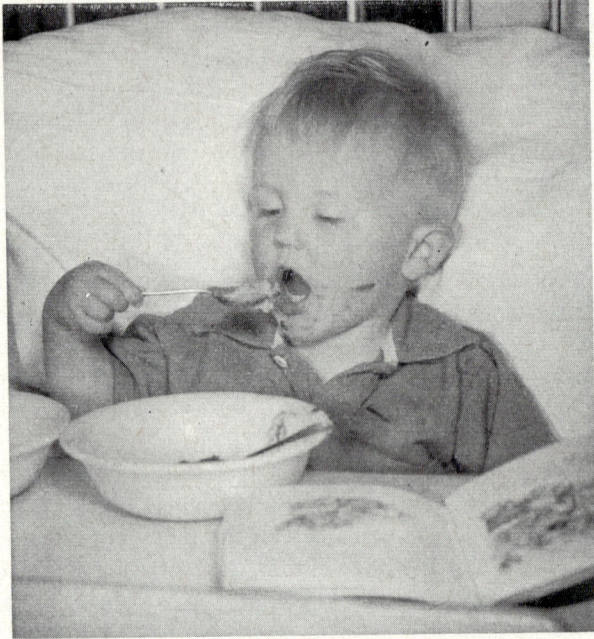

FIG. 74. Children of 15 to 18 months can usually hold a cup two-handed and drink from it without too much spilling. Using a spoon becomes possible a little later. Pouring is uncertain until after the age of 2 years.

When he is 5 he may be expected to dress himself without assistance provided he has not too many difficult buttons and is not expected to tie his laces.

Whilst these activities may give valuable indications of the child's progress, it is possible to assess adaptive skill more formally and accurately by presenting the child with a selection of standard tasks and problems appropriate to his age (Fig. 75). Gesell (1940) has assessed the adaptive behaviour of children under 5 years of age by means of such tasks as building with small one-inch cubic wooden blocks, placing objects in containers and removing them, fitting wooden shapes into their corresponding holes in a wooden square (the Form Board Test), drawing, repetition of digits and sentences, and using a stick or chair to reach an otherwise unobtainable toy.

Using ten 2½ centimetre blocks a variety of tests can be given. At the age of 13 months the attention of most children is fleeting, but about one-third of them will build a tower of two blocks, and by the age of 18 months a tower of three or four blocks will be built in imitation of one constructed by the examiner. By the age of 4 quite complicated structures are being copied and named. By the age of 3 children can make a bridge in which one block is placed upon two others which are separated by $1-1\frac{1}{2}$ cm. if the construction is demonstrated to them, and by the age

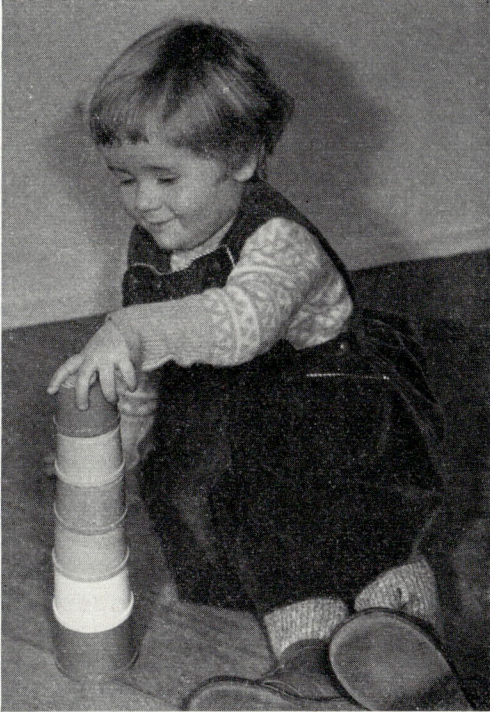

FIG. 75. Characteristic building of a tower of beakers by a $2\frac{1}{2}$-year-old child.

of 4 they can build a bridge by copying the model without having the building demonstrated. By this age too most children can imitate the examiner's representation of a train which consists of three blocks in a row, the forward one of which has another block superimposed.

Similar milestones of adaptive behaviour have been worked out for other simple toys such as a cup and cubes, a pellet and a bottle, box and ball, paper folding, three-holed formboards in which a circle, square and triangle have to be placed. Behaviour with pencil and paper is particularly interesting giving the opportunity for spontaneous drawing in a standard situation. Gesell found that the majority of children aged 13 months marked the paper and by 18 months most of them scribbled. By the age of 3 most drew and often admired their drawings, though these were often unrecognisable to adults. By the time the subjects were 4 years of age their drawings were usually recognised by trained observers. At the age of 5 children would differentiate between parts of objects and people they drew and by the age of 6 their drawings contained much detail and implications of action.

More detailed scoring is possible of tests in which the child is asked to copy forms such as a vertical line, a horizontal line, a circle, a cross, a square, a triangle and a diamond. A particularly valuable test is the 'Draw a Man Test'; at the age of 3 a child may draw a face with appendages but often what he produces is unrecognisable. By the age of 4 he usually represents the head and the eyes and the legs. As he grows older his representation becomes progressively detailed and better proportioned, so that by the age of 5 or 6 years the man has a neck as well as a body, hands as well as arms, and wears clothes. The drawings of a man change and develop in a remarkably predictable way and this has allowed very detailed scoring of the 'Draw a Man Test' (Goodenough, 1926), see Chapter 9. A similar predictable sequence occurs in the development of children to draw a house and complete pictures of men and women in whom parts were missing. Gesell also developed simple tests of number concept in which preschool children were asked to count objects which they could handle, objects they drew and their fingers. They were given tests of immediate memory when they were asked to repeat numbers (digit repetition) and to repeat sentences. Tests of comparative judgement were presented by asking children to compare the lengths of lines and make 'aesthetic' comparisons and to compare weights (Illingworth, 1967).

The principles underlying the constructions of intelligence tests for older children and adults are not different from those described for younger children, though the intellectual functions they test are of a higher order. Digit repetition is one item that is found as a test of immediate memory in scales designed for young children and for adults, though, hardly surprisingly, adults are expected to remember one or two more digits than children aged 5 to 6 years. They also contain items which are designed particularly to test adults' ability to classify, complete analogies, extrapolate series, perceive absurdities and to solve logical and mathematical problems. Thus many aspects of adaptive behaviour are examined (see Chapter 9).

Social Behaviour

At the same time as their motor, adaptive and linguistic behaviour is maturing children make numerous and complex social contacts. Since these can only be made using motor, adaptive and linguistic behaviour, any innate handicap which impairs the development of these aspects of behaviour is likely to impair successful social maturation and the distinction between motor, adaptive, linguistic and social behaviour becomes somewhat blurred. At one time, in fact, Gesell wrote in terms of there being a category of 'persono-social' behaviour in which he described together the development of the child's independence and self-care, his mastery of his environment and the maturation of his social attitudes and relationships (Gesell, 1940).

In particular, language has a very complex and important role in modifying the behaviour of the young child and increasing the range of his social contacts. Luria

(1961) puts particular emphasis on the fact that to decide whether or not an action is socially acceptable is greatly facilitated when the problem can be formulated in words.

Milestones of development of social behaviour are more difficult to define partly because the human interactions which comprise them are so very complex. Moreover, the way in which social behaviour is described depends very greatly on the outlook of the writer describing them. The changing social responses of babies, for example, have been interpreted in terms of conditioning by Pavlov and his followers and by Watson in the United States (Luria, 1961; Kasatkin and Levikova, 1935; Watson and Rayner, 1963; Skinner, 1953); in terms of psychoanalytic theory (Freud, 1946, 1962); and in terms of theories derived from animal experiments (Altman, 1962; Harlow and Zimmerman, 1959; Hinde, 1964).

In his first human relationship after birth which is with his mother, the baby is completely dependent. During infancy, as he becomes more aware of himself and his surroundings, this relationship gradually becomes less dependent and more complex. In early childhood it remains the most important tie though increasing numbers of other social contacts are made, first within the family circle and then outside it. But his relationship with his mother, or for that matter the relationship with other members of the family, is not a static one. It varies in character and intensity at different stages of the child's development and according to the mother's changing role. Piaget has described how interaction between the child and other members of his family only becomes possible after the child has acquired concepts of self and has come to appreciate that people are different. He emphasises the close inter-relationship between higher nervous activity and successful social adaptation (Piaget, 1951).

The earliest response of the human infant which seems to merit the description 'social' is the smiling response (Fig. 76). This response is usually first elicited by the mother within the first 4 to 6 weeks of infancy and shortly afterwards, the child will respond in a rather non-specific way by smiling to any other person, whether familiar or a stranger, who smiles at him. Spitz and Wolf (1946) have shown that the smiling response may also be elicited by a lifeless mask, provided that certain conditions are satisfied. The main important ones are, (a) that there be full-face presentation of the mask, (b) that two 'eyes' be clearly visible, (c) that there be some movement. The child does not smile at the mask which is held completely still. The fact that the response occurs in the presence of certain simple and precisely definable 'key stimuli' makes it seem to resemble a type of response which is common amongst animals and especially birds. It appears that the young of many species are born with built-in tendencies to respond to certain fairly simple collections of stimuli and that crude models or dummies can elicit these patterns quite as effectively as the natural objects. For instance, a pecking response in herring gull chicks, which is normally a response to the lowered bill of the feeding parent bird, can be elicited by a small thin stick, painted with patches of red against a white background and held upright. To human perception this model bears little resemblance to the natural "releaser"—the parent's bill—but the key-stimuli are present so the response appears (Tinbergen and Perdeck, 1950). Whether the smiling response of the human infant is inborn like the pecking sequence of the newly hatched gull is still a very controversial point. It is apparent, however, that the frequency and readiness with which it is elicited and probably the age at which it first appears and the time for which it is present depend very much

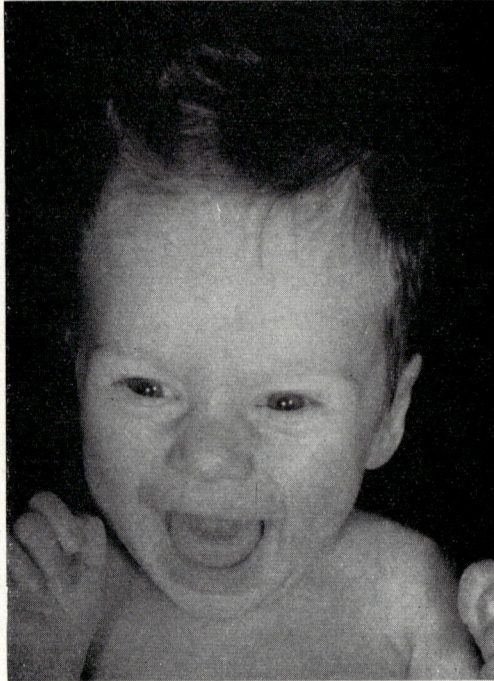

FIG. 76. A baby responding socially by
smiling.

upon the relationship of the mother and her baby. Even in the newborn period conditioning appears to be of great importance in determining patterns of social behaviour. Spitz and Wolf (1946), for example, found that in a few instances where no response appeared and when the child screamed instead of smiling there was evidence of very poor mother/child relationship. Also they report the case of a child born 2 months before term and appropriately retarded in perceptual and motor development who was nevertheless advanced in the smiling response and in social development generally. This advancement Spitz and Wolf attributed to a particularly good relationship with the mother. It is, in fact, not at all uncommon to find prematurely born babies smiling reciprocally to their mothers before they would have been born if carried to term.

From the age of 4 to 5 months, smiling response gradually changes. As the child begins to develop a sense of identity and begins to respond to his mother as an individual he begins to take pleasure in her company without the feeding situation, though feeding and the oral gratification which it brings continue to be of great importance. The child begins to enjoy being fondled, stroked and patted by the mother as he sits on her knee and shows his pleasure by smiling, laughing and babbling back to her when talked to and by biting and sucking her. From the age of 4 or 5 months smiling in response to a mask or any human face known or unknown begins to disappear. The child begins to be selective. He may smile or babble and make grasping and reaching movements when his mother comes, but turn away and be unresponsive with other people. From then on he may be expected to show definite signs of recognising familiar faces but is likely to be shy with strangers. By this age he will often try to engage the attention of people in his activities and will play the game of giving and taking back toys and of hiding and revealing them. There is no doubt, however, that the important relationship of the first year is with the mother or with the person who is caring for the child in the mother's place. There is ample evidence that unless a warm and more or less uninterrupted relationship is established at this time subsequent development may be adversely affected in many ways (see p. 265). It has been demonstrated that if children are deprived of maternal love and care for an appreciable period—say 3 months or more—before the age of 3 years they are liable to be retarded in social behaviour. This retardation may limit their ultimate capacity to form relationships with other people and there is strong evidence to suggest that severe early deprivation is important in the aetiology of delinquency (Bowlby, 1951). Many writers on the subject believe that the effects of deprivation are difficult if not impossible to reverse, but Clarke and Clarke (1960) argue that long-term recovery is not impossible. Also they stress a point which is now widely recognised that some children appear to survive severe social deprivation unharmed. Little or nothing is yet known about the conditions affecting individual vulnerability to maternal deprivation in the early years.

An enormous increase in the child's capacity for social exchange comes when language appears. At the same time the development of motor skills, especially walking and fine manipulation, makes the child increasingly able to explore and master his immediate surroundings. From the age of 18 months he may begin to let his mother know when he needs the lavatory, and he is able to help to some extent in dressing and undressing. His decreased physical dependence has its counterpart in his growing sense of personal identity. He begins to distinguish between what he does and things that are done or happen to him. He is increasingly aware of his relationships with other members of his family and takes the initiative in making social contact with them. He may give his mother and brothers and sisters presents and enjoys playing with them. He likes to help in the house and much of his play imitates what he has observed his parents and older brothers and sisters do. As described in Chapter 10, his relationship with his parents becomes much more complex. Fantasy play is indulged in increasingly (Fig. 77).

The sense of possessing is well developed by the age of 2 years and toddlers of this age find it extremely difficult to share their toys. On the other hand they are frequently direct and violent in their methods of getting toys they want which belong to others. Because of their intensely egocentric attitudes, toddlers find group games without adult supervision virtually impossible. The first stages of social play may be found, however, in the liking two- and three-year-old toddlers have for playing beside, if not with, other children (Parten, 1932). Often, when playing

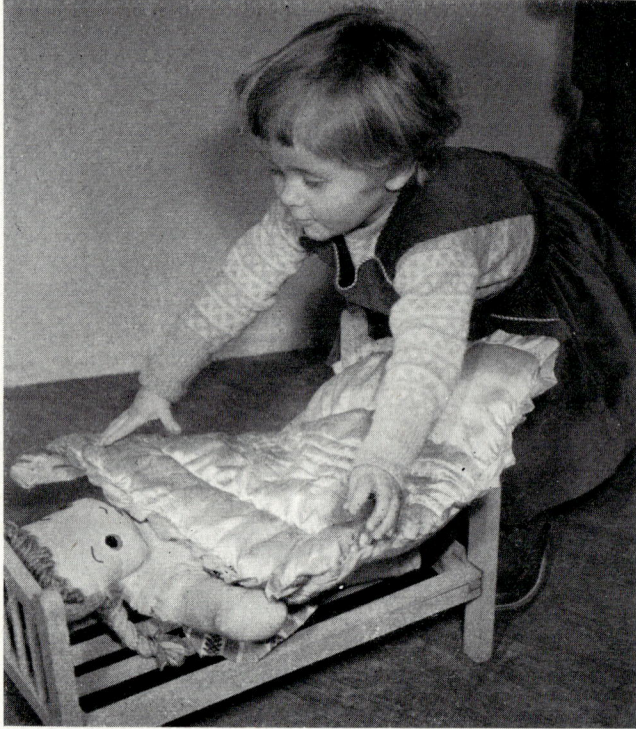

Fig. 77. Fantasy play becomes progressively more important during the latter part of the second year and motor skills are then sufficiently developed for this.

in this way, the child will keep up a commentary on what he is doing, apparently for his companions' benefit, but in fact almost entirely for his own. This so-called 'collective monologue' may reveal very vividly the intensely individual and self-centred world in which the typical three-year-old child lives. The stage of the 'collective monologue' lasts for some months. It disappears gradually as concepts develop of give and take, reciprocity, and joint action to achieve what one child cannot attain alone. As he becomes less egocentric and more able to cope with the competition of other children of similar age and similar desires to his own the child begins to be able to play actively with other children of his own age. Even at this age there are likely to be frequent quarrels which it is difficult for adults to explain about the aims of games or the ownership of toys. But these fights gradually diminish in frequency and by the age of 4 years three or four children may play together for half an hour or more without adult intervention in favourable circumstances.

Between the ages of 4 and 5 years the onset of the 'genital phase' of emotional development occurs. During this phase the child's interest in his or her genitals increases and they become the most important sources of erotic pleasure. The boy shows pride in his penis and the girl tends to show penile envy. There is an awakening of awareness in both sexes that in some way the sexual organs have to do with childbirth, awkward questions may be asked of parents by their three- or four-year-old children as to why a particular woman has 'such a large tummy'.

The genital phase is characterised by a number of important changes in the child's relationships with other adults and children. The differences between the attitudes of boys and girls become accentuated at this time. Boys begin to identify with their fathers and girls with their mothers. Frequently both boys and girls have fantasies of replacing the parent of the same sex in the affections of the parent of the opposite sex. The relationship between boys and their fathers and girls and their mothers tends to become tense and polyvalent; love or hatred; identification or jealousy; admiration or fear may be predominant at different times.

By the time children are aged 4 or 5 imaginative play is usually sufficiently developed for many of these emotional conflicts to be resolved symbolically—a fact made use of by play therapists. Sometimes the symbolic play with dolls or drawings is violent and emotional conflicts are 'played out' with intensity.

It is sometimes said that the child of 4 wants independence, but the independence that he wants is certainly only partial. There is a conflict between the desire for independence and the wish to return to the privileged passive condition of infancy. Similarly parents are often in conflict between their desire to have a mature, competent child advanced in such matters as toilet training and general self-control and their desire to keep him small and dependent. The outcome of these conflicts varies enormously, but by the time the child goes to school the first social crisis is generally over and a more stable pattern of relationships between the child and his family has been established.

When the child first goes to nursery school, kindergarten or school between the ages of 4 and 7 years many of the tense emotional conflicts of the early genital stage have begun to resolve. Even so the independence of a child of 6 years is partial.

He requires adult guidance in his play with other children for anything but a short period, and he is liable to express his distress at any long-term separation from his mother by retrogressive behaviour. For example, he may demand to be cuddled like a three-year-old, to be fed and dressed and undressed though he has already achieved independence in these respects.

Sometimes separations from the mother appear to be more 'traumatic'. A mother who has gone into a maternity hospital to produce a younger sib is particularly likely to be blamed by her older child for having deserted him and the child will punish his mother by refusing to do what she wants, having temper tantrums, being destructive to clothes and, sometimes, showing violence to the new baby. However, separation from the mother after the age of 3 is much less likely to have long-term effects on behaviour development than maternal deprivation before this age. The older child has channels by which he can express his distressed feelings using spoken language or play.

The school years have been called the latent period by psychoanalysts because the intensity of the libidinal drives appears to be less than in the early pre-school years or in later adolescence. But, in fact, they mark a progressive gain in independence, for in school the child is expected to be mature enough to accept codes of behaviour which are different from those which he has previously obeyed at home and he does not have the access to his mother for comfort if he steps out of line. He has to learn to behave in ways which are acceptable to both his teacher and his school fellows. He gradually learns between the ages of 5 and 10 years to subordinate his own wishes to those of the group of children of his own age with whom he plays.

Children form gangs from the age of about 8 years (see chap. 23). Gangs commonly consist of between 5 and 12 children who play together and share the same activities and enthusiasms. Gangs of boys tend to be larger, more cohesive and persist for longer than those of girls. The leaders tend to remain constant, but relationships between individuals in the gang itself change and members of it are likely to find themselves playing different roles at different times.

Much has been written about the delinquent gangs. Much less about the benefits to the child of enlarging his environmental experience and learning to come to terms with other children of the same age in communal pursuits. The gang does give children the experience of taking an active part within a group of contemporaries for a common purpose. Similar experiences may be obtained by older children in the Scouts, Guides or in clubs devoted to specific interests which may vary from mountaineering to philately, or from debating to geology. In all these group activities the child achieves aims which involve much more than immediate emotional self-gratification.

T. T. S. INGRAM

References

D'AJURIAGUERRA, J. and HÉCAEN, H. (1949). *Le Cortex Cerebral*. Paris: Masson.

ALTMAN, S. A. (1962). Social behaviour of anthropoid primates: Analysis of recent concepts. In *Roots of Behaviour*. Ed. Bliss. New York: Harper Brothers.

ANDRÉ-THOMAS, CHESNI, Y. and DARGASSIES, S. ST. A. (1960). *The Neurological Examination of the Infant*. Ed. R. C. Mac Keith, P. E. Polani and E. Clayton-Jones. Little Club Clinics No. 1. London: Spastics Society Heinemann.

BELLUGI, U. and BROWN, R. (1964). The acquisition of language. *Monogr. Soc. Res. Child Devel.*, **29**, No. 1.

BERNSTEIN, B. (1965). A socio-linguistic approach to social learning. In *Penguin Survey of the Social Sciences*. Ed. J. Gould. Baltimore: Penguin.

BIRCH, H. G. (1968). Health and the education of socially disadvantaged children. *Devel. Med. Child Neurol.*, **10**, 580.

BOBATH, K. (1966). The motor deficit in patients with cerebral palsy. *Clinics in Devel. Med. No. 23*. London: Spastics Society Heinemann.

BOWLBY, J. (1951). Maternal care and mental health. *W.H.O. Monogr. Series*, Geneva.

BRAIN, R. and WILKINSON, M. (1959). Observations on the extensor plantar response and its relationship to functions of the pyramidal tract. *Brain*, 82, 297.

BRIMER, M. A. and DUNN, L. M. (1963). *Manual for the English Picture Vocabulary Test.* National Foundation for Educational Research in England and Wales.

BROWN, R. (1964). The acquisition of language. In *Disorders of Communication.* Ed. Rioch and Weinstein. A.R.N.M.D. XLII. Baltimore: Williams and Wilkins.

CARMICHAEL, L. (1954). *Manual of Clinical Psychology.* 2nd edit. New York: Wiley.

CAZDEN, C. B. (1968). Three socio-linguistic views of the language and speech of lower class children—with special attention to the work of Basil Bernstein. *Devel. Med. Child Neurol.*, 10, 600.

CLARKE, A. D. B. and CLARKE, A. M. (1960). Some recent advances in the study of early deprivation. *J. Child Psychol. Psychiat.*, 1, 26.

DARWIN, C. (1877). The biography of an infant. *Mind*, 2, 285.

DREYFUS-BRISAC, C. (1964). The electroencephalogram of the premature infant and full term infant—normal and abnormal development of waking and sleeping patterns. In *Neurological and Electroencephalographic Correlative Studies in Infancy.* Ed. Kellaway and Petersen. New York: Grune and Stratton.

ELLINGSON, R. J. (1964). Cerebral electrical responses to auditory and visual stimuli in the infant—human and sub-human. In *Neurological and Electroencephalographic Correlative Studies in Infancy.* Ed. Kellaway and Petersen. New York: Grune and Stratton.

FANTZ, R. L. (1967). Visual perception experience in early infancy: A look at the hidden side of behaviour development. In *Early Behaviour: Comparative and Developmental Approaches.* Ed. H. W. Stevenson, E. Hess and H. L. Rheingold. New York: Wiley.

FIORENTINO, M. (1963). *Reflex Testing Methods for Evaluating C.N.S. Development.* London: Thomas.

FREUD, A. (1946). *On the Sexual Theories of Children.* Collected Papers, 2, 4th edit. London: Hogarth Press and Institute of Psychoanalysis.

—— (1962). Emotional and instinctive development. In *Child Health and Development.* Ed. R. W. B. Ellis. 3rd edit. London: Churchill.

GESELL, A. (1925). *The Mental Growth of the Pre-school Child: A Psychological Outline of Normal Development from Birth to the Sixth Year Including a System of Developmental Diagnosis.* New York: MacMillan.

—— (1940). *The First Five Years of Life.* London: Methuen.

—— and AMATRUDA, C. S. (1947). *Developmental Diagnosis: Normal and Abnormal Child Development.* London: Hoeber.

GOODENOUGH, F. L. (1926). *The Measurement of Intelligence by Drawing.* New York: World Book Company.

GREGOIRE, A. (1937). *L'Apprentissage du Langage.* Vol. 1. Paris: Droz.

HARLOW, H. F. and ZIMMERMAN, R. R. (1959). Affectional responses in the infant monkey. *Science*, 130, 421.

HINDE, R. A. (1964). Intraspecific communication in animals. In *Disorders of Communication.* Ed. Rioch and Weinstein. A.R.N.M.D. XLII. Baltimore: Williams and Wilkins.

ILLINGWORTH, R. S. (1967). *The Development of the Infant and Young Child: Normal and Abnormal.* 3rd edit. Edinburgh and London: Livingstone.

INGRAM, T. T. S. (1959). Muscle tone and posture in infancy. *Cerebr. Palsy Bull.*, No. 5, 6.

—— (1962). Clinical significance of the infantile feeding reflex. *Devel. Med. Child Neurol.*, 4, 159.

—— (1969). The development of higher nervous activity in childhood and its disorders. In *Handbook of Clinical Neurology.* Ed. P. J. Vinkin and G. W. Bruyn. Amsterdam: North-Holland Publishing Co.

—— et al. (1970). *The Edinburgh Articulation Test for Young Children.* (To be published.)

JACOBSEN, R. and HALLE, M. (1956). *Fundamentals of Language*. The Hague: Mouten & Co.

KASATKIN, N. I. and LEVIKOVA, A. M. (1935). On the development of early conditioned reflexes and differentiations of auditory stimuli in infants. *J. Exper. Psychol.*, **18**, 1.

LABOV, W. (1966). *The Social Stratification of English in New York City*. Washington: Center for Applied Linguistics.

LENNEBERG, E. H. (1966). The natural history of language. In *The Genesis of Language*. Ed. F. Smith and G. A. Miller. M.I.T. Press: Cambridge, Mass.

LEWIS, M. M. (1951). *Infant's Speech*. London: Routledge and Kegan Paul.

—— (1963). *Language, Thought and Personality in Infancy and Childhood*. London: Harrap.

LURIA, A. R. (1961). *The Role of Speech in the Regulation of Normal and Abnormal Behaviour*. London: Pergamon Press.

—— (1966). *Higher Cortical Functions in Man*. London: Tavistock Publications.

McGRAW, M. D. (1943). *The Neuromuscular Maturation of the Human Infant*. New York: Columbia University Press.

NELIGAN, G. A. and PRUDHAM, D. (1969a). Norms for four standard developmental milestones by sex, social class and place in family. *Devel. Med. Child Neurol.*, **11**, 413.

—— —— (1969b). The potential value of four early developmental milestones in screening children for increased risk of later retardation. *Devel. Med. Child Neurol.*, **11**, 423.

PAINE, R. S., BRAZELTON, T. B., DONOVAN, D. E., DRORBAUGH, J. E., HUBBELL, J. P. and SEARS, E. M. (1964). Evolution of postural reflexes in normal infants and in the presence of chronic brain handicap. *Neurology*, **14**, 1036.

PARTANEN, T. J., WASZ-HÖCKERT, O., VUORENKOSKI, V., THEORELL, K., VALANNE, E. and LIND, J. (1967). Auditive identification of pain cry signals of young infants and its sound spectrographic basis. *Ann. Paediat. Fenn.*, **13**, 56.

PARTEN, M. B. (1932). Social participation among pre-school children. *J. Abnorm. Soc. Psychol.*, **27**, 243.

PEABODY WORD RECOGNITION (1959). *Manual for the Peabody Picture Vocabulary Test*. By L. M. Dunn.

PIAGET, J. (1932). *The Language and Thought of the Child*. London: Routledge and Kegan Paul.

—— (1950). *The Psychology of Intelligence*. London: Routledge and Kegan Paul.

—— (1951). *Play, Dreams and Imitation in Childhood*. London: Heinemann.

PRECHTL, H. F. R. (1958). The directed head turning response and allied movements of the human baby. *Behaviour*, *XIII*, 212.

—— and BEINTEMA, D. (1964). The neurological examination of the full-term newborn infant. *Clinics in Devel. Med. No.* 12. London: Spastics Society/Heinemann.

RENFREW, C. (1964). Assessment of late and poor talkers. In *The Child Who Does Not Talk*. Ed. C. Renfrew and K. Murphy. *Clinics in Devel. Med. No.* 13. London: Spastics Society/Heinemann.

SKINNER, B. F. (1953). *Science and Human Behaviour*. New York: Macmillan.

SPITZ, R. A. and WOLF, K. M. L. (1946). The smiling response: a contribution to the ontogenesis of social relations. *Genet. Psychol. Monogr.*, **34**, 57.

STERN, C. and STERN, W. (1928). *Die Kindersprache*. 4th edit. Leipzig: Barth.

TEMPLIN, M. C. (1957). Certain language skills in children, their development and inter-relationships. *Institute of Child Welfare Monographs No.* 26. Minneapolis: University of Minnesota Press.

TINBERGEN, N. and PERDECK, A. C. (1950). On the stimulus situation releasing the begging response in the newly hatched herring gull chick. *Behaviour*, **3**, 1.

WASZ-HOCKERT, O., LIND, J., VUORENKOSKI, V., PARTANEN, T. J. and VALANNE, E. (1968). The infant cry. *Clinics in Devel. Med.*, *No.* 29. London: Spastics Society Heinemann.

WATSON, J. B. and RAYNER, R. (1963). Conditioned emotional reactions. In *Research Readings in Child Psychology*. Ed. Palermo and Lipsitt. New York: Holt, Rinehart and Winston.

WEIR, R. H. (1962). *Language in Crib*. Hague: Mouton & Co.

9   Intellectual Development

IN the very earliest stages of a child's life, the psychologist has little to offer but speculation. He is interested in two main aspects of development. The first is the way a child's behaviour reflects the relationship between growing abilities and the requirements of the social, physical and intellectual world in which he is growing up. The second aspect is the range of individual variations in that behaviour. Most children are brought up dependent on adults who have much the same set of expectations of the child's behaviour and most children follow much the same sequence of development of their abilities; it is because of this uniformity that it is possible to make general statements about children's development and to establish those norms of behaviour which enable the abnormal to be identified and assessed.

Stimulus-Response Behaviour

There are two main lines of approach to the psychological study of children's behaviour. One may be called the 'Behaviourist' or S-R approach. S-R stands for stimulus-response; according to this, behaviour can be analysed into units of responses to stimuli, which are changes in the environment. There are two kinds of S-R units, the relatively small number of innate unlearned units, the reflexes, and the much greater range of learned responses, which are founded ultimately on reflexes, but which extend behaviour far beyond the limited repertoire of human reflexes. The S-R approach is concerned with observable behaviour only, and studies the conditions under which S-R units are acquired. The large amount of experimental work done on learning, both in animals and human beings, has led to various theoretical schemes aiming at interpreting behaviour development in S-R terms. Gagne (1965), for instance, develops a system of levels of learning beginning with the most elementary pattern of classical conditioning, as demonstrated by Pavlov's well known experiments with salivating dogs, and developing into more complex forms of learning by way of operant conditioning, chaining of S-R units, multiple discrimination, concept learning, principle learning to problem solving. Each of these learning processes depends on the establishment of the previous level of responses. Thus the learning of a chain of responses such as eating with a spoon or putting on a coat is not possible unless the child has previously acquired the unit responses which constitute the ordered chain. Nor does the observation of a spoon pushed off a table enable a child to 'discover' the principle embodied in the law of gravity. The necessary foundations are the concepts of mass, force, inverse square and the like. And these concepts are not within the province of young school children.

There is no question but that certain aspects of the development of behaviour can be interpreted in terms of S-R learning. It is probable that much early learning is basically conditioning; the child who responds readily by tears, or by hitting out, or by protective movement has probably been conditioned to respond in these ways. Also, behaviour therapy, which is essentially learning by conditioning, can be successful where the S-R unit is specific and can be identified. Fear responses to such specific stimuli as feathers, dogs or dentists can often be extinguished by such conditioning techniques. The evidence about enuresis is conflicting, and certain other forms of behaviour, like thumb-sucking or nail biting, seem to be rather resistant to such techniques. The old 'cure' of painting the fingers with bitter aloes was usually unsuccessful. General anxiety states and the like do not seem to respond to conditioning.

Cognitive Structures

The inadequacies of the S-R interpretation have recently led to the revival of a complementary scheme, which concentrates on the development of cognitive structures in the child. A cognitive structure is most simply explained as the child's way of representing the world to himself in some kind of organised system. With very young children it is very difficult to translate their behaviour into terms of cognitive structure, but as children grow older their patterns of interpretation and modes of thinking become clearer. Bruner (1964, 1968) suggests that in the first 7 or 8 years, the child passes through three stages in the development of cognitive structure. The first he calls enactive representation, in which the child interprets the world in terms of action. A thing or a situation is what is done with it. A rattle means shaking it, a block means something that is grasped but cannot be put into the mouth. The adult equivalent is tying a knot, which is easy to perform but difficult to describe. The second stage he calls iconic; by now the child can represent the world in terms of imagery, and is no longer dependent on the immediate presence of an object or situation. This stage is where human intelligence leaves animal intelligence behind. Up to about 2 years, methods of animal training are applicable to children. The third stage is called symbolic, in which the child can represent reality in terms of relations and symbols such as words and numbers. The sequence can be illustrated by an experiment with a board with a number of upright pegs on it; a ring is placed on one of the pegs, removed, and the child asked to replace it on the same peg. Young children can do this, but if the board is turned through 90 degrees, the younger children, in the enactive stage, cannot do it. Their difficulty is that their pattern of movement in relation to the board is now different. Older children between 2 and 3 years can do it, apparently by creating an image of the board, rotating the image and adapting their behaviour to the image. More complex rotation, say 180 degrees, makes the ordering of the image more difficult. Finally, about the age of 7 years, the child reaches symbolic representation, using a formula like 'second peg on fourth row'.

A parallel and more influential scheme has been proposed by Jean Piaget (Phillip, 1969), a Swiss biologist turned psychologist. His scheme rests on two foundations, the process of accommodation and assimilation, and a sequence of developmental stages through which all children progress in the same order, though not at the same speed. Accommodation means that the child responds to new experience in terms of his needs and interests; after the first year, or even before, he begins to operate on his environment. He looks in order to grasp, and grasps in order to shake. Assimilation means that his activities are being built into his representation of the world around him. The two processes of accommodation and assimilation go hand in hand in creating the child's interpretation of his experience.

At first the meaning of experience is the action. Thinking and doing are not separate processes, and not till about 18 to 24 months is the child able to internalise his actions in the form of mental processes. This period when the child's thinking is tied to his actions is called by Piaget the period of sensori-motor representation. From 2 years to about 7 years the child is developing his powers of internal representation but has not yet developed a system of operations. He is still essentially ego-centric. If a three-year-old, James, and his six-year-old brother, William, are asked 'Have you a brother?' both will answer 'Yes'. If William is asked if James has a brother, he will answer 'Yes, I'm his brother'. But James, when asked if William has a brother, will tend to answer 'No, there is just William and me'. At this stage also, children can learn to count, but often only specific objects. They can distinguish right from left in themselves, but their left is absolute; it is everyone's left. They can only apprehend one aspect of a situation at a time. Thus, six beads may be apprehended as more if they are spread out, and fewer if they are clustered. It depends on what is perceived at the time. During this period of 5 years, from the age of 2 till 7, children are extending their experiences piecemeal, and at their own pace are working towards the next stage, that of Concrete Operations. This stage lasts from about 7 to 11 years. The child is now freeing himself from the immediate situation, as he previously freed himself from action by internalising. He can now reverse his thinking processes. Water is poured from one jar to another. He can now mentally reverse the operation and apprehend that it is the same amount of water; it does not now change as in a separate new situation. He can see that points of view other than his own are possible, though not easily. But he cannot yet think in general principles; each situation is interpreted in its own context, and the typical method of problem solving is trial and error. Scientific and mathematical principles are beyond his scope. Older children in this stage can appreciate a parabola as representing the flight of a ball, but they have no idea what the co-ordinates are. Drawings of a seven-year-old represent each object as occupying its own space, such that a row of houses are drawn as of the same size and shape. Only at about 11 years of age is there an attempt at perspective, when the houses are drawn from a specific point of view, and distant houses are smaller.

The next stage in the sequence is Formal Operations, which are developing from 12 to 15 years, and is normally achieved about 14 to 15 years. This represents the adult form of logical thought. The main point about Piaget's findings is that the quality of children's thinking is different from that of adults. The logical systems are different, and though the child's thought processes may appear illogical to an adult, they are nevertheless relatively consistent within their own system. A big half and a small half make sense to a child; if a cake is divided equally, he has a real difficulty in choosing. The most probable explanation is that the pieces of cake change size according to which is chosen. The other half always seems bigger, hence the delay and difficulty. A further point that Piaget insists on is that the sequence of stages of intellectual development is invariant; children may vary in their rate of progress through the stages. Thus a very dull child may not reach the level of formal operations; somewhere in the later teens the developmental process comes to an end. A final point is that at each stage children are prisoners of their cognitive structures, and can only organise and interpret their experience in terms of their current thought structures. A nine-year-old cannot order his thinking in formal operations, nor can an adult order his thinking in terms of concrete operations. In other words, the adult cannot re-create earlier interpretations and cannot see through the eyes of a child. Understanding of children comes through rigorous observation and interpretation in the adult system, that is, formal operations.

Despite the value of Piaget's contributions to the understanding of the quality of children's thinking, much of Piaget's doctrine has often little direct reference to the day-to-day behaviour of children and the observation of it. There is a marked parallel here to Freud's views on personality development, where one cannot directly observe the formation of an Oedipus complex or the Super-ego. What is of more immediate importance is the child's intellectual competence, or the level of his intelligence. It is intelligence that largely determines the child's way of living in society, and in that sector which is of great significance to the older child, the school.

Intelligence

The one word, intelligence, refers to a process which is very far from simple, or indeed unitary. There are several distinctions which must be made if differences in intelligence are to be assessed and interpreted clearly. Firstly, the use of the noun 'intelligence' is misleading. The word should be an adverb, 'intelligently', as it refers to a way of behaving. Secondly, the assessment of intelligence involves three components. These are intellectual efficiency, intellectual maturity, and learned knowledge and skills. They are not wholly independent, but at various stages in the child's growth the contribution of each can and does vary. Finally, there are no units of intelligence, such that any absolute statement can be made about the quantity of a child's intelligence; assessments of intelligence are all relative, and the Intelligence Quotient is only an assessment of a child's intellectual competence relative to children *of the same age*.

Some children behave consistently more intelligently than others, but a satisfactory formal definition of this characteristic that distinguishes the more from the less intelligent child has so far eluded psychologists. There is, however, a substantial amount of agreement about what sectors of behaviour can be taken as indicating differences of intelligence among older children at least. In school studies, poor spelling or handwriting are not necessarily considered to indicate low intelligence, but inability to cope with arithmetic 'problems', poor vocabulary or inability to construct coherent sentences are usually taken as indicating a low level of intellectual ability. So too, certain games, like chess, are considered to require more intelligence than others, like tiddlywinks. In the same way, occupations can be ranked in an intellectual order.

Assessing Intelligence of Young Children

A difficulty arises when the children are very young. In terms of the accepted concept of intelligent behaviour, children under the age of 2 show few sectors of behaviour which provide enough evidence on which to evaluate differences in intelligence. Developmental scales, many of them quite adequately standardised, do exist (see also Chapter 8), but it is difficult to estimate for children below the age of 4 years how much of the behaviour being assessed is intelligent and how much developmental. There is only a slight relationship between bodily growth and neuromuscular co-ordination on the one hand, and intelligence on the other.

One such scale, that of Ruth Griffiths (1954) divides the child's behaviour into five sectors, viz. locomotor, personal-social, hearing and speech, eye and head, performance. For example, in the locomotor scale at 12 months the average child can walk when led, and at 24 months can kick a ball without overbalancing. In the personal-social scale the child responds to simple requests like 'Give me the cup', or claps hands in imitation; at 24 months he can point out parts of a doll's body, and should indicate four parts from hands, hair, feet, eyes, nose and mouth. He can also open a door and help in dressing or undressing himself. In the hearing and speech scale, he is expected to say three words clearly at 12 months, and reach twenty words by 24 months; and to be able to name four toys or similar common objects. The head and eye scale is concerned mainly with neuromuscular co-ordination. In the performance scale the one-year-old can, after being shown, tip two cubes from a box; by 24 months he can unscrew a screw top to extract a sweet. Quotients can be obtained from the scale, but the intermixture of physical and intellectual developmental tasks makes any prediction of future I Q hazardous.

A similar scale has been developed by Psyche Cattell (1940). This is on the same lines as the performance scale of Ruth Griffiths. More apparatus is needed. At 12 months, the child copies the tester beating two spoons together, is able to place a cube in a cup and has a speaking vocabulary of at least two words. By 24 months, the child can copy a simple folding of paper, name certain three small objects like a toy chair, a box, a key or a fork, and carry out simple commands, like 'put the spoon in the cup'.

Both these tests require a considerable degree of skill and experience on the part of the tester, and only major deviations from normal or average performance should be regarded as significant or of predictive value. Generally, a high level of performance can be considered as more valid than a low one; but at this early age differences in motor development can easily be confused with differences in intellectual development. Intelligent children can be ham-handed, though less frequently dull children are dextrous.

Intelligence Testing

Between the ages of 3 and 6, the child's behaviour has departed from what Piaget calls the sensori-motor stage, activity is becoming internalised, and thinking of the concrete operational type is appearing. The translation from overt action to internal representation in the form of imagery and thinking makes it more possible to assess what can more properly be called intelligence. Differences in ability are beginning to fan out, and the range of difference in behaviour among five-year-olds is much wider than among five-week-olds. Assessment of differences in intelligence become somewhat more meaningful, and tests of intelligence as distinct from perceptual-motor development have been constructed and used for many years.

The two most commonly used individual tests of intelligence are those developed by Binet and Wechsler. The original Binet scale has been revised several times, the revision in present use being the 1961 (LM revision), usually known as the Stanford Binet (Terman and Merrill, 1961). This is composed of various types of problems presented to the child. He is asked to give the meanings of words; some are easy, like orange and envelope, while others for the older children are more difficult, like mosaic and philanthropy. Children are asked to copy simple designs, like a diamond, to recognise absurdities, such as explaining why it is absurd to find in a grave the skull of Robert the Bruce when he was 10 years old, to do simple arithmetical computations, to interpret pictures or to repeat digits. The range of test items is very comprehensive, and the different items are arranged in groups of six, each appropriate for a year group of children. Thus the seven-year-old group consists of six items—Picture absurdities, Similarities, Copying Diamond, Comprehension, Opposite-analogies, and Digit Repetition. The level of answer accepted varies according to age; for each group the acceptable answer is that which is at least better than that given by approximately 50 per cent of the children of that age. For each acceptable answer the child is credited with 2 months of 'mental age'. This score is then related to his chronological age, and converted, by reference to tables, to an Intelligence Quotient on a scale of mean of 100 I Q and standard deviation of 16 I Q. Any child who is average for his age, therefore, obtains an I Q of 100.

The 1960 LM revision covers an age range from 2 years to adult (defined as 14 plus years of age). The Merrill-Palmer Scale (Stutsman, 1931) is a downward extension of the Binet scale, overlapping the younger end of the Binet. It covers the ages from 18 to 72 months; the items for the younger children are very similar to those in the Griffiths and Cattell scales. The items for the older children contain a number of form board tests and assembly tests, like jigsaw puzzles. There are tests of motor co-ordination, and tests involving the copying of a circle and a star. Vocabulary and comprehension of spoken instructions are also included.

The other commonly used test is the WISC (Wechsler Intelligence Scale for

Children). This was developed from the Wechsler Bellevue test which was devised as a test for clinical diagnosis of the different intellectual functions commonly taken as comprising 'general intelligence' (Weschler, 1958). The WISC test covers the age range of 5 to 16 years and is divided into two Scales, a Verbal and a Performance Scale. The Verbal Scale contains tests of Comprehension, Information, Arithmetic, Similarities and Vocabulary, each set containing items in order of increasing difficulty. The Performance Scale consists of tests of Picture Completion, Picture Arrangement, Block Design, Object Assembly and Coding. In Block Design, for instance, coloured blocks are to be arranged to form a pattern shown to the child, and Object Assembly is a jigsaw type of test. There is a system of scoring for each type of test, and a Verbal and a Performance Scale Quotient can be obtained as well as an I Q for both Scales combined, the Full Scale. It must be noted that if the WISC test is being used to explore clinically a child's intellectual functioning, an I Q cannot be derived from it; on the other hand, if the test is used to ascertain a child's I Q, the test must be presented in the prescribed standard manner and clinical exploration avoided during the administration of the test. The three I Q's which can be derived from the test, namely Verbal, Performance and Full Scale, are all expressed on a scale with mean of 100 I Q and standard deviation of 15.

The Wechsler Preschool and Primary Scale of Intelligence (WPPSI) covers the age range of $4\frac{1}{2}$ to 6 years of age, and is a better test than the WISC for younger children. The contents are very like those of WISC and the scoring follows the same pattern.

All these tests require skill in administration, and the scoring system needs to be adhered to strictly. Besides giving an assessment of a child's intellectual ability relative to children of the same age, such intelligence tests are a fruitful source of information on the development of children's thinking. The acceptable style of answer to the test items is not set by logical or absolute standards, it is determined by the kind of answer given by children. In the Binet Vocabulary test, for example, an acceptable answer to the question, 'What is an envelope?' is 'For a letter' or 'What you send'. Younger children define by description and use. Older children, even if wrong, attempt definition by classifying the term, for example, 'mosaic' is defined as 'Stone—little stones they have over in Italy' or 'limpet' as 'Somebody who has no energy'. Again, in the Binet test, children of age $3\frac{1}{2}$ years are shown a picture of children entering a house for a birthday party. Acceptable answers at this age are 'He's got the candy' or 'going in the door'. At age 6 years, these answers would not be accepted, and such as 'The girl is ringing the doorbell and the boy and girl are bringing packages, there's a Christmas cake in the window' are of acceptable level.

Interpretation of Intelligence Quotient

By the age of 6, assessment of a child's intellectual ability is possible, if the tests are administered individually by a skilled tester. Unskilled testing can lead to error. By this age, most of the items dependent on motor co-ordination have disappeared, and in general, an Intelligence Quotient at age 6 has for most children a substantial predictive validity of later intellectual ability. The figures below are from a Californian study (Honzik *et al.*, 1948), wherein the same children were tested annually from age 6 to 18 years.

TABLE 9

Constancy of IQ from age 6 to 18 years

Age in years	Correlation with I Q at age 10	Correlation with I Q at age 18
6	0·76	0·61
7	0·78	0·71
8	0·88	0·70
9	0·90	0·76
10	(1·0)	0·70
12	0·87	0·76

The correspondence is expressed in terms of correlation co-efficient. This is a measure of correspondence such that a correlation co-efficient of plus one represents perfect correspondence, and a co-efficient of zero a purely chance relationship. All the co-efficients in the table are positive, indicating a tendency for I Q to remain constant; and all are fairly high, indicating that substantial change in a child's I Q over the years is the exception rather than the rule.

The broad conclusion is, however, that the assessment of intelligence below the age of 5 or 6 is of doubtful validity; much that is being assessed cannot properly be called intelligence. Also the younger the child, the narrower the range of differences of behaviour that can be measured. Finally, the figures given above, which may be taken as typical, refer to 'normal' children. Those with *remediable* pathological conditions are more liable to vary in I Q.

The relationship between intellectual efficiency, intellectual maturity and acquired knowledge creates difficulties in interpreting assessments in terms of a child's developmental status. Efficiency and maturity are not necessarily concordant. An efficient crawler can beat an inefficient but more mature walker in competence in locomotion. So, too, the more mature thinker may not have acquired the skills to perform efficiently. An immature child may draw a man efficiently front view, but the more mature child attempting to draw in profile has difficulty with the leg and arm on the far side. An immature child may prattle fluently in simple sentence structure, while the more mature child has difficulty in finding words and structures to express more complex thinking. The less mature word-by-word reader makes fewer literal errors than the child who is reading in larger units of phrases or sentences. Intelligence tests, like the Stanford-Binet L-M and WISC, do not score separately for maturity and efficiency. Certain items are more closely related to maturity than others. The copying/drawing items, for example, are not scored on draughtsmanship, but on the child's concept of what he is drawing, which changes with age. Vocabulary tests reflect maturity in the form (not the correctness) of the definition attempted. The working principle is that the errors a child makes are as revealing as the number of his correct responses, and a pattern of error is often a useful guide to a child's developmental status.

The place of acquired knowledge in assessing a child's intellectual standing has been, and still is, a matter of controversy. The basic fact is that all knowledge is acquired. As a child grows older the kind and range of knowledge he acquires varies with his development. The younger children may join in number games, imitating the older children, but not aware of the need to count to join properly in the game. A year later the same child may appreciate the nature and rules of the game, and set himself to learn to count, so as to be able to play properly. So too with language; the single word may adequately express the younger child's concept of a situation. As he grows older, more words and more complex structures are needed to maintain his developing intellectual processes.

It follows that non-verbal and non-number tests, that is tests based on simple diagrams or on concrete material, are inadequate assessments of a child's intellectual processes. The intelligent child requires language and number to think with; and if deprived of these in a test situation, he has no opportunity to show how intelligent he is. Non-verbal, or performance tests, are therefore in no sense better or 'purer' measures of intelligence than those dependent on acquired knowledge and skills; indeed they are less valid for most purposes.

It also follows that a deficiency of acquired knowledge and skills will in the first instance be most probably due to a corresponding deficiency in intellectual functioning and maturity. If some children in the same families, at the same schools and in the same community can reach a given level of knowledge and skills, it is reasonable to assume that others in the same circumstances have equal opportunity to reach the same level. The observed differences in intelligence cannot be attributed to inequality of opportunity. In fact, within the same family, the differences in I Q between children can be considerable. A Scottish inquiry (Maxwell, 1969) reveals that for families of four or more children, the average difference between the highest and the lowest I Q within the same family is of the order of 26 points I Q ; in half the families, the difference was more than 26 points. It is therefore by no means unlikely that a child, borderline mentally handicapped with I Q of 70, may have a brother or sister in the same home, attending the same school, with an intellectual level above average. The attribution of a low intelligence to poor cultural environment may on occasion be correct, but it must be clearly established by independent evidence. Low I Q may be due to poor environment, but it may also coincide with poor environment. Also, the ability of most children to make up lost educational ground very rapidly after a temporary setback should not be underestimated.

Finally, the term Intelligence Quotient, or I Q , needs to be interpreted with great circumspection. There are no units of intelligence, such as centimetres or kilograms, and therefore there is no zero from which measurement is made. A child's standing height is measured from the floor, but a child's intelligence is measured from the average performance of a representative sample of children *of the same age*. Traditionally, the Intelligence Quotient is a ratio (not a quantity), and is obtained from the fraction Mental Age over Chronological Age. Mental age was defined as the average age of all children who obtained the same score on a test of intelligence. Thus a child of mental age of 12 years, with a chronological age of 10 years would obtain a quotient of 1·2, *i.e.* 12 divided by 10. This was multiplied by 100 to get rid of decimal points, giving an Intelligence Quotient of 120. Thus a child who was of average ability for his age would obtain a quotient of 1, or an Intelligence Quotient of 100. This value of I Q 100 is the point from which I Q's are measured. The concept of Mental Age is now virtually obsolete, and I Q's are expressed on a scale of mean of 100 and standard deviation of 15, or occasionally 16. It must be known what the standard deviation of an I Q scale is before any given I Q can be interpreted. The scores on an I Q scale are distributed on what is known as a normal distribution, and the standard deviation or S.D. is a measure of the extent to which scores are distributed round the mean. If they are widely scattered, the Standard Deviation is large; if they cluster closely round the mean the Standard Deviation is small. The I Q is now best interpreted in terms of a child's standing in a population of children *of the same age*, and this is best expressed in percentile rank. A percentile rank is the percentage of children of the same age who do less well than the child in question. Thus, for I Q, a child with a percentile rank of 25 would be more intelligent than 25 per cent of his contemporaries, and less intelligent than 75 per cent of them. The broad relationship between I Q's and percentile rank is given in Table 10 below (intrapolation is not linear).

TABLE 10

Percentile Rank	2·5	16	25	50	75	84	97·5
I Q (S.D. = 15)	70	85	90	100	110	115	130
I Q (S.D. = 16)	68	84	89	100	111	116	132

The Wechsler series of individual tests and the Moray House series of group tests have a standard deviation of 15, the Binet Terman–Merrill L-M revision has a standard deviation of 16. Children of the same age are normally considered as those within an age range of 1 to 4 months.

The I Q is therefore now not considered as a quotient, though the term, being a familiar one, has been retained. The concept of Mental Age has been found to create more confusion than it resolved. The difficulty was that a difference of 2 years of Mental Age, say between a four-year-old and a six-year-old, represented a very much more significant difference than that between a ten-year-old and a twelve-year-old. A six-year-old with the intellectual level of the average four-year-old would have an I Q of 67, which is low; a twelve-year-old performing on the level of the average ten-year-old would have an I Q of 83. The difference as expressed in I Q is a better reflection of the situation.

Another question in the interpretation of I Q is that of the constancy of a child's I Q. Table 9 (page 255) indicates the tendency for I Q to remain constant rather than to vary over the years, but there is another aspect, the precision of any measure of I Q . This depends on what is technically called the reliability of the test. This is best expressed as the standard error of any test score. If the standard error is 4 points of I Q , a reasonable figure for an individual intelligence test, it means that an I Q of 110 can be interpreted as 110 ± 4, *i.e.* the chance of a second assessment falling within the limits of 106 to 114 I Q is two to one. If the limits are taken as twice the standard error, then the chances of a second assessment falling within the limits 102 to 118 are twenty to one. Few tests have a standard error of less than 3 points I Q ; tests of younger children and performance tests have standard errors of at least 6 points I Q . The standard error represents the part played by chance in the assessment.

Regression to the Mean

It follows that in any test score there is a component of chance which along with other factors leads to a phenomenon known as regression to the mean. The effect of regression is that the scores of children, who on the first test were above or below the average, will on a second or another test tend to be nearer the average of the population they are drawn from. This appears in practice in various forms. If a child is tested and has a clearly below average score, and is tested again, whether after treatment or not, the second score will tend to be higher than the first, and the greater the standard error of the score, the greater will be the apparent improvement. Conversely, children with initially high scores will appear to deteriorate. Another example is the relationship between I Q and school attainment. If a pupil has an I Q of 115, and if the correlation between the intelligence test and a test of school attainment, expressed on the same scale is, r = + 0·7 (again a reasonable figure), the expected quotient on the attainment test would be of the order of 111. Only within fairly broad limits can it be expected that the highest I Q's will be best at school attainment, and the lowest I Q's the poorest. A further effect of regression is shown in such tests as WISC where the I Q's are obtained separately on a Scale of Verbal tests and a Scale of Performance tests. Since the scores on these two Scales do not coincide exactly, there is regression to the mean. Children scoring high (or low) on one scale will tend to score nearer the average on the other scale. The average difference between I Q's on the two scales is of the order of 8 points, half of the children having differences of more than 8 points, half having less. Regression to the mean is a sufficient explanation of such differences, and a comparison of a population of children attending a psychological clinic shows a pattern of differences very similar to that obtained from a population of 'normal' children.

In all such cases, where comparison between two sets of assessment is being made, it must be kept in mind that it is only differences which clearly exceed the limits estimated by regression that can be considered as meaningful. Children selected as educationally backward, for example, will tend to regress to the mean when reassessed. It is too easy to attribute this regression to remedial treatment.

Educational Backwardness

The concept of Mental Age has been discarded in intelligence testing, but it still appears in certain educational contexts. Most tests of reading and arithmetic express the finding in terms of Reading Age or Arithmetic Age. These findings require to be interpreted with great care, with the following points kept in mind. The first is that the name of a test is not an adequate indication of its content. Some commonly used tests are properly called Word Recognition Tests, but are frequently taken as an assessment of reading attainment, which they are not. The nature of the test itself must be examined. Does it require comprehension of the words? Does it stress errors or speed? How many different styles of reading does it encompass? Does it depend on visual or auditory recognition? Few tests of reading in current use add much to the information which can be given by a reasonably observant teacher; most are too short and therefore often very unreliable. Arithmetic tests, particularly the Schonell diagnostic tests, are better and more thorough, though not now directly related to the kind of arithmetic being developed in Primary Schools.

The use of units of mental age in assessment of children contains another pitfall which we have already indicated. A child whose reading age is 2 years behind his chronological age may or may not be seriously retarded, according to what his chronological age is. Retardation of 2 years in the reading attainment of an eight-year-old represents a clear lack of progress in reading and a low standard of achievement. At age 13, 2 years retardation means a performance equivalent to that of an average eleven-year-old, which is by no means illiterate.

The commonest cause of educational backwardness is stupidity. The task of the educational psychologist is in the first instance to distinguish between those children whose educational backwardness is largely remediable, and those who are backward but appear to be functioning at a level compatible with their estimated ability. It must be remembered that, by definition, half the school population is below average. The other task of the psychologist is to distinguish between presenting symptoms and the real causes of the condition. Some deficiencies are more socially acceptable than others. Reading difficulty may be real enough, but be only one symptom of a more serious condition of emotional or personal disorder. Cases showing a simple and clear relation between cause and effect do occur, but they are comparatively infrequent. The commoner situation is a complex of interrelated conditions, and the natural tendency to close the inquiry when one cause has been established is often difficult to resist. It is possible for a child to have infected tonsils, an anxiety condition, and a weakness in arithmetic all in one, and remedy of one condition may not necessarily result in improvement in the others. A co-ordinated team approach to diagnosis and treatment is nearly always necessary.

Learning abilities are as important to the child as security and esteem in occupation are to the adult, with the additional complication that frequently the parents' acceptance and affection for the child can be determined by his educational success.

Often, the prognosis for remedial psychological and educational treatment of learning difficulties is not very good, but if no action is taken, there is a probability that emotional maladjustment may develop. In such cases, the psychologist's attention is directed more to the parent than the child. If, however, there is a real learning difficulty, the psychological approach may take two main lines. If there appears to be a cognitive defect which renders learning difficult, as in genuine cases of specific dyslexia (which are not frequent), the approach is to support and guide the child in learning to live with his disability, and to find and encourage those sections of behaviour in which he can experience success. Any kind of psychological or educational treatment which concentrates on the areas of failure is not effective. On the other hand, when the learning difficulties are remediable, the treatment is usually basically simple. The main working principles are first, that the pupil should clearly understand what he is expected to do, and second, that any teaching method which has been previously used without success is contra-indicated. The application of these principles depends on the skill and experience of the psychologist.

SHEENA MAXWELL
JAMES MAXWELL

References

BRUNER, J. S. (1964). The course of cognitive growth. *Amer. Psychol.*, **19**, 1.

—— (1968). The course of cognitive growth. In *Thinking and Reasoning*. Ed. P. C. Watson and P. N. Johnston Laird. London: Penguin Books.

CATTELL, P. (1940). *The Measurement of Intelligence of Infants and Young Children*. New York: Psych. Corp.

GAGNE, R. M. (1965). *The Conditions of Learning*. New York: Holt Rinehart and Winston.

GRIFFITHS, R. (1954). *The Abilities of Babies*. London: Univ. Press.

HONZIK, M. P., MACFARLANE, J. W. and ALLAN, L. (1948). The stability of mental test performance between 2 and 18 years. *J. Exper. Education*, **309**, 17.

MAXWELL, J. (1969). Sixteen years on: a follow-up of the 1947 Scottish survey. Edinburgh: Scottish Council for Research into Education.

PHILLIP, J. L. (1969). *Origins of Intellect: Piaget's Theory*. San Francisco: Freeman.

STUTSMAN, R. (1931). *Mental Measurement of Pre-school Children*. New York: Harcourt Brace.

TERMAN, L. M. and MERRILL, M. A. (1961). *Stanford-Binet Intelligence Scale L-M (3rd Revision)*. London: Harrap.

WECHSLER, D. (1958). *The Measurement and Appraisal of Intelligence*. 4th ed. Baltimore: Williams and Wilkins.

10   Emotional Development

'Childhood has its own ways of seeing, thinking and feeling; nothing
is more foolish than to try and substitute our ways.'

Rousseau.

Relevance of the Subject

IT is hard to realise that it is just over 200 years since Rousseau published the
first account of emotional development based on the direct observation of children
(Grange, 1963). The above quotation, so reasonable to the informed contemporary ear, signifies an intuitive grasp of the whole subject so far in advance of its
time that '*Emile*' has suffered long neglect. Even his few supporters who were
interested in Rousseau's revolutionary ideas on child development did not seriously
regard them as having any practical significance. It is unfortunately true that
even today it is still necessary in some quarters to justify the study of the beginnings
of the human mind and of human behaviour as a matter of no mean importance
in the practical affairs of man.

At the outset then, let us consider the claims of this subject for our serious
attention. Firstly, there is the 'pure research' attitude which values discovery
for its own sake. Secondly, there is the goal of establishing norms so that the
earliest signs of deviation may be detected, and this has obvious relevance for
clinical practice. Thirdly, what we can learn about the emotional stages of childhood may contribute further to our understanding the factors involved in mental
health at all ages. Fourthly, and in line with the second half of Rousseau's quotation, knowledge about the way children's minds work permits us to deal with
children appropriately. Perhaps the most modest of these four aims, it may yet
prove to be the most significant.

Let us consider each in more detail:

Pure research. The field of psychology has always given rise to the most
intense controversy and schism, possibly because the science is a young one and
established knowledge meagre. It would not, however, be expected perhaps that
opinions would differ radically about what it is we are attempting to study when
we speak of the emotional development of the child. Yet that is, or has been, very
much the case. At one extreme is the approach of Watson and his followers of the
Behaviourist School who declared that human behaviour could be explained
without reference to 'personality' or anything else which is unsubstantial. Freud,
in contrast, was primarily concerned with revealing the invisible and irrational

261

forces in personality. At the present time we have reached a stage of gradual if grudging mutual respect and acknowledgement that each has much of value to offer.

Research cannot proceed without its appropriate methodology, and here there are immense difficulties especially in early childhood studies. It is easy to take refuge in the fact that the infant cannot communicate to the observer feelings, thoughts, or attitudes so that there is a constant danger of making subjective interpretations, but not so easy to explain why until recently there have been practically no systematic studies of, for example, the behaviour of infants. Developments in this field are available to the reader in 'Determinants of Infant Behaviour' (Foss, 1961; 1963; 1965). One pioneer endeavour is worthy of special mention, namely 'The Nursing Couple' (1941) in which Middlemore studied the breast-feeding situation and took the first step in differentiating some main varieties of infant activity *as part of an interactive process*. There are still very few studies of the reciprocal interaction (diadic behaviour) of mother and baby or indeed of parents and children of any age.

Another considerable methodological landmark was the recognition that observational data were constantly available in the *spontaneous play* of children. While this has become an accepted method in clinical child psychiatric practice both for diagnostic and therapeutic purposes, here also there are few research studies comparable in diligence of observation with the pioneer work of Susan Isaacs (1933). It is true that her interpretations of the children's words and actions in a nursery school setting were in line with the theoretical postulates of Melanie Klein, but the data are there, recorded and observed, and available for study and re-evaluation by successive generations of students.

The psycho-analysts, Freud included, have often maintained that every analysis itself constitutes a research project and in the sense of 'clinical research' this is a reasonable claim. As a procedure for eliciting psychological data about childhood it is subject to all the imperfections of a retrospective technique, including the patient's ability to recall. In fact this method has clearly demonstrated that there are laws concerning the retention and loss of childhood memories (*infantile amnesia*). An interesting modification which has been applied in recent years is the simultaneous psychoanalysis of mother and child which is beginning to reveal parallels in the thought processes of each, though refuting a simple cause and effect relationship (Burlingham, 1955; Hellman, 1960).

The work of Piaget is a unique contribution to our understanding of children's thought processes. His critics have rightly observed that the subjects he has studied are (*a*) few in number; (*b*) his own children; and (*c*) without controls. It must be acknowledged, however, that with great originality, especially in the design of experiments, he has revealed probable mechanisms and sequences of thought according to stages of development which others are now testing with all the necessary safeguards of controlled research. Piaget's concern is primarily with the sequence of development and not with age norms. His work is also referred to in Chapters 8 and 9 on the development of behaviour and intelligence, for which it has considerable relevance; here we shall consider some of its implications for child psychology and psychiatry as discussed by Woodward (1965). Piaget's approach serves to bridge the intellectual and emotional aspects of child development which have tended in the past to be treated separately. A few examples will serve to show the importance of his findings for certain theories of psychological development. For example, he states that the infant's inner world and reactions are bound by perceived objects and hence by the immediate present; memory images do not develop until halfway through the second year, nor does the capacity to represent one object symbolically by another. These findings are at variance with theories which attribute to the infant a capacity for recall. Again, although the two-year-old shows some capacity for the recall of past events in action and play the child has not yet the necessary verbal structure for understanding a promise. Before the age of about 11 years concreteness in thinking may be expected. The richness of Piaget's work is matched only by the complexity of his terminology and it is already obvious that time will have to elapse before the full implications of his contribution are grasped.

If the methodological techniques so far discussed are disconcerting to those accustomed to the research methods of the physical sciences this is not necessarily a defect but rather a recognition that this particular field of study has unique features demanding its own methods of investigation.

Ethology, the study of animal behaviour, has developed rapidly as a research discipline in recent years, and already its findings are providing fresh slants on human behaviour. Tinbergen (1951) has paid particular attention to what is termed the *Innate Releasing Mechanism*, a species-specific response to a particular stimulus.

Imprinting is a particular type of innate releasing mechanism whose function is closely linked with a particular type of conditioning (Lorenz, 1956).

In a now famous experiment Lorenz has demonstrated that the newly-hatched greylag gosling responds to the movement and noise of its mother by following her, but will develop the *following response* to any object between the sizes of a bantam hen and a rowing-boat which moves and emits noises of varying pitch. In many different species it has now been demonstrated that certain types of useful biological learning occur most easily at particular ages, and it is likely that such *sensitive periods* remain to be charted in human development.

Establishment of norms

It is tempting to believe that what Gesell has done for psychomotor development, namely establishing age norms from birth to adolescence, demands only comparable enthusiasm and industry to make available analogous standards of emotional maturation. One basic aspect of human emotional development invalidates this belief: the tremendous variation from one individual to another at all stages of emotional growth. Indeed age is only one, and not necessarily the dominant, of several major variables such as sex, social class, historical and cultural setting. This might appear to be a baffling situation when attempting to assess an individual child at a given moment in time, but is in fact not so very different from the difficulties involved in estimating physical growth. In both instances a single set of observations has little value whereas one in a longitudinal growth series, even if relatively short, can be revealing. Admittedly units of height, weight and so forth are reassuringly concrete compared with the intangibles of feeling, attitude, thought and behaviour, but these are the relevant data and we must learn to use them. *Moreover it is likely that instead of pursuing normative values we must learn to recognise characteristic sequences.* Even allowing for the many variables mentioned the human organism does seem to have a unique sequence of unfolding. This is very much in keeping with the approach of Piaget. It is also inherent in psychoanalytic theories of personality growth.

For a presentation of the psychoanalytic view refreshingly down-to-earth in its concern with the practical problems of clinical assessment the reader is referred to a monograph by Anna Freud (1963). Here she develops the concept of 'Developmental Lines' and details the sequence of events in a number of these: (*a*) Dependency to emotional self-reliance, (*b*) towards body independence, (*c*) egocentricity to companionship. Particularly pertinent are the concluding observations about correspondence between different lines of development in a particular child. She points out that in practice we expect a fairly close correspondence so that to be a healthy personality a child who has reached a specific stage in one line will have made a corresponding achievement in another. Yet it is recognised that many children show a very irregular pattern, *e.g.* with high achievement as regards bodily independence such as sphincter control while lagging behind in play-level and vice versa. It is suggested that out task is not to isolate two such lines or aspects of development but to trace their interaction giving special consideration to what is determined by innate, and what by environmental factors.

This is a convenient point to add that even if we are some way from resolving this duality, it is at least apparent that the former mutually exclusive attitude to personality development, the heredity–environment controversy, is meaningless. That being so, in a sense the approaches of Gesell, Piaget and the psychoanalytic school are all too exclusively child-oriented. Each acknowledges the importance but does not record environmental data. A reciprocal pattern of behaviour between mother and child unfolds from birth onwards, possibly earlier, and this is often implicitly recognised in clinical practice. In all cultures and social classes mothers and babies 'play games' such as 'peek-bo' and 'this little piggy' which almost certainly correspond to stages which the child is just about to reach (see later reference to 'body image'). The mother, it seems, is responding intuitively to minimal cues, but neither these nor the infant's response, nor the maternal reaction to the response have been studied systematically. We lack a map of developing inter-personal relationships.

Implications for Later Life

Irrespective of theoretical orientation there are few who would now deny the importance of childhood experiences in shaping the adult personality both with regard to (*a*) *character formation*, and (*b*) *mental stability*. Differences arise, however, as soon as we consider how these factors operate. Eysenck and Rachman (1965) postulate two inter-related inherited tendencies obtained by subjecting to factor-analysis the 'neurotic traits' of large numbers of children. These traits are found to correlate together thus defining (1) a factor of 'neuroticism' (instability), and cutting across this (2) a second factor which divides conduct problems from personality problems, and which is designated 'introversion–extraversion'. The 'introverted, neurotic' child is characterised by personality problems such as a tendency to be depressed, seclusive, absent-minded, irritable, to have day-dreams, inferiority feelings, mood swings and mental conflict. The 'extraverted neurotic' child on the other hand tends to have conduct problems, to be ego-centric, rude, violent, disobedient and destructive and is given to fighting, stealing and truanting. It is claimed that this division applies to girls as well as boys and at varying ages. Evidence is presented suggesting that underlying the 'neuroticism' is an inherent pre-disposition of the autonomic nervous system to react strongly and lastingly to stimuli; whereas the introversion–extraversion tendency depends on the speed and strength with which conditioned responses are formed. Individuals who condition quickly tend to develop introversion personality problems. Symptoms are explained as maladaptation or inappropriate conditioning and, logically, conditioning techniques are used in what is termed 'behaviour' therapy. For those to whom the essence of the human being is the 'inner world' the capacity for self-awareness, for reflection and imagination, the behaviourist approach must inevitably seem incomplete, almost irrelevant, in spite of its insistence on objective observation.

Much controversy surrounds the problem of *how* childhood experiences affect later personality. No less important is the task of identifying *which* particular factors operate significantly. The one about which considerable evidence has accumulated is that of *social deprivation*. For a full review of this subject the reader is referred to Bowlby's classic monograph (1952) and to the *World Health Organization Bulletin* No. 14 (1962). Here we shall deal with a few main landmarks. Spitz (1945) was among the first to draw attention to the fact that human infants if not given sufficient mothering, even though nutritional and hygienic standards are adequate, tend to become withdrawn, listless, apathetic, to succumb readily to acute respiratory or gastro-intestinal infections and often to die. This clinical picture he called 'anaclitic depression', and Bakwin (1942) described its appearance in babies kept in hospital for long periods. There was no information about the children who survived, but other workers such as Goldfarb (1943) following the development of children reared for long periods in institutions began to recognise a typical personality picture which Bowlby termed the 'affectionless character' and which resembled in many respects what we understand by the adult 'psychopathic personality', namely gross impairment in the capacity for human relationships combined with a defective sense of conscience. This aetiological hypothesis not surprisingly has been unpopular with child-care personnel and with some paediatricians but if the case was originally overstated it certainly helped to foster a more consciously humane attitude in the professional handling of young children and especially as regards the rights of their parents. The main facts, however, cannot be side-stepped. From clinical studies there is growing evidence that early bereavement, related to social deprivation, is a highly significant factor in a later tendency to depression, especially suicide (Brown, 1961), as well as to delinquent and psychopathic personality (Gregory, 1958).

Supportive evidence regarding the importance of emotional deprivation has recently come from an unexpected quarter, that of animal behaviour. Harlow (1962), working at the Primate Laboratory, University of Wisconsin, has studied the behaviour of monkeys reared under differing, carefully controlled environmental conditions. Monkeys reared in isolation developed peculiar patterns of behaviour. They sat and stared vacantly, circled repetitively, rocked, chewed and pinched themselves, especially at the approach of a human. Six months' isolation made these effects permanent.

Curiously the presence of an inanimate, soft, warm 'dummy' mother prevented these disturbances from developing in severe form. Intimate body contact appeared to be the primary mechanism. The maternal relationship was significant in facilitating the interaction of the infant with other infants and, surprisingly, opportunities for optimal interaction of the infants with other infants appeared to compensate for the lack of mothering, at least as far as later social and heterosexual relations are concerned.

No less remarkable are the experiments on partial social deprivation: 100 monkeys of each sex were reared in cages where they could see and hear other monkeys but could not play with them during the first 6 to 12 months of life when they normally learn to play with each other. None of these male monkeys so reared has ever made an adequate sexual adjustment to any female monkey. Half of the female monkeys did, after a time, respond sexually to normal males and some did conceive. When in due course these socially deprived females became mothers, without exception they failed to feed their babies, and in fact abused them. The offspring, moreover, displayed precocious sexual behaviour.

While caution is necessary in applying experimental findings on monkeys to the life situations of human beings, nonetheless these results tend to reinforce hypotheses about the pathogenicity of early emotional deprivation. Particularly impressive is the evidence for a connecting link between one generation and the next.

This type of deprivation is but one form of early childhood experience. Others, such as parental attitudes, now await accurate definition and prospective study.

The Understanding of Children

At first glance this is the least ambitious of our goals—to study the emotional development of children in order to understand them. Yet in many ways it is the most challenging. We have seen that the experiences of children from infancy onwards can affect their wellbeing, even their physical health, that these events may have an important bearing on their future emotional lives. There is, however, a danger of setting our sights at too long a range and ignoring the present, of making children insecure or unhappy or afraid, not intentionally or neglectfully but from ignorance or unwillingness to recognise the evidence before us. It is fairly certain that satisfying experiences in childhood do strengthen personality resources later on but there is also a humanitarian aspect in that one should through understanding attempt to make the lives of young people happy. Understanding the ways and methods of communication of children has also important pedagogical significance in that it can help us to use appropriate educational techniques at different age levels, not merely in the sense of formal instruction but of imparting cultural values.

Stages of Emotional Development
Infancy

The life of a young infant may be considered as a constantly repeated cycle of events—much sleeping or near-sleeping and less wakefulness during which occur feeding, eliminating and crying. The infant cannot say what he feels, for example, when his stomach is empty or his surface temperature has fallen or his posture is suddenly changed, but presumably these are situations of unease. In contrast the drowsy cooing and babbling after a feed when clothes are warm and dry, when sensations in general are pleasurable seem to represent the earliest stages of contentment, of enjoyment in just existing. There are many imponderables here but none more curious than the paradox that this creature who is entirely dependent on the mother (or her substitute) for physical survival is yet very frequently in almost complete command of the adult. While fashions change as to whether crying babies should be lifted or left (both extremes are probably ill-advised) it is not difficult to imagine that the dawning mind is becoming aware of the power of its own cry. While child development is often seen as a gradual transition from dependence to independence (or more correctly from relatively more to relatively less dependence) it is equally important to recognise the renunciation of the omnipotent attitude of the infant. Whereas some adults never achieve much independence at all, others remain imperious and demanding throughout their lives. Nearly every child during the second or third year has to live through the painful experience of this renunciation which contributes to the typical negativistic behaviour of a toddler.

Psychoanalytic theory lays great emphasis on the dominance of the mouth in infancy, that is to say as a zone of pleasurable stimulus. It is also at this early stage a principal touch organ, its use for the tactile examination of objects preceding that of the fingers. Thus the lips suck and touch, the tongue tastes and feels, the gums bite and chew—a wide range of sensations are centred in the mouth, during this so-called *oral phase*. In consideration of the most primitive levels of sense-organ activity disproportionate emphasis has almost certainly been placed on the mouth at the expense of the tactile sensibility of the skin surface and of stimuli from the kinesthetic and vestibular systems (see Erikson, 1958). Displeasure also tends to be displayed orally in screaming, biting or spitting but here again there are wide physical concomitants in violent contractions of skeletal muscle. If the adult personality shows the characteristically infantile traits of extreme dependency combined with imperious demands this person has in psychoanalytic terms an 'oral character'. This is an extreme form of immaturity, emotional development having, as it were, been held up or 'fixated' at this stage either because of grossly inadequate nursing or because of a sudden disruption of a satisfying nursing experience. The terminology here does not serve well the quite profound considerations which it is intended to imply. Immaturity of this degree may indeed represent failure to emerge from this very early stage, but the fixation is one not of an aspect of body-erotism only but of the whole circumstances of interdependence with other people which, appropriate to that early stage, have persisted without necessary modifications into later life.

The development of the earliest attachment to the mother ('object relations') is regarded by Bowlby (1960) in a radically different way from that of traditional psychoanalytic theory. On the basis of the ethological concepts of instinctual response systems mentioned earlier Bowlby suggested that the infant's attachment to the mother is a basic component in this earliest reciprocal social relationship and is not secondarily derived from the satisfactions of food and warmth. Clinging, it is postulated, is as fundamental a response as sucking. This is a challenging hypothesis with important theoretical implications regarding the origins of anxiety and depression.

Now let us consider the mother's role in this earliest of human relationships. It is convenient to see in her activities a spontaneously (a) affectionate, and (b) protective attitude. This rather artificial division is useful as we see distortions of each clinically, for example, maternal rejection or ambivalence, 'maternal over-protection' (Levy, 1943). It is much easier to talk about disturbances in mother–infant behaviour than to make any dogmatic statements about what is normal. There is in fact little definite evidence about the long-term sequelae of disorders of mothering but certainly at the time the infant may react with unusual patterns of crying (either too much or too little), of feeding (apathy, vomiting, rumination), breath holding, head rolling, and so on. The infant nursed in tense arms often screams, loses interest and may vomit but rapidly settles to contented sucking when transferred to experienced hands. The rocking chair, the crib, and the lullaby have evolved empirically no doubt because they aid the relaxation of both parties. There is much evidence then that infants require in addition to nourishment and protection, frequent gentle confident handling by a familiar person.

Babies respond to a smile with a smile by the second month (Ambrose, 1961) but this is not necessarily an indication that they as yet recognise people. By 6 to 8 months however the child already reacts to separation from the mother with the characteristic sequence of distress, rage, apathy and grief of the older child (Schaffer, 1958). This stage would appear to represent a crucial 'milestone' in the development of interpersonal relations, the beginnings of attachment specifically to the mother. As Schaffer himself has pointed out there is a danger of this finding being misinterpreted to mean that separation of younger babies from their mothers carries no danger psychologically. In fact, however, there is abundant clinical evidence that the initial 'coupling' process between mother and infant may be disrupted when delayed, for example after a premature birth where the child requires to remain in hospital. It is probable that the father is recognised also long before the first birthday. There is a curious absence of systematic enquiry into any aspect of the father's role in relation to his developing child.

Infant Management and Mental Health

It is now relevant to consider to what extent particular child-rearing practices affect the emotional development of the individual. It has to be acknowledged that there is little solid foundation for the important role in character formation and adult mental health that has been ascribed at various times to, for example, artificial feeding, swaddling, early or sudden weaning, too much or too little lifting and cuddling, and closely related to this, leaving babies to cry; to rigidly organised feeding schedules or toilet training in the first weeks of life; and to the frequent use of laxatives, enemas and rectal suppositories. These are matters on which the advice of the physician in family, health clinic, or paediatric practice is commonly sought and unfortunately there is no trustworthy book of rules, and there probably never will be. This does not mean that all or any of these practices are unimportant; each and every one has demonstrably acted as a traumatic experience for an individual as revealed in the course of exploratory psychotherapy. This, however, is a complex matter because of the tremendous variation from child to child. Innate factors do exist even if we know little about them. For example, one infant may be comfortable only with a well-ordered feeding regimen, a second on a self-demand schedule, a third able to accept either, and a fourth a 'difficult feeder' no matter what is tried. This last baby may, of course, be 'difficult' no matter how skilled and relaxed is the nursing person, or may be responding to the insecure, inconsistent handling of a very nervous mother so that the precise feeding schedule is a relatively minor consideration. This is the second consideration, that it may well be true if unproven as yet that in every example mentioned associated factors, and especially relationship factors, are paramount. Where, for example, in the aetiology of a neurosis inappropriate administration of enemas to a young child is relevant, it may not be the practice itself that has contributed as much as the 'emotional climate' of the transaction, whether, for example, the manipulation of the child had a sadistic or other erotically-toned component. When considering the importance of weaning, Bowlby (1960) pungently comments that 'a mother is more than a pair of breasts' thereby highlighting the too often neglected concomitant experience of the child at this time, such as the birth of a sibling or separation from the mother.

It appears then that within very wide limits all sorts of infant-rearing methods can be employed without detriment to the child's emotional development *provided the mother is orientated to the needs of the child*. Thus her technique may not be identical with all her children. In response to tangible cues from her children she may do things differently or the same things at different stages.

10

Where in contrast a mother—and at a slightly later age this begins to apply with equal force to father—is in child-rearing activities responding primarily to her own inner needs, then we are in the realms of maternal psychopathology. We may be confronted with a psycho-neurosis or acute psychosis in the mother which involves her child and for which treatment is required; a disorder of the mother–child relationship where the mother's personality is basically a sound one, in which the disorder is often 'triggered' by events during this or a previous pregnancy, at the time of delivery or just after, and where psychotherapeutic intervention is often quickly effective; or where the disturbed mothering is but one facet of a profoundly disordered personality in the mother such as a 'character disorder' which is unlikely to be modified by any treatment procedure, and where therefore the professional helper must be content to give support, encouragement, and direct advice on child management.

From this brief survey of the psychopathology of mothering it follows that imparting information is but one aspect of *parent education*, and not always the most important. What the majority of parents want is guidance on how to act in specific situations, and they are often helped in this by group discussions with other parents. The frequent gain in understanding and self-confidence is how-ever not merely from the acquisition of facts, but from sharing their anxieties with others, meeting approval in the process from the other parents and the group leader. An invariable task of parent education is the modification of culturally-determined attitudes and practices. These may be inappropriate in the sense that they do not tally with the facts of child emotional development. Many parents for example are still shocked to find their infant exploring his genitalia and orifices, to witness an erection in a male baby, especially during feeding, or to observe masturbatory movements of young children of both sexes. It is a relief to them to hear that these are common and harmless activities. Many are surprised that disgust is culturally determined and that there is no cause for alarm when a baby plays with his own excreta.

By all means let us give accurate child developmental information to parents so long as we recognise that there are other aspects than didactic teaching.

Early Childhood

As soon as the child begins to walk the beginnings of striving for independence are seen, at first fluctuating with frequent retreats to the safety of the parent's arms. Separation for any length of time as we have seen causes intense distress. With the development of speech the main channel of communication is established and we as observers have our first real access to the child's thoughts and feelings. Long before 'make believe' play is reached early forms of fantasy take shape. Objects are credited with living, human attributes (*animistic thinking*) so that, for example, a hurtful bang on the head leads to reprisals against 'the bad table'. It has been suggested that familiarity with all external objects is achieved in the first instance by seeing in them aspects of the child's own body. Moreover, there is a magical quality in early thinking in the sense that thoughts alone can shape events, and when we consider the intensity of a young child's loving as well as hating these events may be alarming. *Animism* and *thought omnipotence* may return during adult mental illness, and are seen also in primitive societies. In the minds of young children fantasy and reality merge. Childhood thought, as Rousseau sensed, has its own logic which we now begin to comprehend as these mental mechanisms are recognised. Much of the behaviour at these early stages can be seen as the drive to discover new things and experiences and the mastery of the anxieties aroused. This results in frequent flight to what is familiar, and sometimes the deliberate manufacture of what is familiar as in bedtime and other *rituals*. The teddy-bear serves many purposes: when the child is alone as an imaginary companion or something to cuddle in place of mother; as a scapegoat; as a pretended companion to praise or blame, love or reject, as inner needs dictate. On this particular topic the writer A. A. Milne is probably still the most perceptive observer.*

Some children, however, prefer a piece of blanket or fringed material from which they may be inseparable for years, more especially at bedtime or when feeling ill or insecure, and to which they give a special private name. Winnicot (1958), has described this as a 'transitional object'. This he regards as the child's first real possession, an intermediary perhaps between a thumb and a doll. Children are greatly comforted by being allowed to take with them not just toys but especially familiar objects when they go to hospital or other strange places. When the toddler returns again to the security of his own home he may begin wetting or soiling (or these may have appeared during separation and persist for a time), demanding to be fed, refusing to sleep alone or even be separated during the day, may return to baby-talk, and begin thumb sucking. All this behaviour is a typical response to a situation of fear and of insecurity which is or has just been experienced, and represents a *regression* to an earlier emotional level. This can occur in human beings (and probably animals too) at all stages of life though adults hide it better, and bodily functions are not so obviously affected. Regression serves as a safeguard and is almost always temporary. Parents can be greatly helped by being warned in advance about its likely occurrence, and the import-ance of responding appropriately to the child's temporary infantile needs. Another common situation which may lead to regressive behaviour is the birth of a baby brother or sister. Once parents have grasped the reality and intensity of the toddler's feelings of rivalry, jealousy, love and hate they usually have the initiative to deal effectively with the situation. The child acquires socially commendable attitudes but slowly, and there should therefore be no shock at hearing the im-perious demand to 'send the baby back'. Fortunately dolls and teddies are there to take some of the brunt of this intense ambivalence.

Irrational fears of specific things often develop in the early years, fears of flies, dogs, horses—the so-called *phobias*. The dangerous impulses which the child ascribes to these creatures is regarded as a measure of the intensity of feeling being experienced within the child (*projection*).

* 'Now We Are Six'; 'Winnie The Pooh'. A. A. Milne. London: Methuen.

Toilet training has important psychological components. Besides the earlier curiosity and exploration, faeces and to a less extent urine are at various stages regarded with pride and often fear. There is evidence that in neuro-physiological terms conscious sphincter control is not possible till about one year old. The mother who is pleased at 'never having had a dirty napkin' often mistakes her accurate timing of the child's gastro–colic reflex for early mastery of bowel evacuation. When this does become functionally possible the child often refuses to perform on request, and may seem deliberately to 'hold back'. When accidents are ignored and successful defaecation rewarded, regular bowel habits usually form fairly easily; but if much fuss and temper is aroused in the parent a common sequel is 'constipation'. This is often explained as the result of a painful anal fissure but this is more often a result than a cause. Intense parental preoccupation with cleanliness may also inhibit the child's early bowel functioning.

Quite small children often seem to locate accurately the sensitive areas in their parent's make-up, thus providing themselves with retaliatory weapons. For example, towards a mother who is really upset by a child's misbehaving in company, this is clearly a way to punish her; if anorexia makes her distraught as often as not this is the form a behaviour disorder takes, and so on. The acts of defaecation and urination represent aggressive impulses as evidenced by the slang connotation of these terms in our vocabulary. In order to conform with the mores of society represented by the parents' approval, pleasurable interest is converted to disgust (*reaction formation*). Sometimes this transition is exaggerated to one of inhibition of all assertiveness making the child passive, conforming, and lacking in initiative. Quite often this is associated with both oral inhibition such as speech hesitancy and bowel inhibition leading to constipation and encopresis. The wish to indulge in messy play may also be displaced to a 'safer' area so that toddlers often play messily with their food and as this is transient and usually does not interfere with nutrition as such it is best tolerated. Ultimately these impulses are sublimated to socially-approved goals such as sand and water play, clay and plasticine, modelling or painting. Psychoanalytic theory holds that this phase of development is the origin of certain 'anal' character traits such as meanness, excessive preoccupation with orderliness and precision.

Real interest in co-operative activity with other children seldom begins before $2\frac{1}{2}$ to 3 years so that organised group activities in nurseries or elsewhere before that age usually fail. Ego-centricity, ruthless possessiveness, and uncontrolled aggression gradually respond to socialising influences, partly because of the fear of punishment but more importantly from the fear of losing the parent's love. This is how conscience is formed on the basis of the one real parental sanction. It is not difficult to see therefore how closely interwoven are the strands of love and conscience.

If certain questions and situations tend to produce an anxiety-laden response from the parents which the child identifies in the pitch of the voice, evasive tactics, inappropriate anger or laughter and so on, then curiosity is inevitably sharpened and there is a tendency to indulge in speculative fantasy. The anatomical differences in sex may be accepted readily, or become a source of confusion and anxiety, largely depending on family attitudes; the same is true of the facts of reproduction, birth and death. The manner in which such questions are answered is every bit as important as the answers themselves.

Between about 4 and 8 years there is often intense fear of anything which could possibly lead to bodily mutilation, or injury, and especially in boys anxiety about loss of limbs, fingers, or toes, or the penis itself (*castration anxiety*).

This underlies the occasional terror at any surgical procedure in the lower part of the body—not only when masturbation is countered by the threat 'to cut it off'. A related anxiety is the common fear of the hair being cut.

All such fears are commoner in boys than in girls, and have been attributed by Freud (1908) to the imagined retaliation of the father as a result of the boy's erotic stirrings towards his mother. This classical 'oedipus complex' is probably by no means a universal phenomenon though with the associated castration complex it does seem aetiologically important in hysterical conditions in both sexes.

Whether the sexual component is accepted or not there is no doubt about the intense attachment of most small girls to their fathers, small boys to their mothers and ensuing rivalry with the parent of their own sex. Herein lies the prototype of later 'triangular' situations. If the possessive child is tolerated and perhaps humoured, reconciliation is slowly achieved. Rejection or eroticised play on the parents' part, usually unconsciously determined, may lead later to neurotic and psychomatic problems.

Later Childhood—the Emergence of a Person

Mind in an abstraction. In describing its development it is therefore necessary to use abstract concepts. Among the most fundamental of these are the awareness of oneself, essentially of one's own body; a gradually acquired awareness of constancy, compounded of all sensory experience, within and without the body. The awareness of its parts, of their relative proportion is really a neuro-psychological concept, *the body image*. The somewhat analogous but more complex concept is that of the *ego*, the part of the mind which perceives, thinks, remembers, registers the outside world, and which is conceptualised as having a boundary which delineates 'the self' from the 'non-self'. It is useful to the neurologist to regard certain subjective phenomena of his patients as distortions of the body-image; some of the bizarre experiences of a schizophrenic are comprehensible to the psychiatrist as defects of the ego-boundary.

Ego development probably begins in a rudimentary fashion at or before birth and may be dependent upon the integrity of the central nervous system and especially an intact perceptual apparatus. Given this organic matrix, from the start we recognise as interdependent and interacting factors the built-in biological drives and the life experiences out of which personality is forged. The sense of *identity*, of being oneself a unique individual is central to any concept of a person, but we know little of how identity formation is achieved. The resolution of this process in adolescence when the course of personality development is finally set has been extensively studied by Erikson (1950).

However, long before a child goes to school one important facet of personality will ordinarily have arrived, namely a *sexual identity*, the feeling of being male or female. At the present time the medical psychological aspects of the subject are clouded in complexity for 'male–female' has now three possible meanings at least (i) the form of the genitalia and secondary sexual characteristics; (ii) the chromosome appearances; and (iii) the subjective feelings of the individual. With recent advances in the study of inter-sex it was confidently anticipated that personality studies would reveal a link between somatic and psychological sex. But the evidence so far though not final by any means strongly suggests that an individual feels male or female because of the attitudes of others from an early age rather than because of any particular hormonal effect. Though the aetiology of homosexuality remains doubtful, at least one carefully controlled study of males suggests a specific pathogenic family constellation, an assertive mother dominating a detached father whom she denigrates to her intensely loved son (Bieber *et al.*, 1962). Whatever the precise pathogenic influence many psychiatrists and psycho-analysts incriminate disturbed mother–son and father–daughter relationships.

While it is well known that transient homosexual attachments are common in adolescence and usually need cause little concern, it is often a surprise to parents when young children show marked preference for the toys and activities of the opposite sex. We are more tolerant of little girls who wish to be 'tomboys' than of little boys who show a sudden interest in prams and dolls, but neither tends to be a lasting predilection.

This aspect of the child's identification is greatly facilitated when both parents are uncomplicated in their sexual roles. In a one-parent family the child will usually seek out another relative or friend as a substitute.

This is but one of the many roles which grandparents may fill to the child's advantage. When we consider that a child psychiatric clinical study almost invariably involves three generations it is remarkable how little research has been focussed on the role of grandparents. It is a unique relationship with its frequent blend of affection and permissiveness. It affords to the child a sense of continuity, of 'roots' and of belonging.

Certain games are played with such frequency and enthusiasm by young children that they deserve a word of special mention. 'Playing at houses' which usually involves a wedding and offspring with many variations serves to foster identification with a parent of the same sex, to seek answers to questions about reproduction and to master fears of their own parents by acting the parts of the awesome fathers and mothers. Whenever a person or an animal is particularly feared the child tends to play this part in fantasy and to repeat this over and over again. Many a child has played at 'being the dentist', but never the patient—at least voluntarily. 'Playing at doctors' serves the same end as well as the exploration of sexual differences. This is also one of many ways in which the problem of death can begin to be tackled. Children are seldom morbid about this but intensely interested. Most questions—and at this stage they are endless—should be answered with as much of the truth as is appropriate to the child's age and comprehension.

By the time the child goes to school emotional maturation is seen in the gradually acquired toleration of frustration, increasing control of motility, ability to concentrate on tasks set by another, and an acceptance of limits. Given reasonable ability and compatibility of temperament between pupil and teacher information is acquired rapidly whereas awareness of inner instinctual drives has become negligible.

With the first stirrings of puberty the emotionally quiet period is at an end and both feelings and behaviour enter a phase of new turmoil.

FREDERICK H. STONE

References

AMBROSE, J. A. (1961). The development of the smiling response in early infancy. In *Determinants of Infant Behaviour*. Ed. B. M. Foss. London: Methuen.

BAKWIN, H. (1942). Emotional deprivation in infants. *J. Pediatrics*, **35**, 512.

BIEBER, I. *et al.* (1962). *Homosexuality*. Basic Books, New York, Ch. VI.

BOWLBY, J. (1952). Maternal care and mental health. *W.H.O., Monograph Series No. 2.* Geneva.

—— (1960). Grief and mourning in infancy. *Psycho-analytic Study of the Child*, **15**, 9. London: Hogarth.

BROWN, F. (1961). Depression and childhood bereavement. *J. Ment. Science*, **107**, 754.

BURLINGHAM, D. (1955). Simultaneous analysis of mother and child. *Psychoanalytic Study of the Child*, **10**, 165.

ERIKSON, E. H. (1958). The psychosocial development of children. In *Discussions in Child Development*, **3**, 169. Ed. Tanner and Inhelder. London: Tavistock.

—— (1950). *Childhood and Society*. New York: Norton.

EYSENCK, H. J. and RACHMAN, S. J. (1965). The application of learning theory to child psychiatry. In *Modern Perspectives in Child Psychiatry*. Ed. J. G. Howells, Edinburgh and London: Oliver and Boyd.

FOSS, B. M. (1961). (Ed.) *Determinants of Infant Behaviour I*; (1963). *Ibid, II*; (1965) *Ibid, III*. London: Methuen.

FREUD, A. (1963). The concept of developmental lines. In *Psycho-analytic Study of the Child*, **18**, 245.

FREUD, S. (1908). *On the Sexual Theories of Children*. Standard edn., Vol. IX. London: Hogarth.

GOLDFARB, W. (1943). Infant rearing and problem behaviour in adolescents. *Am. J. Orthopsychiat.*, **13**, 249.

GRANGE, K. M. (1963). Rousseau's Emile and its English background. *Acta Paedopsychiatrica*, **30**, 405.

GREGORY, I. (1958). Studies of parental deprivation in psychiatric subjects. *Am. J. Psychiat.*, **115**, 432.

HARLOW, H. F. (1962). Social deprivation in monkeys. *Scientific American*, **207**, 136.

HELLMAN, I. (1960). Simultaneous analysis of mother and child. *Psycho-analytic Study of the Child*, **15**, 359.

ISAACS, S. (1933). *Social Development in Young Children*. London: Routledge.

LEVY, D. M. (1943). *Maternal Overprotection*. New York: Columbia Univ. Press.

LORENZ, K. (1956). Comparative behaviourology. In *Discussions on Child Development*, 1, 108. Ed. Tanner and Inhelder. London: Tavistock.

MIDDLEMORE, M. P. (1941). *The Nursing Couple*. London: Castle.

SPITZ, R. A. (1945). Hospitalism: An inquiry into the origins of psychiatric conditions in early childhood. *Psycho-analytic Study of the Child*, 1, 53; 2, 313.

SCHAFFER, H. R. (1958). Objective observations of personality development in early infancy. *Br. J. Med. Psy.*, 31, 174.

TINBERGEN, M. (1951). *The Study of Instinct*. Oxford.

W.H.O. (1962). *Deprivation of Maternal Care*. Public Health Papers, 14. Geneva.

WINNICOT, D. W. (1958). Transitional objects and transitional phenomena. In *Collected Papers*. London: Tavistock.

WOODWARD, M. (1965). Piaget's theory. In *Modern Perspectives in Child Psychiatry*. Ed. J. G. Howells. Edinburgh and London: Oliver and Boyd.

11   Protection Against Specific Infections

DURING the past century there has been a steady and most remarkable decrease in deaths from infection, and children, particularly those under 5 years of age, have been the principal beneficiaries. Deaths among children (0 to 15 years) from the four main infectious diseases (scarlet fever, diphtheria, measles and whooping-cough) have fallen from rates ranging from 1,250 per million (measles) to 2,500 per million (scarlet fever) in the decade 1850–60 to negligible proportions in recent years. Nonetheless, infection is still the most important contributor to illness among children. For example, in the Thousand Families Study in Newcastle (Miller *et al.*, 1960), there were 8,467 significant incidents of illness among 847 children in their first 5 years of life (1947–52); of those, 6,845 (80 per cent) were infections and 1,622 (20 per cent) were non-infective conditions such as accidents, allergic rashes, surgical operations, squints or speech disorders. Of the infections, more than half were respiratory infections (cold, sore throats, febrile catarrh, bronchitis, etc.), rather more than one fifth were due to the specific fevers (measles, whooping-cough, chickenpox, mumps, etc.), and about one tenth were alimentary infections. Thus these three groups of infections were responsible for 87 per cent of all infective illnesses and 70 per cent of total illness. The only other groups numerically important were staphylococcal infections which contributed 5 per cent and pyrexias of unknown origin causing 3 per cent of the illnesses (see Table 11).

TABLE 11

Distribution of 6,845 Incidents of Infective Illness in 847 Children in Five Years Newcastle upon Tyne, 1947–52

Respiratory infections	3,755	Staphylococcal infections	341
Whooping-cough	392	Acute infections of unknown	
Measles	540	origin	221
Chicken-pox and zoster	240	Herpetic stomatitis	118
Rubella	134	Conjunctivitis	79
Mumps	113	Tuberculous infection	61
Alimentary infection	793	Infective hepatitis	24

The impact of these various infections on the physical and mental development of the young child may be considerable. Colds, catarrh and measles predispose to otitis media and bronchitis; chronic otitis media may cause partial deafness which in turn may retard learning at school; whooping-cough may lead to pneumonia and bronchiectasis and, some believe, to mental retardation; measles and mumps may be followed by encephalitis. The risks of infection are increased by poverty and overcrowding and the various social and environmental factors associated with them: for example, deaths from the pneumonias of early childhood still have a sharply rising social gradient from Class I to Class V, while acute respiratory infections and streptococcal sore throats are commonest in over-crowded communities. Improvements in the nutrition, housing and way of life of the economically poorer classes will continue to be a very important factor in reducing the amount and severity of infection in a community. More specific measures to protect susceptible children will be further discussed here. These measures consist, in the main, of attempts to give the child a specific resistance or immunity against infectious diseases like smallpox, diphtheria, poliomyelitis, whooping-cough, measles and tuberculosis. Little effort has as yet been made to provide protection against the great mass of acute respiratory infections but the steady progress now being made in the identification of respiratory viruses associated with such clinical syndromes as the common cold, croup, febrile catarrh, influenza and the non-bacterial pneumonias gives promise of future success. Again, no specific prophylaxis is available for the hotch-potch of alimentary infections although special control measures (*e.g.* chemoprophylaxis and chemotherapy) may be effective in particular circumstances as is also the case with the acute pyogenic infections.

Acquired Immunity

The term immunity is often used elastically to cover any biological mechanism that gives the body protection or resistance against infection. The physico-chemical barriers of healthy intact skin and mucous membranes with their associated secretions—the unsaturated fatty acids of the skin, the hydrochloric acid of the stomach, the lactic acid of the vagina, the lysozyme of tears and mucous secretions—give the body what is sometimes called natural immunity but which more properly is a non-specific resistance to infection. Similarly, the body's capacity to deal with invading pathogens in the early stages of infection—the phenomena of inflammation, localisation and phagocytosis—exemplifies a physiological and non-specific resistance that should not be equated with immunity. Immunity is an acquired resistance to infection, which develops during the course of a clinical or inapparent infection or can be induced artificially by the injection of ready-made immune substances (antibodies) or of an innocuous suspension of the pathogen or some metabolite or fraction of it (antigens). This immunity is specific for the particular pathogen causing the infection or used artificially as antigen; for instance, a child who has had measles is unlikely to have a second attack but is not thereby protected against whooping-cough.

Immunity may be acquired naturally or artificially; and both forms of immunity may be acquired either actively, that is the antibodies are produced by the host's tissues, or passively, that is the antibodies are supplied to the host ready made. An attack of measles gives immunity to further attacks and this is naturally-acquired active immunity. Most infants are immune to measles for the first 4 to 6 months of life, owing to the 'placental' transfer of antibodies from mother to fetus; this is an example of naturally-acquired passive immunity. Following the injection of an antitoxin, passive immunity is rapid in onset, immediate if the antiserum is given intravenously and requiring only a few hours to reach adequate levels if given intramuscularly or subcutaneously; but it has a short duration of only a few weeks, since the antibody, being a foreign protein, is quickly eliminated by the body. On the other hand, antibody transmitted from mother to fetus is eliminated from the infant much more slowly, *e.g.* diphtheria antitoxin has a half-life of approximately 30 days. In the older child and adult, however, the breakdown and disappearance of injected homologous antibody occurs at a faster rate.

The route by which antibody is transferred from mother to offspring depends on the animal species. In ruminants and pigs antibodies are concentrated in the colostrum and are ingested and absorbed from the gut when the calf or lamb gets its first milk by suckling or feeding. Absorption of undenatured antibody occurs only in the first 24 hours or so of life. With rodents and primates, it has usually been supposed that antibodies pass through the placenta from mother to fetus and the difference in the modes of transfer in ruminants and rodents has been attributed to the number of layers of tissue between maternal and fetal circulation— four or five in ruminants and pigs, one in rodents and primates. However, it has been shown that in certain animals with 'placental' transfer, *e.g.* rabbits and guinea-pigs, antibodies pass from the maternal circulation into the uterine lumen, whence they pass through the entodermal membrane of the yolk sac into the vitelline circulation. It is not known if this mode of transfer occurs in the human species but there is evidence of some selection and concentration of certain antibodies during transfer from mother to fetus. Thus, the titres of antitoxins and viral antibodies, *e.g.* diphtheria antitoxin, staphylococcal and streptococcal antihaemolysins and vaccinial antibodies, are often higher in cord blood than in maternal blood whereas some bacterial antibodies, iso-agglutinins and sensitising 'reagins' are present in much lower concentration in infant than in maternal blood. These variations are important in determining the passive immunity of the infant to different infections and explain why most of the specific childhood fevers rarely occur in infants under 4 to 6 months of age. Whooping-cough is an exception, not because antibody cannot be transferred but probably because there is little or no protective antibody to transfer. The level of antibody transferable from mother to offspring can be raised by antenatal immunisation of the mother and this procedure has been suggested for infections like tetanus and poliomyelitis.

In contrast to passive immunity, active immunity takes time to develop but persists for months or years and, once acquired, is capable of rapid restoration when it has dropped to a low level. There is evidence that the capacity to produce antibody in response to certain antigenic stimuli, *e.g.* pertussis vaccine, is less well developed in the first few months of life than it is in the older infant. However, with potent antigens, *e.g.* tetanus toxoid, infants under 3 months of age respond as well as the older child and poor responses to certain antigens may be due to the interfering effect of passively transferred antibodies, *e.g.* to diphtheria, polio-myelitis and measles.

The Rationale of Immunisation

Before discussing the application of immunisation to the control of communicable disease, it may be useful to summarise some of the basic principles in order to clarify what immunisation may realistically be expected to achieve in different types of communicable disease. The objective of immunisation is to produce, without harm to the recipient, a degree of resistance as great as, or greater than, that which follows a clinical attack of the natural infection. With this objective in mind, those communicable or infectious diseases amenable to control by vaccination may be considered in four main groups: toxic; acute bacterial; chronic bacterial; and viral infections. In the first group, *e.g.* diphtheria and tetanus, the brunt of the infection is due to a specific poison or toxin which can be purified artificially, rendered harmless by treatment with formalin (= toxoid) and used as a very effective antigen or prophylactic. The potency of toxoid antigens can be measured and standardised with great accuracy, and the amount of antitoxin that is produced in the inoculated person gives a reliable indication of the degree of resistance to infection in that individual.

Among the acute bacterial infections, humoral antibodies probably play the predominant role in the acquisition of immunity but there are obstacles, some almost insuperable, to an acquired immunity in certain infections. For example, in the acute pyogenic infections (staphylococcal, streptococcal, pneumococcal), there are many different serotypes within the species and infection with one type of strepto-coccus or pneumococcus does not protect the individual against attack by another type so that repeated attacks of streptococcal sore throat or pneumococcal pneu-monia may occur. Since there are 40 to 50 serotypes of *Streptococcus pyogenes* and some 70 pneumococcus types, it would be very difficult to prepare effective multivalent vaccines against infections with these pathogens. Among other acute bacterial infections *e.g.* whooping-cough and cholera, antigenic variation within the species is much more limited and it should therefore be possible to produce effective vaccines. Whole bacterial cells contain many different antigenic com-ponents, of which probably only one or two are particularly concerned with the virulence of the organism. It is important to try to identify and to preserve these so-called 'protective antigens' in vaccine preparations.

Another difficulty is that in infections like whooping-cough and cholera, the infection affects predominantly the epithelial surfaces so that antibodies produced as a result of vaccination may not gain easy access to the site where the pathogen is producing the infection. For this and other reasons it was essential to test vaccines against whooping-cough and cholera in properly controlled field trials, so that objective assessment of their value could be obtained.

So far the assumption has been implicit that the production of a specific protect-ing antibody is the main requirement for effective immunisation, although it should be noted that immunity may persist long after such antibodies cease to be demonstrable, as in whooping-cough. When the 'continued fevers' or chronic bacterial infections are considered (*e.g.* typhoid, brucellosis, tuberculosis), it must be concluded from knowledge of the clinical course of these infections that the identifiable specific antibodies play little part in overcoming the disease. Thus, antibodies to the specific antigens of the typhoid and brucella bacteria are demonstrable in the blood of the patient within a week of onset of the illness, but the fever may go on for many weeks before clinical recovery. In addition, relapses in these continued fevers are not uncommon despite the presence of high concentrations of specific antibodies. In contrast to the acute bacterial infections, the infecting organisms in chronic infections are for the most part intracellular parasites, and it seems likely that what is called cellular immunity may be more important in overcoming the infection than the presence of humoral antibodies. It may be noted that in tuberculosis and brucellosis a living attenuated vaccine is used to produce immunity.

In the viral infections it is known that humoral antibodies are important but, again, cellular immunity also seems to be important in some diseases; thus, children with hypo- and agammaglobulinaemia can recover from infections like measles, chickenpox and mumps with an apparently good immunity but without detectable circulating antibody, whereas they rapidly succumb to acute bacterial or toxic infections. Such children can be successfully vaccinated with smallpox vaccine and with BCG. These findings indicate that specific humoral antibodies are not essential for recovery from some virus diseases. On the other hand, immunity to certain virus infections seems to be equated with the presence of antibody; *e.g.* human gamma globulin can be used prophylactically to prevent or modify measles and infective hepatitis in those intimately exposed to the risk of infection; killed viral vaccines which stimulate the production of humoral antibody can give good protection against influenza and poliomyelitis.

Immune Response and Duration of Immunity

The newborn baby may contain in his blood antibodies to the agents of certain toxic, bacterial and viral infections according as the corresponding antibodies are present in the mother's blood. This passive immunity gives protection to the infant at a time when he is poorly equipped to produce specific antibodies, but it also interferes to a varying extent with the infant's capacity to respond to the stimulus of toxoids or vaccines in the early months of life. Killed poliomyelitis vaccines elicit poor or nil antibody responses when given to children under 6 months of age and live measles vaccine is ineffective if given before 9 to 12 months of age. However, the newborn infant can be given protection following inoculation of BCG and smallpox vaccines where humoral antibody is non-existent or unimportant.

When a good specific antibody response is being sought to a toxoid or killed antigen, the usual procedure is to give two or three doses of the antigen at intervals of several weeks. The first dose of antigen evokes a poor antibody response after a latent period of approximately two weeks, but after the second dose the amount of antibody produced is multiplied tenfold and after a third dose may be increased a hundredfold. The first or 'priming' dose of antigen will be more effective the larger it is, particularly if it is particulate or is released slowly from a mineral carrier; or if it is mixed with certain bacterial vaccines, *e.g.* tetanus toxoid plus typhoid vaccine, diphtheria toxoid plus pertussis vaccine. The second and subsequent doses are effective in much smaller amounts than the first, and without help of adjuvants. The response is much better if the two doses are spaced out at an interval of 6 to 8 weeks, and, provided the priming dose is adequate, the response to the second dose will still be maximal even if it is given some 6 months after the first. However, where there is reason to believe that a community has acquired a basic immunity from the widespread occurrence of clinical or inapparent infection, as in influenza, one dose of antigen will act as the secondary stimulus.

As regards the duration of immunity after the basic course, this can be measured precisely in the case of toxic infections according to the level of specific antitoxin in the blood or, less precisely, in diphtheria by the Schick test. Recent studies have shown that an adequate concentration of diphtheria antitoxin may persist in the blood of children for 3 to 4 years after primary immunisation in early infancy. After a primary course of three doses of tetanus toxoid, a satisfactory antitoxin titre may be present for 10 years or longer.

The duration of immunity after injections of killed bacterial vaccines may not be equated with the presence of demonstrable antibody; for example, after a course of three doses of pertussis vaccine given to children (average age one year) there was no change in the degree of protection in successive 6 months during a follow-up period of $2\frac{1}{2}$ years, although antibodies were no longer demonstrable in a considerable proportion of the children within a year after immunisation. Again, in typhoid fever there is no correlation between antibody titres and clinical protection, as has been shown by controlled trials of typhoid vaccines. In the viral infections, although antibody titres may serve as a measure of the degree of protection, there are certain anomalous findings: for example, high titres of neutralising antibody have occasionally been found in the early stages of fatal cases of smallpox.

The role of immunisation in communicable disease control is best assessed from the results of carefully-designed field trials with vaccines that have been submitted to satisfactory laboratory assays of potency. Thus, BCG, pertussis and typhoid vaccines have been used for half a century or more, but it was only after large-scale controlled trials of these prophylactics had been carried out that a reliable assessment of their value could be made. Similar field trials have been carried out for poliomyelitis, influenza and measles vaccines, so that public health programmes for the control of these and other infections can now be planned with a reasonable assurance that a degree of effectiveness will be obtained, particularly if the prophylactic agents can be shown to fulfil certain laboratory requirements. In the use of toxoids, for example diphtheria and tetanus toxoids, laboratory yardsticks of antigenic potency are available and mandatory under the Therapeutic Substances Act (TSA) regulations. With bacterial and viral vaccines, attempts are now being made to establish minimal requirements for protective efficacy on the basis of correlated field and laboratory studies. For example, a mouse-protection test for pertussis vaccines has been found to give reasonably good correlation with clinical protection. With smallpox vaccines, the most reliable method of testing potency is to do pock-counts on the inoculated chorio-allantoic membrane of the chick embryo, and this method is now recommended as the International Standard Test.

Immunisation Against Specific Infectious Diseases

The case for prophylactic immunisation of a child community against specific infectious diseases will depend on a number of factors; *e.g.* the prevalence and economic importance of the infection; the relative value of immunisation compared with other control measures; the safety, efficacy and practicability of the immunisation procedure; the control of non-endemic infections which may be introduced from another country, *e.g.* smallpox.

Infectious diseases against which immunising agents are presently available may be conveniently divided into two groups; (i) those in which there is no satisfactory method of control other than by vaccination, *e.g.* smallpox, diphtheria, whooping-cough, tetanus, poliomyelitis, influenza, measles, and (ii) those in which prophylactic vaccination would be useful along with other control measures, *e.g.* tuberculosis and typhoid.

Although prophylactic vaccination is the only reliable control measure in the first group, it is doubtful if in any particular country there is a case for large-scale immunisation against all of them. Each country should therefore prepare its priority list according to its own known needs. At the top of this list for most countries would be smallpox for a variety of reasons. Diphtheria should be high on the list since this preventable infection is still too prevalent in many countries. With diphtheria would be associated whooping-cough because of its high incidence and severity in infancy, and because the two prophylactic agents can be usefully combined. Active immunisation against tetanus is frequently combined with diphtheria and whooping-cough immunisation, in some countries because tetanus in childhood is still a sizeable hazard, in others because active immunisation has advantages over passive protection with antitoxin. Poliomyelitis would be high on the list in the more developed countries where clinical infections are common, but would not yet be required in many developing countries despite evidence of a high incidence of inapparent infection. The case for mass immunisation against measles is considered later. Immunisation against influenza has restricted applications, *e.g.* in school children among whom the first wave of infection during epidemics frequently occurs.

Tuberculosis might seem to be a preventable infection belonging to the first rather than the second group, but some countries, *e.g.* the United States of America, prefer to use other public health measures for its control, while in certain areas with a high incidence of low degree tuberculin sensitivity, the prophylactic value of BCG vaccination is still in doubt. Typhoid fever is a prevalent infection among children in many of the developing countries; *e.g.* in Ceylon with a population of

9 millions it is estimated that some 20,000 cases of typhoid occur annually. The long-term control of this infection depends on good standards of environmental sanitation and household hygiene. Vaccination could play a useful part as a short-term prophylactic measure.

The rationale and procedures for immunisation against some of the specific infectious diseases of childhood will now be briefly outlined.

Smallpox

Although smallpox has ceased to be an endemic infection in the United Kingdom, the risk of its importation has increased with modern swift travel facilities. Air passengers from endemic areas such as India and Africa may arrive in Britain in the incubation stage of the infection, which, if the individual has been previously vaccinated, may appear in a modified and not easily recognisable form. When, after the importation of a primary unrecognised case, a crop of secondary cases occurs, there is liable to be a stampede towards mass immunisation, including the vaccination of many persons for the first time. In these circumstances, the serious sequelae, *e.g.* post-vaccinal encephalitis, of primary vaccinations in schoolchildren and older persons may cause more sickness than the smallpox outbreak itself.

Mass campaigns for the eradication of smallpox in endemic areas are now being planned and executed, and already, in a number of Latin-American countries, these campaigns have been successful in getting rid of smallpox as an endemic infection. Until all endemic areas have been cleared up, however, the official policy in countries such as the United Kingdom must be to encourage primary vaccination and re-vaccination at as high a level as possible. The primary vaccination rate ranges from 40 to 50 per cent of children under 5 years in Britain or may be much higher following importations of smallpox as happened in 1962. Since the risk of complications is greater when primary vaccination is done in infancy than in the age period 1 to 4 years, it is now recommended that primary vaccination should be done in the second year of life, although it is often administratively more convenient to vaccinate infants between 3 and 6 months of age. The method of choice is the multiple pressure technique, as recommended in the Ministry of Health memorandum (1956) on vaccination.

The most suitable site for vaccination is the upper arm, although some doctors prefer to vaccinate girls on the inner aspect of the ankle or on the sole of the foot. Revaccination should be carried out at school entry and after that probably only when the subject is going abroad, particularly to an endemic area or to a country where a certificate of recent vaccination is compulsory.

Diphtheria

Although the spread of diphtheria, unlike smallpox, is associated to a considerable degree with symptomless carriers, it is possible that diphtheria could be eradicated by the maintenance of a high and persistent level of artificial immunisation. The close correlation between the initiation and widespread application of active immunisation and the steady fall of both morbidity and mortality rates, can leave no doubt about the effectiveness of this procedure. In the United Kingdom, many health authorities have not had a single notification of diphtheria for 5 years or more and if infection should occur in an immunised person, it is usually a local non-toxic pharyngitis with exudate or a carrier state. Contrasted with an annual average of 55,125 cases and 2,783 deaths in England and Wales for the decade immediately preceding large-scale immunisation, there was in the 5 years 1962–66, an average of 23 cases per annum with a total of 9 deaths. However, localised outbreaks of diphtheria do occasionally occur in schools or families and the family doctor with the help of the health authority must take prompt action on the recognition of a suspicious case. Advice about appropriate measures for the control of localised outbreaks has been given by Taylor, Tomlinson and Davies (1962).

The failure to control diphtheria in some countries is probably related most often to the failure to carry out the immunisation programme effectively, that is to give some 60 to 70 per cent of pre-school children the primary course of 3 doses at 6 to 8 weeks' intervals and to follow this with a booster dose about the time of school entry. An indication of the effectiveness of an immunisation campaign directed primarily at the pre-school and schoolchildren is the tendency for a shift of both cases and deaths to higher age-groups.

Whooping-cough

One of the most prevalent of the specific childhood fevers is whooping-cough; some 40 to 50 per cent of children are affected before their fifth birthday and 70 per cent by the age of 10 years. Death rates in the first year are 10 times greater than in the one to four-year-olds, and at least 100 times greater than in the five- to nine-year-olds. Although mortality rates in the United Kingdom have fallen precipitously in the past two decades, whooping-cough can still be a protracted debilitating infection in young children with both physical and mental complications such as bronchopneumonia, bronchiectasis and behaviour disorders.

The causative organism, *Bordetella pertussis*, has an antigenically homogeneous basic structure but recent studies have shown that there may be variation in the content of surface-agglutinating antigens and that these antigens in currently isolated strains of *Bord. pertussis* mostly differ from those in the strains used for the preparation of vaccines (Preston, 1965). Large scale controlled trials in the fifties showed that certain vaccines were highly protective for young children aged 6 months to 4 years (Report, 1959) and the subsequent mass use of the triple DPT vaccine was accompanied by a decline in notifications of whooping cough from 92,407 in 1956 to 19,427 in 1966. However, a recent survey organised by the Public Health Laboratory Service (Report, 1969) indicates that vaccines in present use in Britain do not give a high degree of protection. It is not known if this loss of protective efficiency is due to the variation in the surface antigens but this matter is being kept under review by the health authorities.

Because whooping-cough may occur, and is most severe, in early infancy, immunisation should begin at 3 to 4 months of age. Three doses of triple DPT vaccine are given at 6 to 8 week intervals or the last dose may be given 6 months after the second.

Where a good vaccine does not give complete protection, the attack is usually of a mild and modified nature but children with such atypical attacks may be a source of danger to younger unprotected siblings. Because of this risk and particularly when pertussis vaccination is not begun in the first 6 months of life, it may be advisable to give a booster dose to older siblings at school entry.

The prophylactic use of gamma globulin in home contacts has not been found to be an effective means of control (Morris and McDonald 1957).

Tetanus

Tetanus is a very rare disease in Britain, with not more than 140 to 150 cases per annum and on average 30 deaths per annum in the decade 1959–68. However, in developing countries, particularly those with large agricultural communities, tetanus following injuries of various kinds can be a serious problem and in many, neonatal tetanus is still an important cause of infant mortality. As examples of the size of the problem approximately 1,000 cases of tetanus are admitted annually to hospital in Ceylon, while pilot studies carried out in one part of rural India indicated that tetanus was one of the 10 major causes of morbidity and mortality in that area. Again, neonatal tetanus has been shown to occur in over one per cent of births following confinement at home in the Dakar area of Senegal and accounts for 20 to 80 per cent of the deaths from tetanus at all ages in a number of countries. In countries where tetanus is a public health menace, active immunisation begun in early childhood and maintained by booster doses on entering and leaving school, would seem the obvious answer. Tetanus toxoid is a potent and cheap antigen which can be used in combination with other prophylactics such as diphtheria toxoid and pertussis vaccine or with typhoid vaccine.

The problem of neonatal tetanus presents some practical difficulties. Immunisation of the pregnant woman so that the baby would be born with an adequate amount of antitoxin to protect it against neonatal infection might seem to be the obvious answer. There seems little doubt that if this could be done, the problem of neonatal tetanus could be solved. The practical difficulty is that most cases of neonatal tetanus occur following childbirth at home where there has been no antenatal supervision of the pregnant woman. It would obviously be difficult to arrange for these women to have active immunisation during pregnancy. An alternative solution, viz. the administration of tetanus antitoxin to the baby at birth, also presents practical difficulties and it seems that extension of maternity nursing care plus health education may be the eventual answer.

In more developed communities the usual prophylactic procedure against the risk of tetanus following injury has been to give a dose of tetanus antitoxin which will protect for a few weeks. The main objections to this method of control are: (a) the considerable cost of the antitoxin and the cases of serum sickness that still occur after its use; in addition, acute anaphylactic deaths may rarely follow injections of antitoxin; (b) the patient who has already had an injection of antitoxin and requires a second dose within a period of 1 to 2 years, may eliminate the second dose of antitoxin very quickly, so that it ceases to have any protective value. In addition, such patients are more likely to have anaphylactoid reactions; (c) a considerable proportion of the clinical cases of tetanus follow mild injury when the patient has not been seen by a doctor. In recent years, the prophylactic injection of tetanus antitoxin to injured persons attending hospital or doctors' surgeries has become less commonly practised. Instead, if the wound is recent and fairly superficial, it it thoroughly cleaned, the patient is given an injection of tetanus toxoid and a suitable antibiotic (penicillin or erythromycin) may be prescribed for a few days.

There is increasing support for active immunisation against tetanus on a national scale. Experience with this form of immunisation among troops on active service during the second world war demonstrated how effective it was as a prophylactic against tetanus when the incidence was reduced to less than 0·1 per 1,000 wounded. Any individual who has had a course of active immunisation and suffers injury requiring antitetanus treatment, is given a further booster dose of tetanus toxoid. Unfortunately it is often impossible to tell with an injured person whether he has had active immunisation against tetanus and therefore the hospital officer may feel obliged to give a dose of tetanus antitoxin, particularly if the wound is deep, extensive or septic. Some reliable and easily ascertainable method of recording immunisation is needed. The usual arrangement is for the individual to have a personal immunisation card on which his various vaccinations have been recorded but unfortunately these cards get lost or mislaid and are not available when they are most needed. Alternatively, the use of a metal or plastic disc (to be worn round the arm or neck), on which the immunisation history is recorded, has been recommended. It has even been suggested that a small tattoo mark inside the ankle or on the iliac crest could be applied when active immunisation is completed and would be readily noticed by any doctor examining an injured patient. Where a non-immunised individual has been given a dose of tetanus antitoxin following an injury, an effort should be made to give him active immunisation, since further doses of tetanus antitoxin are unlikely to give protection. A first dose of absorbed tetanus toxoid should be given at the same time as the antitoxin to be followed 6 weeks later by a second dose.

Poliomyelitis

The efficacy and safety of killed (Salk type) poliovirus vaccines have now been fully confirmed by large-scale use in many countries. However, a number of objections have been raised against killed vaccines. For example, the response after a course of 3 injections may not persist so that booster doses may be needed. Again infants with maternal antibody do not respond satisfactorily to the vaccine, and in older children the antibody response to the most important component (type 1 poliovirus) was relatively poor with the then current vaccines. From the time that the application of poliovirus vaccines became a practical possibility, several virologists have devoted their activities to the production of an attenuated live vaccine which could be administered orally, and this type of vaccine is now used in many countries.

The relative merits of live and killed poliovirus vaccines are discussed below.

ANTIBODY RESPONSE. The poor response to the type 1 virus in some polio killed vaccines can be overcome by trebling the concentration of the type 1 virus component or using a specially purified vaccine. On the other hand, studies of the antibody response to the live vaccine show that antibody will not be demonstrable if for any reason infection of the alimentary tract is not achieved, e.g. if too small a dose is given or if there is interference by other viruses.

EASE OF ADMINISTRATION. The 3 or 4 injections of killed poliovirus vaccines could be combined with other prophylactics, e.g. diphtheria-pertussis, and some encouraging results have already been reported from such a combined vaccine, provided it is not given too early in infancy. In order to obtain a satisfactory response the oral vaccine has to be given in 3 repeated doses of the trivalent vaccine; or monovalent vaccines, in the order types 1, 3 and 2, may be given in successive doses.

ALIMENTARY TRACT INFECTION. The killed vaccine does not prevent natural infection of the alimentary tract so that poliovirus may persist in a well-immunised community. However, immunisation with the killed vaccine curtails or prevents oropharyngeal infection and the mass use of potent killed vaccine in Sweden has been followed by a disappearance of the polio viruses.

COST. The living vaccine is much cheaper to produce although control of its safety and preservation of its potency may present practical difficulties.

SAFETY. Since the Cutter accident with imperfectly inactivated vaccine in 1955, laboratory standards for safety have been much more rigid and a close surveillance of the vaccinated population for cases of paralytic poliomyelitis following vaccination has produced no evidence of any such risk. With live vaccines the main danger is that the attenuated strain might, during growth in the gut and transmission to new hosts, revert to a more virulent form. There is evidence that some return to neurovirulence may occur after human parasitism but that this reversion is not progressive. A careful follow-up of large numbers of vaccinated children in the U.S.S.R., Czechoslovakia, the Americas and elsewhere gives good ground for believing that the live vaccine is remarkably safe, although in Canada and U.S.A. a few cases of clinical infection due to type 3 vaccine strain have been recorded.

EFFECTIVENESS. There is now a large body of evidence that a course of 3 doses of killed poliovirus vaccine gives a high degree of protection, probably over 90 per cent. The so-called failures of the vaccine in the United States of America and Canada in 1959 occurred in areas where the level of immunisation was inadequate (that is, in overcrowded low income areas, particularly in the negro quarters) and most cases occurred among unvaccinated children. Although there has been no properly controlled assessment of the protective value of live vaccine against paralytic polio there is ample evidence to show that it is effective.

In some areas, however, especially where sanitation and hygiene are poor and other enteroviruses widespread, interference by 'wild' viruses with the live vaccine virus may prevent infection and hence immunisation. This may prove a serious drawback to the use of live vaccine in tropical and subtropical regions where the enteroviruses are common. Vaccination in early infancy may overcome this difficulty although parasitisation of the alimentary tract of the neonate is less successful than in infants a few months old.

HERD IMMUNITY. An apparent advantage of the live vaccine is that it spreads within the community and so protects non-vaccinated as well as vaccinated members. But there is evidence that this spread may be quite limited, for example among close contacts in nurseries, and that only young children are likely to disseminate the virus among family contacts. Again, spread may be inhibited by previous infection of the gut with other enteroviruses. The trivalent oral polio vaccine used in Britain is best given at the same time as the injections of DPT vaccine and may be begun at 3 to 4 months of age, followed by two further doses at 6 to 8 week intervals, or the third dose may be given 4 to 6 months after the second (see schedule, table 12).

Measles

The virus of measles was first isolated in tissue culture from the blood and throat washings of patients in the early stages of infection by Enders and Peebles (1954). After repeated passage the virus was adapted to growth on chick embryo tissue with resultant attenuation in its virulence. Living vaccines prepared from this attenuated strain have given a high degree of protection against measles in field trials but the injection is followed by a febrile reaction, *e.g.* 39° to 40°C (102° to 104°F), in 20 to 30 per cent of the inoculated children. With more attenuated strains, *e.g.* the Schwarz vaccine, the incidence of febrile reactions may be reduced. The febrile reaction can be damped down by the injection of a small dose of gamma globulin at the time the vaccine is given but gamma globulin is expensive and the supply is limited so that this modification is not satisfactory for large scale use.

The large question facing the medical profession is whether or not to recommend the widespread use of measles vaccine. The family doctor and the paediatrician are perhaps not impressed with the need to protect healthy children against measles which nowadays is usually an uncomplicated childhood fever of a few days' duration. From the public health viewpoint, however, the problem looks different. An uncomplicated case of measles needs two or three visits from the doctor and there are upwards of a million cases in the epidemic wave every year. Again, the incidence of complications is not negligible. In a recent analysis of some 53,000 notified cases occurring in the Northern conurbations of England in 1962–63 (it was reckoned that about 80 per cent of the cases were notified), Miller (1964) found that 1 in 15 had rather serious complications of which the most common were bronchitis and pneumonia (38 per 1,000 of the affected children), acute otitis media (25 per 1,000) and neurological disturbance (4 per 1,000), including encephalitis at about 1 per 1,000. Thus, during a measles year there may be some 35,000 children with serious complications, of whom 6,000 to 8,000 will require hospital treatment. This gives measles a rather different complexion as a public health problem and provided the measles vaccine is *safe* and *effective*, there is probably a case for its large scale use, particularly in industrial urban areas, where infection tends to occur early and complications are more common (see Report, 1968).

In many developing countries where morbidity and mortality rates from measles are still very high, there is an urgent need for the widespread use of measles vaccine.

Gamma globulin may be used to prevent or modify an attack of measles in young children intimately exposed to the risk of infection. In children between 6 months and 2 years of age, or in those who are particularly susceptible to infection, it may be thought advisable to aim at complete protection but otherwise a dose of gamma globulin is given which will result in a mild, modified attack if the child does develop the infection.

Influenza

Epidemics of influenza due to virus A occur in Britain at two- to four-year intervals and outbreaks of virus B influenza in less frequent cycles. Incidence tends to be highest among children and in semi-closed communities, for example, boarding schools, secondary day schools, and institutions. These epidemic waves cause a sudden marked increase in sickness absenteeism in schools and industry and although uncomplicated influenza is not a serious infection, its high attack rate may cause considerable dislocation of education and upset the public economy. Obviously any specific prophylactic measure that might lessen this burden would be well worth while.

Since 1951, a committee of the Medical Research Council has organised a series of controlled trials of influenza virus vaccine. These trials have been carried out in industrial communities, universities, the armed services, schools and so forth. Initially the control groups were given a bacterial vaccine but in later trials different virus A and B vaccines have been used on comparable groups of volunteers. The overall results have shown a reduction in sickness absenteeism of approximately 40 per cent among those vaccinated against the prevalent virus infection compared with the control groups. These rather disappointing findings may be due to either (*a*) the failure of the vaccine to give adequate protection or (*b*) the possibility that the method of assessment may be incapable of measuring the true degree of protection against virus influenza.

A clinical diagnosis of 'influenza' is bound to include respiratory infections due to other viruses. However, outbreaks of febrile respiratory illnesses among semi-closed communities, *e.g.* boarding schools, are more likely to be homogeneous and if shown by laboratory investigations to be due to virus influenza, opportunities for a fairer assessment of the protective value of the vaccine may be obtained. A striking example comes from the experience in a sharp outbreak of authenticated virus A influenza in a large residential school where about half of the boys had been given prophylactic vaccine (Hawkins, Hatch and McDonald, 1956). Compared with an attack-rate of 20 per cent among the uninoculated boys, the incidence was only 2 per cent among boys who had been inoculated twice (14 months and 3 months respectively before the outbreak) and it varied from 8 to 12 per cent among boys given one injection either 3 months or 14 months before the outbreak. These findings suggest that 2 injections of an appropriate influenza virus vaccine at one year's interval will give children a high degree of protection against the infection.

In more recent trials with Asian influenza vaccine, the most encouraging results came from a group of public schools where the boys received one injection of the vaccine on reassembly after the summer vacation. Influenza struck a number of these schools at about the time the boys received their inoculations; the groups receiving the Asian virus vaccine developed a considerable degree of immunity about 8 days after their injections, when the attack-rate dropped abruptly to one-third of the incidence in the other two groups receiving respectively a polyvalent A (non-Asian) and a B virus (Report 1958). A technical advance which may result in better and more prolonged protection against influenza is the use of a water-in-mineral oil emulsion in which the vaccine is incorporated. With doses of this oil adjuvant vaccine equivalent to one-fifth of the ordinary saline vaccine, the antibody titres are considerably higher and persist at a high level for a year or more after a single injection. A polyvalent vaccine of this kind containing influenza A and B viruses and adenovirus types 4 and 7 gave a high degree of protection against febrile respiratory infections among troops in training (Meiklejohn, 1962). Russian workers have used live modified virus vaccine instilled into the nostrils with apparent success during epidemics.

Tuberculosis

Despite epidemiological evidence, particularly from Scandinavian countries, of the protective effect of BCG vaccination, there were until recently very few well-controlled trials from which a critical assessment of the vaccine could be made. Now, controlled field trials in different age-groups and communities, e.g. in the United States of America, the United Kingdom and Algeria, have shown that BCG and vole bacillus vaccines can give a high degree of protection (around 80 per cent) to vaccinated infants and adolescents, and that this protection may persist for 10 years or more after vaccination. The protective effect of BCG vaccine in the adolescent, as demonstrated by the British trial (Report, 1963), has been corroborated in controlled trials for infants (Rosenthal, 1955, 1956; Sergent, Catanei and Ducros-Rougebief, 1956), for American Indian subjects in the age-range from infancy to 20 years (Aronson, Aronson and Taylor, 1958), and for schoolchildren (Hyge, 1947, 1956). In contrast, the reports of two large trials under the United States Public Health Service in Puerto Rico and in Georgia and Alabama, in which children and young adults were the volunteer communities, indicated that the benefit to the inoculated groups was only in the neighbourhood of 14 to 31 per cent. This low rate of protection may be related to the occurrence of the phenomenon of low-grade tuberculin sensitivity, associated with infection by mycobacteria other than the tubercle bacillus, which may confer a certain degree of specific antituberculous immunity (Palmer, Shaw and Comstock, 1958: Palmer and Long, 1967). Probably the low potency of the BCG vaccines used in these American trials was also a contributory factor (Hart, 1967).

Among children in the U.K. study who gave strong positive reactions to 3 tuberculin units (TU) on first testing, there was an annual incidence of tuberculosis of 3·5 per 1,000 in the first $2\frac{1}{2}$ years, and 1·67 in the second $2\frac{1}{2}$ years. In contrast, the annual incidence among those with weaker positive reactions to 3 TU or positive only to 100 TU was respectively 0·77 and 0·73 per 1,000 in the first $2\frac{1}{2}$ years and remained at these levels. This interesting finding should act as a warning to medical staff who are engaged in active immunisation of school-leavers to follow up carefully for the first few years any children giving a strongly positive tuberculin reaction. In addition, the age at which BCG vaccination is to be recommended for the schoolchild might be advanced from the present recommended age of 13 years to about 10 to 11 years in the hope that earlier vaccination would protect some of those who become infected at the time of puberty and are likely to develop clinical tuberculosis.

Besides the recommendation that schoolchildren in the United Kingdom should be offered BCG vaccination if they are tuberculin-negative, other groups at special risk, such as babies born into a tuberculous family, should of course be offered this protection.

Combined Antigens

Practically all substances used as prophylactics, whether they be whole bacterial or viral vaccines or bacterial toxoids, contain more than one antigen. The host's tissues respond to these multiple antigens by the production of specific antibodies to each, and seem to have the capacity to respond to a considerable number of separate antigens given simultaneously, provided each antigen is present in adequate amount.

It is important when using combined antigens to see that they are well balanced so that a powerful antigen does not mask the effect of a weaker. For example, tetanus toxoid is a more efficient antigen than is diphtheria toxoid and the usual mixture is 5 flocculation equivalents of tetanus toxoid to 25 flocculation equivalents of diphtheria toxoid. Again, the type 1 polio virus is a poorer antigen than types 2 and 3, and the present tendency is to double or treble the amount of type 1 virus in the killed or live polyvalent vaccines in order to obtain a better type 1 antibody response. A point that may have some practical importance is that if combined antigens, for example, diphtheria and tetanus toxoids, are given to a child who has been immunised already against *one* component of the mixture, say diphtheria toxoid, the booster effect of the latter may be so marked as to interfere with the primary response to the other antigen (Barr and Llewellyn-Jones, 1953).

The advantages of using combined antigens compared with single antigens, for instance, pertussis vaccine plus diphtheria and tetanus toxoids (DPT), are:

(*a*) the reduction in the number of injections; (*b*) the adjuvant effect of the bacterial component on the toxoid; and (*c*) the fact that immunisation against diphtheria and tetanus, which are rare hazards, is acceptable by the public if combined with immunisations against a prevalent or dreaded infection such as whooping-cough or poliomyelitis. Disadvantages are that (*a*) the optimum age for immunisation against whooping-cough is early in infancy and for diphtheria and tetanus rather later; (*b*) if babies are given a course of immunisation of this triple vaccine in the first 6 months of life, a booster dose may be needed a year or two later and this may be administratively difficult; (*c*) if one component of the mixture, say the pertussis vaccine, is a poor antigen, its inadequate protective effect may adversely affect the acceptability of the combined vaccine; (*d*) there is a slightly greater risk of provocation poliomyelitis with combined bacterial-toxoid vaccines than with single antigens. The killed polio-virus vaccine may be added to the other three components but the interfering effect of passively-transferred antibody to polio vaccine in infants under 6 months is a contra-indication to this quadruple vaccine and the present policy in the United Kingdom is not to recommend it for primary immunisation in infancy.

Immunisation Programmes

The aim of immunisation programmes is the control of infection in the community rather than individual protection. A lower level of herd immunity than is necessary for solid individual protection can effectively control the incidence of communicable diseases if a high proportion of the susceptible community is immunised. An exception is tetanus since each individual at risk must be protected actively or passively.

In some areas most of the immunisation work is done at child health clinics and in others a large proportion of it is done by the family doctor or paediatric specialist. Though there are obvious advantages in having the immunisations carried out by the family doctor (and statistics indicate that the proportion of immunisations done by practitioners is steadily increasing), it is essential that there should be a well-organised system for ensuring that the child receives his injections at the appropriate age and time intervals and that there is an efficient system of recording the immunisations. An immunisation campaign carried out without provision for its continuation as a routine procedure will not give satisfactory results.

Limited public health facilities and finance, shortage of trained staff and difficulties in enlisting the co-operation of the community, make it necessary to devise different immunisation programmes for countries in varying stages of economic development. The general aim must be to immunise regularly and economically, with the minimum number of visits and injections, a sufficiently high proportion of the susceptible population.

Knowledge about the duration of immunity following the primary course of immunisation and after booster injection is not yet sufficiently precise in a number of communicable diseases, so that the number and timetable of booster doses must be left rather elastic. The need to use safe and efficient (and if possible standardisable) prophylactics cannot be over-emphasised since the continuance of immunisation programmes with the co-operation and confidence of the public depends on the successful results of these procedures.

TABLE 12

Schedule of Immunisation Procedures in Countries with Adequate Health Services

Age	Prophylactic	Interval	Notes
During the first year of life	DPT and oral polio vaccine. (First dose)		The earliest age at which the first dose should be given is 3 months.
	DPT and oral polio vaccine. (Second dose)	Preferably after an interval of 6 to 8 weeks.	
	DPT and oral polio vaccine. (Third dose)	Preferably after an interval of 4–6 months.	
During the second year of life	Measles vaccination	After an interval of not less than 3 to 4 weeks (see Note 4)	While the second year is recommended for vaccination against smallpox, if special circumstances call for it, vaccination may be carried out during the first year.
	Smallpox vaccination	After an interval of not less than 3 to 4 weeks (see Note 4)	
At 5 years of age or school entry	DT and oral polio vaccine		With the exception of smallpox revaccination these may be given, if desired, at 3 years of age to children entering nursery schools, attending day nurseries or living in children's homes.
	Smallpox revaccination		
Between 10 and 13 years of age.	B.C.G. vaccine		For tuberculin-negative children.

Additional Notes

1. The basic course of immunisation against diphtheria, pertussis, tetanus and poliomyelitis should be completed at as early an age as possible consistent with the likelihood of a good immunological response. Live measles vaccine should not be given to children below the age of 9 months, since it usually fails to immunise such children owing to the presence of maternally transmitted antibodies. Primary vaccination against smallpox should normally be deferred until the second year of life after vaccination against measles.

2. Examples of timing doses of basic course of immunisation:

	1st dose	2nd dose	3rd dose
Age	3 months	5 months	9–12 months
	4 months	6 months	10–12 months
	5 months	7 months	about 12 months
	6 months	8 months	about 12 months
	Interval	Interval	
	6–8 weeks	Preferably 6, and not less than 4, months	

3. In view of the possibility of accidental infection of eczematous members of the family of a child vaccinated against smallpox it would be preferable for all routine smallpox vaccinations to be carried out by or with the knowledge of the family doctor.

4. An interval of 3 to 4 weeks should normally be allowed to elapse between the administration of any two live vaccines or between the administration of DPT vaccine and a live vaccine, other than oral poliomyelitis vaccine, whichever is given first.

TABLE 13

Schedule of Immunisation in Countries with Inadequate Health Services

Age	Prophylactic
0–1 month	BCG and Smallpox vaccination (see Note 1)
3–5 months	DPT vaccine (alum adsorbed) Oral polio vaccine (see Note 2) Smallpox vaccination if omitted at 0–1 month
4–6 months	DPT and oral polio vaccine BCG vaccination if omitted at 0–1 month
1–2 years	DPT and oral polio vaccine Measles vaccine (see Note 3)
5–6 years (school entry)	BCG and smallpox revaccination DT + typhoid vaccine (see Note 4)
11–12 years	Smallpox revaccination Tetanus and typhoid vaccine

Notes: This schedule aims to give protective immunisation in the minimum number of visits.

1. BCG and smallpox vaccination should be done in the neonatal period if the baby is born in an institution.

2. Oral polio vaccine should be given if there is evidence of cases of paralytic poliomyelitis among young children.

3. Measles vaccine may be given in countries where the infection and its complications cause high morbidity and mortality: but it is expensive.

4. If typhoid fever is endemic in the area, one dose may act as a booster at school entry.

A schedule of an immunisation programme for countries with well-developed health services, modified from the schedule in the memorandum *Immunisation against Infectious Diseases*, Dept. of Health and Social Security, November 1968, is set out in Table 12. A simpler schedule for developing countries is set out in Table 13. 　　　　　　　　　　　　　　　　　　　　　　　　　R. CRUICKSHANK

References

ARONSON, J. D., ARONSON, C. F. and TAYLOR, H. C. (1958). A twenty-year appraisal of BCG vaccination in the control of tuberculosis. *Arch. intern. med.*, **101**, 881.

BARR, M. and LLEWELLYN-JONES, M. (1953). Some factors influencing the responses of animals to immunisation with combined prophylactics. *Br. J. exp. Path.*, **34**, 12.

ENDERS, J. F. and PEEBLES, T. C. (1954). Propagation in tissue cultures of cytopathogenic agents from patients with measles. *Proc. Soc. Exp. Biol. N.Y.*, **86**, 277.

HART, P. D. (1967). Efficacy and applicability of mass BCG vaccination in tuberculosis. *Br. med. J.*, **1**, 587.

HAWKINS, G. F. C., HATCH, L. and McDONALD, J. C. (1956). Influenza vaccination in a residential boys' school: Report to the Medical Research Council Committee on Clinical Trials of Influenza Vaccine. *Br. med. J.*, **2**, 1,200.

HYGE, T. V. (1947). Epidemic of tuberculosis in state school with observation period of about 3 years. *Acta tuberc. scand.*, **21**, 1.

—— (1956). The efficacy of BCG vaccination: epidemic of tuberculosis in a state school, with an observation period of 12 years. *Ibid.*, **32**, 89.

MEIKLEJOHN, G. (1962). Adjuvant influenza adenovirus vaccine. *J. Am. med. Ass.*, **179**, 594.

MILLER, D. L. (1964). Frequency of complications of measles, 1963. *Br. med. J.*, **2**, 75.

MILLER, F. J. W., COURT, S. D. M., WALTON, W. S. and KNOX, E. G. (1960). *Growing up in Newcastle upon Tyne.* London: Oxford Univ. Press.

MORRIS, D. and McDONALD, J. C. (1957). Failure of hyperimmune gamma globulin to prevent whooping-cough. *Arch. Dis. Childh.*, **32**, 236.

PALMER, C. E. and LONG, M. W. (1967). Effects of infection with atypical mycobacteria in BCG vaccination and tuberculosis. *Amer. Rev. Resp. Dis.*, **94**, 553.

—— SHAW, L. B. and COMSTOCK, G. W. (1958). Community trials of BCG vaccination. *Amer. Rev. Tuberc.*, **77**, 877.

PRESTON, N. W. (1965). Effective pertussis vaccines. *Br. med. J.*, **2**, 11.

Report (1958) Trials of an Asian influenza vaccine. *Br. med. J.*, **1**, 415.

—— (1959) Vaccination against whooping-cough. *Ibid.*, **1**, 994.

—— (1963) BCG and vole bacillus vaccines in the prevention of tuberculosis in adolescence and early adult life. *Ibid*, **1**, 973.

—— (1968) Vaccination against measles. *Ibid*, **1**, 449.

—— (1969) Efficacy of whooping-cough vaccines used in the United Kingdom before 1968. *Ibid.*, **4**, 329.

ROSENTHAL, S. R. (1955). Standardisation and efficacy of BCG vaccination against tuberculosis. *J. Amer. med. Ass.*, **157**, 801.

—— (1956). The role of BCG vaccination in the prevention of tuberculosis in infancy and childhood. *Amer. Rev. Tuberc.*, **74**, 313.

SERGENT, E., CATANEI, A. and DUCROS-ROUGEBIEF, H. (1956) Deuxieme note d'une campagne de premunition anti-tuberculeuse par le BCG poursuivie a Alger depuis 1935. *Bull Acad. nat. Med.*, **140**, 562.

TAYLOR, I., TOMLINSON, A. J. H. and DAVIES, J. R. (1962). Diphtheria control in the 1960's. *Roy. Soc. Hlth. J.*, **82**, 158.

General Reference

Immunisation against infectious diseases (1969). Ed. D. G. Evans. *Brit. med. Bull.*, **25**, No. 2.

Part II

CHILD CARE & SOCIAL PAEDIATRICS

12 Children in Society

THE attitude of society to children is determined by many influences, such as its general level of cultural development, its socio-economic condition, its past history and the effects of external pressures, its assessment of the future and the life expectancy of its infants and children. The transformation from childhood to adult life entails such far-reaching changes in outlook that it is difficult for the grown man to recall his early impressions of the world around him and his own childish reactions to adults. Thus, although many older children make resolutions in the light of their own experiences about their future attitudes to children, their deepest convictions are changed or lost in the transition to the wider world of the adult. Many people in later life have grown so far from childhood that they neither understand nor like children: moreover, if childhood was an unhappy time for them, they may translate their own past miseries into a positive antipathy to the young and all that youth stands for. Anyone who has attempted to provide better conditions for children recognizes this hostility to the young on the part of some adults, which may have an important influence on the attitude of society in general.

Children and Their Needs

THE QUALITIES OF CHILDHOOD. The general attributes of children are familiar to us all—their adventurous minds and insatiable appetites for knowledge; their lively imagination, loyalty and capacity for affection; their imitativeness and response to leadership; and their capricious activity and energy. We also recognize that children are torn by strong emotions which they find difficult to subdue, so that rage, cruelty and jealousy explode suddenly and unpredictably. These are qualities which all children share to some degree and yet every child is unique, differing in intelligence, personality and physical capacity from his fellows. This individual variation is greater between children than between adults, for they have not yet been moulded to conform with the pattern dictated by the society in which they live.

There is another characteristic of children which is of fundamental importance— they are continuously changing. Everything that happens to a child is incorporated into him as part of his total experience and helps to shape the future adult. In early life apparently trivial incidents may have far-reaching consequences whereas such stimuli have less and less effect as the individual matures, until with full manhood his personality is relatively little influenced by external events.

BASIC REQUIREMENTS. Human society is shaped by adults and its form is dictated largely by the needs and desires of men and women. It is often not recognised that children are also members of the same community and that they too have needs and responsibilities, albeit different from those of their elders. The change which has taken place in recent years in the general attitude to the child is the acknowledgement that his needs are rights which should not be withheld from him.

Six basic requirements of the young child can be identified and failure to satisfy any one of them will prejudice his normal growth and development. First, he needs adequate nutrition and the importance of this has been discussed in Chapter 5. Second, he needs protection, both from environmental hazards and from the consequences of his own inexperience and immaturity. These two requirements are essential to survival. Every child has innate drives to provide for his own nutrition and protection but in early childhood they are not sufficiently directed nor are the child's abilities developed enough to ensure his preservation.

The third need is for education, which increases in importance as society becomes more demanding and as simple ways of earning a living become fewer. Moreover, education is necessary if the individuals is to contribute to and benefit from his cultural heritage. Fourth, the child needs affection if he is to mature emotionally into a well-adjusted adult. The consequences of deprivation of affection are considered in Chapter 10. Fifth, contacts with other children are necessary from the age of 3 or 4 years, to satisfy the instinctive demand for companionship and to allow the child to learn standards of behaviour and tolerance for others. This need is normally easily satisfied but the increasing isolation of the modern family and its small size militate against free and easy social contact, while the growing number of multi-storey flats in our cities is adding to the difficulty. The latter development also restricts the opportunities for play—the last of the six basic requirements of children.

RECREATION AND PREPARATION. Childhood is commonly considered as a time of preparation for adult life. During this period of rapid growth, the mind is at its most receptive, the developing personality can be moulded to the requirements and restrictions of society and activity can be directed towards acquiring the skills needed to earn a living. It is important to realise, however, that childhood is not only preparatory but also a period of time to be enjoyed for itself. Nearly one quarter of the life-span is spent as a child and these years should be lived as fully as any later period—indeed, for many people they will be the happiest part of their lives, though they cannot know this at the time.

In simple societies, when life expectancy is short, the years of growth constitute an even larger proportion of the total life and perhaps it is because of this that children are made to contribute from an early age. In such circumstances, childhood as a period of distinctive activity is shortened almost to extinction and play as we know it hardly exists. In more complex communities, the pendulum has often swung in the opposite direction, with children having no contributory duties but devoting their waking hours to preparation for adult responsibilities, and again little or no time is 'wasted' in play. This pattern was seen in its most extreme form in middle-class nineteenth century Europe, when children worked long hours at school lessons and were the constant targets of admonition and precept designed to force them into the rigid mould of social behaviour expected of adults in that era. It is salutory to remember that in the poorer strata of the same society, childhood was being corrupted by the horrors of rapid industrialisation, with its child labour amounting to slavery, its high resultant child mortality and what Hugo called 'the dwarfing of childhood by physical and spiritual night'.

Today we, in contrast to our predecessors, consider childhood as a time to be lived and enjoyed for its own sake as well as a time of preparation for the future. Though some restrictions must necessarily be imposed in the interests of education and the controlled acquisition of experience, the activities of childhood should not be subordinated entirely to the needs of training. Adequate time must be given for play and other pursuits which have no obvious long-term objective. Such activities contribute to experience and so help to shape the developing mind and body but this should not be considered their primary purpose, since they are an integral part of childhood to be valued as such.

The Attitude of Society to Children

In considering the attitude of adult society towards children, we must distinguish between the feelings of adults for their own children, the way in which they regard other children within their own tribe or group and their attitude to children in general. The ways in which adults think and talk about children may also differ widely from the way they treat them in practice.

The esteem in which young children are held is conditioned to a considerable extent by their prospects of survival to an age when they can make an economic contribution to the common weal. When the main concern of a community is survival or the maintenance of a tolerable standard of living, each infant is an additional burden which may tip the scales adversely and which can only be sustained because of the promise of future economic benefit from the child's work. Thus in agrarian or poor industrial societies, where production is simple and does not require long educational or training processes, children are expected to contribute almost as soon as they can walk, by fetching and carrying, by caring for younger children and later by sharing in manual work. As societies become more complex and work becomes more skilled, the need for education increases and the child's participation is consequently postponed: at the same time, however, improving economic conditions make his assistance less urgently necessary.

Throughout the ages, the probability of any particular infant surviving to contribute significantly to the common effort has been low because of the high infant and child mortality, and this is still true of many communities in the world today. In such circumstances, far more babies must be produced than will survive, and it cannot be expected that parents will form deep attachments to their young or that they will entertain more than instinctive protective feelings towards them. In some aboriginal societies, adults may appear to be affectionate because they seldom if ever punish or maltreat their children, but this permissive tolerance is due to the low status accorded to children rather than to any real consideration for them. Thus men who would never lift a hand to a child to punish him for wrong-doing, may practise infanticide or ritual cruelties with utter indifference. Even in societies where the struggle for survival is not so severe and economic considerations therefore not all-important, the likelihood that the infant will not survive to adult life limits the extent to which parents can allow themselves to become emotionally involved with an individual child. It is only when improving standards of living and better methods of child care result in low mortality rates in infancy and childhood that deep bonds of affection can develop between adults and their young children. Moreover, in societies where the nuclear family is a separate socio-economic entity, the parents are totally responsible for their own children, and in such a single productive unit there can be intense interaction between the individual members. In simple agrarian societies, with a much wider family net-work, responsibilities, interactions and hence ties are diffused and the individual is less important. It is probable therefore that the modern concept of parental love is of comparatively recent origin and that throughout most of history interest in and affection for infants and young children has been at a much more superficial level.

Proof of this is difficult to obtain and indeed the very absence of documentary evidence testifies to the general lack of interest in young children in the past. We can gain some insight from the scanty references in diaries and autobiographies of well-known people. Thus, for example, John Evelyn, the seventeenth century diarist, casually mentions the deaths of his infant sons in a few brief lines between descriptions of life in Restoration England, and only the death of an older son seems to evoke any real grief. All Evelyn's sons predeceased him and this was a common enough experience in Britain in past centuries; not even royalty was immune, for Queen Anne bore many children and buried them all. If the great and wealthy could lose their children so frequently and at such an early age, how much more must ordinary people have been afflicted without leaving any permanent record of their losses. Adam Smith in his book *The Wealth of Nations* states that, in the highlands of Scotland in the eighteenth century, it was not uncommon for a woman who had borne 20 children not to have 2 alive and that in some places half of all the children died before they were 4 years old. With losses such as these, which were commonplace in years gone by, children were likely to be brought up with great austerity. Physical chastisement by beating or whipping was often severe and intended to eradicate innate wickedness as much as to punish for misdemeanours. Young children were accorded a very lowly status in the household, especially the girls who were more likely to be a persisting burden on the family's resources.

If parents were thus unable to develop deep feelings of affection towards their offspring, they would be unlikely to entertain such sentiments towards the children of their neighbours. Indeed, whereas it is instinctive for parents to show solicitude for their own young, there is little natural impulse to nurture or protect other children. Sacrifice of the individual for the sake of the tribe is a deeply ingrained principle of survival and the infant, being the weakest member, is the obvious victim, though the very old are almost equally vulnerable. Among primitive peoples, therefore, and even among more civilised communities such as ancient Sparta and Rome, excessive production of unwanted children, especially females, was controlled by their systematic destruction at birth. This widespread practice of deliberate infanticide served the purposes of restricting the population to that which could be supported by available resources and of maintaining a eugenically sound stock. Nevertheless, it inevitably led to abuse and inequity and came to be associated with many other inhumanities, such as ritual sacrifice and mutilation. Other civilisations, such as ancient Greece and Egypt, while permitting limited infanticide, generally treated their children more mercifully, perhaps because of the greater influence of women in these societies.

Communities which cherish their own children, even if only as part of their economic wealth, may yet be completely indifferent to children from alien groups. The compassion for children in general which is professed in modern western countries owes much to Christianity which is the only one of the great world religions which recognises the rights and needs of children and denounces infanticide. Nevertheless, the practice of Christianity has often not matched its ethic, and at some periods of history children have been cruelly maltreated in the name of Christianity. That compassion for child life is not a basic human instinct becomes apparent in time of war or famine, when lack of consideration for the young often results in their death on a large scale and children may be treated with the utmost savagery. Ideas of sparing children or putting their interests first when danger or great calamity threatens are really quite recent and are seldom implemented in practice, as accounts of past wars show. Examples of what may happen to children in wartime can be found in Froissart's chronicles of European wars in the fourteenth century, in histories of the English wars in Ireland or the extermination of the North American Indians and in recent accounts of war in Africa and Vietnam.

In western society today, it is customary to believe that such pitiless cruelties are things of the past or only occur among barbarous peoples and that modern man is humane and gentle in dealing with children, both his own and those of others. In an abstract way this may be true and there has probably never been such philanthropic interest in children and their needs as is evident in our present society. The increasing awareness of the extent of child abuse and neglect in the United States, Britain, Australia and other affluent countries has therefore come as something of a shock to many people, suggesting as it does that one of our most highly cherished notions about ourselves may be illusory.

Attitudes to Minority Groups of Children

In the struggle for existence, there is little place for the misfit and those who do not fill an accepted role are liable to be eliminated or at best disenfranchised. This has been customary practice throughout history and the concept of equal opportunity and provision for all individuals is relatively new. If the lot of children has generally been a hard one, the fate of the minority who stand apart from the herd by reason of abnormality of form, behaviour or social circumstance has usually been infinitely harsher.

TWINS. In many societies, the attitude to twins differs from that to ordinary children. Often one or both infants are killed at birth, in the belief that they are unnatural or will bring ill fortune. Sometimes this rejection extends to the mother herself, who may be ill-treated, or even to both parents. Thus, for example, some North American Indian tribes imposed restrictions in the form of taboos on the parents of twins. In other societies, twins are believed to possess supernatural powers and are feared or held in awe. They may be thought to be endowed with magical influence over the weather and may be given privileges not granted to single children. Usually the first twin is most highly esteemed but in West Africa the second twin is considered the senior, on the grounds that the first infant has gone ahead to open the way for the second, who must therefore be the more important. The exposure or drowning of the weaker twin, as practised in ancient times, had a certain logic, since it afforded a better chance of survival to the more vigorous infant.

ILLEGITIMATE AND ABANDONED CHILDREN. The fate of the illegitimate child depends to a considerable extent on the view taken of marriage and the organisation of the family or kinship. In most cultures the infant resulting from a casual union is at a disadvantage and is harshly treated, or at least deprived of privileges. Any society which practices extensive infanticide for eugenic or economic reasons is unlikely to be charitably disposed towards infants born out of wedlock. In most western countries, unwanted illegitimate infants have been quietly disposed of for centuries by smothering, drowning or exposure, despite sporadic efforts to stamp out these practices. In the middle ages, a predominantly peasant society was tolerant of such children as survived and they were usually accepted and provided for by the community or brought up in religious houses by monks or nuns. However, as feudalism, and with it the monasteries, declined, destitute children became an increasing economic liability and their treatment grew correspondingly more severe. With the growth of towns and cities, illegitimacy increased: in fifteenth century Scotland, for example, more than one quarter of all children were born out of wedlock and in some towns the rate reached 40 per cent or more. This growing burden, which affected all European countries and all social strata, stimulated strong measures against immorality, often initiated by the Church. Unmarried mothers were forced to do public penance and often punished by flogging or imprisonment. Care was denied to their children because such help was considered to encourage depravity. Nevertheless, despite censure and punitive measures, illegitimate births continued to occur and, in the eighteenth century, workhouses and foundling hospitals were started in many countries to accommodate the mothers and their children. The death rate among infants in these institutions was appallingly high but, since this went some way towards solving the problem, the public conscience was unmoved until well into the nineteenth century.

Unwanted children who survived infancy were likely to be bound as apprentices to masters who had complete disciplinary powers and often abused them brutally. Children were sent up chimneys to brush away the soot and often sustained fatal injuries or burns. Others slaved in collieries and factories for 12 or more hours daily. Many were sold overseas to work in plantations. It may seem strange that countries professing Christian standards should treat children with such callousness but disapproval of the sins of their mothers was stronger than charitable feelings towards the children, who were often considered to be naturally wicked because of their origin. It is only in recent times that people have ceased to condemn the child of an unlawful union and moral disapproval still colours the judgement of some. The development of suitable provision for the illegitimate child and his mother is described in Chapter 17.

MALFORMED CHILDREN. In the animal kingdom, the malformed individual is at such a biological disadvantage that he succumbs quickly and the human child is liable to suffer the same fate unless steps are taken to ensure his survival. In primitive cultures, nearly all abnormal infants die, while the few who live are generally accepted and accorded the lowest status in the community. More sophisticated societies, aware of the eugenic and economic implications of allowing such children to grow up, are likely to dispose of them by exposure after birth or other means. In early Scotland, according to Boece, infants with inherited disorders ran the risk of being buried alive, sometimes with their mothers as well.

The general attitude to the seriously malformed survivor, which persists to this day, may be summed up as one of revulsion or pity while he is a child and rejection when he reaches adult life. As long as the extended family is the social unit, abnormal children can be cared for and their parents sustained by their relatives as a group, but the isolation of the nuclear family which is so common today throws the whole burden of management on to the parents, mainly the mother. While provision is usually made for the child's obvious needs by the state or by voluntary agencies, modern society gives little real support to parents and, if their resources are inadequate, the child becomes the responsibility of the state. The lot of the surviving handicapped child may thus be better in a simple society, with its closely knit social life, than in a complex urban community. Though his status in the former is lowly, he is accepted and his position is secure, whereas in the city, though the concept of help for the handicapped meets with general approbation, there is little attempt at the personal level to integrate the malformed person into the community, and he remains insecure and isolated.

Modern medical care and the abandonment of infanticide on ethical grounds have led to a sharp and continuing increase in the number of malformed children who survive and, although much can now be done to ameliorate their condition, the problems posed by this new trend have not yet been squarely faced.

R. G. MITCHELL

13   Social Influences on Parents and Their Children

PSYCHIATRISTS interested in the causes of mental states and behaviour called schizophrenia now place greater emphasis on the family in which this condition originated rather than the intra-psychic qualities of the schizophrenic. Human behaviour is seen as adaptive, and the characteristic personality symptoms of schizophrenia are seen as responses to particular types of interpersonal contexts rather than relatively fixed and durable properties of individuals. As D. D. Jackson, Director of the Mental Research Institute in California, puts it '. . . the view is not of the individual *in vitro* but of the small or larger group within which any particular individual's behaviour is adaptive. We will move from individual assessment to analysis of the contexts or, more precisely, the system from which individual conduct is inseparable'.

The social sciences, especially social psychology, sociology and anthropology, share the psychiatrist's interest in the effect of social contexts on patterns of behaviour. In the study of child-rearing these disciplines examine relationships between the environment in which parents operate, parental behaviour and the development of children. Anthropological studies of child-rearing practices in non-literate societies suggest, for example, that in general boys are reared with the implicit, and often explicit, aim of making them independent and self-reliant while girls are trained to play more obedient, responsible and nurturant parts in social life. In hunting and fishing societies, however, where there are no means for the storing and accumulation of food, where each day's food comes from the last day's catch, there is greater stress on initiative and independence in the rearing of both boys and girls. In pastoral and agricultural societies on the other hand carelessness and innovation may easily jeopardise the future food supply and the faithful adherence to known routines leads to a premium being placed on obedience and responsibility in the rearing of both boys and girls. Sociologists and social psychologists have mapped out and attempted to account for the variations in child-rearing techniques used by different social classes in the population. Particular aspects of parental behaviour have been studied in more detail. For example the ways by which parents of differing social backgrounds teach their children certain skills, discipline their children and prepare them for important events in their lives such as going to school for the first time. Alongside this work, knowledge has accumulated concerning variations in marital relationships in our society (*e.g.* with regard to differing attitudes to family planning, strength of contacts with extended kin) so that we now have a more rounded picture of the way of life of different groups in the population.

The aims of some of these studies are more easily and adequately achieved than others. While it is a relatively straightforward exercise to document, say, variations in parental aspirations for children, it is more difficult to identify with certainty the variables which influence the incidence of such aspirations because the available evidence can often be interpreted in different ways. Two points should be made however. First, social scientists are aware of such issues and have found that with many problems it is possible to carry out research which will exclude or back up a particular explanation, that it is possible to discuss such problems both rigorously and critically. Second, while social science has still much to discover about the specific *ways* in which social influences operate on parents there is now no doubt that the contexts and conditions in which parents live do exert a considerable influence on their child-rearing techniques. This also implies that the genetic transmission of characteristics or the distribution of different personality characteristics in a parent population will not be sufficient to explain the major variations in child-rearing patterns. The importance of the social perspective in understanding particular aspects of childhood development can be assessed from our later discussion of mental subnormality and language development.

Aims

We shall attempt to do three things in this Chapter:

Firstly, to outline the known differences in child-rearing practices of the different social classes in Britain with reference to pre-school children.

Secondly, to explain the child-rearing practices of parents in the Registrar-General's Class V.

Thirdly, to demonstrate how variations in the social position of the family have implications for the development of children in the particular fields of mental subnormality and language development.

Differences in Child-rearing Practices

The recent major British study of child-rearing in Nottingham (Newson and Newson, 1963), like most other studies of child-rearing, is based on interviews with mothers, but unlike many studies of child-rearing, it is longitudinal in design— the authors interviewed a single group of mothers at a number of points in time after a baby had been born. In subdividing their population into social classes they used a slightly modified version of the Registrar-General's classification of occupations.

Of course not all items of maternal behaviour varied by social class. On the other hand the simple distinction between non-manual and manual groups obscures the distinctive behaviour of a particular class. Thus in the first year of life the wives of unskilled workers seemed fairly distinct from the rest of the manual category in that as a group they breast-fed less, started potty training later (and were less successful in their attempts at training), restricted genital play more and rated their husbands as participating markedly less in the child's upbringing. Unfortunately we do not have such reliable and sophisticated evidence for other areas within Britain. Some evidence can be gleamed from the national sample of children born in Britain during the first week of March 1946 and studied by Dr. J. W. B. Douglas and his group (Douglas and Blomfield, 1958). Their middle

TABLE 14

Items on which there were significant differences in the child-rearing patterns of manual and non-manual workers in Nottingham

Age 1 year
  Manual worker's wife is less likely to breast-feed, more likely to be using a feeding bottle at 12 months, more likely to be using a dummy.
  Manual worker's wife puts her child to bed later and the child is less likely to sleep in a room alone.
  Manual worker's wife is more likely to restrict genital play.

Age 4 years
  Manual worker's wife is less strict about table manners and bedtimes and is less likely to see herself as strict.
  Manual worker's wife is more likely to let children settle their own differences, to threaten her child idly with authority figures, to smack her child (particularly when the child smacks her) and to attempt to influence her child by saying 'I won't love you'.
  Manual worker's wife is less likely to tell her child a story at bedtime.
  Manual worker's wife is less permissive concerning genital play and nakedness, and is more likely to give false explanations as to where babies come from.
  Manual worker's wife is less self critical about her child-rearing practices.
  Manual worker himself is rated by his wife as participating less fully in the child's upbringing.

class parents also began potty training earlier though they do not report the relative success of training among different social classes. At 4 years of age working class children were not only more likely to be sharing rooms but also beds, even where housing conditions did not necessitate this. Unlike the Newsons, Douglas' group constructed an index of maternal efficiency based on the health visitor's report of the cleanliness of the child and home, the adequacy of the child's shoes and clothes and the mother's management of the child. As one would expect working class respondents showed up poorly on this index, but this was demonstrated to be partially a product of the associated larger family sizes, poorer housing and overcrowded conditions.

The evidence is even thinner when one looks for corroboration of the Newsons' work on four-year-olds. The general picture painted in previous studies (see Klein, 1965) of working class child-rearing patterns, for example, was of an early period of attention, warmth and indulgence lasting until about $1\frac{1}{2}$ years of age (or until the next child arrived) which then gave way to a period (lasting at least until school age) in which the child was socialised more by its elder siblings and playmates, in which the control techniques exerted by parents were inconsistent and characterised particularly by more aggressiveness than among middle class parents, and in which parents were most concerned about keeping the children out of trouble and maintaining a workable degree of obedience. Some of this work undoubtedly finds support in the Newson's findings, *e.g.* the finding that working class parents are indulgent in the sense of being less concerned to impart rules of behaviour to their children, *e.g.* the pronounced use of physical control techniques.

Five points should be noted about much of this earlier work however:

Terms like 'warmth' and 'indulgence' are difficult to use because invariably some aspects of behaviour do not accord with these characterisations. Thus the working class according to the Newsons' work are clearly not indulgent concerning sex and genital play in their children.

Especially dubious are studies which claim that any particular social group is using consistent/inconsistent discipline techniques. If inconsistency is intended to imply the use of different control techniques in similar situations then to know this one would have to observe individual families for a period of time and analyse the consistency of the mother's dealings with one type of misbehaviour—no British studies have actually done this. If inconsistency is intended to imply the use of different and varied control techniques in dissimilar situations then there would be slightly more evidence for this to be a middle class characteristic.

The third point is that particularly in Britain we know very little about the upbringing of children aged 2 to 5 years. Most writers have tended to gloss over this period, concentrating slightly more on the child's very early years or ways in which parents influence the child's progress at school.

As child-rearing patterns in America have demonstrably changed in the course of the last 40 years there might well have been genuine changes in British child-rearing patterns during the past 20 years. If this were the case one might expect 'contradictory' findings when comparing studies carried out at different points in time.

Many studies of child-rearing employ the Registrar-General's classification of occupations into five social classes. This classification, whilst perhaps adequate for its initial purpose of distinguishing gross class differences in mortality, was certainly not intended to distinguish child-rearing patterns in our society with the result that it is an insensitive instrument when used for this purpose. Research findings suggest that quite distinct groups are included within the same class and that there are similarities between different classes. Both these points may be exemplified by the Newsons' findings concerning semi-skilled workers (Class IV). On several items these mothers showed patterns of behaviour and belief more similar to those of white collar workers and the findings seem consistent with the argument that within this class there are substantial groups of people with child-rearing practices quite distinct from other semi-skilled families. The importance of variations within social classes is also corroborated by work which suggests that the husband's aspirations and promotion opportunities together with the patterns of contact which working class families have with middle class ways of life influence the educational success of their children. Findings suggest, for example, that those working class children who are successful 11 + examination candidates tend to come from families where one or both parents have either had or been eligible for senior secondary education, where one of the parents has married 'down' the social scale or where one or both have had to switch from clerical to manual occupations in the course of their lives. This not only implies that there will be variations in child-rearing patterns according to such criteria but also that these criteria will distinguish different child-rearing patterns within social classes as defined by the Registrar-General.

Explanation of Child-rearing Practices

What we now intend to do is to map out in some detail the differences between the child-rearing practices of unskilled workers and other manual workers in Britain, and attempt to explain these distinct features in sociological terms. We focus particularly on the unskilled group because many 'problem families' are seen to originate here, because they often underutilise health and welfare services, because children in this group show up poorly on a variety of developmental indices, and because it contains many of the poor and needy in our society who require both understanding and assistance.

TABLE 15
Items on which there were significant differences between the wives of unskilled workers and other manual workers in a sample of children aged 4 years in Nottingham

The wives of unskilled workers are:
  More likely to let children settle their own differences.
  More likely to use physical punishment, less prone to use deprivation of privileges as a control technique, more likely to use the threat of an authority figure in disciplining (and also to use it in a more idle way).
  Less concerned about manners, order and rules at mealtimes and more prepared to provide alternative food for their children.
  Less likely to tell their children stories at night and to participate wholeheartedly in children's play.
  Less likely to be self-critical of their approach to child-rearing.
  Low in permissiveness of aggression towards parents and severe in punishment of this.
  Less likely to tell the child where babies come from and most likely to give false explanations of this, and more restrictive as regards nakedness and genital play.

To explain these characteristics we have derived a number of variables from studies of unskilled workers (see Cohen and Hodges, 1962). Where studies reporting variation among manual workers are not available, however, we rely on research which compares manual and non-manual workers, our assumption here being that unskilled workers constitute the extreme case of such a comparison. Basically our argument is that various aspects of the situation in which unskilled workers' families operate influence the parents to hold certain beliefs and act in certain ways which in turn influence their child-rearing practices. We examine this process by taking three approaches to the handling of interpersonal relationships characteristic of this group and we argue that these become embodied in specific child-rearing practices and are encouraged by the circumstances and sets of relationships which one finds in the milieu of the unskilled worker.

Lack of Planning Orientation

The families of unskilled workers live in a milieu in which there are limited opportunities for upward job mobility and very often instability of job opportunities and income; in which they have little property, possessions or resources to allocate; in which they are encouraged by modern marketing practices to adopt the 'buy now pay later' principle; in which they are frequently dependent on a range of social agencies the workings of which often seem both foreign and arbitrary. These conditions have several repercussions for the life of such families. Immediate goals are likely to supersede long-term goals in importance; the maintenance of a reasonable standard of living and meeting one's commitments in the face of insecurity form a dominant theme of family life. These variables also undermine their assurance concerning the future, the predictability of the future which is such a necessary pre-condition for planning to occur. Long-term strategies (*e.g.* the relatively high aspirations which such groups often hold for their children's future) tend to be expressions of hopeful optimism rather than a systematically thought out series of steps for advancement. Such limited strategies are also a product of other circumstances associated with this way of life; for example parents' own minimal contact with and distrust of the very institutions which could help them to specify and realise such aims and the parent's 'kin-centred' pattern of social life which often serves to insulate parents from a wider sphere of contacts and experiences—as well as the vagaries of economic insecurity.

Partly because of their lack of planning experience we would argue that these parents are less aware of the potential part which they themselves might play in the moulding of both persons and situations with which they come into contact, and that they employ a more limited repertoire of strategies to deal with occurrences in which this is necessitated (see next point on aggressiveness). The child for them develops 'naturally', language is acquired 'naturally', in fact the child after the age of about $2\frac{1}{2}$ is expected to be a relatively independent and self-sufficient being. There seems therefore to be a different conception of the child's overall development, less awareness of the part which might be played by parents in this process and thus fewer attempts to impart the standards which would be appropriate to a more sophisticated and differentiated conception of the child's growth.

This seems congruent with the findings that the mother idly uses the threat of authority figures in disciplining, that she is less self-critical, that she is less prone to use deprivations of privileges and praise, that she is less likely to tell stories to her child at night and a further tendency (not in Table 15) for these mothers to be less aware of the problems which they themselves create for their children. For example, the Newsons write that 'From the way parents talk about bedtime stories, it is clear that middle class parents have a much stronger tendency than working class parents to think of story telling as a part of their educational duty towards their children . . . whereas working class parents are inclined to think of stories merely as a diversion, a childish indulgence, one among many ways of humouring children, but of no particular significance' and this tendency is clearly most pronounced among the wives of unskilled workers. Lastly we should emphasise that we are not implying that these families are less concerned to do the best for their children than some other group. There is little or no evidence to support such a position. What varies between classes is parents' approach to achieving this common aim and this seems to be influenced by the circumstances in which they live.

Aggressiveness in Interpersonal Relationships

Aggressiveness in situations in which difficulties and differences of opinion arise has also been found to be a characteristic working class (especially lower working class) interpersonal strategy in such spheres as husband/wife relationships, in their contacts with official agencies when making complaints and also in child-rearing. According to Table 15 this section of the population is most likely to use physical punishment in disciplining their children and also to be tolerant of it in their children so long as it is directed towards other children. To illustrate the normality of aggressive behaviour on the mother's part in these settings we reproduce a quotation given by the Newsons:

> ("How often do you in fact smack him?") Well, it's just one of those things—he has more one week than he does the next week. On average, he gets the stick about three times a week—on average; sometimes more. (And you sort of smack him with your hand in between?) Yes—Oh, very often; every time he passes me I'm helping him on his way!"

This aggressiveness as a general interpersonal tactic seems to originate in the work experiences of the father. The nature of his work does not involve him in the exercise of influence over other people, or in the making or handling of relationships in non-aggressive terms. He is essentially one who is obedient to others and one who is usually dispensable to any particular employer because he possesses no special skills which would make him difficult to replace. To have any influence at all in situations he is often only left with the option of putting up an aggressive front and, while arising from a position of weakness, such aggressive behaviour patterns are often perceived by unskilled workers themselves as a mark of strength and independence. We would not want to imply too simplistic an explanation here however. Thus child-rearing practices fostering aggressiveness, though possibly rooted in such conditions, themselves independently condition children into aggressive social roles which in turn make them more likely to handle relationships in aggressive terms. Furthermore, and to link this with the last section, the mother's aggressiveness is itself partially a product of the fact that she is not systematically influencing the child in particular directions, thus she cultivates a more limited range of influence strategies to deal with a somewhat different set of issues, and more frequently adopts what she considers the most effective strategy to counteract the immediate consequences of children's actions, smacking. We have already traced back the way in which this approach to influencing the child seems to be influenced by class factors. It is difficult in these circumstances to disentangle what is influencing what, because many agents which influence the parents and the development of the child work towards the same end. Some evidence which does fit with our remarks on work and its influences, however, is presented by McKinley (1964) in the United States who demonstrates, for example, that within all his class groupings workers with a low level of autonomy at work used relatively more physical socialisation techniques.

Orientation to Behaviour Rather Than Mental States

Several writers have noted the tendency for this group to be concerned mostly with the child's overt actions rather than its intentions and purposes; they seem to be most concerned with bringing about conformity in behaviour rather than self-regulation and the internalisation of standards. Where the parents do attempt to influence the disposition of the child, the psychology of the process is simplified and characterised by the kind of hopeful optimism mentioned earlier. Thus some of these parents speak of beating respect into their children so that the children will not get into trouble when they get older. Aside from the spheres of sexual behaviour the mother does not seem concerned with instilling rules into her child—this is suggested by the lack of pressure for manners and rules at mealtimes and lack of concern to arbitrate in children's quarrels.

When she does use rules they seem to be applied to cases where children's actions have deleterious overt consequences and she is less concerned with the intentions and inner state of the child in a given situation and how these relate to any given rule. Thus as regards children's quarrels, mothers who accept the role of an arbitrator make comments like 'I try to be fair', 'Go into it and work out what it was all about','I try to see both sides', whereas the non-arbitrator simply applies a general rule to the situation, *e.g.* 'Take no notice' or 'Wait till the blood comes running under the door'. She only acts when the children's behaviour has had such drastic consequences that involvement is inevitable. Further evidence of this comes from the work of Hess and Shipman (1967) who found that lower working class mothers of four-year-olds were more likely to tell their children to do what their teachers told them when attending school for the first time rather than to stress how school itself would form an extension of the child, an area of interest and self-fulfilment. Here again the parents seemed most concerned about the overt actions of the child *vis-a-vis* the school situation, not so much with outlining the resources which the school could supply which would enable the child to realise itself in the context of the school.

Why should these parents be less concerned with the internalisation of standards and in general with the internal mental states of their children? Broadly this seems to us a product of two sets of factors.

First, there are general influences on parents which do not encourage the facility to detect the intentions, feelings and unique characteristics of others. This tendency is fostered by the familiarity of those they come into contact with (evidence for this being their more intense patterns of contact with extended kin and their relatively low membership of voluntary organisations), and the fewer demands made upon them to develop such facilities (thus husbands' work is limited to the performance of overt, relatively simple manual operations in which the management of interpersonal relationships or the supervision of personnel is hardly a requirement built into the nature of the job). Second, this tendency seems to be entailed by the two previous characteristics of these mothers which we have noted. Thus their reduced concern to influence and mould the child leads to less concern over the transmission of standards and of influence techniques which will encourage the child to adopt these standards as his own, to internalise them. The greater use of physical disciplining does not tend to involve reasoning out the rights and wrongs of an action done at a particular time and for a particular reason. Under these circumstances mothers are less likely to put themselves in the situation of needing to understand their child, and are likely to be less involved in coming to grips with their child's intentions, feelings, and aspirations.

Implications of Social Variations for Mental Subnormality and Language Development

We now go on to consider two aspects of children's development. In the case of mental subnormality we outline the incidence of different types of subnormality in a population, the difficulties involved in explaining this evidence in terms of obstetric complications and the case for considering social variables as promoting the emergence of subnormality among certain groups in this population. In the case of children's language development, we attempt to relate directly the variations in child-rearing practices to different types of language use on the part of both children and their parents.

Mental Subnormality

Many studies have shown a higher prevalence of mental subnormality among working class children. Mental subnormality, however, is a loose diagnostic category, based on the child's ability to perform certain tasks and it might include children with different levels and kinds of ability whose low performance results from a variety of genetic, neurological, psychiatric and social circumstances. It is possible for example that the condition and its aetiology differ between social groups. To disentangle contributory factors greater diagnostic precision is required.

A recent study, undertaken in Aberdeen by Birch and his colleagues, identified all 8 to 10 year old children born and resident in the city who were regarded by the school system as ineducable or requiring special education and who, whilst in ordinary schools, had a measured I Q of 70 or less. These children were specially examined by psychologists, psychiatrists and neurologists. Data were available on the social background and obstetric antecedents of all city children aged 8 to 10 years. The accompanying Table shows that prevalence varied sharply from 3·7 per 1,000 in the children of non-manual workers to 24·9 among children of semi-skilled and unskilled workers.

TABLE 16

Prevalence of Mental Subnormality in a Total Community, by Socio-Economic, Intellectual and Neurological Status

Occupational status of father	Number of mentally subnormal children aged 8–10	Number of children aged 8–10	Prevalence (per 1,000)				All
			<50		50+		
			CNS Positive	Negative	CNS Positive	Negative	All
Non-manual	9	2,405	3·3	—	0·4	—	3·7
Skilled manual	42	3,552	3·1	0·8	2·8	4·2	10·9
Semi- and unskilled	53	2,131	2·8	—	6·6	15·5	24·9

Two further diagnostic criteria were available:

1. Levels of I Q within the subnormal range.

2. The presence of one or more localised signs of central nervous system (CNS) damage or two or more non-localised 'soft' signs, *e.g.* clearly recognisable disturbances of speech, gait or balance.

The prevalence of severe subnormality (I Q less than 50 on the WISC test) does not vary between socio-economic groups. On the other hand milder degrees of subnormality, relatively frequent in the lowest social groups, hardly exist in the upper group. Prevalence is particularly high among semi-skilled and unskilled workers when no signs of CNS damage exist.

These findings may be further interpreted as follows. Among mentally subnormal children in the upper socio-economic group 89 per cent show severe intellectual impairment, whereas in the lower income group 89 per cent have a milder degree of subnormality. Furthermore all subnormal children in the upper group showed signs of CNS damage whereas subnormality occurred without neurological signs in 62 per cent of the lowest socio-economic group. Mental subnormality clearly has neither the same intellectual nor the same neurological connotation in different socio-economic groups. These widely different distributions are suggestive of different aetiologies, of the presence in working class families of factors associated with subnormality which have no recognisable organic basis and which do not occur in middle class families.

Complications of pregnancy, delivery and the newborn period are frequently cited as possible causes of mental subnormality. In the Aberdeen study, moderate and severe pre-eclampsia, antepartum haemorrhage, short gestation, breech delivery, low birth weight and disturbed condition as a neonate were all over-represented in the pregnancy histories of mentally subnormal children compared with the total population. One or more of these complications occurred in 51 per cent of children with CNS signs compared with 32 per cent where no such signs were present. The difference, though suggestive, was not significant. Most of the conditions listed above occur more frequently in the pregnancies of lower class mothers, so that if the hypothesis of birth injury were fully substantiated it might account for the social class gradient in mental subnormality.

The wide differences between social classes in the distribution of clinical sub-types of subnormality raise awkward problems for such an interpretation. The subtype most consistent with the hypothesis of brain injury (severe defect with CNS signs) occurs with equal frequency in all classes; on the other hand the largest concentration of lower class subnormality occurs in that clinical subtype showing no overt signs of neurological damage and the mildest intellectual deficits. Moreover, the mere presence of obstetric abnormality cannot be regarded as a sufficient cause because such abnormalities occur in the histories of a large propor-tion of intellectually average or able children. The almost total absence of upper class children in the 50 to 70 I Q range raises two further possible interpretations. The characterisation of a child as mentally subnormal, made visible by attendance at a special school, carries a stigma for the child and his family which is likely to be felt most keenly in upper social groups whose social milieu places a high value on intellectual attainment; such groups are therefore more likely to resist ascertain-ment and will have more power to achieve this end. The second possibility is that minimal brain damage in upper class children may be sufficiently offset by conditions of upbringing that they fall above the upper level of defined mental subnormality whilst similar lower class children fall below. The familial context, in terms of aspirations, power, facilities for intellectual development, therefore becomes relevant to both identification and the search for causes.

Many studies have shown that parental social class is related on the one hand to pregnancy and labour complications and on the other to the educational achieve-ment and I Q scores both of the parents themselves and of their children (Richardson and Guttmacher, 1967). This relationship is not confined to the mentally subnormal. As indicated in Table 16 the lower social classes are heavily over-represented in mentally subnormal populations; for this reason alone, and without invoking a causal relationship between obstetric factors and mental defect, one would expect to find a high incidence of obstetric abnormalities in the histories of mentally subnormal groups. The obstetric problems, perinatal death, early delivery, low birth weight, etc., can be traced to inadequate maternal nutrition from childhood onwards, poor living conditions, susceptibility to infectious illness, poor physical growth, and the risks are often enhanced by close-spaced frequent childbirth from an early age. The familial context giving rise to these problems, accompanied by the conditions of upbringing described earlier in this chapter, provides the early environment of the pre-school child. Thus different facets of a lower class environment may create physical and cultural outcomes even in the absence of direct birth injury.

Children's Language

Psychologists interested in the development of children's verbal performance report that social class correlates significantly with several measures of speech development by the time children are 5 years of age (Moore, 1968). That is to say there is a high probability that the middle class child will have a wider range of vocabulary than his working class counterpart, that he will enunciate words more clearly, comprehend speech more effectively and display greater maturity and complexity in terms of the structure of his speech by the time he enters the infant school. In fact among girls social class variation in their speech quotient is found as early as 18 months of age. These findings have been replicated in the U.S.A., and have led to the adoption of compensatory education schemes in the pre-school years by some states, particularly when faced by the poor performance and alienation of many negro pupils from the school system.

The sociologist here is interested in the ways that children and adults actually use speech rather than in the children's competence at speaking which is measured by the psychologists' test of verbal intelligence. He is interested for example in the social situations in which the different social classes are involved and how these relate to the topics discussed and the types of speech used in dealing with the range of people and problems encountered in such situations. As an example let us look at the linguistic implications of the ways in which members of different social classes handle children's quarrels. We have already noted the greater tendency for middle class mothers to arbitrate in such quarrels, but aside from the fact that their reaction is more likely to involve prolonged verbal contact with the protagonists, they are also concerned with the judicial function of applying standards of right and wrong to particular cases of social disruption. In such a situation the middle or upper class mother seems more likely to enquire as to the intentions of the participants and the extent to which consequences of an act were foreseen, and she often indicates, if only by implication, what can be rights of appeal against a decision she makes. In so doing she is demanding a rather complex verbal performance from her child—at a minimum it will involve the child in reporting past actions and mental states and attempting to justify such actions while the mother also leaves herself open to verbal influence from the child. Such a procedure is not just characteristic of a whole range of discipline situations in the family, it also seems to pervade other aspects of the life of these children. Other research workers see the middle class mother as more concerned to bring about not only obedience to a wider range of social standards and expectations, but also the internalisation of such standards, and to effect this the middle class person is more concerned to point out the particular advantages and disadvantages of such rules to the child and those with whom the child is in contact. This all tends to entail more complicated language use on the part of the parent, thus creating a more sophisticated set of language models for the child, and the adoption by the child of a less predictable and more complex speech syntax (Bernstein).

We might best illustrate and extend our argument here by returning to the unskilled group discussed earlier and, as these all have implications for language use, the general characteristics which we ascribed to them. The lack of overall planning orientation was associated with a reduced concern over the transmission of standards and a belief that the child's potential would unfold naturally in the years before school. This clearly reduces the range of verbal contact and verbal control which parents see as necessary, and as they hold a less differentiated conception of the child's growth, they are probably less likely to relate to the child in ways designed to be appropriate to, or to promote, the child's level of language attainment. The greater aggressiveness in the type of interpersonal tactic used means that where infractions of rules are censured there will be less use of reasoning, less consideration of the consequences of actions, less basis upon which the child may make appeals against parental authority. This latter point may be associated with the higher incidence of tantrums among children of unskilled workers, tantrums being one means of demonstrating one's opposition when no explicit discussion is countenanced by parents. The relative lack of concern for the intentions and purposes lying behind actions reduces the range of verbal inquiry and concern on the part of parents and limits the variety of speech elicited from the child on any given occasion.

Clearly other conditions associated with unskilled workers' lives will also encourage such restricted language use. The fact that housing conditions are more limited and limiting for the child will mean that there will be more incentive to be out on the street playing with his peers rather than staying in and around the home—and we know that children use less complex speech forms when interacting with playmates. The larger family size and the closer spacing of children in these families will serve to limit the opportunities for parental verbal interaction with any given child. The more limited range of experience of the child in this home will mean that the language he uses will be more proficient at dealing with the familiar and the everyday, vocabulary range is likely to be limited, pronoun usage more pronounced; pronoun usage in turn limits the range of modification and qualification possible within speech.

While we initially made a distinction between language competence as measured by the psychologist and language use, it is important to note that many psychologists now not only maintain that language use is related to language competence, but also that the possession of language itself influences the ability of the child to acquire other skills in much the same way that the pursuit of intellectual disciplines depends on the ability to read and write.

Conclusion

While the structure of our overall argument need not be restated, two major and related implications of this argument should be mentioned. Firstly, if as has been suggested, social and parental factors play such an important part in the distribution of sets of characteristics in a population of children the way in which these factors operate to put a large section of children at risk to any particular deleterious condition must be set alongside other factors (possibly associated with genetic, neurological or personality make-up) in any explanation of the incidence of such a condition. To illustrate our second point let us return to the analogy we first took from the field of mental health. Where the explanatory framework of schizophrenia emphasises the part played by the family context of the schizophrenic the condition of the patient will not be facilitated when, even after therapy, the patient returns to the same context. Thus we currently find more concern in the field of mental health over new intervention techniques such as family therapy. The implication of our own argument is similar in that intervention techniques designed to alleviate the situation of a large group of children at risk to certain conditions must focus on the child-rearing contexts which serve to influence the development of these children. We have also argued, however, that the actions of parents themselves are produced and reinforced by the milieux in which they live, and that these milieux influence child-rearing techniques because of their association with certain types of interpersonal strategy.

A. J. WOOTTON and R. ILLSLEY

References

BERNSTEIN, B. A sociolinguistic approach to socialization with some reference to educability. In *Research in Sociolinguistics*. Ed. J. Gumperz and D. Hymes. New York: Holt Rinehart and Winston (in press).

BIRCH, H. G. *et al. Mental Subnormality: A Community Study*. Baltimore: Williams and Wilkins (in press).

COHEN, A. K. and HODGES, H. M. (1962). Characteristics of the lower blue-collar class. *Social Problems*, 10, 303.

DOUGLAS, J. W. B. and BLOMFIELD, J. M. (1958). *Children Under Five*. London: Allen and Unwin.

HESS, R. D. and SHIPMAN, V. C. (1967). Cognitive elements in maternal behaviour. *Minnesota Symposia on Child Psychology*, 1, 57.

JACKSON, D. D. (1967). The individual and the larger contexts. *Family Process*, 6, 139.

KLEIN, J. (1965). *Samples from English Cultures*. Vols 1 and 2. London: Routledge and Kegan Paul. (With summary of literature.)

McKINLEY, D. G. (1964). *Social Class and Family Life*. New York: Free Press of Glencoe.

MOORE, T. W. (1968). Language and intelligence. *Human Development*, 11, 1.

NEWSON, J. and NEWSON, E. (1963). *Patterns of Infant Care*. London: Allen and Unwin.

—— —— (1968). *Four Years Old in an Urban Community*. London: Allen and Unwin.

RICHARDSON, S. A. and GUTTMACHER, A. F. (Ed.) (1967). *Childbearing: Its Social and Psychological Aspects*. Baltimore: Williams and Wilkins.

14   Historical Development of the Child Health and Social Services

IN eleventh-century Scotland, Queen Margaret made herself personally responsible for the daily care of nine orphans, and during the fourteenth and fifteenth centuries religious hospitals throughout Britain accepted the care of infants of mothers dying in childbirth in these hospitals. In the sixteenth century, baby-farming became an organised trade as, with the practice of wet-nursing steadily increasing, many infants were sent into the country to foster-mothers. Indeed, baby-farming continued as an accepted practice until well into the nineteenth century. Under Elizabethan Poor Law and contemporary Scottish Poor Law, both of which remained in force, practically unaltered, into the nineteenth century, poor children were subjected to harsh, repressive measures, all the emphasis being on servitude. Nevertheless, isolated attempts were made to improve the lot of orphans and foundlings, and Christ's Hospital (founded 1553) and church records in Scotland bear evidence of concern for poor and orphaned children.

By the publication of Bills of Mortality during the seventeenth century some idea of child mortality was gained for the first time. Two-fifths of all deaths were in infants under 2 years and the mortality among farmed-out children was enormous. Factory schools were started for destitute children by Firmin in London (1681) and spinning schools in Scotland (1633). The care and education of deaf children were furthered by such as John Bulwer (1644) and John Wallis (1652), but medical care of children generally was non-existent though efforts were made to regulate midwifery practice by, among others, Peter Chamberlen II in 1616.

No progress was made during the early eighteenth century, though further attempts to improve midwifery practice were made at Edinburgh (1726) and London (Manningham, Smellie and others). Wet-nursing was approaching its zenith and was a profitable career for many women who abandoned their infants so as to be able to hire themselves as wet-nurses. Such abandoned or 'dropt' infants aroused the pity of Captain Thomas Coram and his unremitting efforts finally led to the foundation of the Foundling Hospital in London (1741). Some progress was made in the medical care of children by the publication during the century of many paediatric works by such men as William Cadogan, George Armstrong, and others. Armstrong with the help of his brother John, the poet-physician, opened the first Dispensary for the Infant Poor in London (1769), a pioneer effort which ceased its activities in 1781 (Maloney, 1954). This dispensary was in many ways the forerunner of the modern child health centre. Another similar dispensary was opened in London by Lettsom (1770), and suggestions were made from time to time by such men as Smellie and William Buchan that women and young girls should be trained in child care. By the end of the century, cow's milk was steadily supplanting wet-nursing as an alternative to maternal feeding. During this century also, Thomas Braidwood furthered the training and education of deaf children first at Edinburgh (1760) and later at Hackney, London (1783), and the first asylum and school for blind children was opened at Liverpool (1790). Vaccination was introduced by Jenner (1798) but among the epidemic diseases measles had already begun to supplant smallpox as the major killer of children. Thus, the eighteenth century saw the seeds of modern maternal and child care sown but falling on the stony ground of the Industrial Revolution.

The period from 1800 to 1850 was the grimmest in British social history as far as the child was concerned. The inexorable advance of the Industrial Revolution exposed the child to exploitation and misery; child labour became the rule, but against it philanthropic effort attempted to cope. Schools of Industry and spinning schools were organised throughout the country. Robert Owen opened his Infant School at New Lanark (1816) and the Infant School Society was founded in 1824. These infant schools aimed at providing moral training, amusement, and attention to the general health of children of both sexes between the ages of 2 and 6 years and may be regarded as the predecessors of the nursery schools of today. For the destitute and poverty-stricken child, John Pounds began the Ragged School movement and was followed by Watson, Chalmers and Guthrie in Scotland. Later, Barnardo and Quarrier interested themselves in orphan children. Lord Ashley, later the Earl of Shaftesbury, became the champion of the child in Parliament and very slowly conditions began to improve as successive Royal Commissions reported and legislative action followed. The Poor Law was reformed in both England and Scotland, the new Poor Law remaining in force with various amendments for almost another hundred years, but even this reformed law left the child with a hard lot, as Dickens showed in *Oliver Twist*. Even for the more fortunately placed child, life was difficult in a different way, as portrayed in *Jane Eyre*. Social unrest following the French Revolution, and the development of industry, combined to arouse public opinion to the need for a national system of day schools, but the movement in this direction was impeded by religious differences. In the field of infant welfare, John Bunnell Davis opened the Universal Dispensary for the Infant Poor in 1816 after 10 years of constant effort to interest leaders of the profession in the necessity for such an institution. Davis was far in advance of his time, for he envisaged health visiting and health education by pamphlets couched in simple, effective language.

The year 1870 is, in many ways, an important one in the history of the child in Britain, and much of the development of the modern child health and social services can be traced to events occurring about this time.

Children's Hospitals, Teaching and Training in Paediatrics

Efforts were made to teach paediatrics systematically at Manchester (1829) and

Edinburgh (1837) and about the middle of the century the children's hospital movement (Great Ormond Street, London, 1852) and the development of children's wards in general hospitals (Liverpool, 1857) began. *Pari passu* with this trend came the organisation of outpatient departments, convalescent homes for children, special hospitals, lectureships and facilities for voluntary clinical and systematic instruction in children's diseases, and in 1906 the first chair of Diseases of Children in Britain was founded at King's College Hospital, London. In Edinburgh, in 1931, a chair of Child Life and Health was established which conveyed the broader concept of the study of the child in health and disease, a characteristic outlook of the twentieth century.

School Medical and Dental Services

SCHOOL MEALS AND MILK. Prior to 1870, schools were provided in England and Scotland by voluntary bodies and the church, some education was also given to children under the Poor Law, but the great masses of young children received no education. Compulsory education was introduced into England in 1870 and in Scotland 2 years later. The inclusion of children from the poorest homes within a national educational service made it evident that a considerable proportion were unable to benefit from such educational facilities on grounds of physical defect or malnutrition. Soon, therefore, voluntary bodies began providing meals for necessitous children, this need being recognised in the Education (Provision of Meals) Act, 1906, and the Education (Scotland) Act, 1908, both of which authorised education authorities to provide meals for such children. Since the introduction of these early measures the powers of education authorities have been extended by the Education Act, 1944 for England and Wales and the consolidating Act of 1962 for Scotland respectively. Through the school meals service a daily dinner at a subsidised price, remitted where there is need, is provided for about two-thirds of the pupils in schools maintained by education authorities. In both countries a Milk-in-Schools scheme was introduced in 1934 and from 1946 until 1968 this school milk (one-third of a pint) was given free at all grant-aided primary and secondary schools. The free milk scheme now exends only to nursery and primary schools and to special schools.

MEDICAL INSPECTION AND TREATMENT. In 1884, the Medical Officers of Schools Association was founded with the object of promoting school hygiene. Its members were composed of representatives of children's hospitals, public schools, charity schools and of others interested in the health and welfare of schoolchildren. A year after its foundation the Association published a Code of Preventive Rules dealing with the control of infectious disease in schools. The latest edition of the Code, now called Handbook (1969), deals not only with infectious disease but also with other aspects of school hygiene. In spite of this early interest in the health of schoolchildren, little that was effective was then achieved regarding their general medical supervision and treatment. In 1890, the London School Board appointed a school medical officer and Bradford, 3 years later, made a similar appointment. Uneasiness at the high percentage of rejections of recruits for the South African

War resulted in a Royal Commission on Physical Training (Scotland) and an Interdepartmental Committee on Physical Deterioration (England) being appointed in 1902 and 1903 respectively. From the recommendations of these two bodies, the School Medical Service was inaugurated. In 1907, the Education (Administrative Provisions) Act required English education authorities to provide for the systematic medical inspection of all children attending public elementary schools and empowered them, if they so desired, to provide certain forms of treatment if approved by the Board of Education. Later, by the Education Act of 1918, specified forms of treatment required to be provided. In Scotland by the Education (Scotland) Act, 1908, permissive powers were granted to institute medical inspection, and in 1913, medical treatment was made possible when needed by any schoolchild. Thus, school medical officers and school nurses officially came into being. It soon became apparent that much avoidable damage had already occurred by the time children first entered school, and child welfare schemes were instituted under the Notification of Births (Extension) Act, 1915, and the Maternity and Child Welfare Act, 1918. Since then there has been an increasingly close liaison between the two local authority medical services. All previous powers and duties of education authorities were incorporated in the Education Acts of 1944 and 1962 for England and Scotland respectively. Under the 1944 Act, the Board of Education became the Ministry of Education and in 1964 this Ministry was combined with the Ministry of Science to form a Department of Education and Science with a Secretary of State. Under both the 1944 and 1962 Acts the school medical services in England and Scotland became the school health services and provided schemes for medical inspection and free treatment of pupils attending any school, county college or junior college. Whereas formerly there was no obligation on a parent to submit his child to medical inspection, these two Acts make such inspection obligatory. The conduct of medical examinations and inspections are governed by Regulations (1953). Special arrangements are made for handicapped children. In 1967 there were 920 special schools provided by local education authorities and voluntary agencies in England and Wales and in Scotland 163 similarly maintained schools in 1968. Child guidance clinics are provided for the maladjusted (see Chapter 20). These clinics were not officially recognised until 1935, and in 1967 there were 359 clinics in England and Wales associated with education authorities. In Scotland 24 out of 35 local authorities provided child guidance services in 1968.

SCHOOL DENTAL SERVICE. From 1870, dentists began to be appointed to some of the bigger schools and by 1890 a few dentists, notably Fisher of Dundee, had got to work in a small way in a number of Poor Law schools. By 1898 there were sufficient dentists working among schoolchildren to form the School Dentists Society, affiliated since 1921 with the Society of Medical Officers of Health. Dentists got a firmer footing in schools with the introduction of medical inspections and since then, and especially since 1930, the school dental service has expanded. A few pioneer authorities had also employed dentists in their maternity and child welfare schemes (e.g., St. Pancras, 1911). The recent Education Acts have ensured that the school dental service becomes an established part of the school health service and the National Health Service Acts have enforced priority dental facilities for expectant and nursing mothers and for children under 5 years. This work is often undertaken by school dental services locally. The full development of the school dental service has been impeded by lack of recruitment. The Dentists Act, 1956, permitted the training of dental auxiliaries and an experimental scheme was introduced in 1960 by the General Dental Council to ascertain the value to the community of this new type of dental ancillary. Such a person when trained must be employed in the public dental services under the direct personal supervision of a registered dentist. By 1965, 132 dental auxiliaries had been trained and employed in dental services of local authorities and the experiment seems to be justified by the encouraging results so far obtained.

Infant and Pre-School Services

PRACTICE OF MIDWIFERY. After the introduction of the registration of births and deaths in England (1837) and Scotland (1855), the first scientific inquiry of statistical importance relating to maternal care and infant mortality was carried out by William Farr in 1867–69, in collaboration with the Obstetrical Society of London and Dr. William Stark of Edinburgh. This survey revealed that between 50 and 75 per cent of births in England and 33 per cent in Scotland were attended by midwives with little or no training. The *Lancet* (1868) added its weight to the agitation for the proper training and control of midwives as did the Institute of Midwives (founded 1881, and now the Royal College of Midwives) but no legislation was forthcoming until 1902 when the Midwives Act was passed for England, and 1915 when a similar Act was passed for Scotland. Under these first Acts the training and standard of practice of midwives, and consequently their status, have been raised to a high level. Present-day legislation governing midwives is embodied in the Midwives Acts, 1951, for the two countries. The importance of antenatal care and its direct bearing on infant mortality were emphasised by J. W. Ballantyne of Edinburgh during the last decade of the nineteenth century. The first bed in the United Kingdom for antenatal purposes was endowed in 1901 at the Royal Maternity Hospital, Edinburgh. Thus, antenatal care is essentially a twentieth century development.

BABY-FARMING AND THE PROTECTION OF CHILD LIFE. Shortly after the Farr inquiry, public conscience received a rude shock by the trial and execution in 1870 of Margaret Waters, a notorious baby-farmer. In spite of previous efforts by J. B. Curgenven and Lord Shaftesbury to control the evil, nothing was done until the Society for the Protection of Infant Life (founded 1870) agitated successfully and was largely responsible for getting the Infant Life Protection Act, 1872, passed. A series of Acts dealing with protection of child life followed and all their provisions were incorporated in the consolidating Children Act, 1908, the 'Children's Charter', which among other provisions set up juvenile courts. This great Act has been superseded since by a series of amending and improving Acts. With the end of the Poor Law (between 1930 and 1948 called Public Assistance) in sight, the government in 1945 appointed the Curtis Committee in England and the Clyde Committee in Scotland to review and report on existing arrangements for the care of children deprived of a normal home life. These two committees reported in 1946 and made similar recommendations for the two countries. As a consequence of these recommendations, which were accepted by government, the Children Act, 1948, was passed under which the responsible central government departments were designated—the Home Office (England) and the Scottish Education Department—to undertake the supervision of all deprived children. Peripherally, each local authority was required to appoint a children committee and an administrative officer, the children's officer. Recent legislation in Scotland has altered this administrative machinery and proposals for reform of certain local authority functions relating to child care in England have been presented (see Chapter 17).

ADOPTION. The problem of the unmarried mother and her child has always been a difficult one and with the development of infant welfare services before and during World War I the problem of the illegitimate child became increasingly important. Mainly through the energies of voluntary organisations, e.g., the National Council for the Unmarried Mother and her Child (founded 1918), an agitation was set afoot to put adoption of children on a legal basis. First the Hopkinson Report (1921) then the Tomlin Report (1925) were published dealing with the problem. Finally, in 1926 the first Adoption Act in Britain was passed and applied to England and Wales, a similar Act for Scotland following in 1930. These Acts, proving inadequate to prevent undesirable adoptions, were succeeded by the Adoption of Children (Regulation) Act, 1939, the application of which was deferred, owing to the outbreak of World War II, until 1943. Even after a national consolidating Act was passed in 1950, problems still remained and a departmental committee, the Hurst Committee, was appointed in 1953 to review the existing law of child adoption and recommend any necessary changes in policy and procedure. Following this committee's report (1954) new adoption legislation was introduced (1958) which is currently operative. In 1967, in England and Wales 22,802 children were adopted and 2,140 in Scotland (see Chapter 17).

HEALTH VISITING. Nothing immediate seemed to come from Davis's suggestion (1816) of home visiting of infants. The first organised health visiting movement came from the Manchester and Salford Ladies Sanitary Reform Association which initiated a system of home visiting in 1862, a lead which was followed by other organisations in the country. Buckinghamshire became the first local authority to employ full-time salaried visitors, trained under a scheme inspired by Florence Nightingale (1892). Official steps towards setting up a standard of proficiency for health visitors came in 1908 and extended in 1919 in both Scotland and England. In 1925 the Royal Sanitary Institute (now the Royal Society of Health, 1955) became the examining and certifying body for the health visitor certificate and in 1933 the Royal Sanitary Association of Scotland became the corresponding body there. So successful was the health visitor in her work in infant welfare that gradually her training was extended to cover school health, tuberculosis, family health and welfare, etc., and local authorities began to employ health visitors in these services. The National Health Service Acts greatly affected health visiting, making provision of such a service obligatory on all local health authorities and defining the duties 'for visiting of persons in their homes for the purpose of giving advice as to the care of young children, persons suffering from illness and expectant and nursing mothers, and as to measures necessary to prevent the spread of infection'. Home visiting to give advice and to educate on health matters is the primary function of the health visitor, who is now concerned with the family as a whole. In recent years she has worked more and more closely with the family doctor and systems of attachment and liaison with groups of practitioners are rapidly developing. Following the report of the working party on the field of work, training and recruitment of health visitors (Jameson Report, 1956), the Health Visiting and Social Work (Training) Act, 1962, set up the Council for the Training of Health Visitors which was constituted in the same year. The Council soon drew up a new syllabus of instruction, since 1965 has approved courses and training schools, and has laid down conditions of admission to such schools. It grants a health visitor certificate after examination, and it conducts research. In 1969 there were 33 training schools in England and Wales and 4 in Scotland.

INFANT WELFARE. Infant mortality in Britain, far from declining during the advances of the sanitary reform movement initiated by Chadwick and others during the nineteenth century, showed a tendency to rise. At the beginning of the present century this wastage of infant life, combined with a declining birthrate, focussed public attention especially on the ravages of epidemic diarrhoea which annually claimed its thousands of victims. Newsholme emphasised the importance of clean cow's milk in artificial feeding and pointed to the success attendant on Budin's *Consultations des Nourrisons* at Paris (1892) and the *Gouttes de lait* of Variot (1893) at the Belleville Dispensary, Paris, and of Dufour at Fecamp (1894). These French organisations had three main objectives, viz., the systematic medical supervision of infants, the encouragement of breast feeding, and the provision of sterilised cow's milk for artificially fed infants. St. Helen's (1899) opened the first infant milk depot in Britain and in succeeding years an increasing number of similar centres was opened throughout the country by both voluntary bodies and municipalities. At some centres free meals were provided for nursing mothers also. These depots rapidly developed into infant consultation centres with health visitors in attendance to give advice on feeding and problems of infant hygiene. Sometimes courses of systematic instruction on child hygiene were given to mothers at these centres, of which the first was at Winchester (1906), and which were often spoken of as 'Schools for Mothers'. Thus began the association of health visiting and advice to mothers on infant care at centres which are now called child health centres (Sheldon, 1967).

Although registration of births was in force throughout Britain, the time lag was considerable before medical officers of health received information concerning these births, and many of the infants were dead before the health visitor had visited. Huddersfield (1906) pioneered a system of early notification of births and in 1907 the Notification of Births Act, a permissive measure, was passed requiring that all births, live and still, after the twenty-eighth week of pregnancy should be notified to the medical officer of health within 36 hours of the birth. The Notification of Births (Extension) Act, 1915 enforced the 1907 Act throughout Britain and in Scotland gave local authorities power to organise schemes for the health and welfare of expectant and nursing mothers and of children under 5 years. In England, similar powers were conferred by the Maternity and Child Welfare Act, 1918.

THE PRE-SCHOOL CHILD. The bringing up of young children presents problems that tax even the most resourceful of parents. For those who are already burdened by other problems or who are less well equipped to meet the stress of managing children in difficult circumstances the strain can be well-nigh intolerable and the risk of family breakdown a very real one. In contrast to the general good standard of physical and medical care afforded to young children, organised provision for their social and emotional needs lags far behind. The case for providing various forms of day care is a pressing and urgent one and the present is a period of intense activity and interest in this field. Official action has been tardy for a variety of reasons and some of the well established forms of day care have not been developed and expanded to the extent both needed and desired. Recently (1968) the government has declared certain urban parts of the country as areas of educational priority and entitled to certain funds for day nursery, nursery school, and nursery class expansion.

DAY NURSERIES. The day nursery is an agency which provides for the care of pre-school children as well as for infants. Day nurseries appear to have originated in France after the Napoleonic Wars when large numbers of women entered industrial or other employment. In England a day nursery was established in London in 1860 and in Scotland one was opened in Edinburgh in 1876 but it was not until the National Society of Children's Nurseries was formed in 1906 that the modern concept of a day nursery as an institution which would benefit both mother and child gained any general acceptance. A great impetus to the day nursery movement was given during World War II, when the government sponsored a wartime day nursery scheme, and at the peak period of the war there were some 1,600 nurseries in Britain. In 1946 the wartime nursery scheme came to an end, but government circulars sent to local authorities recognised the continued necessity for nursery accommodation. It was therefore clear that day nurseries had not only proved their wartime value but that they formed an essential item in post-war planning. Many local authorities, however, closed down most or all of their day nurseries, on a variety of pleas. From 1950 when there were 866 day nurseries maintained by local authorities in England and Wales and 84 in Scotland, the numbers had declined to 445 and 65 respectively by 1968.

NURSERY SCHOOLS. The nursery school is another useful agent for the care and supervision of pre-school children. They may be provided by education authorities or voluntary bodies and are autonomous institutions under the control of nursery school teachers. The prototype of this institution as a separate entity is to be found in Owen's work at New Lanark and the Dame Schools which flourished during the nineteenth century. The kindergarten movement of Froebel was introduced into Britain in 1854 and greatly influenced the growth of infant schools and the nursery school in its modern form. Froebel's work was popularised by Dickens, the first of the modern-type nursery school opening at Salford in 1873. Nursery schools were first recommended in Britain in 1908 by the Consultative Committee of the Board of Education. A beginning was made on a voluntary basis with nursery schools in slum areas, followed by the establishment by Margaret McMillan in 1911 of a large open-air nursery school at Deptford. No legal or administrative action was taken until the passing of the Education Acts, 1918, for England and Scotland respectively, when legislative powers to supply or aid the supply of nursery schools was granted for the first time to education authorities. Dr. Maria Montessori greatly influenced nursery school development, especially in the matter of equipment, including furniture and play material. The nursery School Association of Great Britain (founded 1923) has done much to further the nursery school movement. The Education Acts, 1944 and 1962 (Scotland) recognised the need for further provision but little has yet been achieved in this direction.

NURSERY CLASSES. A nursery class is a less intensive form of nursery school, similarly staffed but conducted, not as an autonomous organisation, but as part of the ordinary infants' division of the primary school.

The Plowden Report (1967) made a plea for expanded nursery education, mainly of a part-time nature, for young children in the 3 to 5 year age group in 'nursery groups' of 20 places, two or three groups making one unit or nursery centre. It recommended ways and means of overcoming some present-day difficulties in nursery expansion.

PRE-SCHOOL PLAYGROUPS OR PLAYCENTRES. These organisations were pioneered in Edinburgh by a local voluntary association. In 1914, to judge the value of home visits by health visitors, this organisation, now called the Edinburgh Toddlers Playcentres Association, arranged for an intensive visitation of some 400 homes in districts where conditions were known to be bad. The results of this investigation revealed that the babies were well enough cared for 'but the ex-baby, the toddler, sat on the fender or on the stairs, or sometimes in the street often unwashed, listless, flabby, with nothing to do'. It was evident that something less deliberately educational than nursery schools and more definitely for health, *per se*, was urgently required. The first toddlers playcentre was opened by the Association in 1915 to provide opportunity for exercise, fresh air, happy occupation and companionship in safe surroundings for children living in the crowded parts of the city. Within recent years other voluntary organisations have entered this field, notably the Save the Children Fund (founded 1919) and the Pre-School Playgroups Association (founded 1962).

WELFARE FOODS. To safeguard the nutrition of pregnant women and children under 5, a National Milk Scheme was introduced in 1940 under which these two classes of the community became entitled to one pint of milk daily, free or at a reduced rate. Later that year a national full-cream dried milk was made available for infants under one year for whom liquid milk was considered unsuitable and in 1941 a national half-cream dried milk was produced. In 1941 also a vitamin scheme was launched to provide pregnant women and children under 2 years with fruit juices and a cod-liver oil compound. The milk and vitamin schemes were merged in 1942, and the vitamin supplements were extended to all children under 5. In 1943, pregnant women were supplied with fish-liver oil capsules or Vitamin A and D tablets instead of the cod-liver oil compound, and later only the tablets were supplied. The British Paediatric Association (1944) recommended the fortification of national dried milks with vitamin D and this was then commenced. With the family allowances scheme coming into operation in 1946 the milk and vitamin service was merged with it to become the Welfare Foods Scheme. In 1954 the distribution of welfare foods, other than liquid milk, was placed on the shoulders of local health authorities where it still remains. On the recommendation of the Joint Sub-Committee on Welfare Foods (1957) the issue of orange juice concentrate was restricted to children under 2 years and the vitamin D content of national dried milk and cod-liver oil compound was reduced. In 1961 changes were made in the conditions of issue of the vitamin supplements. Special tokens were required only for liquid and national dried milk, the cod-liver oil compound, concentrated orange juice and vitamin tablets becoming purchasable at cost price and without surrender of tokens. At the same time the cod-liver oil compound and orange juice concentrate became purchasable for children up to 5 years of age and longer if they were handicapped.

The present vitamin content of the welfare foods is: national dried milk, full and half-cream varieties, 50 i.u. vitamin D as a minimum, with an average of 100 i.u. per 1 ounce of powder; cod-liver oil compound, 3,000 i.u. vitamin A and 400 i.u. vitamin D per fluid drachm; concentrated orange juice, not less than 60 mg. ascorbic acid per 1 fluid ounce of concentrate; each vitamin tablet, 4,000 i.u. vitamin A, 400 i.u. vitamin D, 250 mg. dibasic calcium phosphate, and 0·13 mg. potassium iodide. Arneil (1967) advocated that a palatable combination of vitamins C and D attractively packaged should be sold instead of the present cod-liver oil compound and orange juice concentrate for children.

Family Planning

Family planning, formerly called birth control, is now an accepted part of family welfare. It has a long and chequered career in our history. All the nineteenth century pioneers in the movement to gain recognition of birth control in Britain— Place, Drysdale, Bradlaugh and Mrs. Annie Besant among others—drew their inspiration from Malthus. Contraception as a check to overpopulation was first openly advocated here by Francis Place (1822). In time, through the efforts of individuals such as Marie Stopes and of groups, several bodies were formed to give information and advice on birth control and voluntary clinics were established in the 1920s. In 1926 the House of Lords introduced a motion calling for public health provision for family planning but the measure failed. In 1930, five voluntary bodies amalgamated to form the National Birth Control Council, renamed the Family Planning Association (1939). Further attempts were made to induce successive governments to persuade local authorities to give information on birth control but these were only partially successful. In 1966, circulars were sent by the respective Health Ministers to all local health authorities in the country enquiring about their existing arrangements for family planning services, recommending that these be reviewed and suggesting how they might be developed. Three suggestions were made—a programme of public education, provision of advice and treatment for women to whose health pregnancy would be detrimental, and financial and other help for voluntary bodies. The response to the circulars showed that of 174 local health authorities in England and Wales, 156 provided some form of family planning facility either directly or more commonly (114 authorities) by supporting voluntary bodies such as the Family Planning Association. Following these enquiries came the National Health Service (Family Planning) Act, 1967 (England and Wales) and the Health Services and Public Health Act, 1968 (Scotland) extending local authority powers to include social cases and enabling these authorities to give advice on contraception, to provide medical examination of persons for the purpose of determining what advice to give, to supply contraceptive substances and appliances, and to recover charges, except in medical cases or in non-medical cases for advice or examination only. Local health authorities were also requested to plan their services jointly with representatives of hospital authorities, general practitioners and the Family Planning Association or other voluntary body to ensure the availability of a comprehensive family planning service in all areas.

Abortion Act, 1968

After much controversy this Act was passed and became operative in the same year. Briefly the Act permits the termination of pregnancy under stringent conditions on the following grounds: that the continuance of a pregnancy would involve risk to the life of the pregnant woman, or of injury to the physical or mental health of that woman or any existing children of her family greater than if the pregnancy were terminated; or, that there was a substantial risk that if the child were born it would suffer from such physical or mental abnormalities as to be seriously handicapped. In forming any opinion under the first condition account was to be taken of the woman's actual or reasonably foreseeable environment.

Recent and Proposed Changes and Developments in the Child Health and Welfare Services

The present is witnessing major changes, some already taking place, some contemplated, in the fields of child health and social welfare. During 1968 Green Papers on the reorganisation of the health services of England and Scotland were published. The English Green Paper was subsequently withdrawn and fresh proposals incorporated in Green Papers for England and for Wales respectively (1970). The proposals are tentative and presented as bases for discussion and consultation. The central theme of these papers is that there should be unified administration of the medical and related services in an area by one authority, an area health board, instead of the present multiple authorities. The child health service is an example cited as one which would greatly benefit from unified administration. The report of the Sheldon Committee (1967) expressed the view that the child health service of the future would become part of a family health service provided by family doctors working in groups from purpose-built health centres. The committee also advised that the organisation of the child health service called for a highly trained medical administrator. The Green Papers suggest that if the present local health authority service for young children became part of a comprehensive service administered by an area health board this would provide a good framework for implementing the recommendations of the Sheldon Committee. Discussions on the Green Papers are currently proceeding and will be influenced by the reports of the Royal Commissions on Local Government for the countries concerned. Meantime, in England, the Ministries of Health and of Social Security were merged in November 1968 to form a Department of Health and Social Security with a responsible minister, the Secretary of State for Social Services. In 1969, health functions in Wales were transferred to the Secretary of State for Wales, acting through the Health Department of the Welsh Office.

Changes in the social services for children are discussed in Chapter 17.

Child Health and Welfare in some Other Countries

FRANCE. It has already been seen that France was a pioneer in providing day nurseries, and developing infant health centres (Budin, 1892, Variot, 1893, Dufour, 1894). Today, each *département* of the country has a full-time director of health who is responsible, either through his own organisation or by delegation to semi-public or voluntary bodies, for the provision of a network of child health centres, day nurseries and other group activities. France is particularly rich in benevolent institutions which play a prominent part in the organised child health and welfare services of the country. A school health service provides close medical supervision of students at all educational establishments. The system of public assistance offers special provisions for children deprived of material and moral support and for those who are physically or mentally handicapped. An important field worker in the organisation of child health services is the *assistante sociale* broadly comparable to the health visitor in this country.

UNITED STATES OF AMERICA. In America the development of child health centres (Well Baby Conferences) was largely due, in the first instance, to the efforts of the milk reformers who, in the last decade of the nineteenth century, were divided into the advocates of the 'certified' milk movement, founded by H. L. Coit, and those who supported compulsory pasteurisation of all milk supplies. Nathan Strauss of New York was a leader of the latter group, and realising that the high infant mortality in that city was largely due to gastro-intestinal disease, he opened a milk depot in one of the poorer parts of New York city in 1893 with the active encouragement of Abraham Jacobi, the father of American paediatrics. In 1908 a municipal Bureau of Child Hygiene was established in New York, the first in the country. The following year a conference on the prevention of infant mortality was convened by the American Academy of Medicine, out of which developed the American Child Hygiene Association which, in 1922, fused with another voluntary body, the

Child Hygiene Association of America to form the American Child Health Association (dissolved 1935). A Federal Children's Bureau was founded in 1912 with general advisory, co-ordinating and research functions. Following legislation passed in 1921 there was a rapid development of state bureaux of child hygiene.

The Social Security Act (1935) gave a fresh impetus to the child health and welfare movement which was further advanced by the Social Security Amendments Act, 1965. The Amendments Act made additional provisions specifically designed to benefit children and included (a) increased authorisation for maternal and child health, crippled children and child welfare services; (b) increased funds for grants to help colleges and universities to train more professional personnel to work with handicapped children, especially the mentally retarded and those with multiple handicaps; and (c) a 5-year programme of special project grants to provide comprehensive health care and services for pre-school and school children, particularly in areas with concentrations of low income families. It was estimated that in 1966, some 35 million United States citizens were living in poverty (Van Orman, 1967), and that $3\frac{1}{2}$ million poor children under 5 years of age needed medical help but were unable to get it (Cohen, 1967). The Comprehensive Health Planning and Public Health Services Amendments Act (1966) called for a strengthening of state health agencies and for broadening and increasing the flexibility of support for health services in the community (Stewart, 1967). The problems involved in developing comprehensive paediatric care have become so challenging that part of the American Pediatric Society's Annual Conference (1968) was devoted to a symposium on the subject. In essence the present day administration of the child health services of the United States is based on state and local (county and city) health departments. Health visiting is carried out by public health nurses who combine curative with preventive and educative nursing duties. Voluntary organisations also play a prominent role in community paediatrics.

NEW ZEALAND. The development of child health services in this country is inseparably associated with Sir F. Truby King. Impressed by the considerable wastage of infant life, yet by contemporary standards a moderate wastage, he was instrumental in founding (1907) the New Zealand Society for the Health of Women and Children, given a Royal Charter in 1915, and now conveniently known as the Plunket Society. The Society is a voluntary organisation, subsidised by the State and considered an integral part of the National Health Service of New Zealand. It undertakes the provision of a national service of health visitors (Plunket nurses) who are also trained by the Society; of child health clinics, both static and mobile; of mothercraft teaching at these clinics; of courses of training for nursery nurses (Karitane nurses). Infant health work among the Maori population is largely carried out by the State Department of Health. The health services of New Zealand resemble in some respects those obtaining in Britain. In 1959 a consultative committee on infant and pre-school child health services (Finlay Report) recommended *inter alia* that a child health council should be established to regulate all agencies in the field of child health and that the Plunket Society should continue to provide Plunket and Karitane nurses. A chair of paediatrics and child health was founded at Otago Medical School on the recommendation of the committee and the first incumbent was appointed in 1966.

New Zealand pioneered a school dental service in 1920, providing free dental care for all schoolchildren and employing successfully, in the face of much opposition from dental surgeons, specially trained dental nurses to carry out treatment (Porritt, 1967).

INTERNATIONAL CHILDREN'S CENTRE. This centre, established at the Chateau de Longchamp, Paris, in 1950, was the result of a suggestion made by the French government to U.N.I.C.E.F. The centre exists to encourage study throughout the world of problems relating to childhood, to disseminate information about child welfare, and to give guidance and help to paediatricians and to paramedical and social workers by means of seminars, colloquia, study days, postgraduate courses and research scholarships. These educational activities are conducted both at the centre and in other parts of the world. The centre thus has regional activities in South America, Africa, the Eastern Mediterranean region and Asia, in association with the regional offices of W.H.O., which is represented on the centre's technical advisory board. The centre publishes the 'Courrier' a monthly periodical on medico-social problems of childhood (1950), and 'L'Enfant en milieu tropical' specially for workers in developing countries (1961). The first Director-General of the centre was Professor Robert Debré.

H. P. TAIT

References

Official Publications (H.M.S.O.)

CENTRAL ADVISORY COUNCIL FOR EDUCATION (ENGLAND), (1967). *Children and their Primary Schools.* 2 volumes. (Plowden Report).

CENTRAL HEALTH SERVICES COUNCIL, (1967). *Child Welfare Centres.* Report of sub-committee of Standing Medical Advisory Committee. (Sheldon Report).

CENTRAL OFFICE OF INFORMATION, (1967). *Children in Britain.* Pamphlet No. 34.

—— (1968). *Health Services in Britain.* Pamphlet No. 20.

DEPARTMENT OF EDUCATION AND SCIENCE. *Reports of Chief Medical Officer, 'The Health of the School Child'.* Latest report deals with 1966–8 (1969).

GREEN PAPER, (1968). *Administrative Reorganisation of the Scottish Health Services.*

—— (1968). *National Health Service.* Administrative structure of the medical and related services in England and Wales. (Withdrawn)

GREEN PAPER, (1970). *Future structure of the National Health Service.*

MINISTRY OF HEALTH, (1956). *An Inquiry into Health Visiting.* Report of a working party on the field of work, training and recruitment of health visitors. (Jameson Report).

—— *Reports of the Chief Medical Officer, 'On the state of the public health'.* That report for 1967 (published 1968) is the last from the Ministry before merging into Department of Health and Social Security. The first report from the new Department covers 1968 (1969).

SCOTTISH HOME AND HEALTH DEPARTMENT, *Health and Welfare in Scotland.* Annual reports.

—— (1964). *Children and Young Persons, Scotland* (Cmnd 2306). Kilbrandon Report.

—— (1967). *Dietary Study of 4,365 Scottish Infants, 1965.* Study by G C. Arneil. Scottish Health Service Studies, No. 5.

SEEBOHM REPORT, (1968). *Report of the Committee on Local Authority and Allied Personal Social Services* (Cmnd 3707). Committee set up by Secretaries of State for several government departments.

WHITE PAPER, (1965). *The Child, the Family and the Young Offender.* (England and Wales).

—— (1966). *Social Work and the Community.* (Scotland). (Cmnd 3065).

—— (1968). *Children in Trouble.* (England and Wales). (Cmnd 3601).

Other Publications

FAMILY PLANNING ASSOCIATION. *Family Planning.* Published quarterly, contains numerous articles on development of family planning both in Britain and overseas.

MALONEY, W. J. (1954). *George and John Armstrong of Castleton.* Edinburgh: Livingstone.

McCLEARY, G. F. (1905). *Infant Mortality and Infants' Milk Depots.* London: King & Son.

—— (1933). *Early History of the Infant Welfare Movement.* London: Lewis.

—— (1935). *The Maternity and Child Welfare Movement.* London: King & Son.

POLITICAL AND ECONOMIC PLANNING, (1948). *Population Policy in Great Britain, a Report.* Chapter 3 gives good history of family planning movement in Britain.

France

WORLD HEALTH ORGANISATION, (1956). *Health and Social Workers in England and France.* Report by Laroque, P. and Daley, W. A. Regional Office for Europe. (Not for sale.)

New Zealand

PORRITT, A. (1967). History of medicine in New Zealand. *Med. Hist.,* 11, 334.

ROYAL NEW ZEALAND SOCIETY FOR THE HEALTH OF WOMEN AND CHILDREN (Plunket Society) (1953). *Origin and Development of the Work of the Society.*

—— (1968). *Annual Report of Council for 1967–68.*

United States

AMERICAN PEDIATRIC SOCIETY, (1968). Future forms of medical care for children. A symposium. *Am. J. Dis. Child.,* 116, 458.

COHEN, W. J. (1967). Meeting the health needs of the nation. *Public Health Rep.,* 82, 565. U.S. Dept. Health, Education and Welfare.

GARDNER, J. W. (1966). Welfare provisions of medicare. *Public Health Rep.,* 81, 11. (annotation). U.S. Dept Health, Education and Welfare.

STEWART, W. H. (1967). Partnership for planning. *Public Health Rep.,* 82, 395. U.S. Dept. Health, Education and Welfare.

International Children's Centre

INTERNATIONAL CHILDREN'S CENTRE, (1960). *Structure and Activities.* Paris: I.C.C.

—— (1968). *Report for 1967.* I.C.C.

15 The Infant and Pre-School Child Health Services

MENTION has already been made of the suggestion in the Green Papers on the reorganisation of the National Health Service in England and in Wales that the present child health services of local health authorities might provide a good framework on which to build a comprehensive child health service administered by an area health board. The Sheldon Report (1967) visualised the eventual disappearance of local authority child health services as separate entities and their absorption into family health services provided by general practitioners working in groups with local authority nursing staff attached and all operating from purpose-built health centres. There are now signs of a more rapid growth of health centres. In England and Wales in 1968 there were 83 centres in operation, 69 in the process of building, 68 approved and 104 being planned. In Scotland, progress is being made towards developing family health services by various systems of family doctor/local authority nurse attachments operating from purpose-built health centres and other premises. Both in its present form and its future form the aim of any health service for children must always be the integration of all fields of endeavour in the curative and preventive spheres, giving due place to the many voluntary organisations active in the child health and welfare fields, and working closely with the social services.

The existing medical facilities now provided are shared by three statutory bodies.

REGIONAL HOSPITAL BOARDS. These boards provide a hospital service, which includes outpatient departments and convalescent home facilities. In addition, a consultant service for hospital and domiciliary care is provided. There are 14 regions in England and Wales and 5 in Scotland. All save one—the northern region of Scotland—include the medical school of a university, with which the consultant and hospital service is linked.

LOCAL EXECUTIVE COUNCILS. A medical practitioner service is provided by these councils, as well as dental, pharmaceutical and general ophthalmic services. General practitioners may be employed by local health authorities on a sessional basis for child health clinics; other practitioners who conduct child health sessions at their own surgeries or at health centres may receive the assistance of health visitors from the local health authority. Approved doctors provide domiciliary maternity services for women on their own lists, and such doctors work closely with the midwives employed by local health authorities. In addition, in the area of each local executive council in England and Wales there is a local obstetrics committee which keeps a list of local practitioners specially experienced in obstetrics (general practitioner obstetricians) and who are prepared to respond to any emergency calls by midwives.

LOCAL HEALTH AUTHORITIES. Each local health authority must provide a health visiting service. The functions of health visitors include the giving of advice on the care of young children, expectant and nursing mothers, and on measures to promote health and prevent the spread of infection (N.H.S. Acts). In addition, the local health authority must 'make arrangements for the care, including in particular dental care, of expectant and nursing mothers and of children who have not attained the age of 5 years and are not attending primary schools maintained by a local education authority'. The local health authority is the local authority to which notification of births is made. The extent and scope of a local health authority's service for the infant and pre-school child depend on the nature and needs of the area to be served. In larger authorities a senior medical officer, experienced in child health work, is usually appointed in administrative control of the service, in smaller areas the medical officer of health or his deputy assumes administrative responsibility.

The following may constitute part of such a service.

Health Visiting

The Council for the Training of Health Visitors in a pamphlet (1967) on the functions of the health visitor defines them thus: 'The health visitor is a nurse with post-registration qualification who provides a continuing service to families and individuals in the community. Her work has five main aspects—(1) the prevention of mental, physical and emotional ill-health and its consequences; (2) early detection of ill-health and the surveillance of high risk groups; (3) recognition and identification of need and mobilisation of appropriate resources where necessary; (4) health education; (5) provision of care; this will include support during periods of stress, and advice and guidance in cases of illness as well as in the care and management of children. The health visitor is not, however, actively engaged in technical nursing procedures.' This comprehensive list of her duties might be modified regarding her non-engagement in technical nursing activities for in many rural areas the health visitor combines the duties of home nurse and even domiciliary midwife with that of health visitor. But, whether engaged in health visiting alone or in combined duties, the pivot around which her work revolves is home visiting.

Her predominant activities are still concerned with maternal and child health. In many areas the health visitor is responsible for both the pre-school and school-age periods and so continuity of supervision of the child is assured. Where the pre-school and school health services are separate the closest contact must be maintained and arrangements made for the transfer of records and information. By reason of her close contact with families in which there are young children the health visitor is particularly well placed to recognise early signs of failure in the family which may lead to disruption of normal home life. The health visitor also has important functions in carrying out simple screening tests to aid the early diagnosis of handicapping conditions, *e.g.* taking blood for the Guthrie test for phenylketonuria, testing for congenital dislocation of the hip, for deafness, for squint, etc., and in the supervision of children on the vulnerable or 'at risk' register and of handicapped children. Following the early diagnosis of a disability in infancy or childhood the health visitor, in concert with the family doctor and by reason of her liaison with hospital or assessment centre, can do much to help and encourage the parents of such children by creating a favourable atmosphere in the home.

The closer association of the health visitor with the family doctor is being advanced rapidly. Oxford city was one of the first local health authorities to pioneer a general practitioner/health visitor attachment scheme (1956) and Warin (1968) described the results of complete attachment of all local health authority nursing staff to general practices there. A Scottish Home and Health Department circular (H. & W.S. 29/1967) urged local health authorities to develop general practitioner/ local authority co-operation including the attachment of health visitors, home nurses, domiciliary midwives, etc., to practices. Anderson *et al.* (1967) dealt fully with the subject of attachments, and Ambler *et al.* (1968) presented a detailed account. Confusion has arisen, however, over the use of terms. Anderson *et al.* (1967) defined 'attachment' as the situation where the health visitor is responsible for all the patients on the lists of specified general practitioners within the local authority boundary (*i.e.* traditional geographical districts have been given up), and 'liaison' where the health visitor is responsible both for a geographical district and for the patients on the lists of specified general practitioners. Where patients live outside the health visitor's district, though within the local authority boundary, she does not herself visit them but is responsible for liaison between the general practitioner and the appropriate health visitor. Lewis (1968) used the term 'linkage' to denote the situation where groups of health visitors work in geographically defined areas of high density in urban areas and have as their bases health centres or local authority clinics. At these centres local practitioners can always get in touch with the health visitors by telephone or by visiting so as to discuss problems with each other. Parish (1968) described the evolution in his practice from linkage to attachment, and Brewin (1968) and Clow (1968) described developments in the north of England. Abel (1969) published an important study on nursing attachments to general practice. Thus some progress is being made towards the goal of the general practitioner providing a family health service as envisaged in the Sheldon Report.

Two recent problems face the health visitor. The first is the reappearance of rickets both in immigrant and indigenous children in this country. Arneil's dietary survey of Scottish infants (1967) served to emphasise the urgent need for more intensive and continued health supervision of young children and the better education of their mothers, particularly on nutritional matters. The second is the need for advice and help for the immigrant population of the country. There is a real urgency about this and greater opportunities must be afforded to health visitors, social workers and others to learn something of race relations, cultures, and the difficulties facing immigrants (Galloway, 1967). In many areas there are voluntary committees and specially appointed officers who are knowledgeable and experienced in the field of social and health work among immigrants (Peppard, 1964). Gans (1964) stressed the value of the health visitor working in a district with a high immigrant population and recommended that more coloured health visitors should be employed in areas where the coloured population was high.

Home Nursing

The National Health Service Acts require local health authorities to provide a nursing service for those, including infants and young children, who need nursing in their own homes. The Committee on the Welfare of Children in Hospital (1959) recommended an extension of special nursing facilities for the sick child at home. Gillet (1954) pioneered a special children's home nursing unit at Rotherham in 1949, and Jerman (1965) described the work of a Home Care Unit associated with St. Mary's Hospital, Paddington, London. Such schemes have served to emphasise the need for the closest association between family doctor and local health authority services with the help, as necessary, of hospital and specialist services (Parish, 1968).

Community Nursing Service

The Royal Commission on Medical Education (1968) foresaw the future development of general practice taking the form of large group practices, *e.g.*, with up to 12 doctors, working from health centres with well-trained and organised staff including nursing staff. But manpower and finance affect development and plans of every kind and so within the local health authority nursing services it is important to ensure that skills are concentrated where most needed. Ministry of Health and Scottish Home and Health Department circulars (L.H.A.L. 3/67 and H. & W.S. 1/1968 respectively) urged local authorities to consider the employment of ancillary help in their nursing services and subsequent attempts to use such help have proved fruitful, although some authorities appear reluctant to employ less skilled staff (NASEN, 1968). Extension of the general practitioner/health visitor attachment system is rapidly developing for home nurses and domiciliary midwives as well as for ancillary staff so that forms of family health services are being organised. A recent example of a family health service team in one local authority area consisted of 5 general practitioners in a group practice, 2 health visitors, 2 home nurses, 1 midwife, 2 part-time nurses, bath attendant and 2 relief nurses for emergencies.

The Social Work (Scotland) Act, 1968 and the proposals made in the Local Authority Social Services Bill (1970) make it imperative that the functions of the health visitor be reviewed, for both the Act and the Bill clearly indicate that the main functions of the health visitor and the social worker are distinct and their roles incompatible in the same person. The idea, therefore, of the health visitor becoming also an all-purpose social worker in general practice is misplaced. In the light of these views, Draper *et al.* (1969) discuss four different roles that the health visitor of the future may play as a member of the community nursing service.

Domiciliary Care of the Infant of Low Birth Weight

Recent studies (Warkany *et al.*, 1961, Gruenwald, 1965) have emphasised the need to distinguish between infants of low birth weight who are born prematurely and those born near term. In the former group of infants problems of immaturity are paramount, including liability to respiratory distress syndrome and susceptibility to infection, in the latter group hypoglycaemia is a particular risk which may result in serious neurological complications. The influence of low birth weight as a factor in perinatal mortality has been emphasised by Brimblecombe *et al.* (1968), and Butler and Alberman (1969). Some local health authorities provide a particular service for the domiciliary care of these infants including facilities for immediate resuscitation, the loan of special equipment, feeding bottles, mucus extractors, etc., as well as the attendance of specially trained midwives or health visitors capable of teaching the mothers the special care required. For infants needing transfer to hospital specially equipped ambulances or cars are used, and, where possible, the mother is admitted to hospital along with her infant. The closest liaison must exist among hospital, family doctor and local health authority on such matters as discharge home of the infants and the need for their continued supervision by doctor, midwife or health visitor. Since infants of low birth weight come under the category of infants 'at risk' to handicapping conditions, efficient long term follow-up is important (see Chapter 4).

Protective Inoculations

The preliminary report (1966) of the Medical Research Council's Measles Vaccines Committee on the large scale trial of measles vaccines was followed by a report (1968) covering a total period of 2 years and 9 months, which confirmed the earlier findings that a substantial protection against measles was given by the two vaccine schedules adopted in the trials. These schedules comprised (1) live vaccine given alone, one injection, and (2) inactivated vaccine, one injection, followed by an injection of live vaccine. There was a greater protective effect from the live vaccine given alone and the report (1968) concluded that there was a strong case for its use, particularly as it had a relatively low reaction rate and only one injection was needed. The follow-up study is being continued so as to determine the possible need for the administration and timing of reinforcing doses of vaccine. The Central Health Services Council's Joint Committee on Vaccination and Immunisation, after considering all available evidence on measles vaccination, including the M.R.C. trials, recommended the introduction of measles vaccination and steps were taken to do this in the spring of 1968.

Meantime, the Joint Committee on Vaccination and Immunisation endorsed the recommendation of an advisory group set up to consider schedules of immunisation that a single schedule could with advantage replace the alternative schedules previously suggested. This schedule, modified to include measles vaccination during the second year of life, was introduced in 1968 (see Chapter 11).

It is important that parents should be properly informed of the inoculations given to their children and the diseases against which these measures are designed to protect. A medical record card is issued to N.H.S. patients for the use of medical practitioners in which are entered the various immunisations carried out and this card is kept in the possession of the parents of the child. No personal record card of inoculations is officially available to local health authorities but most use one. Health visitors also keep a careful note of the immunisation histories of all young children in their districts.

Local health authorities also make arrangements for BCG vaccination of susceptible (tuberculin-negative) young children who are contacts of known cases of tuberculosis, and the newborn infants of tuberculous mothers. Newborns may be vaccinated in the maternity hospital or admitted for the purpose to residential homes provided by the local authority. Older children may be vaccinated at chest clinics and, if home conditions are unfavourable, temporarily boarded-out with foster-parents until immunity develops. Some of these children may not be able to return home after converting to a positive skin test owing to adverse home conditions and so must remain with their foster-parents until circumstances improve. Such boarding-out arrangements are usually made by the medical officer of health in consultation with the children's officer, the family doctor concerned being kept fully informed of all developments. Special record cards are kept for BCG vaccinations but general practitioners are precluded from using BCG vaccine in contra-distinction to other prophylactics.

Since no form of immunisation or vaccination is compulsory, continuous endeavour must be made by health visitors and doctors to persuade parents to have their children protected. Constant propaganda by talks, newspaper articles, magazine features, leaflets, films, posters and the like is required to keep the need for protection constantly before parents.

Child Health Centres

The size and staff of a child health centre depend upon local circumstances and whilst in sparsely populated rural areas it may be only possible to hold a session once a week or even less frequently, in a borrowed building, in urban areas it is desirable to have a specially constructed building and to have the centre open more frequently. Mobile clinics are used by some local health authorities for use in rural areas and in outlying housing estates of towns and cities. The Sheldon Report (1967) was rightly critical of the unsuitability and unattractiveness of some rented premises such as halls and similar buildings. Some centres are adapted for the purpose but others, in increasing numbers, are purpose-built. Wherever the centre is, however, the premises must be clean, as attractive as possible, adequately heated, ventilated and lighted, and a friendly welcoming atmosphere must pervade so that mothers will be encouraged to bring their infants and young children to the centre.

Some centres may be attached or adjacent to district general hospitals and so in close proximity to consultant services but in most instances will be separate from hospitals and situated in the areas they are designed to serve. For any centre the site should be large enough to permit of future expansion to meet new needs. The approaches must be good, conveniently accessible by public transport, and access to the centre itself easy. Car parking facilities are necessary and an outdoor paved or grassed play space for toddlers should be available adjacent to the playroom and fenced or otherwise guarded. In planning the layout of a centre, as a separate entity, or as part of a health centre, provision should be made as outlined in the Ministry of Health's Local Authority Building Note No. 3 (L.H.A. Clinics) (1965, amended 1968). The basic accommodation is as follows:

1. Pram shelter, situated near entrance path and within sight of waiting hall.
2. Entrance lobby. This should be large enough to permit people to pass freely to reception office, waiting hall and other parts of the centre.
3. Reception/Records office. Should be a separate room if the centre is large but in a smaller centre a table and chair in waiting hall will suffice for the clerkess.
4. Food sales and storage space. The Sheldon Report viewed the sale of dried milk, proprietary infant foods and cereals at child health centres with disfavour and recommended that if a local authority decided to undertake such sales it should be organised as a separate activity and staffed by paid clerical staff or voluntary workers.
5. Kitchen. This should be small to provide light refreshments for those attending the centre. It may be linked with the food sales room for service by one person. It can be used for cookery demonstrations and should be planned so that one side can be opened to allow a small group seated in the hall to watch the demonstration.
6. Sanitary accommodation for clientele should be within easy reach of waiting hall and fixtures for disposable towels are needed.
7. Waiting hall. Formerly this was the largest room of the centre but modern trends are towards reducing it in size to release a larger area for the health education room. Nevertheless, it still remains the hub of the centre. It is advantageous if the hall and health education room can be separated by movable walls so that the two rooms can be used as a single large hall for meetings, etc. The records office, kitchen and health education room should open directly off the waiting hall. There should be facilities for poster displays and demonstrations. The waiting hall either alone or with the health education room may also be used as a play-centre or creche when not required for clinic sessions.
8. Health education room. The main activity here, in the room formerly called the weighing room, is health education. It can also be used for weighing children and expectant mothers and should be suitable for relaxation classes for some 8 to 12 mothers.
9. Storage space for health education material—deep cupboards or small store should be supplied near (8).
10. Playroom. Useful for toddlers playing during mothercraft and health education talks. It adjoins the waiting hall and should have access to outdoor play space.
11. Health visitor's/midwife's room. This should adjoin (8) and serve a dual purpose, being used by health visitor or midwife during clinic sessions for individual interviewing.
12. Clinical room and waiting bay. This should be close to (8), (11) and (13). It should have access to a subsidiary exit for use during immunisation sessions, and cubicles for mothers attending antenatal sessions. Good ventilation is particularly necessary throughout the area.
13. Doctor's consulting room.

14. General purpose room which may be used for other local authority activities at the centre, e.g. chiropody.
15. Storage accommodation for linen.

Office and staff accommodation should include one or more health visitor's rooms for interviewing, consultations and home visiting records storage, a common room where staff, general practitioners and others working together may meet, staff cloakroom and sanitary accommodation, etc. The centre should be planned with a minimum of corridors, and with adequate central heating and water supplies. A separate dental unit may with advantage be incorporated in the layout.

Staff

Medical sessions at child health centres are held at stated times, usually in the afternoons and sometimes in the forenoons. Gans (1964) showed the value of evening sessions for the children of immigrant working mothers and the importance of the attendance at these sessions of the health visitors of the district in which the centre is situated. The medical staff may be general practitioners engaged on a sessional basis, registrars from children's hospitals, or medical officers of the local health authority. In some areas these local authority medical officers are engaged in both the pre-school and school health services and this is most advantageous but where this is not the case, arrangements should be made for the interchange of medical officers so that they may gain experience in both branches of child health supervision and so establish a co-operative spirit between these two services of a local authority.

The training of a doctor working in the child health services has become of increasing importance and special vocational postgraduate study is essential particularly in child development, screening techniques and ascertainment of subnormality, and assessment. Courses are offered in this field by the Society of Medical Officers of Health, university child health departments and other establishments.

The nursing staff consists of one or more health visitors whose districts the centre serves. These health visitors will be in attendance during the medical sessions at which mothers and young children for whose home visiting they are responsible are due to attend. In some centres, especially large ones serving wide areas, a senior health visitor will be in attendance daily for advising mothers and arranging appointments for the medical sessions. Sometimes health visitor sessions are held at stated times other than those when medical sessions are held and appointments are not usually made in these instances.

A dental officer and attendant, usually from the school dental service, may be present daily or on a sessional basis if the centre is equipped with dental facilities. Dental care is a priority service which local health authorities must offer for the benefit of pre-school children, and so suitable arrangements must be made for this service to be readily available.

Clerical help is required for keeping attendance registers and filing case-records, for distributing welfare foods, and for the preparation of teas. Sometimes voluntary helpers assist in or undertake these duties.

The Functions and Work of a Child Health Centre

These were fully discussed in the Sheldon Report (1967). Basically the functions are supervisory, diagnostic and educational, with prevention the theme. The centre, however, does not supply the answer to all the problems of child health and care. The prevention of home accidents, for example, can only be tackled adequately by the health visitor in her home visiting when she is aware of the conditions prevailing in the home. Consequently, the child health centre must be kept in proper perspective.

SUPERVISORY FUNCTIONS. (a) Routine medical examinations of children presumed healthy. These examinations should be designed to enable the doctor to estimate the child's physical, mental and emotional development and should coincide with the ages of the child at which tests for certain specific handicaps are most suitably performed. The examinations should, therefore, be carefully spaced, for to make them too frequent might detract from their thoroughness. An appointment system is essential but elasticity must be allowed for a mother to bring her child to the centre at other times when she feels in need of advice.

The first examination should take place between 2 and 6 weeks of age, preferably not later, and the examination should include screening tests for congenital dislocation of the hip, talipes, spinal curvature, etc. The second examination is best made about 6 months of age when the first screening test for hearing should be carried out and a third examination could profitably take place about 9 months. Thereafter, regular examinations should take place at the second, third and fourth birthdays when, in addition to the overall examinations and discussion with the mother, the cover test for squint should be performed. Tests for hearing should be repeated at the third and fourth examinations when dental inspections could profitably be included also. The fourth birthday examination should be regarded as the pre-school examination and the findings, including visual acuity, made available to the school health service. All measurements of height and weight at these regular medical examinations should be accurately recorded and entered in the metric system, although conversion tables may be available to render readings into inches and pounds if desired. The former ritual of frequent weighing so characteristic of the early days of the child health movement is no longer necessary or desirable. All weighing should be in the nude. Increments in height are more significant than gains in weight. Height measurements may with advantage be combined with measuring of the heights of the parents.

(b) Advice on nutrition and hygiene. This is still of great importance and the need has been emphasised by Arneil (1967). Immigrants present special problems with language, cultural and other difficulties as mentioned previously. In many instances it will be essential for the health visitor to pay follow-up visits in the home to ensure that the advice given at the centre is both understood and put into operation.

(c) Immunisations. The recommended schedule of immunisations should be followed. It is a matter of choice whether special immunisation sessions are held or the inoculations performed for limited periods before or after the appointment sessions.

DIAGNOSTIC FUNCTIONS. The early detection of physical, mental and emotional defects is vitally important. Not only should children on the vulnerable or 'at risk' children's register be carefully examined but also children with no known precipitating factors, as they may develop defects. The danger, too, of defects being multiple must be borne in mind. All defects discovered or failure to pass screening tests necessitate referral, through the family doctor, to hospital or assessment centre for comprehensive diagnosis and treatment.

Case-records are important. There is an urgent need for a standardised national record card for entering the findings at examination. The Sheldon Report recommended that a national card should be devised. Meantime the record card designed by the Society of Medical Officers of Health should be used which enables the centre medical officer and the general practitioner to record the developmental progress of infants and young children on four parallels of development—locomotion and posture; vision and hand and eye co-ordination; speech and hearing; and social behaviour and play, as well as the physical examination findings.

EDUCATIONAL FUNCTIONS. Not only is individual teaching of mothers carried out by the doctors and health visitors during consultations but group teaching is also undertaken. Short talks may be given by the health visitor to small groups of mothers during a clinic session. Series of weekly or fortnightly meetings may be arranged by the senior health visitor of the centre at which talks, films, and demonstrations are given on subjects ranging from breast-feeding, protective inoculations, accident prevention, sleep, common infections and behaviour problems to cookery and practical garment making. Some of these meetings may be held in the evenings when fathers can act as baby-sitters at home. Discussion groups for fathers should also be organised, and where practicable, joint meetings with mothers and fathers. These last are particularly helpful for the parents of handicapped children, for they are in especial need of help and support and benefit from the interchange of experiences with others having similar problems. For talks, free use should be made of blackboard, charts, film-strips, flannel-graphs, and films.

With so many general practitioners organising child health sessions at their surgeries or at health centres, health visitors may, if the doctors so desire, attend these sessions and assist the doctors in their work. With attachment systems, this is already a feature.

Day Care of the Pre-School Child

The present is a period of considerable experiment in and expansion of various forms of day care, part-time and full-time, for young children. This has been brought about by the progressive closure of day nurseries by local health authorities and the virtual cessation of nursery school expansion as part of governmental economic policy since 1945. Egan (1966) discussed the need for a revision of views on the present role of local health authority day care facilities for young children. The Plowden

Report (1967) dealt at length with the need for nursery education, especially part-time, of children before compulsory school age, the Seebohm Report (1968) endorsed these views, and Yudkin (1968) in a revealing report showed the inadequacy of statutory provision and the dangers of uncontrolled growth of unsupervised forms of day care throughout the country. The trend among women which already exists towards continuing to work after marriage will probably continue and even increase as will the tendency to return to work when the children are older. Government has conceded (1968) that certain parts of the country are urgently in need of day care facilities such as day nurseries and nursery schools and has allocated funds to improve facilities in these areas. Failure on the part of the authorities to provide adequate facilities for infants and especially for young children has led to increasing interest in forms of day care on the part of parents and voluntary organisations. The type of provision made for such care has been determined by the needs of the children in a particular area.

The home backgrounds of children vary greatly and this is reflected in the variety of group activities now in operation, all of which are designed to help the mother and supplement the home by meeting the needs of the children whatever these needs may be. For some children the most urgent need is for the companionship of other children of the same age, e.g. only children, for others living in confined housing conditions, high flats, etc., space in which to play safely and in freedom but under supervision. For yet others, e.g. children from culturally deprived backgrounds, a daily period in the care of persons who understand their needs and whose relationship with the children is helpful and understanding. The needs of handicapped or backward children as also those of immigrant children must not be forgotten. Thus we have organisations such as the Save the Children Fund (founded 1919), the Pre-School Playgroups Association (founded 1962) and the National Society for Mentally Handicapped Children (founded 1950) which organise and help with the promotion of nursery groups. The Pre-School Playgroups Association has drawn up an admirable Code of Standards for playgroups. In addition to these there are many local organisations which assist in the provision of such groups for pre-school children, e.g. the Camden (London) Committee for Community Relations which has organised three multiracial playgroups in the borough.

Over the years considerable controversy has raged on the part played by and value of various forms of day care for young children but in particular day nurseries. It is generally conceded however that all forms of properly supervised day care have a positive value. The children attending them are given a sense of security and communal living, freedom, and a friendly but firm and unobtrusive control exerted by the staffs who understand and respond to the children's needs. Day nurseries were never intended to cater for the mass of young children. Indeed, their role has always been a modest one. Day nurseries are required for a small proportion of young children—those of single parents, of separated parents, those from families where the mother must work because of the father's disability, and those from homes where the mother is ill or in hospital or where conditions are such that break-up of the family seems imminent unless the children are admitted to a nursery, or where the home conditions are overcrowded or otherwise unsatisfactory. Children requiring supervision and care for physical, emotional or other conditions may be cited as further suitable candidates for day nursery care. The period of stay at the nursery obviously depends upon the circumstances surrounding each child—some may need only part care, others full day care, and for varying periods of time. Realisation of these various situations has led local authorities to devise systems of priority for admission to day nurseries largely based on the above types of case. Two universities at least, Manchester and Edinburgh, provide day nursery services for staff members and students.

The various forms of group day care may be classified as follows:

Day Nurseries

The National Health Service Acts gave powers to local health authorities to provide or to aid the provision of day nurseries and permitted a charge to be made only for meals or food supplied at the nurseries. Amending legislation (1952) empowered authorities to make a comprehensive charge for all the services provided at day nurseries. Recommendations concerning day nurseries, whether provided by local health authorities or privately administered have been issued from the Department of Health and Social Security and the Scottish Home and Health Department and the following is based on these recommendations.

Location

A day nursery should be situated as centrally as possible in the area it is required to serve; it should be within easy reach of public transport; and may, with advantage, be sited close to or form part of a health centre.

Premises

The number of children should not normally exceed 40 to 50 but as an economy measure larger nurseries (up to 110 children, Edinburgh) may be planned, designed to accommodate several such groups cared for separately but making use of communal staff rooms, kitchen and laundry. Standards of accommodation have been laid down officially and the following is based on these recommendations.

1. Entrance hall with facilities to display health education material.
2. Matron's office for interviewing parents. This should have an annexe to serve for medical or isolation purposes if separate accommodation is not provided for these.
3. Nurseries. Generally three have been recommended (infants, 1 to 2 year olds, 2 to 5 year olds), allowing as minima, 40 sq. feet per infant, 30 sq. feet per 1 to 2 year old, and 25 sq. feet for each 2 to 5 year old. Recent experiments with grouping children of mixed ages from infancy to 5 years, centred round one or more members of staff to whom the children in the group can look as 'mother' figures, have been pioneered by Epsom (1969) at Southwark, London, and Harding (1969) at Camden, London. The results achieved have been most encouraging. Such a scheme facilitated more flexibility in admissions, contact between children from the same

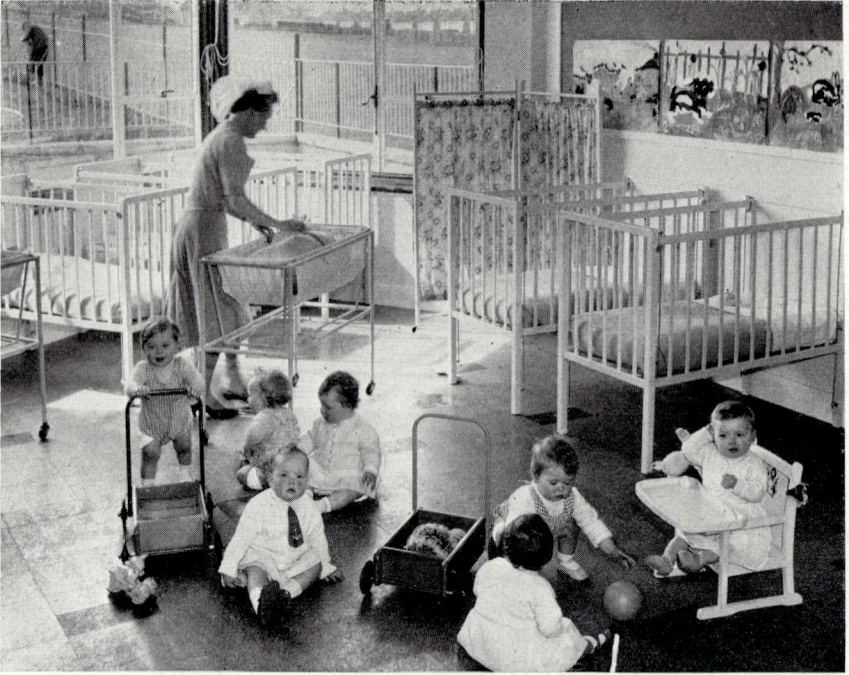

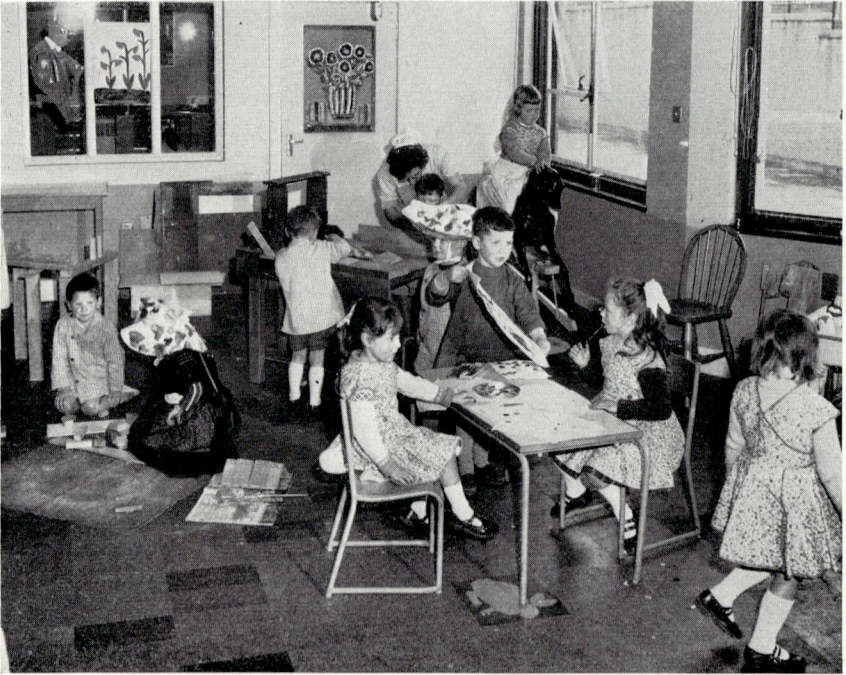

FIGS. 78 and 79. Infants and pre-school children in a
purpose-built day nursery.

families, and between handicapped children and normal children in the same setting.

4. Cloakroom and toilet facilities should include arrangements for keeping children's outdoor clothing and drying them in wet weather. Toilet requirements should be fitted as follows: For each unit of 10 babies and younger children—1 bathing sink, rack for chamber pots, 1 lowest level water-closet, slop hopper, fixtures for individual towels. For each unit of 20 older children—4 low level water-closets, 5 low level washhand basins, bath can be shared by 2 units, fixtures for towels, storage for toothbrushes. In both units a washbasin and towelmaster fitment are needed for staff.

5. Kitchen, scullery, larder and dry-store room. Dishwashing machines are advantageous but the facilities must conform to the Food Hygiene Regulations.

6. Milk feed preparation room.

7. Laundry and drying facilities. Separate boiler for napkins is essential and covered sterilisable containers for soiled garments.

8. Linen and airing cupboards.

9. Housemaid's cupboard.

10. Staff accommodation, including cloakroom with individual lockers, toilet facilities, based on 1 water-closet and 1 washhand basin per 8 staff, and an incinerator. Dining and sitting room with study room if the nursery is a training centre. To emphasise the importance of hand hygiene after use of the toilet, notices should be put up in the toilets with the caption 'Now wash your hands'.

11. Covered pram store.

General Requirements

Windows should be low enough for the children to see out and French windows are useful. Care must be taken to safeguard the children against swinging doors. and jutting open windows. Central heating or underfloor heating should be provided but supplementary heating is useful in the playrooms. Fixed fire or radiator guards are necessary and sun-blinds are desirable. Adequate hot water and drinking water supplies are essential, all hot water taps used by the children being thermostatically controlled at a safe temperature. Proper means of fire-escape are necessary. A garden play space and a hard surface playground for dry and wet weather respectively, and protection from hot sun should be provided. Storage place for toys and equipment both indoors and outdoors should be provided. Howard and Pank (1968) outlined design standards and criteria for nurseries for use by the Save the Children Fund in their work.

Staff

The matron must be trained and experienced in the care of healthy children She may be a state registered nurse or certificated nursery nurse previously experienced as a deputy matron. In a training nursery, the matron must have teaching ability. A warden or play-mistress is required especially if the nursery caters for 2 to 5 year olds. The remainder of the staff consists of: a deputy matron, who should be a certificated nursery nurse of at least 2 years' experience since qualification, certificated nursery nurses, nursery assistants, and nursery nurse trainees if the nursery is a training establishment recognised by the National Nursery

Examination Board or the Scottish Nursery Nurses Examination Board. Exclusive of domestic staff, the ratio of full-time staff to children must not be less than 1:5, three students in training being regarded as equivalent to one full-time member of staff. The domestic staff should include an experienced cook and a sufficient number of full-time or part-time workers.

The nursery staff by their friendly attitude should seek to establish cordial relations with both children and their parents. They should be able to help the children's own mental development without undue interference and, while recognising the children's limitations, to give the necessary help when required. They should be able to provide or improvise materials and stimulus for the children's growing mental needs. The children's wellbeing is provided for through proper feeding arrangements, adequately regulated warmth, clothing and activity, a high standard of cleanliness in kitchen, bathroom and playroom, and an understanding of their needs for fresh air, outdoor play and proper ventilation.

Daily Nursery Routine

Briefly, the nursery day includes time for play both indoors and out of doors; for music, rhymes, stories and games; for washing, and use of lavatories without hurry or crowding; for informal and more formal meals; and for sleep, rest and quietness.

Staff Contacts with Parents

Regular contact with parents is essential and the matron or her deputy should personally receive each child daily from the parent and hand him over again in the evening. Mothers' meetings or clubs organised in connection with the nursery are valuable in that instruction, help and advice may be offered to the mothers and discussion take place on matters pertaining to child health and care. Fathers may also be interested in the nursery and their help enlisted to make and repair equipment and toys.

Health Measures

All children must be medically examined on admission to the nursery and at regular intervals thereafter, records of each child being kept. The record card used at child health centres suits admirably and permits of more uniform record-keeping as regards development, physical, mental, social and emotional. Examinations are usually carried out by medical officers of the local health department and these doctors visit the nurseries frequently, *e.g.* once weekly. For emergencies, arrangements may be made for the services of a neighbouring general practitioner. Any child thought to be suffering from an infectious disease should be excluded from the nursery, or isolated there until seen by the doctor. Hence the importance of the matron or her deputy receiving the child in the morning and knowing where the parent may be found during the day. The diet for the children must be adequate and suitable, including the full allowance of milk and supplementary vitamin preparations as provided under the national scheme. It is also useful to display the week's menu in the nursery entrance hall so that parents may see the type of diet given to the children. Arrangements for the midday rest by the provision of stretcher beds and of blankets are also necessary. The health of the staff, both nursing and domestic, requires supervision and all members of staff should be examined once yearly by mass miniature radiography.

Private Day Nurseries, Child-Minders, and Daily Guardians

Private day nurseries, run by factories and by individuals, must be registered and inspected by local health authorities under the Nurseries and Child-Minders Regulation Act, 1948 as amended by the Health Services and Public Health Act, 1968. Child-minders, who must also be registered, are persons who for reward look after one or more children, to whom they are not related, for 2 hours in the aggregate in any day or for any longer period not exceeding 6 days. Some local health authorities have adopted an arrangement whereby the authority (a) pay child-minders a small weekly sum in return for their willingness to accept children in the local authority's priority groups and placed with the minders by the authority and, in appropriate cases, pay the minders' charges for caring for such children and (b) arrange and pay a reasonable charge for children in the authority's priority groups to receive day care in nurseries or part-time nursery groups run by private or voluntary bodies. There has been a considerable increase within recent years in the number of private nurseries and child-minders. In 1968 there were registered under the Nurseries and Child Minders Regulation Act, 1948, in England and Wales, 5,849 nurseries with 146,098 places, and 5,802 minders caring for 47,208 children. This compares with 339 private nurseries and 468 child-minders providing places for 9,872 and 3,506 children respectively in 1951. Special training and experience are now required of local authority staff charged with enforcing the amended provisions of the Nurseries and Child-Minders Regulation Act, 1948.

NURSERY SCHOOLS AND CLASSES. These are described in Chapter 16 on the School Health Service.

Toddlers' Play-Centres or Clubs, Nursery Play-Centres or Play-Groups, Part-Time Creches

There is a bewildering series of names given to these groups of pre-school children. Voluntary bodies as well as churches and organised groups of parents are particularly active in the field of part-time care of young children. Local health authorities may provide play-centres or part-time creches at child health centres at times other than the regular clinic sessions. Some play-centres are held at community centres in connection with new housing estates, in the social or recreation room of a block of high flats, or for very small groups in the homes of the mothers. The objects of the play-centres, clubs, creches or whatever name may be given to them, is to afford companionship for the children, to give mothers 'an afternoon off' for shopping, visiting, hospital attendance, just 'a rest' or to enable mothers to undertake part-time work. The centres are usually open on one, two or more mornings or afternoons a week for two or more hours. Health visitors give valuable help in advising those responsible for the group on health and other matters. Many of these forms of group-care for young children require to be registered under the amended Nurseries and Child-Minders Regulation Act, 1948, but exemption is granted to those which are maintained or assisted by local authorities. An interesting development of recent years is the opening of play-groups in children's hospitals and units, the first being started at the Brook Hospital, Woolwich, in 1963, under the aegis of the Save the Children Fund (Harvey, 1965).

Staff of many kinds are found in the varied types of establishments registered under the Act. Some have professional qualifications in child care or education but, as often happens, may have been out of the practical field for so long as to have lost touch with modern views on child health and care. Child-minders are frequently, however, housewives whose experience is limited to bringing up their own children and this may be insufficient to equip them to look after other people's children. In consequence of these situations it is most desirable that opportunities for some training should be offered to all those who care for children in private groups. Local health and education authorities should be encouraged to organise jointly simple courses combined with observation visits to well established nurseries and nursery schools.

Nursery Nurse Training

The examining body in England and Wales for the nursery nurses' certificate is the National Nursery Examination Board. In Scotland the corresponding body is the Scottish Nursery Nurses Examination Board which grants a separate certificate. In both countries the training course lasts 2 years and includes infant and pre-school child care (in England and Wales up to 7 years of age), experience in the care of the latter being obtained at nurseries, both day and residential, and nursery schools and classes. The National Nursery Examination Board's examination is a written one, together with an assessment throughout training of the candidate's practical work and her record of observation which each student must produce; the Scottish Board's examination is currently both written and practical but will soon be along parallel lines to the N.N.E.B. procedure. The Plowden Report (1967) recommended modification of the N.N.E.B's course for nursery assistants, many of whom would be older women, in view of the greatly expanded pre-school nursery-group education suggested by the Report.

Mother and Baby Homes

Local authorities together with religious and voluntary organisations receiving financial support from local authorities, provide homes to which mainly un-married mothers are admitted during the later stages of pregnancy. They may remain with their infants for several weeks after confinement which may take place in the home or in hospital. Nicholson (1968) reviewed critically a representative sample of homes in England and Wales and concluded that much re-thinking was needed on the scope and purpose of these homes. Mother and baby homes require to be registered by a local authority but the authority may exempt any home either conditionally or unconditionally on an annual basis.

Holiday Homes

Local authorities usually give financial support to voluntary organisations providing these homes. The homes are very useful for affording an opportunity to mothers accompanied by their infants or young children, to spend a fortnight's rest in the country or at the seaside. Young children after pneumonia or other respiratory infections benefit greatly from such holidays.

Domestic Help Service

This service, presently permissive under the National Health Service Acts, became obligatory on local health authorities under the Health Services and Public Health Act, 1968. The service is one which the Local Authority Social Services Bill (1970) proposes should be transferred to new social services departments of local authorities in England and Wales; in Scotland the social work departments have already assumed responsibility for the administration and provision of the service. Infants and young children benefit from the service in that it allows them to remain at home during the illness or confinement of their mothers in preference to other arrangements, *e.g.* placing with foster-parents, etc. A charge is made for the service.

Accident Prevention (see also p. 469)

Paradoxical though it may seem home is not the safest place for young children. A Scottish Home and Health Department circular (3/1964) and the British Medical Association report on Home Accidents (1964) both emphasised the mounting toll of children's lives from accidents in the home and called for greater effort by local authorities and voluntary home safety committees acting together to publicise preventive measures. The B.M.A. report recommended a system of statutory notification of accidents in view of the lack of accurate national statistics. In 1967, of 7,909 deaths in Britain from home accidents no less than 874 were in children under 5 years of age, and 115 were in the age-group 5 to 14 years.

The Ministry of Housing and Local Government (1966) issued a Design Bulletin, *Safety in the Home*, containing comprehensive advice on the safety measures which should be provided in new homes. The British Standards Institution has laid down many standards of safety for children's toys and playthings (Code, B.S.3443, 1968), and under the Consumer Protection Act, 1961, numerous regulations are in force dealing with heating appliances, including colour coding of flexible cords attached to domestic heating appliances, children's nightdresses, stands for carry-cots, and children's toys, to mention but a few. The dangers of plastic bags when in the hands of young children are well known. Colebrook (1970) has reviewed British Standards concerned with children's safety. Fireworks constitute a particular hazard. Although agreement was reached between the British Firework Manufacturers Association and the Home Office (1963) on several major

matters concerning their manufacture, government did not see fit (1969) to introduce legislation limiting the sale of fireworks for organised displays only, as
urged by the Royal Society for the Prevention of Accidents (RoSPA). Poisoning
from drugs, domestic cleaning materials, and other toxic substances demands
that these materials be stored in properly constructed cabinets. Standards have
been developed by the British Standards Institution specifying the type of
fastening device necessary. Warley *et al.* (1968) drew attention to the danger of
accidental poisoning from lead contained in cosmetics used by immigrant Indians
and Pakistanis. It is estimated that some 12,000 children are the victims of accidental poisoning in the home including some 4,000 requiring hospital treatment.
The National Poisons Information Service is increasingly called upon for advice
on preventive measures. The Report on Hospital Treatment of Acute Poisoning
(1968) recommended that the prevention of poisoning was so important as to
warrant special study by government. During its Care with Medicines Campaign
(July–September, 1968) RoSPA produced a striking poster (HS/133–1) illustrating
the similarity between drugs and sweets to demonstrate the serious risk. In babies
the danger of cot deaths is ever present and sudden death in infancy was the subject
of a special report (1965). The 'battered baby' syndrome, too, deserves mention
here (B.P.A. 1966).

Legislation will not make people safe any more than it will make them healthy or
moral, but early training will. From an appreciation of the fact that safety is
awareness of danger arise the increasing activities of local authorities working in
conjunction with local voluntary home safety committees to educate the public
and children in safety measures. Through its *Safety News* (monthly), *Home Safety
Journal* (quarterly), and the assistance it gives in the organisation of local campaigns
RoSPA plays a valuable role. Some local authorities either themselves or through
voluntary home safety committees (Edinburgh) have schemes for issuing on loan
fireguards and other safety devices to parents with young children. Apart from
national campaigns, local activities include competitions, films, talks and demonstrations using models, posters, flannel-graphs, etc., given at child health centres,
day nurseries, nursery schools, women's guild meetings, young mothers' and
parents' clubs. Above all are the personal advice to and education of parents in
their own homes by family doctor, health visitor and others.

Outside the home the greatest danger to children is the road. Table 17 shows
the magnitude of this danger on Britain's overcrowded roads.

Between 1964 and 1968 Britain's population increased by 1,173,000 (2·2 per cent)
and the number of motor vehicles licensed rose by 2,058,000 (16·7 per cent) (Lain,
1969). In an attempt to promote road safety measures for under five year olds,
RoSPA inaugurated the 'Tufty Club' scheme (1961). The number of such clubs
now exceeds 3,000 with a membership of over a million. By joining such a club
children can be taught the rudiments of road sense and kerb drill either in groups
or individually. Full details of the scheme are obtainable from RoSPA. The
national cyling proficiency scheme was begun for the juvenile cyclist and many
local authorities have appointed road safety officers to increase the extent of road

safety training of the young. Two further risks out of doors to which preventive measures are directed deserve mention. These are agricultural accidents especially from tractors, and drowning. As a consequence of the latter the 'Learn to swim' scheme was launched.

TABLE 17

Children under 15 years

Year	Killed	Seriously injured	Slightly injured	Total casualties
1964	823	13,644	45,090	59,557
1965	900	13,965	47,139	62,004
1966	879	14,789	46,280	61,948
1967	885	15,186	46,945	63,016
1968	890	15,697	47,375	63,962

The personal factor is paramount in accident prevention and this was brought forcibly home by the slogan of the national road safety campaign (1965)—'Road Safety Depends on YOU'.

Vulnerable or 'At Risk' and Handicapped Children

A handicapped child has been defined as one who suffers from any continuing disability of body, intellect, or personality which is likely to interfere with his normal growth, development and capacity to learn. The early diagnosis of handicapping conditions is thus important so that full assessment and periodic assessment, immediate treatment, parental guidance and support, appropriate education and training, and later vocational training and placement in the community can be undertaken. Local health authorities keep registers of handicapped children to ensure that the children concerned and their parents may be afforded every opportunity of receiving the fullest benefits of the specialist services and of the facilities offered by both voluntary and statutory bodies working in this field. Various simple screening tests have been evolved to diagnose early such conditions as congenital dislocation of the hip, phenylketonuria, deafness, cerebral palsy, squint, etc. The concept of the child vulnerable or 'at risk' to handicapping conditions by virtue of hereditary factors or adverse antenatal, intranatal or postnatal conditions has been developed within recent years, by *e.g.* Fisch (1957), Howorth (1958) relating particularly to deafness, and Sheridan (1962) from a wider standpoint.

The idea behind the 'at risk' concept was economy of medical effort in early identification of handicap. Local health authorities therefore began to keep registers of infants and children 'at risk' to handicap. Various criticisms have been voiced over the value of keeping such registers, the criticisms being based on administrative and scientific difficulties. Walker (1967) found a wide variation in the percentage of infants born who were placed on the 'at risk' registers of local health authorities in Scotland, the range varying from as low as 7 per cent to as high as 42 per cent. Hughes (1964) found that 20 per cent of infants born at Reading were placed on the 'at risk' register, and this has been a generally accepted proportion. While it is known that this 20 per cent of infants are more likely to turn out to have handicaps it is also known that among the 80 per cent not on the register there will be a number who will develop handicaps. It is for this reason that the Sheldon Report (1967) recommended that local health authorities should keep registers of healthy infants and children under 5 years so as to ensure that so far as possible these children would be presented for regular periodic examinations and developmental assessment. Forfar (1968) and Thomas (1968) dealt very fully with 'at risk' registers, their pros and cons, and the early detection of handicap in children has been comprehensively described by Hamilton (1968). A working group of W.H.O (1967) on early detection and treatment of handicapping defects in young children suggested the name 'special care register' rather than 'at risk register'.

Registers of congenital malformations observable at birth are also kept by local health authorities under the voluntary scheme of notification. The main purpose of this notification is to bring to light unexpected trends and the observation of any unusual concentration of malformations requiring epidemiological investigation.

Movement within these registers can take place in a number of ways. The healthy child will remain in the same category till he enters school but at any time he may develop a condition which necessitates his transfer to the category of 'at risk' or handicapped children, either direct or after assessment. A child originally on the 'at risk' register may be found healthy and transferred to the register of healthy children; alternatively if a handicap is revealed in time he will be transferred, after assessment, to the handicapped children's register. A malformation observable at birth may be curable or of such minor consequence that no treatment is required or it may give rise to serious handicap. The handicapped children's register will therefore be built up mainly from children with congenital malformations, from those on the 'at risk' register, and to some extent from the healthy children's register. Close co-operation with the school health service is essential in dealing with handicapped children.

Recognition of the importance of child development is evidenced by the foundation of a chair in that subject at London University (1964) and introduction of the various postgraduate courses in the subject held for doctors engaged in the child health services. A unique study in child development is the First Report of the National Child Development Study (1958 cohort) involving 11,000 children who were studied originally at the time of their birth. This first report deals with them at the age of 7 years, and it is hoped that these same children may be studied when aged 11 years, and even later.

The organisation of assessment centres is a necessary step in furthering the diagnosis and care of the handicapped child. This may include a period in a centre for day care. A playgroup can offer a useful supportive service to the handicapped child and his family. Comprehensive schemes of ascertainment of children with hearing and visual defects were recently outlined by working parties of the

Scottish Education Department (1967, 1969). Whitmore (1969) discussed an operational assessment service for handicapped children.

The problem of the young chronic sick, 'perhaps the most unfortunate group in any community', was the subject of a report (1964) by a special sub-committee of the Scottish Health Services Council. The report drew attention to the lack of knowledge of the true extent of chronic sickness among the young. It urged that measures should be taken to ensure early diagnosis; that no gap occurred in the supervision of the children's health, especially in the transition between the child health and school health services; that a register of such children should be kept by the local health authority; that counselling centres for the guidance of parents, and day care centres should be set up; that a residential unit to serve Scotland was needed for those with multiple handicaps.

The most encouraging recent trend in the field of childhood handicap has been the increased provision for the care and training of the mentally subnormal young child. Special advisory centres for these children and their parents, training or occupation centres run on day nursery lines, and short-term residential units are examples of developments in this direction. Much stimulus to these developments has originated from the National Society for Mentally Handicapped Children (1950).

Preventive Advice Centres

Short (1968) described the establishment in Edinburgh of a centre by the health and social services department in an area with a high incidence of social and medico-psychological problems. The aims of the centre were to provide a simple, integrated service with a particular bias towards early intervention at crisis periods; to encourage positive community action; and to conduct operational research. A joint committee of representatives of health, welfare and children committees was responsible for administering the centre. The staff included a co-ordinator and director of research; a medical social worker; health visitors; district nurses; several child care officers; two district mental health officers; district probation officer; Citizen's Advice Bureau personnel; receptionist; clerical staff. In addition, marriage guidance was provided at evening sessions. A senior registrar in psychiatry and a senior psychiatric social worker were attached part-time to the centre. Owing to difficulties of accommodation it has not been possible to provide rooms for the local general practitioners but the experimental centre has already proved a useful adjunct to the area concerned.

H. P. TAIT

References

Official Publications (H.M.S.O.)

CENTRAL ADVISORY COUNCIL FOR EDUCATION (ENGLAND) (1967). *Children and Their Primary Schools*. 2 vols. (Plowden Report).
—— *First Report of the National Child Development Study* (1958 Cohort), by Butler, N. R., Pringle, M. L. K. and Davie, R. (1966). Submitted to Council. Vol. 2.

CENTRAL HEALTH SERVICES COUNCIL (1967). *Child Welfare Centres.* Report of Sub-committee of Standing Medical Advisory Committee of Council. (Sheldon Report).

—— (1968). *Immunisation against Infectious Disease.* Memorandum prepared by Standing Medical Advisory Committee for Council.

—— (1968). *Hospital Treatment of Acute Poisoning.* Report of the Joint Sub-Committee of the Standing Medical Advisory Committees. Consumer Protection Act, 1961.

COUNCIL FOR TRAINING OF HEALTH VISITORS (1967). *The Functions of the Health Visitor.* Health Services and Public Health Act, 1968.

DEPARTMENT OF HEALTH AND SOCIAL SECURITY (1969). *Nursing Attachments to General Practice.* By Abel, R. A.

MEDICAL RESEARCH COUNCIL (1966). Vaccination against measles. Report to Council by Measles Vaccines Committee. *Brit. med. J.*, 1, 441.

——(1968). Vaccination against measles. Second Report to Council by Measles Vaccines Committee. *Brit. med. J.*, 2, 449.

MINISTRY OF HEALTH (1965). *Enquiry into Sudden Death in Infancy.* Reports on Public Health and Medical Subjects, No. 113.

—— (1968). *Local Authority Building Note,* No. 3. (Local health authority clinics, 1962, amended). National Health Service Acts. Nurseries and Child-Minders Regulation Act, 1948.

ROYAL COMMISSION ON MEDICAL EDUCATION, 1965–68. (1968). Cmnd 3569. (Todd Report).

SCOTTISH EDUCATION DEPARTMENT (1967). *Ascertainment of Children with Hearing Defects.* Report of a working party.

—— (1969). *Ascertainment of Children with Visual Handicaps.* Report of a working party.

SCOTTISH HOME AND HEALTH DEPARTMENT (1967). *Dietary Study of 4,365 Scottish Infants,* by Arneil, G. C. Scottish Health Service Studies, No. 6.

—— (1967). *Assessment of the Current Status of the 'At Risk' Register,* by Walker, R. G. Scottish Health Service Studies, No. 4.

SEEBOHM REPORT (1968). *Report of the Committee on Local Authority and Allied Personal Social Services.* Cmnd 3703. Committee set up by Secretaries of State for several government departments. Social Work (Scotland) Act, 1968.

WORLD HEALTH ORGANISATION (1965). *Domestic Accidents.* By Backett, E. M. Public Health Papers, No. 26.

—— (1967). *Report of Working Group on Early Detection and Treatment of Handicapping Defects in Young Children.* EURO 0332 (not for sale).

Other Publications

AMBLER, M., ANDERSON, J. A. D., BLACK, M., DRAPER, P., LEWIS, J., MOSS, W. and MURRELL, T. G. C. (1968). The attachment of local authority staff to general practice. *Med. Officer,* 119, 295.

ANDERSON, J. A. D., DRAPER, P., AMBLER, M. and BLACK, J. M. (1967). The attachment of local authority staff to general practices: a follow-up study. *Med. Officer,* 118, 249.

BREWIN, P. H. (1968). Contact between general practitioners and public health nursing staff in the West Riding: a three-year comparison. *Med. Officer,* 119, 171.

BRIMBLECOMBE, F. S. W., ASHFORD, J. R. and FRYER, J. G. (1968). Significance of low birth weight in perinatal mortality: study of variations within England and Wales. *Br. J. prev. soc. Med.,* 22, 27.

BRITISH MEDICAL ASSOCIATION (1964). *Accidents in the Home.* Report of special committee. London: B.M.A.

BRITISH PAEDIATRIC ASSOCIATION (1966). The battered baby. A memorandum. *Brit. med. J.*, 1, 601.

BUTLER, N. R. and ALBERMAN, E. D. (1969). *Perinatal Problems: Second Report of the 1958 British Perinatal Mortality Survey*. Edinburgh: Livingstone.

CLOW, J. T. (1968). Attachment of health visitors to general practitioners. *Med. Officer*, 119, 173.

COLEBROOK, P. (1970). How do British Standards help? *Mother and Child*, 42, 11.

DRAPER, P., AMBLER, M., LEWIS, J., ANDERSON, J. A. D. (1969). The health visitor after Seebohm. *Nursing Times*, 65, 40, 82, 114.

EDITORIAL (1968). Public health nurses and their future. *Med. Officer*, 119, 169.

EGAN, D. F. (1966). The future role of local health authorities in the day care of the young child. *Public Health*, 80, 233.

EPSOM, J. E. (1969). Personal communication.

FORFAR, J. O. (1968). 'At risk' registers. Annotation. *Develop. Med. Child. Neurol.*, 10, 384.

GALLOWAY, J. (1967). Some aspects of immigration. *Med. Officer*, 118, 69.

GANS, B. (1964). Experiences in a coloured children's welfare clinic. *Proc. R. soc. Med.*, 57, 327.

GRUENWALD, P. (1965). Terminology of infants of low birth weight. *Develop, Med. Child. Neurol.*, 7, 578.

HAMILTON, F. M. W. (1968). The early detection of handicap in children. *Med. Officer*, 120, 167.

HARDING, W. G. (1969). Personal communication.

HARVEY, S. (1965). A hospital playgroup. *Mother and Child*, 35, 15.

HOCKEY, L. (1968). *Care in the Balance: A Study of Collaboration between Hospital and Community Services*. London: Queen's Institute of District Nursing.

HOWARD, R. and PANK, P. (1968). Design standards and criteria for nursery building. *Nursery Journal*, 57, 5.

HUGHES, E. (1964). The 'at risk' child. *Practitioner*, 194, 534.

JERMAN, B. (1965). Home nursing: daily care of a home care unit. *The Guardian*, 19 May.

JOHNS, J. (1967). A university nursery (Manchester). *Mother and Child*, 39, 9.

JOSEPH, M. and MAC KEITH, R. C. (1966). *A New Look at Child Health*. London: Pitman Medical Publishing Co.

LAIN, J. A. (1969). Road casualties down by over 20,000. *Safety News*, No. 393, p. 6.

LEWIS, J. T. (1968). Attachment, liaison, linkage. *Med. Officer*, 119, 323.

NASEN (1968). *The State Enrolled Nurse in the Public Health Services*. London: National Association of State Enrolled Nurses (NASEN).

NICHOLSON, J. (1968). *Mother and Baby Homes*. London: Allen and Unwin.

PARISH, P. A. (1968). Health visitor attachment in general practice. *Nursing Times*, 64, 256.

—— (1968). District nursing attachment in general practice. *Nursing Times*, 64, 292.

PEPPARD, N. (1964). Health of the coloured child in Great Britain: social aspects. *Proc. R. Soc. Med.*, 57, 323.

PHENYLKETONURIA, (1968). Population screening by Guthrie test for phenylketonuria in South-east Scotland. Report by consultant paediatricians and medical officers of health of the South-east Scotland hospital region. *Brit. med. J.*, 1, 674.

PRE-SCHOOL PLAYGROUPS ASSOCIATION, (1968). 1,020 *Playgroups: A Survey*. London: Pre-School Playgroups Association. (This organisation produces an admirable journal, *Contact*, at regular intervals.)

SHORT, R. (1968). An Edinburgh preventive advice centre. *Med. Officer*, 120, 114. Report of conference.

SOCIETY OF MEDICAL OFFICERS OF HEALTH, (1967). *The Doctor and the Child Welfare Clinic*. Tunbridge Wells: The Medical Officer.

THOMAS, G. E. (1968). The registration of children at risk of handicap. *Med. Officer*, 120, 162, 177, 191, 208.

WARIN, J. F. (1968). General practitioners and nursing staff: a complete attachment scheme in retrospect and prospect. *Brit. med. J.*, **2**, 41.

WARKANY, J., MONROE, B. B. and SUTHERLAND, B. S. (1961). Intrauterine growth retardation. *Amer. J. Dis. Child.*, **102**, 249.

WARLEY, M. A., BLACKLEDGE, P. and O'GORMAN, P. (1968). Lead poisoning from eye cosmetic. *Brit. med. J.*, **1**, 117.

WHITMORE, K. (1969). An assessment service for handicapped children. *Med. Officer*, **122**, 263.

WILSON, G. (1967). *The Hazards of Immunisation*. London University: Athlone Press. (Heath Clark Lectures).

YUDKIN, S. (1968). 0–5: *A Report on the Care of Pre-School Children*. 2nd edit. London: Allen and Unwin.

16   The School Health Service

Administration

A STUDY of the framework of school health services in other countries shows much variation in historical development and in forms of administration. In the Netherlands the beginnings of a school health service are early discernible, two school medical officers having been appointed as early as 1868 by the municipality of Haarlemmermeer. The promulgation of the Compulsory Education Act in 1901 was a strong stimulus to municipalities to organise the medical supervision of schools, in most cases through the part-time employment of general practitioners, but it was not until 1942 that the first legal regulations were made covering the school health service. Responsibility for the service in the Netherlands remains in the hands of the municipalities, except in one province where a voluntary organisation is in charge of school health work. There are some 400 full-time medical officers who supervise all nursery and primary and an increasing number of secondary schools.

In the U.S.A. development appears to have been haphazard. In most areas, including large towns, the service is provided by boards of education; in rural areas and in some large cities the county or city health departments are responsible; and in at least one city, the health department is responsible for the school health work in the elementary schools and the board of education is responsible for it in the secondary schools. General practitioners or paediatricians may be employed on a part-time basis for routine inspection while in many areas parents are asked to have their children examined by their own doctor. In some areas the school health service is still in the earliest stages of growth, and this is the case in Chicago where a school medical officer was for the first time appointed in 1950.

In England in 1907 and in Scotland in 1908, responsibility for the establishment of a school medical service, as it was then designated, was placed upon the local education authorities. The introduction of the National Health Service did not affect its status and the school health service remains a responsibility of the local authority.

From the beginning, the importance of full co-operation with the public health service was emphasised and the association was more closely cemented when in 1919 the Chief Medical Officer of the Board of Education became also Chief Medical Officer of the newly constituted Ministry of Health. Locally, also, this co-operation has developed after the same pattern, and today the school health service is an integral part of the local health department.

Staff

In England, local education authorities must appoint a principal school medical officer with the function of administering the service and, as already indicated, this official is the medical officer of health. In Scotland, under regulations made in 1946, the medical officers of health are chief administrative school medical officers, and the day-to-day running of the service is in the hands of a Chief Executive School Medical Officer and a Chief Dental Officer; in the case of smaller authorities the medical officer of health may act as both chief administrative and chief executive school medical officer. Under these senior officials is a staff of medical officers in department, dental officers, health visitors and nurses, physiotherapists, speech therapists, chiropodists and others. In order that these officers may be most profitably employed they should, as far as possible, be relieved of clerical work, and clerical assistants are therefore employed, not only centrally, but also in treatment centres, specialists' and dental clinics, and also, in some areas, in the medical rooms of the schools during the medical officers' routine visits.

In only a minority of areas, however, has the school health service its full complement of full-time staff. The number of school doctors is not keeping pace with the increasing population of school children. In many areas school health work is undertaken along with their other work by medical officers of the pre-school child health service or by those engaged in general public health duties. The trend towards a closer partnership among the various sections of the nation's health services, especially the child health services, has resulted in the increasing practice among local authorities of employing general practitioners part-time at inspection sessions. Indeed, from the very inception of the school health service general practitioners have been employed in its work by some authorities, notably Oxfordshire. The increasing employment of general practitioners nowadays is entirely compatible with an efficient, forward-looking service, provided that the role of the general practitioners is planned as an integral part of the service. In the opinion of the Chief Medical Officer to the Department of Education and Science, the future of the school health service undoubtedly lies in the sessional employment of selected family doctors and married women doctors, and the whole-time employment of a small number of doctors specially trained and experienced in child development and health. The former will be largely responsible for the day-to-day medical work in the schools assigned to them and the latter for the overall administration, the promotion of health education, and the medical supervision of deviant and handicapped pupils. A closer working partnership must also be fostered between the school health and hospital paediatric services. Increasingly, the school health service is concerned with the earlier identification of children with mild disabilities which may nevertheless interfere with growth and especially with development and learning in school; a wider functional assessment of children as they reach school age; a more comprehensive assessment of each individual handicapped pupil; and a greater participation in the management of incipient maladjustment and its prevention. It is for these reasons that specially designed postgraduate courses in child development, assessment of handicap and sub-normality are provided for local health authority medical officers and interested general practitioners. Medical examination for the ascertainment of the education-ally subnormal child may only be undertaken by a medical officer holding one of the prescribed qualifications for such work. The most recently published figures for England and Wales show that there were 2,914 medical officers equal in whole time service to 930 employed in the school health service.

The school health visitor should, wherever possible, have the assistance of a registered or enrolled nurse and a suitable assistant since she will also be engaged in health visiting duties in other spheres, *e.g.* in the infant and pre-school child health service. She must keep in close touch with the school, act as a link with the school, the home, the local authority and the family doctors. She carries out most of the home visiting and it is desirable that she is present at the medical examination of 5 year old entrants but not necessarily throughout every other examination. She should provide any necessary information about the child or his home background and should attend for consultation with the school medical officer towards the end of examination sessions. Active participation by the health visitor in health educa-tion programmes in schools is very desirable. Registered or enrolled nurses should be employed for clinics where nursing duties are performed and for carrying out hygiene inspections of the pupils and assisting at medical inspections, *e.g.* weighing and measuring of children, simple vision screening, and record-keeping. The latest published figures for England and Wales show that 8,823 school health visitors and nurses were employed, equal in whole-time service to 2,889 nurses.

The various activities of the school health service are described in the subsequent sections of the chapter.

Accommodation

SCHOOL MEDICAL ROOMS. Suitable medical rooms are often lacking in older school buildings and the school doctor and nurse may be constrained to work in a class-room, staff room, or other makeshift accommodation, but in every school of modern design there is, or should be, a medical room where privacy can be assured; of a size adequate for the testing of vision and hearing; and having in its immediate vicinity a waiting-room or waiting space for mothers and children. In Building Bulletin No. 25 (1965) diagrams of three different arrangements for a medical suite in a secondary school are given which show what can be achieved in a small amount of space.

SCHOOL CLINICS. A school clinic supplies, as a minimum, a consulting room in which the school medical officer may hold his diagnostic session and a minor ailments treatment room. Accommodation for dental treatment, consisting of a surgery and recovery room, is, as a general rule, incorporated and there may be provision for specialists' clinics (Fig. 80). Extra rooms would be required for physiotherapy, speech therapy, and other specialised treatments.

Inspection

Periodical medical inspection was the principal, and almost the only, employment of the school medical officer when the service was first constituted. It continues to be an important activity and the most recent Education Acts have made this inspection compulsory. There is no doubt that, in the earlier years of the

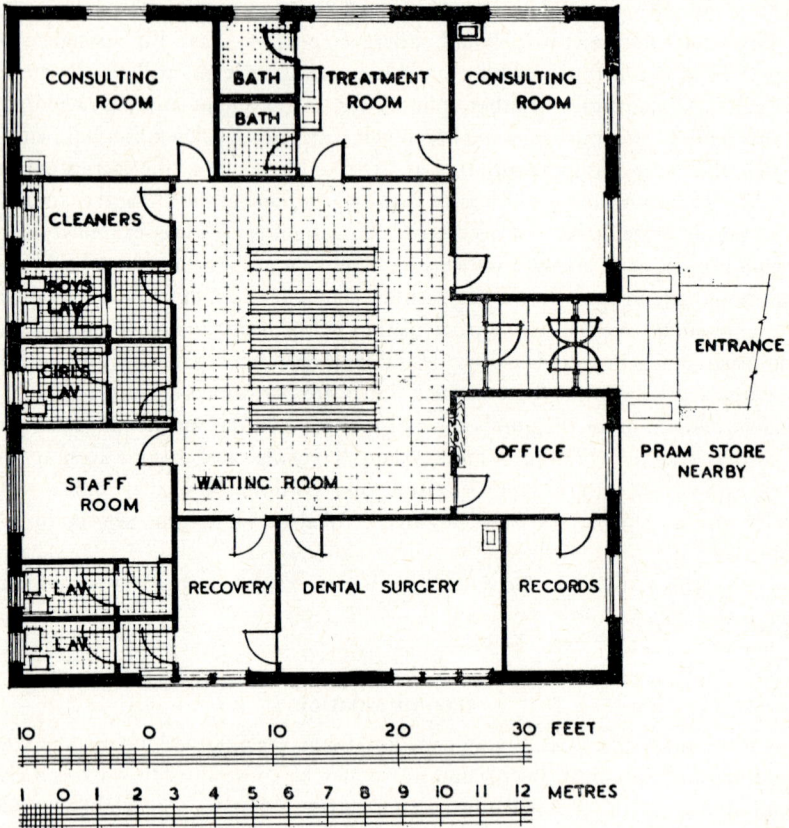

Fig. 80. Plan of a School Clinic.

(*Courtesy of the City Architect, Edinburgh*)

service, periodical inspection of whole groups of children at specified ages was the best procedure for ascertaining defects in the school population. Since then conditions, medical, social and educational, have greatly changed and the value of repeated inspection has been seriously questioned. The central departments today, therefore, not only allow but actively encourage local authorities to look for more efficient procedures. A large number of authorities, while retaining the entrance and leaving inspections have amended their programmes so as to omit the intermediate inspection and introduce a more continuous health supervision of the child by close contact among medical officer, school health visitor, parent, teacher and family doctor, reinforced by clinical examination when such examination is required.

The basic record of the school health service is the School Medical Record Card which provides space both for clinical observations and for information about the child's environment. The record cards used in England and Wales and in Scotland differ considerably in format and in information obtained. In 1967 a new form of school medical record card was introduced by the Scottish Home and Health Department, allowing for fuller clinical reporting. Instead of listing a limited number of specific diseases, the new card provides for the diagnosis to be classified according to the International Classification of Diseases code. Part of the information can be processed mechanically to obtain statistical analysis. There is hope that the new card will provide not only more accurate but also more interesting information on the health of school children.

Medical inspection is, as a general rule, carried out in the medical room in school, but where such accommodation is not available the inspection is carried out at the nearest school clinic or treatment centre. The school health visitor or nurse is in attendance, and in some places it is the practice for the teacher to be present also. Supervision and follow-up are the responsibility of the school health visitor.

Parents must be notified of the time of the inspection and this is often done by sending a letter of explanation which, in addition to inviting the parent to attend, contains a list of questions about the child's health history which the parent is asked to complete and return. Although the presence of parents tends to slow down the session, it is a great advantage if they can be present to supplement the medical history, receive advice from the school doctor and have explained to them the need for any treatment or investigation that may be recommended. Each child on his first inspection may have his card made out by the teacher or by the school secretary, but information of a confidential nature, such as family history, should be obtained and recorded by the doctor or nurse. Height and weight should be measured by the nurse and not by the teacher, and children should be weighed wearing vest and pants without footwear. The children are presented to the doctor for examination and those found to be in need of treatment or further investigation are referred to the appropriate agency, or put down for special examination later either in school or at the doctor's diagnostic session at an appropriate clinic. Every child requiring special care in school is notified to the teacher. Special examinations are conducted at any age in the child's school life either on account of some condition found or suspected at routine inspection or at the request of parents, nurses or teachers.

RECORDS. Liaison with the medical officer in charge of the pre-school child health service should be such that the records of his department are made available to the school health service when a child reaches school age. Entries on record cards should be accurate, legible and adequate, and reports from specialists, hospitals, etc., should be attached. In some areas co-operation with hospitals is such that a report is sent to the school medical officer on every schoolchild discharged after treatment. The record card provides for the school doctor and nurse information which they require throughout the child's school life, and it furnishes the statistical information incorporated in the school medical officer's annual report to the central government department. There is no standard procedure for the filing of record cards but full confidentiality must be preserved. In some areas they are kept in the office of the principal school medical officer and are taken out by the school medical officer on each occasion on which a visit is paid; in others, information about exceptional pupils is available at the school health service office but the record cards are kept in the individual schools. Under the latter arrangement, special care must be taken to prevent access to them by unauthorised persons. For the school health service to function effectively the teacher must receive sufficient medical guidance about the physical and mental disabilities of his pupils and the Scottish Home and Health Department (1969) recommended that more use should be made of the pupil's progress record card, which is maintained for each child by the education service, to record such information as required. The medical record card follows the child as he moves from school to school and, it may be, from place to place, securing a continuity of record not affected by any change of family doctor, and when completed at the end of the child's school career is a source of information which is often not to be found elsewhere, and which can be made available to the general practitioner, the factory surgeon, or other medical persons with the permission of the individual concerned. Inquiries about a pupil's medical history while at school may be made years after school-leaving age has been passed and records should, therefore, remain in the custody of the school health service and should not, as sometimes happens, be transferred through the local executive council to the general practitioners.

Treatment

In the Netherlands, Denmark, and other European countries, prevention and cure are entirely separated in school health work. No treatment whatever is provided and every child who requires it is referred to the family doctor. Conditions are different in Britain where the National Health Service Acts have not relieved local education authorities of the duty laid upon them by the Education Acts of 1944 (England and Wales) and 1962 (Scotland) to make arrangements for securing the provision of free medical treatment for pupils attending all schools which they maintain.

SCHOOL TREATMENT CENTRES. School health services, therefore, continue to provide clinics for eye refractions, orthoptics, physiotherapy, chiropody and for the treatment of minor ailments such as skin infections. The Scottish Home and Health Department report on the school health service (1969), while accepting that the continuation of minor ailments clinics was sometimes justified on the grounds that they saved absence from school through a child being taken to the family doctor, nevertheless suggested that as and when circumstances permitted, local authorities should consider the closure of these clinics and provide instead facilities in schools for treatment of minor cuts and bruises only. Speech therapy and child guidance (see Chapter 20) are organised as part of the school health service in England and Wales and as part of the educational service in Scotland.

SPECIALIST CLINICS. Under the National Health Service Acts the provision of specialist clinics became, in the main, the responsibility of regional hospital boards. Over previous years the school health service had built up its own organisation of specialist clinics for certain disabilities in its treatment centres, in schools, or in other premises, and, where practicable, these clinics have been continued under the charge of specialists provided by the regional hospital boards. Where these arrangements have not been continued, special clinics for school children may be held in hospitals. If it appears desirable to do so, local authorities still have power to provide and pay for any specialist service for school children.

Specialists engaged in school clinic work are the paediatrician, paediatric neurologist, orthopaedic surgeon, cardiologist, and child psychiatrist, but the specialist clinics most frequently provided are those of the ophthalmologist and the otologist. Indeed the great majority of children with visual defects and squints and very many with hearing defects and unhealthy tonsils and adenoids obtain treatment through the school health service.

'CLEANLINESS' CLINICS. This euphemism is officially applied to delousing centres. The Education Acts take full cognisance of the problem of infestation and provide powers for compulsory inspection, for compulsory treatment at cleanliness clinics, and for the prosecution of parents through whose negligence re-infestation occurs. Useful though such powers may be in individual cases, they will not eliminate infestation, for the schoolchild most frequently acquires his vermin from reservoirs beyond the reach of these powers, from brothers and sisters, and from the parents, especially the mothers, themselves. Thus infestation with lice is often a family affair, indicating ignorance, apathy and defective social conscience, not lack of medical care. The rate varies considerably from district to district, but the incidence in England and Wales as a whole, for school children, was 1·7 per cent in 1967. There is some evidence of a recent increase in head lousiness associated with the present-day cult of long hair among boys and adolescents.

THE SCHOOL HEALTH SERVICE AND THE FAMILY DOCTOR. Except when treatment can be most suitably and conveniently provided in the clinics and centres previously described, the curative care of diseases diagnosed by the school medical officer is the responsibility of the family doctor to whom such cases are therefore referred. Close co-operation with general practitioners is of fundamental importance to the success of school health work. To foster such co-operation a recommendation was made by responsible medical bodies that a child found by a school medical officer to need special investigation or treatment, should be sent to a consultant only after prior consultation with the child's own doctor, to whom a copy of all reports from the consultants would be sent. This is almost universal practice now, and co-operation is still furthered by personal discussion between school medical officer and family doctor on problems affecting individual children.

13

Pupils Requiring Special Educational Treatment
(Handicapped Pupils)

Over the years the pattern of disease and disability in schoolchildren has changed, particularly during the past few decades. Diseases that once caused the death of many children and disabled more have now been brought under control. As a result, emotional and behavioural disturbances, speech and language disorders, learning difficulties, including those arising from defective vision and hearing, respiratory disorders particularly asthma, epilepsy, and physical handicaps from trauma, congenital and hereditary conditions are the chief disabilities in children with which the school health service has to deal. The problem of multiple handicaps is a particularly difficult one. Many children with congenital defects, especially those who are severely handicapped, often have more than one disability, especially educational retardation. Almost 40 per cent of the cerebral palsied children in the special schools in England and Wales in 1964 were considered to be educationally subnormal; other additional handicaps included defects of hearing, speech, vision, and emotional disturbance which all increased the teaching problems presented by the children.

Under the Education Acts, it is the duty of an education authority to ascertain what children in its area require special educational treatment (in Scotland called special education). In forming a judgment the education authority is called on to consider not only the school medical officer's advice, but also any reports or information which can be obtained from teachers or other persons with respect to the ability and aptitude of the child. Among the 'other persons', the educational psychologist is most often the source of information and his assessment is required in Scotland since 1969. It is also the duty of the education authority, having ascertained what children in its area require special educational treatment, to make appropriate provision for them, and the general categories of handicapped children have been laid down by the Secretary of State to the Department of Education and Science and the Secretary of State for Scotland. It must be borne in mind that the canon applied to the handicapped pupil is primarily neither a medical nor a social, but an educational one.

The regulations pick out for special mention two categories, the blind and the deaf, who must be educated in special schools for the blind or the deaf, even if one or more of the other handicaps is also present; other handicapped pupils are to be educated in ordinary schools, special schools, hospital classes or at home, as the case may be. Whenever it is possible, a child should remain in an ordinary school, where, among other advantages, he may enjoy those activities of school life which are additional to, and as important as, the formal work of the classroom. To do so, the child with a disability may need such special treatment as the provision of a hearing aid, exemption from strenuous games, or some particular seat in the classroom. But if his handicap is educationally too great to be overcome in an ordinary class, special classroom instruction must be provided. In the U.S.A. provision for the handicapped child is made largely by means of special classes in ordinary schools but in this country, though many such classes do exist, provision to a large extent is made in special day or residential schools. If, after a period of special educational treatment a pupil is found to be fit for ordinary education, he ceases to be a 'handicapped pupil' and returns to the normal stream of education.

In some municipal areas the provision of special educational treatment may be considered as adequate, and transport difficulties are overcome by delivering children to and from their homes by ambulance or bus, but in many rural areas provision is inadequate or even unobtainable and over the country as a whole there is a shortage of day and residential schools, particularly for emotionally disturbed pupils of secondary school age.

EARLY ASCERTAINMENT. Early ascertainment of handicap is of great importance to the child and also to the parents, and as soon as a child has entered upon school life, the school doctor should be vigilant to suspect and detect handicap. But ascertainment before school age is reached is important in every kind of handicap and in certain categories, notably the deaf, it is absolutely essential if the child is to benefit fully from special educational treatment. For this reason an education authority has powers to secure the examination by the school medical officer of any child who has attained the age of 2 years. In Scotland this examination must include both a medical and a psychological examination (1969). Such early ascertainment may secure for the child preventive or curative treatment which has not yet been furnished through the channels of the National Health Service. It may make available to the parents specialist advice on the training and management of the pre-school handicapped child, and it may make possible admission to a special nursery school, for there is some, limited, nursery school provision for the blind, deaf, educationally subnormal, and for children with physical handicap. Even if special nursery school provision is not available, admission to an ordinary nursery school or day nursery may be possible and of benefit to the handicapped child. The upper limit of compulsory school age for the handicapped child is 16 years at present.

The pattern of work of the pre-school child health service is now such that very early ascertainment of handicaps in infancy and the pre-school period is a practical proposition. When there is, as there always should be, close liaison between the pre-school and school health services, the information given to the school medical officer is a valuable aid in his task of early ascertainment.

The categories of handicapped children defined in the Handicapped Pupils and Special Schools Regulations, 1959, and amending regulations are:

Registered Pupils

(*a*) *Blind Pupils*, that is to say, pupils who have no sight or whose sight is or is likely to become so defective that they require education by methods not involving the use of sight . . . . . 0·2 to 0·3 per 1,000

(*b*) *Partially Sighted Pupils*, that is to say, pupils who by reason of defective vision cannot follow the normal regimen of ordinary schools without detriment to their sight or to their educational development, but can be educated by special methods involving the use of sight . . . . 1·0 per 1,000

Registered Pupils

(c) *Deaf Pupils*, that is to say, pupils with impaired hearing who require education by methods suitable for pupils with little or no naturally acquired speech or language . . . . . 0·7 to 1·0 per 1,000

(d) *Partially Hearing Pupils*, that is to say, pupils with impaired hearing whose development of speech and language, even if retarded, is following a normal pattern, and who require for their education special arrangements or facilities though not necessarily all the educational methods used for deaf pupils. . . . . 1·0 upwards per 1,000

(e) *Educationally Subnormal Pupils*, that is to say, pupils who, by reason of limited ability or other conditions resulting in educational retardation require some specialised form of education wholly or partly in substitution for the education normally given in ordinary schools . . . . 10 per cent (1·5 per cent requiring transfer to a special school)

(f) *Epileptic Pupils*, that is to say, pupils who by reason of epilepsy cannot be educated under the normal regimen of ordinary schools without detriment to themselves or other pupils . . . 0·2 per 1,000

(g) *Maladjusted Pupils*, that is to say, pupils who show evidence of emotional instability or psychological disturbance and require special educational treatment in order to effect their personal, social or educational readjustment . . . . . . 5·0 to 10·0 per cent

(h) *Physically Handicapped Pupils*, that is to say, pupils not suffering solely from a defect of sight or hearing who, by reason of disease or crippling defect cannot, without detriment to their health or educational development, be satisfactorily educated under the normal regimen of ordinary schools . . . . . 5 to 8 per 1,000

(i) *Pupils suffering from Speech Defect*, that is to say, pupils who on account of defect or lack of speech not due to deafness require special educational treatment . . . . . . 2 per cent

(j) *Delicate Pupils*, that is to say, pupils not falling under any other category in this Regulation, who by reason of impaired physical condition need a change of environment or cannot, without risk to their health or educational development, be educated under the normal regimen of ordinary schools . . . . . 1 to 2 per cent

Under the Special Educational Treatment (Scotland) Regulations, 1954, the term 'Mentally handicapped pupils' is used instead of 'Educationally subnormal pupils' and there is no category of 'delicate pupils'.

BLIND AND PARTIALLY SIGHTED PUPILS. The two frontiers separating blind children from partially sighted, and partially sighted from normally sighted children, cannot be defined with precision or in terms of strict objective criteria. The decision that a child is fit for one kind of education rather than another depends upon several factors of which his vision, albeit important, is only one. Age or maturity, ability to learn, school progress, emotional and social disposition, and home environment, as indeed with all handicapped children, are factors other than the specific handicap present which must be considered in the assessment. The decision, therefore, rests on a balanced judgment in which the whole child is considered. For further details on blind and partially sighted pupils the reader is referred to special reports of the Department of Education and Science (1968) and Scottish Education Department (1969).

BLIND PUPILS. The critical question is whether the child has sufficient sight to be of educational use. In practice this means a decision must be reached on whether he can, or is likely to be able to, read ordinary or enlarged print, or must rely on braille. A visual acuity, as measured by the Snellen test, of 6/60 with correction, or worse, in the better eye is the usually accepted standard for blindness. The Scottish Education Department report (1969) cast some doubt on this standard and recommended that a child with a visual acuity below 3/60 should, subject to the results of other tests such as near vision and field of vision, be regarded as blind. Available statistics show that there has been a steady decrease over the years in the number of children needing special education in schools for the blind and partially sighted. Most such children suffer from congenital or hereditary defects of vision. At the same time it should be remembered that injury is a still too common cause of blindness and the danger to the eye should be stressed in safety campaigns.

Facilities exist for the education of blind children from the age of 2 years. There is some day-school provision, but the greater number of blind pupils attend residential schools where they remain until the age of 16. The majority then proceed to training for employment as blind persons, while those of good intelligence with an aptitude for study may enter one of the two residential senior secondary schools where they remain until the age of 19. In Scotland almost all blind children remain at school until they are 18.

The blind child receives a general education by special methods involving sound and touch, and he learns to read with his finger tips, the letters being represented not by a raised letter type but by patterns of raised dots known as Braille type, a system invented by a Frenchman of that name who was a teacher of the blind in Paris in the first half of the nineteenth century.

It is hoped to establish a research centre for blind education at the university of Birmingham very soon. Among the aims of this centre will be research into the learning problems and processes of blind children, the in-service training of teachers, and the encouragement and control of experiments in schools for the blind.

PARTIALLY SIGHTED PUPILS. Since the beginning of the present century many workers considered that a number of children who were not blind were nevertheless so handicapped by defective sight that they could not profit from ordinary schooling. For these children, then called 'partially blind' but now, more appropriately 'partially sighted', schools and classes were established. Many of the pupils were myopic and so the schools and classes were spoken of as 'sight-saving', 'sight conservation', or 'myopia schools' in the belief that the use of the highly myopic eye in the work of an ordinary school caused deterioration of vision. It is now accepted that, save in rare cases, pupils do not harm their sight by using it. When the vision of a myopic child deteriorates at adolescence this is normally the result of growth but not of eye strain. While medical views have changed there are children so handicapped by defective sight that they require special educational treatment.

The frontier between partial sight and normal vision is even more difficult to define than that between blindness and partial sight. Where the Snellen rating is 6/18 with correction or worse in the better eye the child should be considered for special schooling. The assessment of near vision is very difficult and it cannot be adequately measured except in tests dependent on reading of print. For this reason final diagnosis may not be feasible until the child has started school and been given the chance to learn to read. If the field of vision is seriously contracted special schooling is indicated.

The group of partially sighted children is not homogeneous. The defects of vision differ in kind and in intensity. In most cases near vision is more useful than vision at distances exceeding 3 or 4 feet. In general, objects at a moderate or greater distance are so blurred as to be completely unrecognisable even with maximum help from glasses. These children will therefore miss the significance of changes in facial expression during conversation and teaching and will fail to profit from the use of the blackboard, wall diagrams, etc. Some may be able to read ordinary print, although keeping the pages very close to their eyes, others can only read enlarged print. It is evident that some partially sighted children may make some progress in the infant classes of an ordinary school where the readers in use at that stage are printed in large clear letters. These children may fail, however, to make progress further up the school when ordinary print is used and at this stage special educational treatment becomes necessary. Others may require such special provision from school entry. It is important, therefore, that ascertainment of partially sighted children should be achieved at as early a stage in their school career as is educationally necessary.

CHILDREN WITH DEFECTS OF HEARING. The number of children ascertained as having impaired hearing has been rising over the past decade, both in absolute terms and as a proportion of the total school population. Some of this rise is due to a real increase in incidence, *e.g.* children born after the rubella epidemics of 1962–64, but much may be ascribed to better and earlier diagnosis and assessment. It is noteworthy that the number of young children under 5 years of age in special schools for the deaf has more than doubled over this period. The trend towards providing more education for very young children and the big expansion in peripatetic services—one of the functions of which is to give guidance on speech and language training to parents of children too young to attend school—may help to account for the increase of children now being educated as partially hearing in ordinary schools, either in ordinary classes or in partially hearing units, as compared with those in schools for the deaf.

Ascertainment. Children have a surprising and at times disconcerting ability to conceal defects of hearing and this is often because they have unknowingly acquired skill in lip-reading. The clinical methods commonly used in ascertainment are the watch, the voice used at minimum level but not as a whisper, and the performance test in which the child carries out simple repetitive activity using toy material in response to various sound stimuli. All are liable to error, however. What is known as the 'Sweep Frequency Test' has superseded other forms of testing designed to screen out children with defective hearing in ordinary schools. In this test which is administered to children individually, the pure-tone audiometer is used with the intensity control set at a predetermined level (usually 15 to 20 decibels). The operator 'sweeps' through those frequencies known to be of the greatest importance in listening to speech (usually 250 or 500 in octave steps to 4,000), testing each ear separately. Children who fail to respond to any one or two frequencies on either side are adjudged to have failed the test and are, therefore, referred for further investigation.

The classification of children with hearing defects in general use is that recommended by the former Board of Education's report on children with defective hearing (1938). A recent report (1967) of the Scottish Education Department on the ascertainment of children with hearing defects concluded that the earlier classification was outdated and recommended a grading according to the educational needs of the child, based on his language development rather than on his hearing loss. Since the earlier classification is still in use, however, some comment is necessary on it.

Grade I. The children in this grade can hear and understand conversation at 20 feet and over in ordinary classroom conditions. They have a hearing loss up to 15 decibels (G.A.) or 35 decibels (P.T.A.). They can be educated in an ordinary school without any special adjustments being made. This group also includes some children with greater hearing loss whose speech and language development is good and who lip-read well. The hearing of many of the children in this grade would benefit from medical treatment, but they do not require the use of hearing aids in school.

Grade II (A and B). The children in this grade can hear and understand conversation between 20 feet and 2 feet away in ordinary classroom conditions. They have a hearing loss between 15 and 40 decibels (G.A.) or 35 and 60 decibels (P.T.A.). By reason of their defect they cannot be properly educated without special arrangements or educational facilities. At the same time their hearing defect is not sufficiently severe for them to need education by the methods used for deaf children without naturally acquired speech or language. Into this grade come those children whose hearing defect is worse than that described above but whose speech and language development are not seriously defective. The hearing of a certain proportion of the children in this grade would benefit from medical treatment, and most of them can be helped by the use of hearing aids.

Grade III. The children in this grade can hear and understand conversation at not more than 2 feet, if at all, though they may be able to hear vowels, with or without distinguishing between them at distances greater than 2 feet. Their hearing loss is over 40 decibels (G.A.) or 60 decibels (P.T.A.) and may be total. Their speech and language, if any, are seriously defective, and, because of their loss of hearing, cannot be developed except by the methods of teaching applicable to deaf children who have not acquired speech and language naturally. This grade does not include any children, no matter what their hearing loss, whose speech and language development are not seriously defective. The hearing of few children of this grade can be improved by medical treatment, but many can be helped by the use of hearing aids.

Deaf pupils (*Grade III*). Though educationally deaf these children often have some hearing which may be useful, of which advantage is increasingly being taken by means of hearing aids. Approximately two-thirds are congenitally, and one-third adventitiously, deaf.

The most important years in the deaf child's education are those before the age when compulsory education begins. The defect of hearing must, therefore, be discovered at the earliest possible age and the number of diagnostic and advisory units throughout the country is rapidly increasing. At these 'audiology units', which may be sited in hospitals, in clinics of a local authority or in schools for the deaf, diagnosis is established and auditory training for the child and guidance for the parents are provided. Nursery school accommodation, too, is available and is of the greatest value to the deaf child. The history of the evolution of the teaching of the deaf is the history of a struggle, protracted, stubborn, and often bitter, between those who advocate manual methods and the protagonists of oral teaching. The manual method makes use of finger spelling and a conventional vocabulary of hand movements or signs whereas in oral teaching meaning is conveyed by speech and obtained by lip-reading. A recent report of the Department of Education and Science (1968) accepted that there was a place for manual media in the instruction of some deaf children and recommended that studies should be undertaken to determine whether or not and in what circumstances the introduction of manual media would lead to improvement in the education of deaf children. Oral teaching is practised in all schools in this country, but a proportion of the children fail to make progress with speech and lip-reading. The majority, however, can understand and to some extent employ oral speech; a knowledge of the manual method is acquired by all in their leisure time; and all children, therefore, leave school able to communicate with other deaf persons, with the officers of the voluntary associations responsible for their after-care, and, to a widely varying extent, with members of the general public. A general education is provided to the age of 16 in special day-classes and day-schools and also in special residential schools, and in the older classes vocational instruction is given. Senior secondary education is available for the relatively small number capable of profiting from it.

The child who has already acquired speech and language in the normal way before the onset of deafness does not present the same educational problem as the deaf child without speech. The former needs special educational treatment which will maintain and develop the natural speech already possessed and this can often best be done in a school or class for the partially hearing.

Partially hearing pupils (*Grade II*). These children have at least the rudiments of naturally acquired speech and language and are accustomed to the use of words. The education provided for them is, therefore, quite different from that devised for the deaf child. There are cases of severe partial deafness for whom immediate transfer to a special school is justified but many should pass a probationary period in an ordinary school during which not only the degree of hearing loss, but the quality of speech and knowledge of language, the ability to lip-read, and the educational progress can be studied. A favourable position in the schoolroom should be provided for all. Emotional disturbance resulting from feelings of frustration and inadequacy is not uncommon in Grade II children and is a strong argument in favour of transfer to a special school.

Instruction in lip-reading should be made available to Grade II children during this probationary period either by gathering them together at a convenient centre or by the appointment of an itinerant teacher who should be either a teacher of the deaf or a speech therapist skilled in lip-reading. In the last few years hearing aids in increasing numbers have been issued to Grade II children, but by no means all are willing to wear them or able to profit from them. With suitable placing in class, instruction in lip-reading, and the provision of hearing aids, the majority of Grade II pupils can be suitably educated in ordinary schools (Grade IIa). The others should be transferred to special classes or schools (Grade IIb).

Particular attention is given in classes and schools to speech and language and to lip-reading, and use is made of group hearing aids, or of individual aids in conjunction with the loop system of communication. Many of the pupils are, or should be, able later to return to ordinary schools as Grade IIa pupils. For those remaining, provision is made in the higher classes for practical activities related to vocational needs and some pupils pursue academic courses.

Delicate children. The substantial improvement in the health of children and in social conditions during the past recent decades has lessened the need for special schools for delicate children. Some of the day and residential special schools which were once used for these children are now occupied by educationally subnormal children. Respiratory conditions, especially asthma, are the chief causes for admission to these special schools. There is still a place for special schools for the delicate but the need is steadily diminishing.

Epileptic pupils. Children with petit mal and those with major epilepsy whose fits are only nocturnal or occur infrequently during the day can and should be retained in ordinary schools and every effort must be made to persuade headmasters and class teachers to accept such children and make suitable provision for care during a seizure. On the other hand, a child who frequently has major fits or fits of long duration is almost impossible to manage in an ordinary class. The child whose epilepsy takes the form of psychomotor attacks involving anti-social or even dangerous acts is also unfit for ordinary schooling and so is the epileptic child with personality disorders the result of his own reaction, or more often the reaction of other people, to the affliction. The incidence of epilepsy is difficult to judge but it is perhaps 1 to 2 per 1,000 schoolchildren but less than 1 in 5 of these needs special educational treatment and the number diminishes as therapeutic control of the disorder becomes more and more effective.

Some epileptic children can suitably be placed in day-schools for the physically handicapped where the tempo of school life is slower and more flexible and the teachers and attendants are accustomed to the management of such children. Some who are at the same time educationally subnormal may most appropriately be taught in schools for children of that category. For a few the handicap is so great that they must remain at home and such tuition as they are capable of receiving is given by a visiting teacher. Provision for the remainder of those requiring special educational treatment is best made in residential schools for epileptic children.

The purpose of these schools is to provide a general education designed to suit a very considerable range of ability; to control the seizures by appropriate treatment; and to re-establish the emotional life of the child if this has been disturbed. After a period of residence some children are able to return home and resume day-school education. For those who remain, vocational instruction is given in the later years of schooling, in gardening, wood, leather and metal work and domestic science; and this enables some at the end of their school life to face employment outside. Those who still need care may be admitted to colonies for adults with epilepsy.

Educationally subnormal pupils (*Mentally handicapped*, Scotland). The Scottish Education Department report on pupils with mental or educational disabilities (1951) allocated them to the following categories:

(*a*) pupils requiring special education because of absence, frequent change of school, faulty teaching and other similar causes;

(*b*) pupils with specific disabilities in reading, arithmetic, spelling and other school subjects;

(*c*) pupils who are retarded, but who are capable of making some progress in the school arts, normally with intelligence quotients ranging from approximately 50 to 70;

(*d*) pupils who are unable to make much progress, if any, in the school arts but who are capable of being trained, normally with intelligence quotients from approximately 30 to 50;

(*e*) pupils who have defects of personality to such a degree that they cannot profit from educational services or who have a harmful influence on others.

Group (*a*) and many of group (*b*) remain in ordinary schools where their educational difficulties should be met, if circumstances permit, by individual attention from the class or head teacher, or by the provision of adjustment classes such as are now organised in many areas to serve the needs of individual schools or groups of schools. The teachers of these classes are advised and visited by the educational psychologist; the classes are small with a roll of 9 pupils or less, allowing individual tuition; and pupils remain in the adjustment class for instruction in the subjects in which they require assistance, returning to their regular classes for other studies and activities. Individual tuition and special educational treatment may also be provided for these children by the local authority's child guidance service.

Groups (*c*), (*d*), and (*e*) are very much the concern of the school medical officer and their ascertainment must now be considered. Educationally subnormal children are brought to notice either at medical inspections or by the school nurse in the course of her inspections, or by the teacher because of failure to make progress in school. Not infrequently these children react to their handicap by behaviour disturbance or truanting and may be referred by the parents, teachers, or the school attendance department for those reasons also. This may take place only after several years have been spent by the child in an ordinary school and in order that ascertainment may be early effected it is the practice in some areas to subject all pupils to a group intelligence test, made by the class teacher with a non-verbal (picture) scale, usually at the age of 7 when promotion takes place from the infant department of the primary school. All pupils who appear to be mentally retarded for one or other of the reasons mentioned are further investigated by means of an individual test or tests, the Terman Merrill revision of the Stanford Binet Scale being that most often used. In other areas the policy is for all seven-year-olds with a reading age of 2 years or more less than their chronological age to attend an adjustment class for a year; if the response is unsatisfactory full psychometric assessment is carried out. This assessment is performed by educational psychologists of the local authority's child guidance service and in areas without such a service by school medical officers carrying out standard tests. A decision is reached on the reports of the school medical officer's medical examination and the educational psychologist's tests, the teacher's estimate, records of school achievement, information concerning social environment and any consultant's report available.

Transfer to a school for the educationally subnormal is best made between the ages of 7 and 10. Before 7 years the child can generally be coped with in the infant department of an ordinary school. After 10 years there may be difficulty in adjusting the child to the methods of the special school. Past experience has shown that pupils with intelligence quotients between 50 and 70 are suitable for transfer to a school for the educationally subnormal, but in some cases this figure is extended to 75. It must be borne in mind that the numerical result of an intelligence test is only one of several factors which must be considered and that ascertainment on the strength of an I Q alone is never justified. Indeed, in the assessment of any handicap the whole child, his strengths as well as his weaknesses, must be considered.

In areas of large population, educationally subnormal pupils are best taught in day-schools of their own. In smaller areas an all-age special class attached to an ordinary school is a better arrangement than that of leaving the mentally retarded in ordinary classes, but it is not an ideal form of organisation and as a general rule it is better that mentally retarded pupils in smaller urban and rural areas should be sent to residential schools, each serving the needs of a number of authorities. Such residential schools, too, provide the best education for any educationally subnormal child who is disturbed in his behaviour or whose home is broken or grossly unsatisfactory.

Pupils in these schools acquire the elements of numbers, reading, writing, and speech, by methods fitted to their need and their capacity, from teachers who have an appropriate extra teaching qualification. In their latter years at school the children receive vocational training in homecraft, gardening, etc., as a preparation for employment when they leave school.

The situation of a child unable to profit from instruction even in a school for educationally subnormal pupils is not the same in Scotland as in England and procedure in each country must be considered separately. Many such children, having intelligence quotients between 30 and 50 and often described as 'ineducable but trainable', are capable of training in personal habits, good behaviour, simple handicrafts, homecraft, and similar activities, and so profit from admission to an occupational centre. In Scotland these children remain the responsibility of the education authority on whom the Education (Scotland) Act, 1962 lays the duty of providing occupational centres which are, in law, special schools. Attendance at these centres is, therefore, compulsory between the ages of 5 and 16. Children found to be unsuitable for enrolment in an occupational centre are reported to the social work department of the local authority which is then responsible for supervision and care of these children.

In England and Wales children are reported to the local health authority at a higher level of intelligence than reporting to the local authority in Scotland, viz. when they are incapable of attending a school for educationally subnormal pupils. The provision of training in an occupational centre or of supervision and care is then the responsibility of the health authority. Government has accepted the principle, however, that responsibility for the education of these mentally handicapped children in England and Wales should be transferred to the education service and legislation is presently being prepared for this transfer.

When a child, leaving school, is considered by the education authority to need care and guidance because of mental handicap the authority must in Scotland send a statutory report to the social work department of the local authority. This is not a statutory duty in England and Wales where, instead, informal passage of information takes place between the local education and health authorities.

Maladjusted pupils. The incidence of maladjusted pupils is difficult to estimate but it probably lies between 5 and 10 per cent of children of school age. Maladjustment displays or betrays itself in many forms. It may be by such clinical signs as tics, pica, enuresis or encopresis; by failure to make progress in class or a sudden deterioration in school work; by truanting; by temper tantrums; or by dishonest, aggressive, or destructive actions, which may end in delinquency. Full discussion on the maladjusted child is given in Chapter 20. It is sufficient here to mention briefly the various forms of special educational treatment which may be provided by an education authority and which is in general under the supervision of an educational psychologist.

When maladjustment is associated with retardation in one or more subjects of study, individual help by the class teacher or a period of study in an adjustment class may enable the child to resume his proper level of school work and so restore his self-confidence. The cause of the child's maladjustment may, wholly or in part, lie in the school situation. Explanation of the cause by the psychologist may enable the teacher to collaborate in removing emotional stress. If, however, the association between the maladjustment and the school is too intimate and too powerful, transfer to another school may be the correct treatment. In some cases children who cannot be adjusted while they remain at home may be boarded-out with foster-parents and attend an ordinary school near the foster-home. For those whose emotional disturbance or anti-social behaviour is of severe degree there are day and boarding schools where constant observation, full investigation and intensive treatment can be given. By reason of their training the school doctor and school nurse are qualified to play an important part in the prevention of maladjustment and in its treatment in the earlier stages and more use might be made of their services than is at present the practice in many areas.

Autistic children constitute a small but important group among the maladjusted. The Society for Autistic Children (founded 1962) is active in promoting greater attention to this obscure condition.

Physically handicapped pupils. The majority of children with physical handicaps necessitating special educational treatment suffer from congenital malformations or hereditary diseases, from infections and their sequelae or from accidental injuries. In England and Wales in 1968, cerebral palsy stood first in the list of conditions necessitating special education, followed by spina bifida. Advances in the treatment of spina bifida and the increasing survival of these babies has led to a considerable increase in the number subsequently requiring special educational treatment (D.E.S. Circular 11/69). Already children with spina bifida constitute the second biggest group attending schools for the physically handicapped. Heart disease comes third in the list, most of the children suffering from congenital malformations; rheumatic heart disease, formerly high on the list of disabling diseases, has dramatically fallen within the last two decades. Muscular dystrophy, haemophilia, and a miscellaneous group of conditions, some rare, some not so rare, form the remainder of the causes of physical handicap.

In the larger urban areas those who are fit to live at home and are not too gravely disabled attend special day-schools. For the homebound or bed-ridden, education is provided by visiting teachers who work under the direction of the head teacher of one of the schools for the physically handicapped. Co-operation by the parents is essential if full advantage is to be taken of the visiting teacher service. Those who require extra medical or surgical treatment or who, because of adverse home conditions, cannot receive the care they need, as well as those for whom special day-school education is not available, go to residential schools where, in addition to teaching staff, nursing, medical and specialist staffs are also provided.

When children are likely to spend some time in hospital and where the nature of their disability does not make teaching inadvisable, education is provided through hospital schools or classes. For children confined to bed, individual methods are used. Others, who are mobile, are collected into small groups or classes. Hospital schools are maintained by the local education authorities of the areas in which the hospitals are situated and not by the regional hospital boards.

The 300 or so thalidomide-handicapped children born between January 1960 and August 1962 are now entering a critical phase of their lives from an educational standpoint, for most have entered school. The Lady Hoare Thalidomide Trust has allocated funds for a study, currently proceeding, of a compact group of 120

Scottish families with thalidomide-affected children, to investigate the I Qs of these children and their social needs in order to estimate the educational requirements of all such children in the United Kingdom.

Children with cerebral palsy. The incidence of this group of disorders is estimated at about 2 per 1,000 of the school population. Many of these children whose disability is of lesser severity can be suitably educated in schools for the physically handicapped; for the educationally subnormal; or in ordinary schools; but others must be considered as a special group of physically handicapped pupils having needs of their own. A number of them, by the use of specialised educational methods, physiotherapy, speech therapy, and occupational therapy, develop their faculties, mental and physical, in a manner not dreamt of some years ago.

Children with speech defects. The child normally achieves mastery of speech by the age of 5 years. If he fails to do so he enters school with a defect which may be a cause of considerable social maladjustment and an embarrassment to his educational progress. Defects in articulation are of many kinds and may be associated with other handicaps. In a considerable number of children the condition is a nervous disorder—stammering—and for some of them special educational treatment should be given, appropriate to the emotionally disturbed child. A still larger group includes the lispers, the clutterers, those whose speech is marred by one or several consonant substitutions, and those with nasal speech, open or closed. In a substantial number of these, investigation shows that mental handicap or a defect of hearing is the cause, and educational treatment appropriate to those handicaps should be provided. There are other cases in this large group which result from malformation of some parts of the speech mechanism and surgical or dental treatment may be required.

Lesser defects of articulation are often amenable to the speech training which should be part of the class curriculum in every school, but for the child with a more serious defect, unless the cause is deafness or mental handicap, therapy should be provided by speech therapists of the local education authority either in the school attended or in a special clinic. It is estimated that one speech therapist is needed for every 8,000 to 10,000 on the school roll but few authorities as yet employ an adequate staff of therapists and smaller areas may have none. Speech therapists should be under the direction of the school medical officer through whom all cases requiring therapy should be referred to the speech therapy centre.

Developmental dysphasia is a rare cause of delay in acquiring speech which needs further research to determine the appropriate treatment. Some children with this disability are referred to the speech therapist, others are found to be best treated by methods appropriate to the deaf child. Until recently there were only two special schools, both in the south of England, for children with severe speech defects of central origin and the pressure on places was acute. Moreover because of cultural and linguistic differences these schools were not ideally suited to deal with speech-handicapped children from other parts of the country, *e.g.* the north of England. In 1968 the Ewing Special School for children in the age range 3½ to 11 years was opened in Manchester with 12 residential places.

For full details of all special schools, day and residential, for handicapped pupils the reader is referred to the lists of special schools issued by the Department of Education and Science and Scottish Education Department respectively.

Prevention of Infectious Diseases

EXCLUSION. The hopeful confidence of past generations that closure of and exclusion from school would effectually control infectious diseases is no longer entertained by medical officers of health. Schools and departments are, therefore, rarely closed because of infections. The exclusion of individual children, of course, is required when they are suffering from infectious maladies but less importance is now attached to exclusion of contacts. This latter action is largely at the discretion of the school medical officer.

IMMUNISATIONS. If no immunisation or an incomplete basic course has been given before school entry, the full basic course of triple vaccine and oral poliomyelitis vaccine should be given. When the basic course has been given before school entry a booster dose of diphtheria/tetanus vaccine and poliomyelitis vaccine should be given on school entry, followed by a further boosting dose of tetanus vaccine and poliomyelitis vaccine just prior to leaving school or between 15 and 19 years in senior pupils. If smallpox vaccination has been performed in the preschool years it is recommended that revaccination should be carried out at school entry and before leaving school or between 15 and 19 years. In view of the possibility of accidental infection of eczematous members of the family of a child, it is preferable for all smallpox vaccinations to be carried out by or with the knowledge of the family doctor. Full details of immunisation procedures and programmes will be found in Chapter 11. The written consent of parents must be obtained before any immunisation procedure is carried out. Apathy towards protective inoculations must be constantly combated by patient, personal persuasion by school and family doctor, nurses and teachers.

Tuberculosis

CASE FINDING IN SCHOOL. The presence of a case of active pulmonary tuberculosis in a school may endanger the well-being of the pupils and, when co-operation between the chest clinic and the school health service is good, the school medical officer is appraised of every such case. Risk of dissemination from a young pupil is rare for at this time a pulmonary lesion most often appears as a primary complex. Older pupils may develop lesions more dangerous to themselves and to others. The greatest danger arises from an open case of tuberculosis in an adult employed at school whether such adult be teacher, ancillary staff or member of a residential school or home. The Department of Education and Science (circular 3/69) stresses this danger and the need to protect schoolchildren against infection by adults. Specific requirements are laid down for the examination of staff before employment, their periodic examination including X-ray of the chest every 3 years, their suspension from employment if found to be suffering from tuberculosis, and the follow-up of cases among schoolchildren.

When a case of tuberculosis is reported in a school, the school health service should carry out a survey of the contacts who, according to the circumstances of the case, may include a single class, a group of classes or a whole school. Tuberculin testing by the multiple puncture method is applied and is followed by radiographic examination of the positive reactors. In some areas this procedure has been extended for the purpose of case finding to children not at risk and testing is offered to school entrants, to other age groups or to whole school populations.

BCG VACCINATION. In 1953 sanction was given by the then Ministry of Health and the Department of Health for Scotland for any local authority to make BCG vaccination available to secondary school pupils for the purpose of fortifying them for their encounters with infection after leaving school, and, in order to allow of subsequent supervision in school, the age group selected was the thirteen-year-olds. The signed permission of the parents must be obtained and in most cases is willingly given; a tuberculin test is applied to the skin by the multiple puncture method and negative reactors are vaccinated. Positive reactors whose sensitivity is the result of previous exposure to infection and not of previous vaccination may have active tuberculosis at the time of testing or may develop it later. All such reactors should be X-rayed, and the examination repeated annually throughout school life.

In 1961 permission was granted by the central authorities to advance vaccination to as early an age as 10 years if, in the opinion of the medical officer of health, circumstances in his area made this action advisable (see Chapter 11).

School Dental Service

The statutory duties of this service are laid down in the Education Acts (1944, England and Wales, 1962, Scotland) as amended. The service concerns that branch of dentistry which is aimed at preventing dental disease and maintaining dental health in the schoolchild. The functions, broadly, are examination and treatment, prevention and dental health education. Recruitment of dental officers to the service suffered considerably following the introduction of the National Health Service when many entered general dental practice. More recently, however, recruitment to the school dental service has improved and the latest figures show that there were the equivalent of 1,364 whole-time dental officers in the service in England and Wales and 198 in Scotland. Partly on account of better staffing and partly because more schoolchildren receive dental treatment from general dental practitioners, school dental officers are now not under the same pressure which formerly presented them with the problem of dealing with so many dentally neglected children requiring treatment for acute pain and long established oral sepsis. Nevertheless, staff shortage still haunts the school dental service.

EXAMINATION AND TREATMENT. It is a statutory duty under the Education Acts that all school children must be dentally inspected. Ideally this inspection should be carried out every 6 months but under existing manpower shortage in some areas this inspection is only possible once in every 2 years. Inspections are carried out in the schools and determine whether a child requires dental treatment. If a child is found to require such treatment the parents are advised that this is required. There is freedom of choice where the treatment is carried out, either to accept treatment from the school dental service or from a dental practitioner under the National Health Service.

Treatment through the school dental service may be carried out in a health centre, in a surgery within a school, or in a surgery in a maternal and child health centre. In rural areas and some urban areas use is made of mobile dental vans, the surgery literally being taken to the children.

DENTAL HEALTH EDUCATION AND PREVENTION. Education has been undertaken through the medium of dental health campaigns, both large and small. Large, national campaigns have been found to achieve results for a short time only and concentration now is on smaller groups and at more frequent intervals. The Scottish Home and Health Department in 1966 arranged with local authorities that all children starting school for the first time would receive a dental health 'pack' free of charge. This pack consists of a plastic pouch containing a letter about dental health to the parents from the local authority's chief dental officer, a 'Happy Smile' club card, which, when completed, would earn a club badge for the child, a card for the bathroom giving the basic rules of dental health, a tooth brush, and a small tube of toothpaste. Distribution of these packs is made by the ancillary personnel and at the time of distribution a short talk is given on the importance of dental health. The idea behind this scheme is to promote dental hygiene and encourage parent participation in dental care.

The school meals service, too, offers opportunities for reinforcing instruction in dental health, particularly as regards good eating habits and cleansing of the mouth after meals. Hence local authorities should have regard, in planning menus, to the effects of food on the teeth, and should encourage dental hygiene after meals in school.

Prevention also includes the fluoridation of water supplies where necessary to raise the level to 1 part per million but progress in this direction is regrettably very slow. Sweden was one of the first nations to adopt large-scale use of topical fluorides in the prevention of caries. At first this was carried out by applying topically, solutions varying in strength from 2 per cent sodium fluoride to 8 per cent stannous fluoride in the surgery but this was found to be too time-consuming to be employed routinely in school dentistry and simpler means had therefore to be sought. After careful laboratory tests and clinical trials it was shown that worthwhile reductions in caries could be obtained by both brushing and by mouth-rinsing with fluoride solutions. Mouth rinsing with weak solutions of sodium fluoride (0·2 per cent) has now become commonplace in Swedish and Danish schools, and subsequent published caries reduction figures lie between 30 and 50 per cent. This method of fluoride mouth-rinsing at fortnightly intervals has since been introduced on a trial basis into some areas of the country, *e.g.* Edinburgh, 1968.

Dental ancillaries. In order to assist in the control of dental disease, two types of dental ancillary have been introduced. These are dental hygienists and dental auxiliaries.

DENTAL HYGIENISTS. This group of ancillary dental workers was established under the Dentists Act, 1956. The course of training lasts for at least 9 months and the curriculum is comprehensive. The training centres are at dental hospitals and in the armed forces. The scope of the hygienists' work is to scale and polish teeth and to use topical applications of stannous fluoride. Much of their work is concerned with dental health education by chairside and group teaching. Knowledge of dental health, the cause and prevention of caries, is imparted to the children in school and to the parents at parent meetings. The facts that teeth are an asset and the dentist is a friend are points emphasised. The hygienist must inspire those to whom he speaks to act for themselves and to realise that dental health is a part of physical health of all people. Hygienists are employed in private dental practice, in the general dental service and in the school dental service.

DENTAL AUXILIARIES. The Dentists Act, 1957, made provision for this type of ancillary worker. The present training was started in 1960 at New Cross Hospital, London, and 60 students are accepted each year. The training is based on the New Zealand scheme of dental nurses and occupies 2 years. The scope of the work which the students are taught embodies the carrying out of simple fillings in both temporary and permanent teeth, the extraction of temporary teeth under local infiltration anaesthesia, cleaning and polishing teeth, scaling teeth, applying to the teeth solutions of sodium or stannous fluoride, and dental health education measures. Talks to schoolchildren are given in school and use is made of visual aids, flannelgraphs and film strips. The work to be carried out by dental auxiliaries is given in writing by the dental officers. Under recent regulations operative from September 1969, the dental auxiliary does not require to work under the direct supervision of a dental officer. This will permit more use of the auxiliary in rural areas which have previously been denied the services of such auxiliaries but direction still requires to be given to them by the dental officer in writing.

The use of ancillary personnel increases the time available to the dental officers to carry out more advanced work. Consultant services are available to the school dental service for orthodontics and oral surgery through the agency of regional hospital boards.

The school dental service must obviously work in close partnership with the general dental service and to this end it is the practice in many areas that the chief school dental officer is co-opted as a member of the local dental committee. The future of the school dental service lies in the use of dental teams comprising dental officers, dental auxiliaries, dental hygienists and dental surgery assistants, this last group of ancillary workers receiving a training at dental hospitals or under further education schemes.

Environmental Activities

The School Premises Regulations and School Building Codes prescribe standards for sites, playgrounds and playing fields, classrooms, ancillary accommodation, such as staff rooms, sanitary and washing accommodation, and kitchens. Lighting, heating, ventilation and water supply and drainage are also dealt with. The school building modernisation programme has made encouraging progress but many older schools in both town and country areas still present grave deficiencies interfering with the well-being of pupils and stultifying the teaching of the elementary rules and habits of health.

School medical officers are especially concerned with those factors in environment which have a direct influence on the health of the pupils. As early as 1908 the Board of Education suggested that school medical officers should report annually on the hygienic conditions prevalent in schools in respect of ventilation, lighting, warming equipment, sanitation, etc., and the Education (Scotland) Act, 1962, lays a statutory duty on them to inspect and report on school premises, furnishing and equipment, having special regard to lighting, heating and ventilation and to sanitary arrangements. A particular problem which closely concerns the school nurse, and of which the importance has been greatly increased by the raising of the school-leaving age, is the supply and disposal of sanitary towels and the personal hygiene of girls in secondary schools and in the higher classes of primary schools. Much discomfort and unhappiness result to the adolescent from inadequate provision.

Provision of school meals. The Education Acts make it obligatory for local education authorities to provide meals and refreshments for pupils in attendance at maintained schools. The school dinner is, as a rule, a cooked meal. In most areas it is prepared in a central kitchen and sent out by motor van to be consumed in the dining centres of neighbouring schools, and the delay between cooking and serving, inevitable under such a system, affects both the palatability and the nutritive value of the food. This is avoided if each school has its own kitchen and for a time the provision of school kitchens instead of central kitchens proceeded with promising speed. Later, however, the need for economy slowed down this development.

The Department of Education and Science circular (3/66) dealt with the nutritional standard of school dinners and recommended an average calorie provision of 880 calories per meal and planned to contain 29 gm. protein (including 18·5 gm. animal protein) and 32 gm. fat. Special provision for the adjustment of these nutrients was not thought necessary as the variations in the size of the portions served to children of different age and sex would automatically regulate the protein and calorie value of the meals served. The circular also recommended that the number of meals at which meat was served should be reduced from the equivalent of 4 to 3 each week and that the portion of meat should be increased and the variety and quality improved for these meat meals. To cater for the extra non-meat serving day, other protein foods such as eggs, cheese, and fish should be increased and potatoes and cereals reduced. It was further suggested that flexibility and variety within the recommended nutritional and food standards were necessary and that more and improved communication between the Department and local education authorities as well as between authorities and their kitchen staffs was necessary so that advice and guidance would be more readily available. Finally, the circular suggested that there should be increased provision of training courses for school meals staff at both national and local levels.

In addition to supplying a very considerable part of the daily food requirements the school dinner introduces the children to a variety of wholesome foods which many of them never taste in their homes. Much opposition, the result of preformed food habits, has often to be overcome, but in the end those pupils who take school meals acquire a knowledge of and liking for a considerable range of food dishes, an experience which, it is hoped, will help to fit them as parents in the years to come to provide for the proper feeding of their families. A school meal, too, provides a valuable opportunity for health and social education.

A charge is made to the parent which covers part of the expense of the meal, the remainder of the cost being met out of the rates. If the family income is below a certain level the meal is provided free of cost to the parent. In England and Wales in 1968 pupils taking dinners numbered 5,020,000 representing 70 per cent of those in attendance. In Scotland 388,856 or 46·4 per cent took dinners. There is some evidence that some parents consider that the school dinner is sufficient to meet the child's daily nutritional needs (Lynch, 1969), and little else need be given at other times of the day.

Dining accommodation of a high standard is found in schools of most recent construction. In the older schools meals may have to be taken in assembly halls, gymnasia, classrooms or even corridors but the number of schools so inadequate in accommodation and facilities is rapidly diminishing.

Milk in Schools scheme. Pupils, whether boarders or not, in public, grant-aided and independent primary schools are entitled to one-third of a pint of milk per day free of charge, and all pupils in schools for handicapped children to two-thirds of a pint per day free of charge. The school milk is provided by the education authority and paid for centrally. Most of it is pasteurised but full cream dried milk, reconstituted, may be supplied where circumstances make the provision of liquid milk impracticable, *e.g.* where schools are isolated in island communities or scattered over wide tracts of hill country. Under the Public Expenditure and Receipts Act, 1968, from September of that year free milk ceased to be available for pupils at secondary schools.

Clothing and footwear. Under powers conferred by the Education Acts, a child whose clothing or footwear is inadequate may be clad and shod by the education authority to enable him to take full advantage of the education provided at school. The parent may be required fully or in part to reimburse the authority for the expense incurred.

Spectacles. The National Health Service provides free spectacles for children but will not replace them if they have been lost or broken through lack of care. Under the Education Acts which lay on local authorities the duty to secure the provision of free medical treatment for schoolchildren, some education authorities pay for spectacles needing replacement responsibility for which is not accepted by the National Health Service.

Games and physical education. These have long been recognised as essential elements in the educational programme. Responsibility for their provision rests on local education authorities under the terms of the Physical Training and Recreation Act, 1937, and the Education Acts, but voluntary bodies are also encouraged by grant aid to contribute towards such opportunities. In primary schools physical education is based on the natural activities of running, throwing, leaping, crawling and climbing and use is made of small apparatus such as balls, ropes, hoops, etc., and of large climbing apparatus of various kinds. Minor playground games and informal versions of the national team games are included. Wherever facilities permit swimming is included. A daily period, taken by the class teacher, is usual in primary schools. In secondary schools a wide range of activities is available—gymnastics, games, athletics (track and field), dancing and swimming. For the more senior pupils outdoor pursuits such as camping, canoeing, sailing and expeditions, activities such as judo, fencing, cycling and skating are available, whilst games such as tennis, badminton, volley-ball and golf are often included. In boys' schools football, rugby, and hockey are the main winter games with cricket in the summer; for girls, hockey, lacrosse and netball are the winter games with tennis in the summer. Games and athletics for secondary pupils are, for the most part, organised and coached by specialist teachers with some help from the other teachers of the school.

A paved playground and a small playing field (1 acre per 100 pupils) are statutory requirements for primary schools. All new primary schools have indoor accommodation for physical education. This usually is a multipurpose hall equipped with climbing frames and ropes. In secondary schools playing fields are of such an extent that all pupils may play field games once a week; a hard paved or porous area on which tennis courts can be laid out is also a statutory requirement. Indoor accommodation is related to the size of the school. It may be a dual purpose hall/gymnasium for smaller schools (up to 360 pupils), but for larger schools a separate gymnasium is required, while in schools with over 750 pupils additional indoor space is required, e.g. a sports hall or indoor heated swimming pool.

The advice of the school medical officer is frequently required with regard to exercise and particular activities, such as swimming, in individual cases, and also as to physical training generally in the school curriculum. It may be necessary for him to satisfy himself with regard to the cleanliness of swimming baths, and take steps to prevent the spread of epidermophytosis and plantar warts in bath houses; to make sure that tinea and impetigo are not being spread by the indiscriminate use of towels and changing clothes; and to exclude from swimming children with running ears or other infective discharges. When the school has a gymnasium he should be satisfied that it is kept clean and properly ventilated. Attention should be paid to under-developed and weakly children who are liable to be over-exercised by a too enthusiastic instructor.

The doctor should not be too anxious to exclude children from physical activities unless he is certain that their condition warrants it. For example, a child who has had 'growing pains' and has a systolic murmur may be turned into a real invalid, with the classical picture of 'effort syndrome', by a doctor who has played for safety by excluding him from all activity even though he has no organic heart lesion. In cases where a physical disability is present, the aim should be to encourage the full range of activity which the child can carry out without suffering further injury. Thus in certain cases of well-compensated heart disease graduated activity under careful supervision will give a better functional result than complete rest.

Accident prevention and first aid provision. In his general supervision of school premises the school medical officer concerns himself with such matters as fire precautions, the guarding of machinery in technical workshops and the prevention of burns and scalds in laboratories and domestic science rooms. He also supervises the provision and maintenance of first aid boxes, and advises head-masters, janitors and groundsmen on the procedure to be followed if an accident occurs in the school, playground or playing field.

Residential camp schools. The purposes of these camps are three in number. The first is to provide for children, mainly from the towns, the chance of becoming acquainted with the countryside and its way of life; the second is to improve health and well-being by residence in wholesome surroundings with good food and regular hours; and the third is to afford the experience of membership of a community and so to develop right qualities of mind and character.

The term 'Camp' tends to mislead, for, in fact, the buildings are substantial wooden chalets with classrooms, assembly and recreation halls and a dining room and kitchen and each accommodates up to 240 children and some 15 teachers and attendants. Camp schools are owned and managed by the education authorities in whose areas they are situated. It is true that a few are occupied for periods of 9 months to a year at a time by delicate or educationally subnormal pupils and in them provision is made for 100 or 120 children only, but the primary concern of the camps is with ordinary pupils and they should not be looked upon as special schools for the handicapped. Where classes or whole schools are sent to them for periods varying from some weeks to a year, the improvement gained in body, mind, character and social training, is often very great. When not occupied by schools, the camps may be used as holiday centres or for conferences by national or international youth organisations. In Scotland camp schools are owned and managed by the Scottish National Camps Association, from which they are rented for residential purposes by local education authorities.

Councils of physical recreation. These have as their purpose the encouragement of young people all over the country to spend part of their leisure time in games, sports, outdoor activity and other forms of physical recreation. The Central Council maintains four, and the Scottish Council two, national recreation centres where, in addition to instructional and holiday courses for students and other adults, school courses are provided for pupils between the ages of 14 and 18 years. These are concerned with a very wide range of games and athletics and with such outdoor pursuits as field studies, rock and snow climbing, pony trekking, sailing and camping. Under powers given to them by the current Education Acts, education authorities may send groups of pupils for periods, usually of a week, to these centres, paying part or the whole of the expense involved.

Other extra-curricular activities. Much has been done in recent years to make school education less purely 'didactic' by introducing into it some of the varied elements—social, recreational and cultural—of outside life. School cruises during term time as well as during school holidays have been regular features since they were resumed in 1961. Some schools organise visits of pupils and teachers to places abroad, especially France, during school vacations, and it is an important function of school medical officers to examine these children before going abroad on these visits and to ensure that they are adequately vaccinated against the usual infections prior to departure.

Duke of Edinburgh's Award for boys and girls. This scheme, when initiated in 1956, was restricted to a small number of experimental local authorities but it has now been extended to cover the whole country. The Award Scheme is not a competition and the standards for each test are intended to match average abilities; perseverance is one of its keynotes. No-one need be debarred because of physical or material handicap. The purpose of the scheme is the encouragement of young people to find happiness in new interests; the development of their talents for the service of the community; and, above all, the building of character. Boys and girls may enter for the awards between their fourteenth and twentieth birthdays, and there are three stages—the preliminary, which leads to a bronze, the intermediate, which leads to a silver, and the final, which leads to a gold Award Badge. In each stage there are four sections—for the boys: Fitness, Rescue and Public Service Training, the Expedition, Pursuits and Projects; and for the girls: Design for Living, Interests, Adventure, Giving Service. Many education authorities have introduced the scheme into their schools and they are empowered to help participants by the loan of camping equipment; by payment of fees for residential training; by the provision of instructions for specialist courses; and in other practical ways.

Health Education (see also Chapter 21)

Ever since the inception of the school medical services in 1907–08, the need for health education in schools has been repeatedly stressed and the numerous reports and pamphlets published on the subject have all recommended that teachers should instruct their pupils at least in the basic requirements for healthy living. Many excellent syllabuses have been suggested but their implementation has always been the main problem. Within recent years world-wide realisation of the need for health education has helped to focus attention more forcibly on the subject in this country. Obviously the health needs of a developing, economically poor country are very different from those of an affluent one. Thus programmes of health education vary within wide limits according to climatic, cultural, educational and economic conditions of different countries. As national programmes vary according to need so it has been found that there are different levels of need in our own country, even in schools of different areas and this must not be forgotten in devising programmes of health and social education.

School gives children the education necessary for their future careers. This is and always has been so but over the years the school syllabus has undergone many changes in content and offers much more now than mere preparation for a career. School attempts to prepare pupils not only for work but for living, for home life, for leisure and for play. But school can only successfully play a limited part in this wide field. The parents, the home and the environment are all involved and ideally all must make their contribution for the greater good. In organising courses of health education the support of the parents must be sought by every possible means. The school environment, *i.e.* classrooms, playgrounds, dining room, toilets, etc., must uphold the health message and all the school staff must participate directly or indirectly by precept and example. The actual instructors in health and social educational matters should be teachers well grounded in the basic principles of health but the school medical officer, health visitor and nurse must always be ready to help with special talks, lead discussions, advise on visual aids, and, above all, help to maintain enthusiasm.

Much of our health education is offered to individuals. Such individual teaching will always be necessary on appropriate occasions but the advice and help given are often corrective and proffered in comparatively short and infrequent sessions. These more intensive sessions are important but can never cover a deliberate programme and are not an alternative to this.

To ensure a structured approach for a meaningful health and social educational policy in its schools of all grades, ideally including further educational establishments, the forward looking education authority makes the best use of the varied knowledge and experience of the staff of its education and school health services. Interesting pilot experiments based on this are currently under way throughout the country. Thus, in some primary schools, class teachers pursue a regular definite programme of health education, the topics for which are supplied in guidelines, provided by the school or local authority experts, to ensure that all aspects of health education are covered simply and adequately, for this age-group of children. In secondary schools with their subject teachers this form of programme is more difficult to follow nor is time so readily found for it. Nevertheless, courses can be devised with the emphasis changing towards social education and mental hygiene. A team of teachers from many departments of the secondary school is required to develop a plan of broad concept and continuing impact. To achieve these desiderata a co-ordinator is required. Such courses should ensure that each pupil gains the knowledge, skills, values and attitudes that make for full and healthy development, that he realises his personal responsibility, and that he develops a worthy sense and positive concept of self. Group discussions with trained leaders are necessary for all secondary school pupils and individual counselling is frequently required. The school medical officer or health visitor may very successfully fulfil the roles of co-ordinator, discussion leader and counsellor.

Education authorities attach increasing importance to the teaching of homecraft to older girls, and in many secondary schools, in addition to cookery, laundry and sewing classrooms, a model flat is attached to the homecraft department where older girls take turns to stay in residence and learn home management under a resident mistress. Education authorities may also make arrangements for the teaching of mothercraft to senior girls, either by female medical officers, health visitors or school nurses, instruction being given to the girls in small groups by talks and demonstrations in school and by visits to day nurseries. Teaching of mothercraft is supervised by the school medical officer.

Instruction in accident prevention. Injury resulting from accidents is a common cause of absences from school, and accidental deaths now form at least a quarter of all deaths in childhood. Of the total number of accidents reported 25 per cent occur in the home and 50 per cent on the roads and health education in schools is, therefore, directed to the prevention of accidental injury in both of these places.

Avoidance of home accidents is rarely the subject of formal instruction but it is incorporated in the ordinary work of the homecraft classrooms, the technical workshops and the science laboratories in secondary schools, where pupils are taught the prevention of burns and scalds, the precautions needed to avoid accidental poisoning with cleaning agents and medicinal substances and the proper use of edged or pointed implements and of electrical and other equipment. When a 'flat' or 'house' is part of the homecraft department there is a still wider field for teaching the secondary school pupil to avoid mishaps in the home.

Training in road safety on the other hand is suitably given by more formal methods and it is recommended that in primary schools a few minutes be given to this instruction by class teachers once a week for older children and thrice weekly for younger children, for whom the instruction includes 'kerb-drill'. In many areas playground demonstrations are regularly staged, equipment being provided by the education authority, the demonstrators being traffic policemen with motor cycles and the children themselves playing an active part. Accidents to child cyclists most often occur about the ages of 12 or 13 years, the ages at which a bicycle but not always the skill to ride it properly are acquired, and education authorities may arrange in their schools for traffic policemen or other instructors to examine bicycles, point out defects, advise on maintenance, and give instruction to young cyclists in the school playground. In 1959, RoSPA inaugurated a National Cycling Proficiency Scheme for training young cyclists who, after passing a test, are awarded a badge. Since that year almost 2 million young cyclists have been trained for the badge.

Instruction in safety precautions and accident prevention at work, at play, on the roads, when swimming or boating, should be included as topics recurring throughout the school programme. It is equally important to ensure that basic and simple first aid instruction is also given especially to secondary pupils.

Instruction in health education. In some countries, notably the United States of America, specialist health educators, trained in the principles of health and hygiene, in the methods of presenting these principles to children and adults, are employed. At present in Britain there are relatively few health educators but the Institute of Health Education has been formed to promote the fuller development of professional full-time health educators. All student teachers in training colleges and university training departments receive instruction in health education (see p. 472). Health visitors also receive both theoretical and practical instruction in the subject during their course of training leading to the Health Visitor's Certificate. In 1954 the University of London Institute of Education initiated a comprehensive course on the content and method of health education, leading to a diploma of the Institute and which is intended for doctors, nurses, teachers and other suitable students.

Employment of School Children

In general the effect of the provisions of the Children and Young Persons Acts, 1933–63 (England and Wales) and 1937–63 (Scotland) as amended by the Education Acts, is that a child may not be employed until he is 13 years of age. From then until he reaches the upper limit of compulsory school age, presently 15 years, he may engage in part-time employment out of school hours but not in an industrial undertaking. In the eyes of the law a person is employed when he assists in a trade or occupation carried on for profit and the provisions, therefore, apply as much to the child helping a parent or relative to carry on a business as to the child earning payment for his services.

The delivery of milk and newspapers and miscellaneous duties in shops and on farms provide employment for the great majority. The provisions of the various Acts and of byelaws issued by local authorities define and restrict the nature, hours and conditions of work done outside school hours. For example, a child is prohibited from being employed during school hours or before 7 a.m. or after 7 p.m.; and no person under 17 years can be employed in street trading. Many pupils earn money by part-time occupation without detriment to their health or their education, but if, after part-time employment has been undertaken, it appears that the child's health or education is adversely affected by it, the local authority has power to prohibit the child's employment.

Restrictions are also imposed on children under 16 years taking part in public performances except under licence granted by the local education authority. No licence may be granted unless the local authority are satisfied that a child is fit to perform, that provision is made for his health and welfare, and that his education will not suffer. The child must also be examined by the school medical officer before being licensed and thereafter at 3-monthly intervals. The licence must specify the times during which the child may be absent from school for the purposes authorised by the licence. Restrictions are also placed on the granting of licences for performances by children under 13 years, for training children between 12 and 16 years for performances of a dangerous nature, and for performing abroad. The Children (Performances) Regulations, 1968, deal in detail with licences, their conditions, restrictions, etc.

EMPLOYMENT OF YOUNG PEOPLE. Under the Employment and Training Act, 1948, the Youth Employment Service may be operated locally either by the education authority or directly by the Ministry (see Chapter 19). The purpose of the Service is to help boys and girls as they pass from school life into the world of work. Its main functions are to collect and disseminate information about careers and opportunities of employment for young persons under 18 years of age or over that age if they are still attending school; to advise such young people on choice of career; to assist them in finding suitable employment; and to provide employers in industry, commerce and the professions with facilities for filling vacancies for young workers.

Nursery Schools and Classes

The earlier history of the nursery school movement has already been described in Chapter 14. Nursery schools first became eligible for grant in 1919 but growth has always been slow although World War II gave nursery schools a temporary boost. Many schools admitted children to infant classes before the age of compulsory attendance; in other schools nursery classes were formed in association with infant departments of primary schools. The Education Acts established nursery education as an integral part of primary education and put nursery schools and classes on the same footing. Any development of nursery education provision, however, was soon checked by economic considerations and the present distribution of nursery schools and classes is somewhat haphazard throughout the country. In only two respects has government been prepared to relax this post-war freeze. In 1960 local authorities were officially encouraged to organise nursery schools and classes on a two-shift basis. This followed the success of various experiments in the organisation of nursery education on a part-time basis later described by Goldsworthy (1964). The second concession came in 1964 when local education authorities were empowered to extend nursery provision, but in existing accommodation, if they were satisfied that a pool of qualified married women teachers was available locally and that these teachers were anxious to return to teaching but were prevented from doing so 'only by the absence of nursery provision for their children'. More recently local education authorities are permitted to open additional nursery accommodation but under rigid conditions of control. At present most maintained nursery school and class places are given to children who suffer from some kind of social handicap, or on medical grounds, or because their mothers are working, or they are teachers' children.

There is a wide measure of agreement among informed observers that nursery provision of a substantial scale is desirable not only on educational grounds but for social, health and welfare considerations. The Plowden Report (1967) recommended that nursery education should be available to children at any time after the age of 3 years until they reached compulsory school age and that nursery education should be predominantly part-time. The report further recommended that day nursery and nursery educational facilities should be integrated into a unified service and suggested measures for obtaining and training nursery assistants for the day-to-day work of nursery groups which would be under the general supervision of qualified nursery school teachers. Current figures for the whole country show that only about 4 per cent of two- to five-year-olds are provided for in maintained nursery schools and classes.

Accommodation and administration. Some nursery schools and classes reach a high standard in building and equipment, others are accommodated in adapted premises which may or may not be altogether suitable for nursery educational purposes. The accompanying plan of Calderglen Nursery School (Fig. 81), makes accommodation for two classes of 40 pupils each. By means of light, rigid

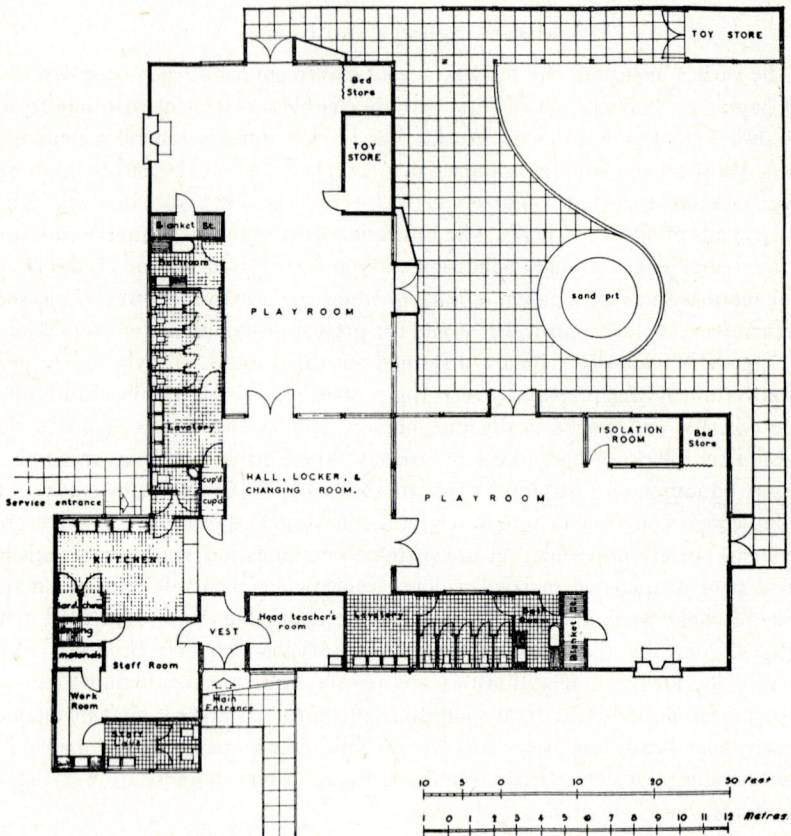

FIG. 81. Plan of a Nursery School.
(*Courtesy of the City Architect, Edinburgh*)

movable screens, each classroom can be divided into two equal or unequal sections and the classes can be broken up into groups. Ample outdoor space for a garden provides many interests with steps, bushes, hard-surfaced paths where the child can push his wheeled toys, patches of grass, trees for shade, and simple gardening equipment such as trowels, watering-cans, etc., to help the child to satisfy his curiosity in growing and living things. Furniture and equipment should be designed to meet the needs of children, with door handles, hand basins and water closets all low enough for children to use comfortably. Tables and chairs should be light-weight, shelves for toys, books and play materials easy to reach, and floors covered with washable material and everything kept fresh and clean.

A nursery school is under the charge of a headmistress who must be certificated and who holds an extra qualification for nursery school work. She is assisted by other, similarly qualified teachers; by nursery assistants, usually young women holding the certificates in nursery nursing, and by nursery students. The last are girls between 15 and 18 years following a 2 years' course of training for the nursery nurses certificate.

A nursery class is a component of a primary school, is normally housed in the same building and is under the immediate charge of the infant mistress and ultimate charge of the head teacher. In accommodation, amenities, and staffing, it should conform as closely as possible to nursery school standards. Nursery classes should have their own playgrounds, lavatories and washrooms. In England the age of the nursery school child is 2 years to 5 years, and of the nursery class child, 3 years to 5 years, but if there are exceptional circumstances, a child may be admitted to a nursery school before 2 years and to a nursery class before 3 years and may be retained after 5 years. If a nursery school is approved for the purpose, children may be retained up to the age of 7 years. In Scotland, children enter both nursery schools and classes at the age of 2 years and may remain until $5\frac{1}{2}$ years.

The daily or sessional programme is flexible, permitting periods of activity and some rest and helping the child to feel settled and safe. For much of the time the child is left free to find his own occupation and to play where and with whom he chooses. At intervals a group activity is arranged—singing, a story, moving to music, percussion band, etc.

The equipment need not consist of expensive toys. There is, on the contrary, much virtue in ordinary things of common household use and in simple robust objects such as waste material from timber yards and factories. The equipment should provide the things which make play possible in many forms and this play may be grouped into three main categories.

PLAY IN WHICH USE IS MADE OF THE MUSCLES, especially the large muscles, in which experiments are made in large movements of trunk and limbs, and which necessitates the surmounting of some obvious physical difficulty. Planks, logs, old motor car tyres, barrels, and large wooden boxes provide inexpensive material for this kind of play. Steps, slides, safety swings, and 'jungle-gyms' are also often supplied.

CONSTRUCTIVE PLAY, which requires materials such as water, sand, and clay, and objects such as bricks, boxes, beads, string, buckets and spades. Older children make use of toys such as motor cars, aeroplanes, farm animals, etc. In satisfying his desire to make, create, and manipulate, the child develops concentration and experimentation, gains manual dexterity and discovers the properties of his material.

IMITATIVE PLAY AND IMAGINATIVE PLAY. Much time is spent in playing at being other people: fathers, mothers, teachers, nurses, doctors, postmen and other well-known persons, and in reproducing the activities of home life; cooking, mending, looking after dolls, shopping, etc. With equal enjoyment children assume the part of animals or birds, of motor cars or aeroplanes, or lose themselves in such imaginative play as cowboys and Indians. It is held by many that a young child can fully grasp an idea only by acting it out in this way for 'what he tries to represent or do, he begins to understand'.

Younger children, and older children when they first join the school or class, prefer, generally, to play by themselves. Later they like to play beside one another and finally to play with one another in pairs or small groups. Larger groups, with the help of adults, form to enjoy singing, dancing, or story-telling, and to take some part in communal activities outside the precincts of the school, such as a walk through streets or park. This can be full of interest and enjoyment if it has some definite objective and is made under the care of a sympathetic teacher or nursery nurse.

It is a fundamental principle of nursery education that the child should be left to do, and encouraged to do, as much for himself as possible. The capacity to do so varies according to the age as well as the personality of the child. Members of the staff must know when not to proffer help and advice and they must also be ready to lend a sympathetic ear, a patient answer to questions and practical help with activities when this is really needed. The child's fundamental need of movement and play both for happiness and for learning as well as for physical and social development is now recognised by all nursery school workers. The methods employed in most nursery schools and classes are founded on a study of the work of earlier educationists in this field, notably Friedrich Froebel, the German educational reformer, and Dr. Maria Montessori, the Italian physician and educationist, combined with the more modern researches of educational psychologists, and the individual teacher adapts these methods to suit the needs of her own little charges.

Co-operation with parents. This is essential for the success of the school and the welfare of the individual children. There is usually daily contact between teachers and mothers who bring and fetch their children. Meetings of the mothers' club, held regularly and frequently, are, as a rule, well attended and give opportunity for discussion of the management and welfare of the child. At these meetings, and at home, mothers participate in the work of the school by cleaning, and by making and mending garments, towels, clothes, equipment, etc. At these meetings, also, the mothers get to know one another and parties and social outings are regular activities of such clubs.

Fathers are also encouraged to participate in the work of the school and many of them willingly give a helping hand by digging, gardening, carpentry and repairing of toys and equipment.

Promotion of physical health. The whole of nursery school life is, by its nature, an education in healthy living for the child, more specific training being given in hand-washing, tooth-brushing, regular elimination and proper feeding habits. Moreover, through the association between parents and nursery staff the lessons of health and hygiene are conveyed to the home. At parents' meetings, as well as in the medical room during inspection of the individual child, instruction is given as to clothing, feeding, sleep, ailments and behaviour difficulties by school doctors and nurses.

Emphasis is rightly laid on the value of activities out-of-doors but extremes must be avoided. If the nursery school or class is a whole-time one, meals will be supplied through the school meals service. Preferably these meals should be cooked

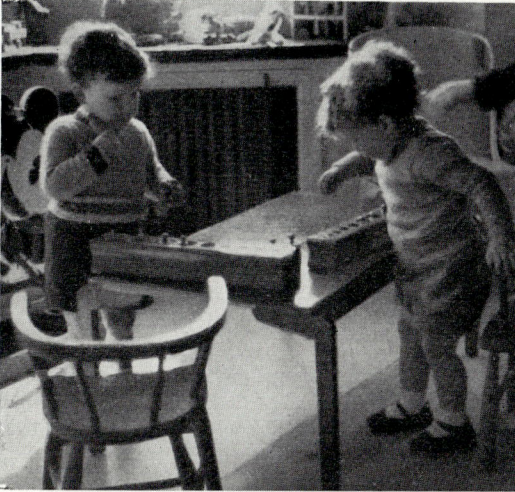

FIG. 82. Nursery school furniture should be of appropriate size and play material suitable for the intelligence of the children.

on the premises and, as a rule, consist of a mid-morning drink of milk, a midday dinner, and a snack at the end of the school day. The meals are planned to introduce the children to a variety of wholesome foods and should be served as attractively as possible. Practice is acquired in the use of forks, spoons and crockery, and in good table manners, and the serving of their fellows is looked upon as a prized privilege of the older children.

A brief rest period is part of the daily routine in the part-time nursery school or class, but in the whole-time school an after-dinner sleep is the constant rule. The risk of infection is minimised by the division of a school into units, by the use of individual face cloths, towels, combs, tooth mugs and brushes; by the provision of adequate floor space; and by insistence on fresh air.

Medical supervision is the responsibility of the school health service whose consultative and treatment facilities, including those of the dental service, are available to nursery pupils. Frequent visits are paid to the schools and classes by the school health visitors or nurses and frequent inspections are made by the school medical officer.

Residential nursery schools. A number of education authorities maintain residential nursery schools in country surroundings. Others make use of holiday homes in which pupils from day nursery schools or classes in town spend holidays of duration varying from a few days to 4 weeks under the charge either of their own teachers or of the staffs of the homes. Medical supervision is provided, either by the school health service or by local practitioners.

Nursery special schools and classes. Early training in expert hands is necessary for children with certain handicaps, *e.g.* blind, deaf, physically handicapped, maladjusted and educationally subnormal, and provision is made for nursery schools and classes for these groups of children by some authorities.

H. P. TAIT

References

Official Publications (H.M.S.O.)

CENTRAL ADVISORY COUNCIL FOR EDUCATION (1967). *Children and their Primary Schools.* 2 vols. (Plowden Report).

CENTRAL HEALTH SERVICES COUNCIL (1964). *Health Education.* Report of a joint committee of the Central and Scottish Health Services Councils. (Cohen Report).

—— (1968). *Immunisation Against Infectious Disease.* Memorandum prepared by the Standing Medical Advisory Committee for the Central Health Services Council.

DEPARTMENT OF EDUCATION AND SCIENCE. *Education and Science.* Annual Reports.

—— *Health of the Schoolchild.* Biennial reports of the Chief Medical Officer of the Department.

—— (1969). *List of Special Schools for Handicapped Pupils in England and Wales.* List 42 (1969).

—— (1968). *Blind and Partially Sighted Children.* Education survey No. 4. By Fine, S. R.

—— (1968). *A Handbook of Health Education.*

—— (1968). *The Education of Deaf Children: The Possible Place of Finger Spelling and Signing.*

—— (1969). *Protection of Schoolchildren against Tuberculosis.* Circular No. 3/69.

—— (1969). *Peripatetic Teachers of the Deaf.* Educ. Survey No. 6.

MINISTRY OF EDUCATION (1955). *Report of Committee on Maladjusted Children.* (Underwood Report).

SCOTTISH EDUCATION DEPARTMENT. *Education in Scotland.* Annual reports.

—— (1949-52). *Reports by the Advisory Council on Education in Scotland on the Various Categories of Handicapped Pupils.*

—— (1968). *Handicapped Pupils in Scotland.* List G. Being a list of the special schools in Scotland.

—— (1967). *Ascertainment of Children with Hearing Defects.* Report of a working party.

—— (1969). *Ascertainment of Children with Visual Handicaps.* Report of a working party.

SCOTTISH HOME AND HEALTH DEPARTMENT. *Health and Welfare Services in Scotland.* Annual reports.

—— (1969). *The School Health Service.* Report of a study group.

WORLD HEALTH ORGANIZATION (1951). *Experiment in Dental Care: Results of New Zealand's use of School Dental Nurses.* By Fulton, J. T. W.H.O. Monograph series No. 4.

—— (1960). *Teacher Preparation for Health Education.* Technical Report Series No. 193.

Other References

ATKINS, C. (1969). Grow straight, grow tall. *Med. Officer,* **121,** 109.

BARBER, D. (1969). Pre-school screen audiometry. *Public Health,* **83,** 75.

BRITISH TUBERCULOSIS ASSOCIATION (1967). Control of tuberculosis; the management of contact groups at places of employment and education. *Med. Officer*, **118**, 171.

FISCH L. (1969). Causes of congenital deafness. *Public Health*, **83**, 68.

FRANCIS, H. (1968). School health service work in the ordinary day schools. *Med. Officer*, **119**, 195.

GOLDSWORTHY, G. M. (1964). *Part-time Nursery Education*. London: Nursery School Association of Great Britain and Northern Ireland.

HOLLINS, F. R. and DICKS, S. (1968). A personal relationships project in senior schools. *Med. Officer*, **120**, 261.

INGRAM, T. T. S. (1964). *Paediatric Aspects of Cerebral Palsy*. Edinburgh: Livingstone.

—— (1967). Specific retardation of speech development. *Public Health*, **81**, 109.

IVES, L. A. (1969). Development of personality and emotional-social adjustment in deaf and partially hearing children. *Public Health*, **83**, 78.

KERSHAW, J. D. (1967). Handicapped school leavers. *Public Health*, **81**, 300.

—— (1968). Individual roles in health education: the medical aspect. *Public Health*, **82**, 153.

LUNN, J. E. (1967). School health service work in the ordinary day schools. *Med. Officer*, **118**, 303, 313, 329.

LYNCH, G. W. (1969). Food intake and the education of children. *Med. Officer*, **121**, 41.

MEDICAL OFFICER (1969). Children going hungry. *Med. Officer*, **121**, 39.

MENZIES, M. P. (1968). Educational television in health education. *Med. Officer*, **119**, 333.

MORRISON, J. B. (1966). Comparison of screening types used in vision-screening of young children. *Med. Officer*, **115**, 45.

NOSEWORTHY, C. A. P. (1968). Individual roles in health education: the education aspect. *Public Health*, **82**, 158.

PARRY, W. H. (1967). Infectious disease in school: an epidemiological review. *Med. Officer*, **118**, 79.

ROBERTS, C. J. (1968). Screening for defective hearing in infancy. *Public Health*, **82**, 173.

SHEARD, A. V. (1968). A survey of cardiac disorders in a school population. *Med. Officer*, **119**, 71.

SIMPSON, E. E. (1967). The hearing-handicapped child at school. *Public Health*, **81**, 126.

SMITH, C. S. (1968). The educationally subnormal child. *Med. Officer*, **119**, 146.

SOCIETY OF MEDICAL OFFICERS OF HEALTH (1969). The needs of handicapped children. Evidence submitted by Society to working party of National Bureau for Co-operation in Child Care. *Public Health*, **83**, 136.

SPEIZER, F. E., DOLL, R. and HEAF, P. (1968). Observations on recent increase in mortality from asthma. *Brit. med. J.*, **1**, 335.

WARD, B. (1968). Congenital heart lesions and education. *Med. Officer*, **119**, 69.

WATSON, T. J. (1967). Techniques for testing the hearing of schoolchildren. *Public Health*, **81**, 118.

WILSON, T. S. and MENZIES, M. P. (1966). The Keystone school vision screening test. *Med. Officer*, **115**, 46.

WORLD MEDICINE (1968). How thalidomide children see themselves. *World Medicine*, **4**, 15.

17　Social Services for Children

The Growth of Social Services for Children

Social services change as the organisation of society changes. As patterns of employment, or education, or leisure alter, new information becomes available about the underprivileged, the inadequate, the anti-social. When social change is associated with growing social wealth the collection and utilisation of information may be made more effective through increased allocations of time, skill, and material resources. As the various findings are circulated, public attitudes are likely to be affected. Forward looking policy makers seek to incorporate into legislation proposals based on the growing body of knowledge. Men and materials are made available to improve the condition and prospects of the newly identified socially disadvantaged. Appropriate skills and patterns of service are developed. Additional information accrues from the extended contacts and leads to further changes in service. Such has been the pattern of growth in Britain for social services concerned with children.

The Nineteenth century. At the beginning of the nineteenth century the number of children whose welfare was seriously at risk was unknown. Children found destitute received some form of care under Poor Relief, but many avoided notice, and many more lived in acute need with their parents. The early 1840s saw two official enquiries, one into the conditions of children's employment, the other into the sanitary conditions of the labouring poor, both of which contributed towards society's involvement in the lives of children. With the growth of educational and public health services to the poor, more information became available about the condition of deprived and distressed children, and consciences were moved to establish services to further their welfare. School meals and clothing were provided by voluntary organisations to the more ragged of the children revealed by compulsory education. Homeless boys and girls sleeping out in the open drew the attention of Charles Booth and others. Reformers such as Barnardo, Coram and Stephenson made provision for the homeless and neglected. Mary Carpenter established the first reformatory school for delinquents in 1854. Seebohm Rowntree's 1899 Survey of the poor in York shed light on the effect poverty had on children living with their parents, perhaps inevitably with an emphasis on the material aspects of life.

The Twentieth century. During the twentieth century legislators have increasingly concerned themselves with the general welfare of children. Certain Acts have applied with minor variations to Britain as a whole, for example, the

Children Act, 1948, as amended by the Children and Young Person's Act, 1963. Other legislation has related specifically either to England and Wales, or to Scotland. Where legislation has not been mandatory there have sometimes been considerable variations in outcome. The Children Act, 1908, which applied to England, Wales and Scotland alike, sought to focus the treatment of juvenile offenders on education and reform and to protect children from parental ill-treatment and neglect. In England and Wales these endeavours led to the development of juvenile courts attached to Justice of the Peace Courts. Despite the recommendation of the Children and Young Person's (Scotland) Act, 1932, that a parallel approach be attempted in Scotland, a committee under the chairmanship of Lord Kilbrandon could say in 1964 ". . . even allowing for the special juvenile courts in (the) four areas, the J.P. Court has not taken extensive root in Scotland, and (that) in this respect the situation is very different from that prevailing in England and Wales."

In 1939 mass evacuation of children brought to public notice hitherto unsuspected realms of material and emotional deprivation. The bulk of children deprived of a normal home life came under the provision of the 1930 Poor Law Act, and although material conditions had improved since the Acts of the nineteenth century, there was still little or no official recognition of their need for personal care and affection. An enquiry into the death in January, 1945, of a boy boarded out with foster parents recommended that 'administrative machinery should be improved, and informed by a more anxious and responsible spirit.' A Home Office committee, under the chairmanship of Dame Myra Curtis, was currently enquiring into the care of children deprived of a normal home life. The committee's report (1946) drew attention to the wide variety of agencies involved in the provision of care and to the many types of care to which a child could be subjected. The report revealed an acute shortage of staff, of buildings, of money, of training, and of co-operation. Its recommendations were concerned with recognising the needs of the deprived child, particularly his need for family life. This last aspect of child care led the committee to ask 'whether this deprivation (of home life) might not have been prevented?' Following on an interim report on training, the Central Training Council in Child Care was established in 1947 to raise standards in, and develop opportunities for, training and recruitment.

The Children Act, 1948, sought to provide a framework within which the concern and understanding of the Curtis Report, and of the corresponding Clyde Report in Scotland, might be translated into action. Each local authority was required to appoint a Children's Committee which would have the duty towards the child in care 'to exercise their powers with respect to him so as to further his interests, and to afford him opportunity for the proper development of his character and abilities'. An executive Children's Officer was to be responsible for the prescribed services, in the provision of which he was to be assisted by residential care staff and boarding out officers (later renamed child care officers).

In 1951–52 the Select Committee on Estimates was led by rising costs to recommend that more attention be paid to preventing the need to receive into care. At the same time many child care officers were becoming unhappy about receiving into care, particularly on a long term basis. Evidence accumulated to show that the effects on a child of removal from home were often far from beneficial. Bowlby's 1951 monograph on Maternal Care and Maternal Health provided a focus for the spreading uncertainty and dissatisfaction. The 1948 Act itself supported the view that children should remain with their parents whenever possible by giving the local authorities the duty to return a child to his parents if this was consistent with the welfare of the child. There was growing recognition that the family circumstances which had once justified boarding out a child until he was old enough to look after himself no longer obtained in the case of many children coming into care.

In 1950 the Home Office, the Ministry of Health, and the Ministry of Education issued a joint circular concerned with the need to co-ordinate the services offered to children in their own homes. Concern for the child in his own home was further emphasised by the Children and Young Persons (Amendment) Act, 1952, which required the local authority to take the initiative in causing enquiries to be made if it 'receives information suggesting that any child or young person may be in need of care or protection'.

In 1960 the Ingleby Committee recommended that local authorities should have the power 'to prevent or forestall the suffering of children through neglect in their own homes'. A preventive service would need to be family-centred, and would entail special provisions, such as preventive caseworkers, family advice centres, and early notification of families at risk. The evidence on the existing state of co-ordination led the committee to suggest as a long term aim the setting up of a unified social work service.

In Scotland, the 1963 McBoyle Report analysed the causes of child neglect in terms of problem families, families subject to circumstances beyond their control, and families suffering from personal or domestic difficulties. The main points made were that situations of child neglect can arise at all levels of society and are not simply a matter of material provision; that neglect is frequently a symptom of problems within the family, and can therefore only be dealt with by working with the whole family; that most families, whatever the appearance to outsiders, wish to hold together, and 'reproach, moralising, and punishment often reduce their (the parents') ability to do so'; and that often parents, particularly the unmarried mother, will not seek aid, and must therefore be sought out. Four solutions were proposed: a comprehensive preventive service, a family advice service, material assistance where necessary, and the power of local authorities to conduct or assist in research.

The 1963 Children and Young Persons Act incorporated a number of the Ingleby Committee recommendations. Section 1 of the Act made explicit three principles which have informed recent developments in the case of children in distress: first, that the child's welfare might be best promoted by diminishing the need to receive him into, and keep him in, care; second, that his welfare might be promoted by diminishing the need to bring him before a juvenile court; and third, that the pursuit of these aims might include giving assistance in kind, or in exceptional circumstances, in cash. The potential benefit of research into child welfare and delinquency was brought to the notice of local authorities, who were empowered to spend money on research: in general, however, authorities do not seem to have realised that research would contribute to the professional effectiveness of the child care service, and might even save them outlay in the long run.

Contemporary views. The case for a family-centred approach to the welfare of children leads to arguments that the organisation of such a service would extend beyond traditional child care boundaries. In 1965 a committee was appointed under the chairmanship of Frederick Seebohm 'to review the organisation and responsibilities of the local authority personal social services in England and Wales, and to consider what changes are desirable to achieve an effective family service.' In its report, published in 1968, the committee proposed that every county and county borough council should be obliged to set up a social service department which would take over virtually all social work done by local authorities. They argued the case for an extensive rationalisation of the care provided to children under 18. Children are taken into care for lack of day nurseries or home helps; are in approved schools when early identification might have led to their attending special schools; are in schools for the physically handicapped or delicate when a school for the maladjusted would have been more appropriate; are in hospitals for the mentally subnormal when they could be living at home if their parents were given more support, or in hostels if there were sufficient places. Amongst the committee's recommendations were a national policy for the care of young children with working mothers, and the development of social work based on the school. Although their terms of reference did not include social work in the courts, a government White Paper published in 1968 proposed that 'all children under 14 and as far as possible young persons under 17 will be dealt with through the medium of their family, and where this is not practicable because of some form of family failure they will be dealt with in a manner similar to that employed for children suffering from family deprivation. Those requiring continuing treatment away from home will be placed in the care of local authorities, and the separate approved school order will cease to exist'.

In Scotland, a White Paper 'Social Work and the Community' published in 1966 put forward the case for a unified and comprehensive social work service. Accessibility to the public and effectiveness of provision were major considerations. In its observations on the treatment of offenders it followed the earlier Kilbrandon Report (1964) and recommended a system of children's panels to deal with all offenders under the age of 16.

The Social Work (Scotland) Act, 1968, requires each county council and large burgh local authority to appoint a social work committee. A single social work department under a Director of Social Work provides the organisation and administration of the authority's social work services. An Advisory Council in Social Work advises the Secretary of State on matters connected with the performance of his functions and those of local authorities in relation to social welfare. The importance of research and training in developing an effective and efficient service is emphasised.

In the main the services to be provided are those previously covered by legislation separately concerned with the care of children at risk, the probation and after care of offenders, and the welfare of such persons as the elderly infirm, the handicapped, and the homeless. Certain functions hitherto the responsibility of other bodies are transferred to the new department, for example, the home care of the mentally handicapped, and approved school after care.

A further major administrative re-organisation relates to the treatment of offenders. Local authorities take over from probation committees responsibility for probation and after care. Children under 16 who commit an offence become classified under the Act as 'children in need of compulsory measures of care'. This category in the main covers children who in the Children and Young Persons Act 1963 are described as being in need of 'care, protection or control'.

Children in this category are to be dealt with by means of a Children's Hearing which 'shall consist of a chairman and two other members, and shall have both a man and a woman among the members'. It must be held in suitable accommodation dissociated from criminal courts and police stations, and be conducted in private. An officer of the local authority, known as the Reporter, has responsibility for a wide range of functions, including deciding whether (*a*) to arrange for a hearing on the grounds that the child appears to him to be in need of compulsory measures of care; (*b*) otherwise to refer the case to the local authority with a view to their making arrangements for the advice, guidance, and assistance of the child and his family; (*c*) otherwise to take no further action in the case. Whatever his decision, the Reporter needs to observe principles of child care quite as much as of legal practice. When specific legal disagreements have to be resolved the case must be referred to a sheriff sitting in chambers.

The functions of the Reporter and the procedures of the children's hearing both give expression to a positive attitude towards preventive measures. Concern to prevent is also displayed in the recommendations of the Act regarding the circumstances under which assistance in cash or kind may be provided. These apply, in the case of a child under 18, when the giving of assistance appears likely to diminish the need to receive him into or keep him in care, or to refer him to a children's hearing; and in all other cases, when the giving of assistance in either form would avoid the local authority being caused greater expense in the giving of assistance in another form. The intention to replace remand homes by assessment centres may also facilitate prevention.

The Act is concerned to increase community involvement in the provision of social welfare, and with this end in view a strong case may be made out for basing the provision of welfare on the local authority. However, the proposal has two possible shortcomings. First, it may be that some authorities do not command the resources essential for an efficiently organised and administered service. There has been little research to determine the size of population on which an efficient unit of social welfare might be based. What is clear is that certain specialist field services and most forms of residential care will not be available to the smaller authorities unless they engage in joint financial outlay with other authorities.

Small units of service may also be unable to provide attractive career prospects to resourceful and ambitious staff.

Second, there is some reason to expect that local authorities may not provide the best foundation on which to base programmes of care for certain marginal members of society. The persistently indigenous and the persistently criminal are two instances. Although children may not be directly affected, for most societies can be moved by the plight of the under-sixteens, they may suffer in their late teens, when many are still extremely immature, and at all ages children may be affected indirectly if they are the offspring of parents who are themselves socially unacceptable. Certain features of child poverty, for example, arise as a consequence of society's unwillingness to allow to certain adults in special need additional forms of social welfare.

The emphasis on prevention must require extensive consultation between the social work department and other departments of the local authority. The Director of Social Work must be able to 'sell' his department's policy to his fellow chief officers. He must also be able to give an acceptable account to the public. In the end, however, the department will be treated as the performance of its staff deserves. In this regard the need for training is paramount.

The Local Authority Children's Department: Its Responsibilities and Powers

The local authority has the responsibility to provide certain services for children whose welfare might otherwise be at risk. Under the 1948 Children Act the authority is given the power to receive children into care, and is encouraged to make arrangements for boarding out. Under the 1963 Children and Young Persons Act the authority is required to engage in such preventive measures as will 'diminish the need to receive children, or keep them in care'. In Scotland, the Social Work (Scotland) Act, 1968, incorporates the Acts of 1948 and 1963, and emphasises the preventive aspects of child care.

Reception into Care. Section 1 of the 1948 Children Act specifies the circumstances under which 'it shall be the duty of the local authority to receive the child into care under this section'. These are essentially concerned with the inability of the child's parents or guardian to provide for his 'proper accommodation, maintenance, and upbringing.' Children's departments vary over the interpretation they place on the circumstances as prescribed. Some treat reception into care as a last resort; others encourage parents to make application rather than leave a child at risk in his own home. The child most likely to be received into care is one whose mother is temporarily or permanently unable to care for him; the child whose mother has died, or deserted, or been admitted to hospital, or rendered homeless.

The majority of children are 'received' from a parent or guardian. Section 1 (3) of the 1948 Act states 'Nothing in this section shall authorise a local authority to keep a child in their care under this section if any parent or guardian desires to take over the care of the child'. The parent or guardian is thus protected from unwanted intervention by the local authority. An unavoidable consequence of protecting parental rights in this manner is that the child may be placed at risk by a parent or guardian who decides to remove him from local authority care on grounds which do not have due regard to the child's welfare.

Powers. Although Children's departments have no powers under the 1948 Act to 'take' children from their parents, they may under certain prescribed circumstances 'resolve' to take over all the rights and powers of a parent or guardian. Section 2 of the 1948 Children Act as amended and extended by section 48 of the Children and Young Persons Act, 1963, defines the grounds on which such a resolution may be taken. These provide criteria for determining the long term inability or unsuitability of a child's parents or guardian to care for him.

The parents must be formally notified when the local authority resolves to assume parental rights. If they object then the resolution lapses unless the authority's decision is upheld by a juvenile court. In the event of agreement by parents or court, the local authority retains parental rights until the child's eighteenth birthday, or until the resolution is rescinded. The child may be placed with his natural parents whilst the resolution is in operation.

The local authority may also be made a 'fit person' in respect of a child. The Children and Young Persons Act, 1963, provides that a fit person shall 'have the same rights and powers as if he was his parent'. A fit person order may be made in respect of certain delinquent children and in respect of children who have been found to be in need of care, protection, or control.   This last group includes those who have been neglected, or illtreated, or who are exposed to moral danger, or are beyond the control of their parent or guardian. A parent cannot bring his own child before the court as being beyond control: he must request the local authority to do so. In this way parents are prevented from a precipitate entry into proceedings they may soon regret, and the Children's department has the opportunity to set a more constructive programme into operation.

Whatever the procedure by which a child enters care, his parents are liable to contribute towards his maintenance until he is 16. The local authority assesses the amount to be contributed, and may apply to the magistrates for a contribution order if regular payment is not forthcoming.

The 1948 Children Act sought to minimise the separation of child from parent, but it did not give the local authority powers to contribute positively towards maintaining the family unit. The 1963 Children and Young Persons Act places on the authority the duty 'to make available such advice, guidance and assistance as may promote the welfare of children, by diminishing the need to receive children into, or keep them in, care . . . or to bring children before a juvenile court; and any provision made by a local authority under this subsection may, if the local authority thinks fit, include provision for giving assistance in kind, or in exceptional circumstances, in cash'.

Financial aid. The 1963 Act directed the attention of local authorities to the fact that the prevention of reception into care involves positive measures, and that one such positive measure is the disbursement of financial aid. Departments were encouraged to explore a wide range of preventive measures. A number of statutory and voluntary bodies have established Family Advice Centres (Leissner, 1967). These are a development out of the recommendation of the Ingleby Committee that parents in need of help and advice should have 'some door on which they can knock, knowing that their knock will be answered by people with knowledge and capacity, and with the willingness to help'. An effective programme of prevention requires an early warning system: to have due notice of families at risk the Children's department must be in constant touch with such other departments as police, education, health and housing. Service may have to be taken into the home at a very practical level: the temporary absence of a mother need not entail receiving a child into care if the home can be maintained by a peripatetic service of home helps and child minders. Some parents may need to learn how to run a home of their own: there are a number of residential establishments where they can do so.

In recommending special disbursements of cash, the Act moves away from the principle that financial aid shall be granted only on grounds of strict equality between applicants. Each department must develop its own policy with regard to the outlay of cash and kind. Among families whose ongoing stability may require a special outlay are those subject to material problems not readily covered by standard sources of assistance. Also included are families seriously deficient in the ability to handle the financial side of daily life. Such families may need to be told, and encouraged to exercise, their rights with regard to publicly available resources. They may also need to learn how to cope as well as possible with the resources they have available.

Social considerations. The emphasis on preventive work in child care derives much of its authority from an underlying belief in the importance of maintaining the link between the child and his parents. When this is not possible, the alternative forms of care tend to be valued in terms of further assumptions about how to ensure the welfare of the child. The first is that the most effective substitute for a child's own family is another family unit. This belief naturally encourages an enthusiasm for boarding out. When there is no prospect whatsoever of the child returning to his family of origin, adoption may be seen as an even more acceptable form of care.

The second approved principle of child care to be noted here is the importance ascribed to a child remaining in contact with the community. A placement which enables him to move about in the socially normal context of daily life is favoured over one which remotes him from everyday society. Living at home, or in a foster home, satisfies this criterion the best. Failing these, residence in a 'family group home' or a hostel, with schooling or employment pursued in the outside world, would be the preferred alternative. Services which enable a child to remain in the community are increasing. Day schools are available for children who are mentally retarded or emotionally disturbed, and who would otherwise have to go away from home to be educated. Child guidance clinics and adolescent counselling services enable troubled children to function relatively well under difficult home conditions.

Some of these services may be provided by the Children's department, some by other departments of the local authority, and some by voluntary organisations.

Research into the effects of separating the young child from his parents and placing him in some kind of institution have exercised a great deal of influence over thinking about the care of children at risk. The interest in preventing the child from coming into care has drawn much of its strength from the findings of Bowlby and others. Ainsworth (1962) summarises these in part as follows: (i) recovery from a single brief separation will be fairly prompt, although possibly leaving a vulnerability to future stress; (ii) relief from fairly prolonged deprivation in infancy may result in rapid improvement, although socialisation, and possibly other aspects of personality functioning may be retarded; (iii) severe deprivation beginning early, and lasting as long as three years, usually has serious adverse effects; (iv) in the first year, the earlier that deprivation is relieved the better; (v) language, the ability for abstract thinking, and the capacity for affection seem to be more permanently affected than other functions.

According to Dinnage and Kellmer Pringle (1967) 'The ordinary family setting not only provides surprisingly much more stimulation when measured in time studies, it also provides one, or a few people, who are regularly present and deeply interested in the infant, and who respond to his communications, so giving him an opportunity to learn early to distinguish, recognise, and enjoy specific individuals, to make sense of the environment, and to acquire the sense of being able to influence it'. This perspective in the link between family life and personal development would seem to have fundamental implications for the experiences which must be available to the younger child in care if he is to have the opportunity to develop in a manner reasonably similar to a child living with his natural parents.

Children in Care

On the basis of approximate figures arrived at by the Curtis Committee, Packman (1968) estimates that rather more than 48,000 children were in care in England and Wales at the time of the 1948 Act. The new legislation extended the range of children and adolescents for whom a service had to be provided and these changes, coupled with a tendency on the part of certain departments to increase the scale of boarding out, resulted by 1953 in growth of numbers in care to 65,309, or 6·2 per thousand children under 18 years. By the early 1960s the number of children in care per thousand had declined to 5·1, to rise to 5·2 by 1968. The numbers in care at any given time vary considerably between local authorities. In 1963 the rate per thousand population under 18 ranged from 12·4 for the county of London to 1·8 for Anglesey and Southport. For all boroughs the average figure was 5·7, for all counties 4·8. Among factors influencing these variations Packman suggests mobility of population, the presence of socially depressed communities, local authority child care policy, the effect of local tradition on policy enactment, and the availability and quality of alternative services.

The Home Office in its returns distinguishes between two categories of care, short stay (under 6 months) and long stay (over 6 months). Short stay care accounts for over 50 per cent of children admitted to the care of Children's departments. However, by far the greater proportion of children in care at any one time are there on a long term basis. In general, short stay care provides a service to the less troubled child and his family—for example, during a mother's confinement it can sometimes facilitate preventive work. Long stay care tends to be associated either with the break-up of the family, or with serious official disquiet over the family's way of life.

Foster Care

The 1948 Children Act specifies the responsibilities of the local authority with regard to boarding-out, adoption, and residential care. The authority is advised to board out children whenever possible in preference to placing them in residential care.

The Boarding-out of Children Regulations, 1955, define fostering in terms of the child living with foster parents in their dwelling as a member of the family. The Memorandum on Boarding-out issued by the Scottish Home Department in 1959 states 'Boarding-out is a great deal more than the finding of a house in which a child may be given a bed and board, kept reasonably clean, and sent regularly to school, it is, in its essential meaning, the creation of a home for the child'.

Creating a home for the child depends on the length of the foster placement, on the attitudes of the child and his natural parents, on the ability of the foster parents to live with the child—and on his ability to live with them—and on the approach to fostering adopted by the local authority children's committee and their staff of child care officers. The child in short stay care should not become greatly attached to the foster parents, even if he is so inclined. The child in long stay care is nowadays likely to arrive after a history of attempts to keep him in his family of origin. Frequently he will be deeply disturbed, when the foster parents may find themselves confronted with behaviour which only a trained adult could handle without upset.

The demands for foster placements, and the resources available, vary over the country as a whole. Placements tend to be more readily available in rural areas, whilst children in need of foster care are most frequently found in communities with a fairly rapid population turnover. Children's departments in industrial areas may therefore have to foster at a considerable distance, or establish alternative forms of care. Fostering may be impracticable for lack of placements in the case of certain children, such as the coloured immigrant. The percentage of children in care who are boarded out has remained fairly constant for a number of years. In 1963 the figure for England and Wales was 52 per cent; in 1966 it was 51 per cent. In Scotland the figure stands in the region of 60 per cent, the higher percentage originating in the boarding-out policy of the old Scottish Poor Law. Local variations in fostering may be illustrated with reference to the 1966 figures for England and Wales (H.M.S.O. Command 3204, 1966).

The Boarding-out of Children Regulations (1955) and the Scottish Regulations (1959) govern all boarding-out by both local authorities and voluntary organisations.

They require that before boarding-out a Child Care Officer shall make a written report on the physical conditions of the foster home, and on such characteristics of the foster parents as their religious persuasion, their physical and mental health, and any findings of guilt which might indicate their unsuitability to associate with a child. Authorities vary over the extent to which they pursue references and check with such departments as police, education, and health. Children's departments are required by the Regulations to visit the child at set intervals, to review his progress at least once every 6 months, and to arrange for regular medical and dental care. The agency has authorised access at all times to any placement which is expected to last more than 8 weeks, and is required to move the child at once if his health, safety or morals are thought to be at risk.

The Boarding-out Regulations may be a source of insecurity to the foster parents. They are expected to commit themselves to the care of a child even though he may be removed from their home without warning. If the child is in care under section 1 of the 1948 Act and the parents insist on their right to have him returned the Children's department must comply. The essential vulnerability of the foster parent renders many prone to fantasies concerning the loss of the child and the motives of child care officials.

The child care officer. The relation between the foster parents and the Child Care Officer is replete with danger points. The officer represents the department and therefore becomes associated with whatever feelings the foster parents have about the Regulations. His power to enter the home, and to comment upon the foster parents' style of child rearing can be a ready source of negative attitudes. His acquaintance with the child's natural parents may lead the foster parents to treat him as an ally of the natural parents, to be rejected or manipulated in accordance with the problems they have about fostering another person's child. Interviews which he holds with the foster child in the absence of the foster parents may encourage them in the conviction that he is 'spying on' or 'setting the child against' them.

A skilled approach by the Child Care Officer can, however, make constructive use of these factors. The foster parents can be helped to face their fantasies. They can examine their feelings about the natural parents, and the officer may be able to facilitate productive meetings between foster and natural parents. The officer can use his extensive knowledge of the child's history and social background to make more understandable to the foster parents the child's otherwise easy to misunderstand behaviour. His interviews with the child can serve to help the child come to terms with his foster parents. Provided the foster parents can be helped to feel involved, these interviews may result in a greater harmony between child and foster parents.

For many children breakdown of a foster placement can be catastrophic, uncertain as they are of their natural parents' feelings for them. Often it is the child who most needs a stable foster home who does the most to ensure that his placement will break down. The Child Care Officer requires substantial competence if he is to help all the parties involved to make a success of the venture.

Successful fostering seems to be associated with such factors as the following. The foster parents must be able to value the child 'for himself'. Fostering in order to resolve one's own family problems is unlikely to achieve anything but distress for all concerned. Ideally, the fostered child will receive satisfactions within the foster family's overall experience of satisfaction at having him live with them. It is sometimes suggested that the foster parents' expectation of payment for boarding out may contraindicate suitability for the care of children. If we remember that foster parents chiefly come from the lower socio-economic classes, then what is important is not so much their concern over payment as the reason why they are willing to earn a relatively small sum by means of an often very demanding method.

Under the Children Act, 1948, the local authority is given the responsibility to oversee the well-being of children whose care and maintenance are undertaken for reward for a period exceeding one month by a person who is not a relative or guardian. Under the Adoption Act, 1958, the authority has similar responsibilities and powers with respect to the 'protected child', that is, any child of compulsory school age or under who is placed by a third party with adults who are not relatives or guardians, and who do not receive any form of reward for the child's care and maintenance. In the case of children placed by their parents with adults without payment, the authority has no powers or responsibilities. At 31st March, 1968, over 10,000 children were in private placements in England and Wales, whilst over 7,000 were awaiting adoption.

Research

A number of useful guides to research in the field of child care are available under the imprint of the National Bureau for Co-operation in Child Care (Kellmer Pringle, 1967: Dinnage and Kellmer Pringle, 1967). Research into child care may be exemplified by selected studies relating to foster care. These tend to be concerned either with the critical examination of practice in specific agencies, or with attempts to correlate elements in treatment with subsequent outcome. The dynamic characteristics of treatment are particularly difficult to isolate and identify. A basic element of interest is the concept of interaction. It is generally agreed that many instances of disturbed behaviour on the part of children can be related to their experience, past or present, of insufficient, inconsistent, or distorted patterns of relationship with significant others. The findings of Bowlby on the effects of maternal deprivation would appear to be concerned in particular with the effects on children of insufficient interaction in the absence of the mother. In fostering, the Child Care Officer can try to ensure that the foster placement does not deprive the child of essential relationships with adults. A research project which compared foster mothers with similarly placed non-fostering housewives found that the former had fewer children and had less outside interests whilst wanting larger families (Wakeford, 1963). A number of research findings indicate that fostering is more likely to be successful if the child and his foster family are in touch with his family of origin. In part this success may be the outcome of consistent treatment originating through the link-up in interaction of the various parts of his life.

Parker (1966) studied 209 placements carried out over a five year period in a single area. On his definition of success he found that boarding-out seems more likely to be successful: (i) the younger the child is at the time of fostering (preferably under 3); (ii) the younger the child is at the time of separation from his mother (however, death of the mother is strongly associated with failure); (iii) if the child has spent less than 2 years in institutions; (iv) if the foster parents have no children of their own (the presence in the home of a child of the foster parents is significantly associated with failure if he is under 5 or within 5 years of the age of the foster child); (v) if the child has had a previous experience of successful short-term fostering.

Trasler (1960) compared 86 foster placements which broke down with 81 placements judged by two or more assessors to be very successful.   His findings were in line with those of Parker in respect of the greater success attending the placement of younger children, the detrimental effect of the presence of a child of the foster parents when of the same age and sex, and the detrimental effect of an extended history of institutional life. He found that the child's emotional reaction to previous rejection made the most significant contribution to foster placement breakdown. The strength of the reaction could be diminished by maintaining contact with his natural parents, and by discussing his experiences of separation. A second major factor contributing to breakdown was the unrealistic expectations of the foster mothers. Pre-placement investigation should be particularly concerned with motives. In line with this recommendation Jenkins (1965), in a study of the needs of foster parents, found that the most satisfactory homes had foster parents who were able to show compassion for children in need, who experienced fostering as a repetition of a previous rewarding relationship, or who were using fostering as an alternative to adoption. Most unsatisfactory were foster parents compensating for guilt feelings.

Adoption

Prior to 1926 in England and Wales, and 1930 in Scotland, there was no legal control in those countries over children taken into private families. The Adoption Act of 1958 defined legal adoption as a process whereby 'all rights, duties, obligations, and liabilities of the parents or guardians of the infant in relation to the future custody, maintenance and education of the infant . . . shall be extinguished, and all such rights, duties, obligations, and liabilities shall rest in, and be exercisable by and enforceable against the adopter, as if the infant were a child bound of the adopter in lawful wedlock'.

Children may be placed for adoption by their own parents or legal guardian, by a third party, by a registered adoption society, or by the Children's department of a local authority. However, only a local authority, or an adoption agency registered by a local authority, may actually arrange for the adoption of an 'infant' (i.e. a person under 21 years of age). Adoption Orders may be made by a Juvenile, a County, or a High Court (or in Scotland, by a Sheriff Court).

Before placing a child for adoption, adoption agencies must provide a detailed report on his health. A serological test for syphilis is required once the infant is 6 weeks old. A full medical report must be submitted to the court dealing with the application for the adoption order. The adopters are thus informed of all known risks to the future health of the infant.

The 1958 Adoption Act specifically empowers Children's Committees to act as adoption agencies. Practice varies greatly, some committees employing specialist adoption staff, others leaving adoption entirely to a local adoption agency. In a sample of adopters studies by Goodacre (1966) local authorities acted as the adoption agency for 39 per cent of adopters in the Registrar General's classes IV and V, and for 16 per cent in classes I and II; voluntary societies on the other hand served 42 per cent of adopters from classes I and II, and only 7 per cent from classes IV and V.

The 1958 Act states that except when the 'infant of school age or under' is to be adopted by a parent, the applicant for an adoption order must, at least 3 months before the date of the order, give notice in writing to the appropriate local authority of intention to apply to a court for an adoption order. The Children's department then has the responsibility to arrange for the adoptive home to be visited and for the child to be supervised until the order is made. This responsibility can lead to complications. In the majority of cases the adoptive parents have already developed a good relation with the adoption agency, and the child care officer can easily become an unwanted third party. Skilled intervention can help in certain instances, however, as when the adoptive parents welcome the opportunity to discuss matters they feel unable to raise with the adoption agency, although here again, such discussion may lead to problems between the Children's department and the adoption agency.

The Adoption Rules require the court to appoint a person who has the duty to safeguard the interests of the infant before the court. This 'guardian ad litem of the infant' (in Scotland the 'curator ad litem') is required to investigate the circumstances of the adoption, to ascertain the physical and economic state of the applicants and their home, to interview all the people concerned, to make sure that all the necessary consents have been freely given, and whenever possible, to ascertain the infant's attitude towards the adoption. The court normally appoints the children's officer as guardian ad litem, although not when the Children's department acts as the adoption agency.

The child for adoption is usually, but not always, illegitimate. The mother's feelings about retaining him or placing him for adoption are likely to be very mixed. Often the future is obscure and particularly if she is young, she may be unable to see her way to maintaining herself with a fatherless child. Alternatively, her youth and lack of experience may encourage undue optimism concerning her ability to bring up her child on her own. The parents of such young mothers may be deeply offended and refuse to help: however, the intelligent intervention of a skilled social worker can frequently tap latent reserves of family goodwill. The mother must explore these and other relevant aspects of her situation with the social worker, and must be helped to appreciate the irrevocable nature of adoption.

If she decides on adoption, then when the child has been placed, and always after he is over the age of 6 weeks, the mother is asked to complete and sign a witnessed form of consent. The child cannot be placed officially for adoption until the 6 weeks have elapsed. The signed form of consent must be produced in court during the adoption proceedings. The mother may specify the religion in which she desires the child to be brought up. She may withdraw her consent up to the time the adoption order is made.

In law, only the mother of an illegitimate child has parental status, although the granting of an Affiliation Order renders the putative father liable for financial assistance, normally until the child is 16. The Adoption Act, 1958, gives the father the right to be heard in court proceedings relating to adoption. Under the Legitimacy Act, 1959, the father has the right to apply to the court for custody of or access to his illegitimate child.

In favour of separating the child for adoption from his natural mother as early as possible is the argument that it prevents the formation of a bond between them which both will in due course find extremely painful to break. However, adoptive parents who accept a child before he is 6 weeks old may find that the mother eventually decides not to give her formal consent. If the child is placed with foster parents during part or all of the proceedings, or is subjected to some form of care for a period before the commencement of proceedings, he may suffer serious distress as a consequence of the several changes in caring adult.

Frequently adoptive parents reach the decision to adopt only after a long history of failure to have children of their own. Successful adoption requires that they come to terms with their own infertility, and the consequent deprivation of natural parenthood. In a society where the birth of children plays a major part in self-fulfilment and self-respect, they must learn to accept themselves according to rather different principles. They must also beware of any tendency they may have to treat the child as the victim of rejecting parents. As adoptive parents they must. work with officials who are seemingly assessing their suitability for child rearing. Traditionally, acceptance has been based on middle class standards relating to age, level of income, duration of marriage, and religious persuasion. More recently some agencies have begun to take account of the emotional elements involved. The rejected applicant may feel that he is the victim of illfounded judgments: at the same time he will almost certainly experience doubts about his own worth. A supportive follow-up period may be required in certain instances.

Adopting the older child may present special difficulties. He will already have a 'family background' whether it be of natural parents, foster parents, or a children's home. Adopters may be especially hard to find for children with special handicaps, including emotional handicaps. Where adoption is unlikely, or strongly contra-indicated, it is incumbent on the adoption agency to view the infant's future as comprehensively as possible. Local authorities are perhaps best placed to do this, although the large voluntary agencies such as Dr. Barnardo's and the National Children's Homes are also able to make use of a wide range of alternative forms of care.

Residential Care

The 1948 Children's Act suggests that a child shall be placed in a children's home when it is 'not practicable to make arrangements for boarding out'. The 1963 Children and Young Persons Act requires the local authorities to '. . . promote the welfare of children by diminishing the need to . . . keep them in care'. Although neither of these proposals is intended to suggest that an alternative to residential care is always to be preferred, they do lend themselves to a devaluation of residential-based services relative to community-based ones.

It is important to remember that there are many children for whom an alternative to residential care is not available either because of the nature of their needs or because of the expectations of society. Numbered amongst these children are those who are severely disturbed emotionally, who are severely handicapped physically or mentally, who belong to a socially stigmatised section of the community (e.g. coloured immigrants), who have parents who intervene excessively in any placement provided, or who require to be placed with a number of siblings. Children admitted to care under emergency conditions, or who require a period of rest and quiet, may best be served by a specially designed residential unit, as may children who experience foster home breakdown. Children who appear before the courts are frequently remanded in custody for reports which are most efficiently prepared in an appropriately designed assessment centre; subsequently they may be committed to approved schools, which traditionally have been seen as the only form of 'residential care' suitable for the majority of delinquents.

There are two conflicting sets of principles impinging on residential care. On the one hand there are the persistent themes of contemporary child care: to facilitate relations between children and their parents, to participate as far as possible in the everyday life of society, and to diminish the period spent in residence. On the other hand there is the responsibility to the handicapped and disturbed child to provide him with a regimen suited to his nature; there is also the obligation to satisfy the expectations of a society that classifies certain children as being in need of a form of care which is based on discipline and social deprivation and which is aimed at rehabilitation. A reasonably comprehensive system of residential care must include establishments concerned with assessment; establishments concerned with providing 'the opportunity to live' to children whose nature prevents them from getting such opportunity in open society; establishments concerned with the care of children who, although not fostered or adopted, are perfectly capable of living in open society; and establishments designed to abate the anxiety and aggression felt by society against those children who break the law, or contravene certain strongly upheld customs.

Children who are classified as chiefly needing a caring regimen in which to grow up may be accommodated in hostels or in children's homes. *Hostels* enable the child to go out into the community for schooling or employment, and for leisure. The adolescent can benefit from hostel life, for he is at a stage of development which especially draws on experience in open society. Such accommodation is currently provided by certain local authorities and voluntary bodies for working boys and girls in care, and for adolescents on probation. On a somewhat similar basis the adolescent unmarried mother may enter a mother and baby home and there spend a number of weeks before and after the birth in a supportive atmosphere, where such difficult problems as whether to have the baby adopted and how to relate to parents can be explored and, hopefully, resolved.

Children's Homes may variously offer the opportunity to participate in the life of open society. The *Family Group Home* is located in a residential neighbourhood and is either purpose built, or adapted from one or two council houses. Between 6 and 12 children are accommodated, normally in the charge of a married woman with a husband who goes out to work and who provides some 'masculine influence'; alternatively one or more housemothers may run the unit. A shortcoming of this fairly intensive type of care is that staff turnover can have an acute effect on the family group; and for a variety of reasons, staff turnover may be frequent.

The *Large Children's Home* may be purpose built or consist of a converted private dwelling house, often of substantial proportions. Up to 50 children may be accommodated, and regimens vary: some emphasise small group living, with units of 6 to 12 children being allocated a part of the building as their own, with a housemother in charge; others utilise the entire building as the child's basic unit of living. Contact with the community at large depends upon the type of child in residence, the geographical location of the establishment, and the principles of residential work observed by the staff, and in particular by the superintendent or warden in charge. Homes of this type are suited to children who need specialist regimens of care. They are being used increasingly to accommodate the seriously disturbed child who can thus be 'distributed' over a wide range of staff. The larger children's home offers staff a more varied way of life than the family group home, a promotion structure, and less stress in the event of staff sickness or resignation.

The *Grouped Cottage Home* consists of a number of separate dwelling units each housing between 8 and 20 children, and with a total population of as many as 300 or more. This pattern of residential life permits a family type atmosphere in the separate units, and may thus to some extent resemble the family group home. In general, grouped cottage homes have their own playing fields, assembly halls, sick bays, and sometimes chapels and swimming baths. The centralisation of facilities may have two unfavourable consequences. First, the children are often almost wholly out of touch with the conditions of life in open society; and second, it is becoming increasingly difficult to find able staff who are prepared to live under the continuous oversight of senior officers, and to accept the restricted opportunities for social life which the isolation of the establishment so frequently entails.

Children under the age of 5 who cannot be boarded out have tended to be treated as a special group. They may be placed in residential nurseries provided by local authorities or voluntary organisations. In the case of the infant and very young child no other setting may be able to provide the intensity of care needed. In general, however, the nursery approach has come to be regarded as too specialised for the somewhat older child: he benefits from contact with children of all ages, and the principles of nursery nursing are not always appropriate to his needs. Many are instead being placed in family group homes which provide whatever additional facilities are necessary.

Many children come into care at short notice. It is therefore not always possible to have a suitable foster placement ready for them. Children's homes also have their problems about taking on children at short notice. A home with a basic population of 'long stay' residents would be seriously disturbed by a continuous turnover of short stay children. The Children Act, 1948, states that a local authority's residential accommodation must include separate provision for the temporary reception of children. Furthermore, facilities must be available for observing their physical and mental condition.

The Children's Reception Home is intended to fulfil these requirements, although the use to which it is actually put varies with local policy. Some authorities place the majority of short stay children directly into foster homes, whilst others, perhaps because of a different admission procedure, perhaps because of a shortage of foster homes, base their temporary reception on the Reception Home. Others again seek to leave the Reception Home free for more specialist functions by establishing short stay children's homes. As the practice of residential care acquires a more systematic foundation of tested theory and practice, with links being established between forms of care and quality of need, the assessment facilities of the Reception Home will come to play an increasingly central part in the comprehensive service. Such a development will be furthered by current proposals to abolish Remand Homes, which have traditionally provided assessment services to the Juvenile Courts. Children who have come into care under conditions of acute crisis may need special forms of care rarely available to those living in children's and foster homes. The Reception Home can in principle provide a suitably protected environment, with the children being able to receive special schooling and psychiatric attention within the building.

Delinquent children and others who comprise the population of *Approved Schools* find themselves in a rather different type of organisation. In structure the schools have traditionally resembled the large single building type Children's home, with a population of between 30 and 150. They are grouped according to junior, intermediate and senior grades and are single sexed. The remit of training and education tends to inform the entire pattern of daily living with the result that life outside the classroom shows less of the quality of child care than would be expected in a Children's home. However, during the 1960's and chiefly in England and Wales, an extensive rebuilding programme has been pursued. Separate units of housing for between 20 and 30 children have introduced into boy's approved schools the possibility of a form of 'family type' care. Each house unit has at least one child care oriented housemaster in charge, and if he is married his wife normally acts as housemother in charge. Approved schools for girls tend to be smaller than those for boys and to have an almost exclusively female staff: in Scotland, however, some advance has been made towards employing male staff at senior level. The majority of girls are committed as being 'in need of care, protection, or control'.

Current thinking about the residential care of delinquents, as exemplified by the Social Work (Scotland) Act, 1968, the Report of the Seebohm Committee 1968, and the Children and Young Persons Act, 1969, (which proposes for England and Wales a system of 'Community Homes' organized on a regional basis), tends to favour setting up a unified system of 'in care' provision to cover all children unable to reside with their natural parents. It is argued that so far as effective care and treatment are concerned the child who commits an offence, and even more so the child in moral danger, is in no essential respect different from other categories of child in care. The distinctions that are emphasised at present rest on society's reactions towards those features of each case that are immediately visible, and which may in fact mislead radically as to the true condition of the child and the meaning of his act.

It is, for example, difficult to justify in terms of the principles of child care, the case for depriving an adolescent girl, found to be in moral danger by a court, of all male company, adults as well as peers. The case is made even more difficult to argue by the fact that had the girl's parents shown the responsibility of approaching a Children's department she might well have avoided a court appearance and instead been fostered or placed in a children's home. It is equally far from clear how to justify the fact that an emotionally disturbed boy who both persistently truants and has night fears may end up in an approved school if the former feature of his behaviour gains the attention of certain authorities, and in a children's home or school for maladjusted children if the latter feature is noted by other authorities.

On the other hand, it should not be forgotten that the persistent delinquent may have acquired anti-social habits which resist the style of life natural to the generality of foster or children's homes. This is particularly true when violence is involved. Some children 'beyond parental control' may be chiefly reacting to their particular family background, and once they are away their problem behaviour may largely abate. Others may have generalised their parental antipathy to cover all adults, so that no measure of straightforward foster care or care in a children's home is likely to reduce their predilection towards public misbehaviour. Adolescents in particular who display behaviour of this nature will require special forms of residential care. Education authorities have the responsibility of providing appropriate teaching for children who are handicapped physically, or who are of limited intelligence, or who are classified as being maladjusted. Authorities may provide facilities which enable the child to live at home; some children must however attend residential schools. Such schools have, like Approved Schools, the dual responsibility of meeting standards in education and standards in child care. Many schools are provided by voluntary organisations under the supervision of the education authorities.

A few especially disturbed children may be sent to psychiatric hospitals. Ideally such a placement should be in a children's unit. A recent development has been the introduction of psychiatric units for disturbed adolescents.

Research into the outcome of residential care suggests that two factors have some causal association with lack of success: early entry into care and the absence of good family (or substitute family) contacts. Within residential living itself three possible sources and outcomes of deprivation have been noted by Dinnage and Kelmer Pringle (1967): (i) Lack of psychological nourishment resulting in retardation and impoverishment; (ii) Positively painful experience with form of ill-treatment or separation leading to a reaction; (iii) Lack of experiences which offer the opportunity to belong to a social group, to achieve a sense of personal identity.

After-Care

Eventually the child in residential care returns to his parental home, or failing that enters some form of lodgings. The residential establishment he leaves has the responsibility of supporting him during this period. Some have set up a 'halfway house' where the adolescent may lodge until he has accommodated himself to life in open society. If the child or adolescent is in the care of a Children's department then he will have been in touch with a child care officer throughout his time 'in care', including his time in residential care. Ideally the officer will have been working with both child and family to facilitate reintegration. Hopefully he will have become a point of reference for them all. This approach to after-care as simply one part of a comprehensive family service is presaged in the Social Work (Scotland) Act, 1968. Whilst after-care remains relatively self-contained, however, it inherits many negative feelings associated with family separation and residential regimens.

The Practice of Child Care

Introduction

The social worker provides a service to adults and children who are experiencing difficulties over living in society. He may concentrate on helping them through a short term crisis; alternatively he may seek to modify significant features of their way of life. In pursuance of these ends, he may engage in activities ranging from: 'the giving of material assistance, through listening, suggesting, advising, and the setting of limits, to the making of comments that encourage the client to express or suppress his feelings, to examine his situation, or to seek connections between his present attitudes and behaviour, and past experience' (Brown, 1966).

The problems which engage the social worker's attention may be roughly classified under four headings. There are first, those which involve a deficiency in such essential components of daily life as food, housing, education, employment; second, those which arise from an inability to use essential components effectively; third, those which are connected with a failure to observe certain basic social norms, such as respect for property rights or for the personal well-being of others; and fourth, those which express stress internal to the individual or family. Many problems which at first sight appear to fall into the first group in fact fall into the second: thus a great deal of child poverty is the outcome not simply of the family lacking material resources, but also of their inability to use resources effectively. The social worker, in recognising how far the family 'makes' its style and condition of life, is concerned to help the members learn how to use resources. The second and third groups have in common the inability of a child or adult to observe certain socially approved standards of behaviour. In the second group this inability is associated with material conditions; in the third group it is associated with 'mental ill-health', 'crime and delinquency', 'immorality', and so forth.

The fact that social work is concerned with fundamental aspects of personal experience and interpersonal behaviour means that it must always raise questions about the propriety of following one course of action rather than another. An effective service may require the social worker to intervene in a person's life in a manner which is contrary to society's norms; whilst a socially acceptable form of service may be both ineffective in respect of socially desired goals, and offensive with regard to the recipient's sense of personal worth. Moral issues are especially pressing when the recipient is compelled to receive the service. The position of children in this regard is particularly delicate.

The social worker who is employed by a local or central authority cannot expect to practice in a manner seriously at variance with public standards. However, his specialised experience inevitably leads him to develop an understanding of the principles of effective care which differs from lay assumptions and attitudes. At present the social worker is not able to make full use of his specialist competence because of the relatively low status he is afforded within the hierarchy of local and central authority decision making. An effective and efficient social work service must rest on a body of practitioners to whom society has granted certain rights and privileges in connection with the ends and means of their practice. The professionalisation of social work is an essential step in the development of a caring society.

Agency Care

The 1948 Children Act established a local authority based service with a remit to work with children, parents, foster parents, and other persons significant to children at risk. Social workers were consequently faced with the need to acquire special competence in work with troubled people functioning under conditions of stress. A disciplined approach to certain types of person living under stress was already available, chiefly in the practice of medical and psychiatric social work. This discipline, known as *social casework*, was gradually adapted to the conditions of child care, as the caseworkers learned to function within the ever-changing yet consolidating framework of local authority services.

As experience lengthened, arguments for prevention came increasingly to the fore. The goals and methods of social casework began to be adapted accordingly. At the level of primary prevention, caseworkers became concerned to maintain family functioning at a standard adequate to the basic needs of children; at the level of secondary prevention they sought to develop means whereby a child's period away from his family of origin might be shortened to a minimum; and at the level of tertiary prevention they became concerned to control any ill effects which being in care might have on a child particularly during the period following on residential care. Residential care workers themselves also began to contribute to secondary and tertiary prevention.

An account of the structure and function of the child care service must give due weight to the philosophy of human relations which informs it. There has been a steady movement away from the nineteenth century view that parents who treat their children with cruelty or neglect are to be excluded from respectable society, whilst their children are to be 'rescued' from the depraved parental influence and initiated into a more acceptable form of belonging to society, through certain procedures of training and discipline.

The contemporary view expresses a belief in the over-riding value of parent-child relations. Even in the case of acute parental neglect or cruelty, a positive element of caring between parent and child is usually apparent to the discerning eye. To ignore it, or to seek to extinguish it, is regarded as an offence against the nature of the child and the parent. The changing philosophy does not, however, entail any relaxation in accepting responsibility for providing children with the basic necessities of a stable upbringing, in the absence of parental competence. What is different is the approach to admitting into care and in the interpretation placed upon the need for care and the attendant child-parent behaviour.

Once it is recognised that the child who needs to be admitted into care belongs to a family where the parents themselves have problems over functioning in a family or in society, then it follows that effective child care must take the form of a case-work service to the family as a whole. The parents of troubled children who see child care as being concerned only with children are unlikely to reach a happy resolution of their own children's problems. A local authority department which focuses simply on admitting children into care is unlikely to find much reason for returning them to their home of origin before they are of age for discharge.

Depending on the nature of the case the caseworker may concentrate his attentions on the child, on one or both of the child's parents, on the interaction of child and parents, or on the interdependence of all family members and persons significant to the family. An essential quality of the service he provides lies in his readiness freely to establish an individualised relationship with the socially deprived, or disadvantaged, or deviant, and to maintain it irrespective of consequent stress for himself. Effective help is closely related to the caseworker's ability to 'bear with' his client until together they achieve a true account of the problem in hand. Frequently it is only at times of crisis, when stress is high, that the individual or family is prepared to take up the caseworker's offer of service.

The ability to live even reasonably effectively in society may be beyond the personal resources of certain children and parents. The caseworker must somehow reconcile the standards of society with the social competence of his clientele. When he cannot realistically aim to get a child or parent to the point where they can observe the required social standard he may try to modify the expectations society holds of them. At times society compounds their difficulties. Officials, professionals, and the general public may take for granted levels of social competence which are just not available to many socially marginal families. Many families live under conditions of poverty such that no ordinary measure of personal competence could enable them to avoid periodic crises of child deprivation and neglect. There are, for example, local authority housing departments that have rent collecting policies which present serious problems of long term saving to the very poor. A truly effective programme of preventive child care must involve the caring services in decision making about the control of such sources of family crises as rent arrears. It is quite possible for a family to be evicted without any reference to the short or long term effects on children, or to the capacity of the family to hold together.

Social workers are now beginning to question the sufficiency of casework when clients are subject to clear discrimination and deprivation by social conditions and policies. They are seeking to develop a method of social work practice which will allow them to intervene directly at the level of environmental impact. *Community work* may be roughly divided into three procedures: first, neighbourhood work which seeks to enable clients with similar problems to work together in order to achieve some measure of control over certain aspects of their difficulties—for example local mothers may be helped to set up a nursery group; second, extending existing social work services with the help of interested members of the community —for example a welfare department establishing a new service for the mentally handicapped with the co-operation of parents and local school children; and third, policy making at local and regional level which incorporates the views and concerns of the prospective clientele and other interested citizens.

Community work as a form of social work is essentially concerned to help clients use more effectively resources which are either currently available, or available given a moderate amount of enquiry and complaint. When the client's predicament points to the need for a radical reallocation of society's resources, then social action would seem to be called for. In the field of community change and action it is important to keep clear the distinction between community work as a form of social work, and social action, which operates more in accordance with the principles social and national politics.

Community work inevitably involves the purposeful use of groups. *Group work* is a form of social work in which members of a group learn to use the group to improve their capacity for social functioning. The group worker focuses either on the development of each member as an individual whose social problems lie elsewhere—as with group discussions of alcoholics, or unmarried mothers, or the parents of delinquent adolescent boys; or on achieving a group which can effectively pursue a social end—as when 'street corner boys' form a youth group, or a number of parents become an effective pressure group regarding local educational or leisure facilities for their children.

Residential Care

The goals of residential care tend to fall into one of three categories, protection of the child, disciplined education (which may be associated with protection of society) and social learning. As a residential establishment becomes committed to a given goal it assumes an appropriate form of organisation. A setting concerned with child protection may provide a way of life which fails utterly to prepare the growing child for the self-sufficiency he will be expected to display upon departure. Disciplined education when it denies expression to immature ways of behaviour, and maintains social order through adult supervision, can easily produce a child committed to a double system of values, a 'public self' skilled in the art of conformist performances, and a 'private self' which reflects experiences of adult rejection and denial by means of negative attitudes towards authority and social restraint.

Social learning under conditions of residential care calls for certain preconditions. The residential establishment must be based on forms of interpersonal relationship which reasonably accord with those holding in everyday society. At the same time, given the positive learning requirement, and remembering that the children involved are in general less than normally adequate in this sphere, the system of relationships must be such that the children are protected from serious consequences if they make mistakes, and are encouraged whenever they are right. Enabling a child to assume responsibility for his own actions in the context of residential life can produce stress in establishments chiefly committed to control by constraint. The appropriate controls for social learning may only operate effectively under certain conditions of physical layout and staff organisation. The staff themselves need the support of skills which can only be acquired and exercised under favourable conditions. To the trained worker every feature of daily living can be used to strengthen a child's social competence. What is called for is sensitivity to the meaning for the child of each separate incident, and the ability to heighten his awareness of those features of his experience which illustrate his capacity to achieve and be accepted.

As a child settles into residence, a special type of relationship has to be established between him and the surrounding adults. Their ways of behaving are not built into his identity as are those of his natural parents. A fine scepticism must be applied to the notion that they can serve as 'substitute parents' except in a very special sense. The child knows that in reality they are not his parents, and indeed if he were to treat them as such he would be functioning in the realm of fantasy. He will almost certainly transfer to them feelings and attributes which he learned in relation to his parents. Such behaviour may be quite inappropriate to his present circumstances. Part of the art of residential care (and of child care as a whole) lies in being able to identify unhelpful forms of 'transferred' attitudes, and thereafter to show the child how other approaches to the world are more realistic and rewarding.

In recent years, residential child care has frequently been linked with the concept of the 'therapeutic community'. A major benefit from the link has been an increased awareness of the need to deal with interpersonal problems at all levels. Effective residential care is particularly dependent on high staff morale. When the caring regimen focuses on the needs of the residents without due regard to the needs of the staff, it ensures that unproductive conflict will appear both within the body of staff, and between staff and residents. Sometimes, however, the concept has been used to justify the indiscriminate promotion of intensive care and has contributed towards avoiding thought about the nature and control of socially deviant behaviour.

It seems unlikely that a single set of principles for residential care could satisfy the needs of all children. Future developments may make it possible for the child coming into care to join a regimen appropriate to his condition, and thereafter graduate by controlled stages to a form of care involving as much contact as possible with open society.

Training and Staffing

Reports from Curtis to Seebohm and Acts from the 1948 Children Act to the 1968 Social Work (Scotland) Act have all placed emphasis on the central part training plays and must continue to play in the growth of an effective caring service. Notwithstanding the enthusiasm however, the current training scene is so unsystematic in its organisation and administration that only a few major features can be indentified here.

A great many child care officers enter the service from other employment. It is possible to obtain a post without preliminary training. The Mallaby Committee found that in a sample of local authorities 43·6 per cent of child care officers lacked qualifications of a standard thought to be desirable by the authority employing them. There are Children's departments where virtually every officer possesses a professional qualification: there are others without any staff thus qualified. However, in recent years a considerable growth in the availability of two-year courses of basic professional training has given rise to the hope that in the relatively near future only staff who have attended an approved course of training will be fully accredited. Opportunities for graduate training are not expanding at anything like the same rate. This fact is likely to have serious consequences for leadership, for the development of a sustained body of theory, and for the general standing of the profession amongst other professions.

A report prepared in 1967 by a committee under the chairmanship of Lady Williams found that less than 15 per cent of staff involved with the child care side of residential establishments had received any directly relevant training. In those establishments concerned primarily with education and character training it is unusual for teaching staff to have undergone any formal preparation in the art of living with children. In general, training has not been thought necessary for foster parents, although a number of local authorities have introduced short courses.

The most widespread form of training for residential child care comprises a one-year basic course. The academic standard demanded of students is not high, but considerable attention is paid to their ability to relate constructively to children. Advanced training is available on a limited scale. There is little integration between the training of agency based workers and residential workers, despite the growing emphasis on a family centred approach to child care. The Williams Committee has proposed that all students of residential work, irrespective of their final field of practice (i.e. with the elderly, the handicapped, the delinquent child, the child in care, etc.) should train on two-year generic residential work courses. However, many authorities in the child care field argue that there is a more urgent need to link the training of child care officers with that of residential child care workers. They support their case by pointing out the often severe ill effects of discontinuity in care. The two views on development in training do not necessarily conflict, but in the short run it seems almost impossible to avoid giving priority to one.

Child Care is being reoriented to require ever increasing numbers of staff and, as the work becomes more complex, staff are being required to possess greater resources of intelligence and sensitivity. Staff shortage and turnover is being accentuated by women marrying earlier and in larger numbers. There is likely to be a growing need to employ married women and to base the service at least in part on career-minded men. Part-time employment and residential posts which do not involve living-in may become other prerequisites of growth.

In commenting on satisfaction in child care Dinnage and Kellmer Pringle (1967) note: 'A common problem for both residential staff and child care officers appears to be that three quarters of their work is fairly routine, while the other quarter demands the most exceptional skill and personal qualities.' Jefferys (1967), in her study of social work in Buckinghamshire, remarked that much of the work did not appear to demand university training. From such material two requirements seem to follow: first, training must come to show how reward may be obtained from a wider range of practice; and second, practice needs to be re-examined in the light of the opportunity it provides for using resources of personal competence. At present, turnover of staff is high throughout child care but especially so in residential care—about one fifth leave this branch of the service annually, and another fifth change jobs within the service.

Future Developments

The trend of social work is towards an ever more comprehensive network of care. It is increasingly difficult to consider services to children at risk without constant reference to a broad spectrum of social work. As the underlying principles of social work come to include consideration of personal distress, family stability and the ability to function in complex systems of social relations, the readiness of the public to make use of social work extends correspondingly. There are prospects of drawing on the competence of professional social workers in the fields of marital counselling, industrial relations, leisure and education, to name a few possibilities. Modifications in casework and extensions in the use of group work and community work are likely to play a central part in these and other developments. A major contribution can be expected from voluntary social work organisations, and other organisations outside social work.

Increased awareness of the personal and social condition of certain children and adults will encourage the growth of services focussing on special needs. The maladjusted, handicapped child, or the homeless adolescent offender are examples of persons for whom appropriate forms of service are almost totally lacking. An effective and economically efficient service to such persons is likely to require a catchment area rather larger than that currently thought to be necessary for the majority of statutory social work services.

Social work has tended to focus on the recipient's needs as they are revealed during the provision of care. As a result the long term social consequences of being the recipient of care have in general been overlooked. The child on probation may be subject to cumulative suspicion on the part of neighbouring parents; the children of families receiving financial help under section 1 of the 1963 Children and Young Persons Act may be the subject of antipathy and discrimination. They may find themselves unacceptable to teachers, youth leaders and foremen. The reactions of society may lead to counter reactions on the part of the child: the delinquent may carry out further acts of delinquency, the socially insecure may collapse into total inadequacy or breakdown. Services which can control the social consequences of receiving care may have to be re-evaluated on that count and developed accordingly. If a child suffers social discrimination by remaining with his natural parents, this fact must be weighed against the effects of deprivation if he enters residential care. Residential care may offer the older child the advantage of regulating public reaction to his deviant behaviour until he can live in society in a less provocative way. To do so effectively, residential care must come to have a social meaning which minimises the stigma of 'being in residential care'.

It is to be expected that in the future social work will make increasing use of public interest, for example, by involving the natural enthusiasm of the young. When interest does not exist, it must be created. Social work is already moving to the awareness that the exercise of specialist skills in relation to persons in distress is only one stage in the pursuit of welfare goals: a further stage is to inform the spirit of society with the values which already, if imperfectly, inform the spirit of social work.

J. D. HOUSTON

A Note on Further Reading

Several useful guides to the literature on social services for children are published by Longmans in association with The National Bureau for Co-operation in Child Care (see 'References'). General accounts of the work of Children's Departments are provided by Pugh: *Social Work in Child Care* (Routledge) and Stroud: *An Introduction to the Child Care Services* (Longmans). In *Child Care: Needs and Numbers* (Allen & Unwin), Packman analyses policy variations over a broad sample of departments and shows the determinants of specific decisions. A more general analysis of administration in social work is provided by Warham: *An Introduction to Administration for Social Workers* (Routledge). Donnison and Chapman's *Social Policy and Administration* (Allen & Unwin) contains case studies in the administration of the social services.

The literature on social casework tends to be piecemeal. The most systematic text is probably Perlman: *Social Casework* (Chicago). Timms: *Social Casework* (Routledge) illustrates rather unevenly the application of theory to the practice of specific agencies. Biestek: *The Casework Relationship* (Heinemann) adumbrates a number of principles which have more ethical than instrumental validity. The confusion about the principles of casework is discussed and exemplified in Halmos:

The Faith of the Counsellors (Constable). A number of worthwhile papers are collected by Younghusband (ed.) in: *New Developments in Casework* and *Social Work With Families* (Allen & Unwin). Winnicott: *Child Care and Social Work* (Codicote Press) and Stevenson *Someone Else's Children: A Book for Foster Parents of Young Children*, and *An Approach to Family Social Work* (both Routledge), present the views of two perceptive social workers.

A detailed, if unadventurous, account of residential child care is Brill and Thomas: *Children in Homes* (Gollancz). Balbernie: *Residential Work with Children* (Pergamon) provides a more questioning approach to selected areas of work. Two collections of *Papers on Residential Work* (Longmans) Edited by Tod give a helpful, if at times rather slight, account of important issues: *Children in Care* and *Deprived Children*. Burmeister: *The Professional Houseparent* (Columbia) is a sensitive account of the basic requirements of effective practice. Employing a more comprehensive viewpoint, valuable insights are provided by Goffman: *Asylums*, and Maxwell Jones: *Social Psychiatry in Practice* (both Penguin Books).

References

AINSWORTH, M. D. (1962). In *Deprivation of Maternal Care: A Reassessment of its Effects*. Public Health Papers No. 14. Geneva: W.H.O.

BOWLBY, J. (1951). *Maternal Care and Mental Health*. Geneva: W.H.O.

—— (1965). *Child Care and the Growth of Love*. London: Penguin Books.

BROWN, M. A. G. (1966). A review of casework methods. In *New Developments in Casework*. Ed. E. L. Younghusband. London: Allen & Unwin.

Children in Trouble (1968). Command 3601. London: H.M.S.O.

Children and Young Persons Scotland (Kilbrandon Report) (1964). Command 2306. Edinburgh: H.M.S.O.

DINNAGE, R. and KELLMER PRINGLE, M. L. (1967). *Residential Child Care—Facts and Fallacies*. London: Longmans and National Bureau for Co-operation in Child Care.

—— —— (1967). *Foster Home Care—Facts and Fallacies*. London: Longmans and National Bureau for Co-operation in Child Care.

GOODACRE, I. (1966). *Adoption Policy and Practice*. London: Allen & Unwin.

JEFFERYS, M. (1967). *An Anatomy of Social Welfare Services*. London: Michael Joseph.

JENKINS, R. (1965). *The Needs of Foster Parents*. Case Conference 11, 211.

KELLMER PRINGLE, M. L. (1967). *Adoption—Facts and Fallacies*. London: Longmans and National Bureau for Co-operation in Child Care.

LEISSNER, A. (1967). *Family Advice Services*. London: Longmans and National Bureau for Co-operation in Child Care.

PACKMAN, J. (1968). *Child Care: Needs and Numbers*. London: Allen & Unwin.

PARKER, R. A. (1966). *Decision in Child Care*. London: Allen & Unwin.

Prevention of Neglect of Children. Report of the Committee of the Scottish Advisory Council on Child Care (McBoyle Report) (1963). Edinburgh: H.M.S.O.

Report of the Care of Children Committee (Curtis Report) (1946). Command 1922. London: H.M.S.O.

Report of the Committee on Children and Young Persons (Ingleby Report) (1960). Command 1191. London: H.M.S.O.

Report of the Committee on Local Authority and Allied Personal Social Services (Seebohm Report) (1968). Command 3703. London: H.M.S.O.

Social Work and the Community (1966). Command 3065. Edinburgh: H.M.S.O.

TRASLER, G. (1960). *In Place of Parents*. London: Routledge.

WAKEFORD, J. (1963). Fostering: A sociological perspective. *British Journal of Sociology*, 14, 335.

WILLIAMS, G. (1967). (Chairman) *Caring for People*. Report of a Committee set up by the National Council of Social Service. London: Allen & Unwin.

18   Present Aims and Problems in Education

OUR view of man's nature and destiny, our religious, political, and social allegiance, our economic status in the community, whether we work with hand or brain or both, the technological advances and the political and international tensions of our age—all these influences will have some bearing on our aims when we consider the education of our boys and girls. Very often, therefore, the educational aims of a particular individual are by no means the result of a cold examination of community needs; too often they are the offspring of subjective thinking tinged with class and personal prejudice. Nevertheless, in all modern democratic communities there is one principle concerning the education of the young that has now won general acceptance; this principle is summed up in the phrase 'equal educational opportunity for all'.

The almost universal acceptance of this principle, adopted by every political party in Britain as essential for ensuring the full use of the human resources of a democratic community, was the result of what Sir Fred Clarke has described as 'the massive social movement' generated by the First World War. The principle was reaffirmed in the White Paper of 1943 on *Educational Reconstruction*, issued to stimulate discussion on the momentous Education Bill of 1944:

> 'The Government's purpose in putting forward the reforms described in this paper is to secure for children a happier childhood and a better start in life; to ensure a fuller measure of education and opportunity for young people; and to provide means for all of developing the various talents with which they are endowed and so enriching the inheritance of the country whose citizens they are'.

In this brief statement of a nation's educational purpose two characteristics are to be noted: it is 'child centred'; and the child is recognised as a potential citizen.

But what kind of world is the child to inherit and serve? It is important to answer this question for the sort of world we live in profoundly affects our educational aims. To-day children are born into a very disturbed and disturbing world. We have exchanged social stability and spiritual certainty for social mobility and intellectual uncertainty. We know so much but we doubt so much. Scientific and technological advances have brought us closer together but they have also made us more dangerous to each other. In the sphere of government the tentacles of the state have steadily invaded areas of our existence once regarded as private enclaves of personal judgment and behaviour. In the realm of social and industrial organisation, units tend towards hugeness; the conveyor belt has superseded the craftsman's tool; the individual is removed steadily further away from the centre of decision; men are treated increasingly in categories rather than as individuals. These are conditions by no means conducive to the exercise of personal responsibility but rather to the increase of tension and frustration. Finally, it cannot be said that the prevailing relativity in morals provides adults with the solid moral convictions that would enable them to steer their children confidently through the snags awaiting them when they leave school. A student of the juvenile courts will have noted that to many parents and children morality is merely a device for keeping out of the hands of the police.

But we must count our assests. First among these is the increased awareness among all sections of the community of the paramount importance of education. Central and local governments, with perhaps varying intensity of zeal, are determined to rid national education of its 'trail of cheapness'; and the child stands four-square in the picture. There is our vastly increased knowledge, not of the human heart but of the human body, of the human mind and of human society. And there are all the resources of science, potentially good even if open to abuse, close at hand for the service of children, not least television, radio and the cinema. That, then, is the sort of world in which we plan for the welfare of our children.

When we discuss the aims and means of education in a democratic society we are in fact attempting to interpret the now generally accepted principle of 'equal educational opportunity for all'. The only way in which we can have equality in education is in terms of opportunity. We therefore recognise the fundamental equalities and inequalities in children by trying to provide, not the same education for all, but the most appropriate education for all. But owing to the extreme difficulty of discovering what is the appropriate education for any individual child we can never be sure of truly judging the individual case. All that the administrator can do is to do his best with the means available. Apart from the problems of selection, which in themselves are the source of much anxiety and unhappiness in both parents and children, we must accept the fact that the ideal of equal educational opportunity is in part illusory, simply because we cannot choose our parents. Equal educational opportunity sometimes leads to social inequalities. If a miner's clever son marries a miner's clever daughter they may produce a future cabinet minister. And does not the son of a cabinet minister enter life with a flying start compared with the son of a miner? Nevertheless the principle of equality remains; we have to be as certain as we can that its operation ensures the same *care* for all; for the 70 per cent less gifted as well as for the rest. That was the object of the Education Act of 1944.

The System in England and Wales

It was the intention of the Education Act of 1944 to re-form the structure of educational provision into a unified and progressive system. Education during childhood and adolescence was divided into three stages; *primary*, to cover the years 5·0 to 11·0 (the non-compulsory period in the nursery school is 3·0 to 5·0); *secondary*, to embrace the compulsory period from 11+ to 15+ (later to be extended to 16+) but also including the non-compulsory period up to 18+; and 'further education', for young people under 18·0 not receiving full-time schooling. This was a revolution in our provision for educating the nation's children; secondary education is now free and universal; every child between 5·0 and 18·0 comes within the provisions of the Act. The magnitude of the change can be measured by the fact that whereas in 1913 there were only 174,000 children in grant-aided secondary schools and in 1938 500,000, in 1965 there were over 2½ million. It is estimated, moreover, that between 1966 and 1980 the secondary school population will increase by 1½ million due to the increasing birth rate, to the tendency of secondary school pupils to stay longer at school and to the proposed raising of the leaving age to 16·0. In 1964 there were 7 million pupils in primary and secondary schools; in 1974 there will be 9 million and in 1984 probably 10 million, which represents a doubling of the school population since 1954. In 1960 there were just over 4 million children in primary schools; in 1974 there will be well over 5 million. Briefly, we are planning for a school population twice as big as it was when the 1944 Act was passed; and incidentally, also, for a university population 10 times greater than it was in 1938 and also much more costly per student.

The above figures indicate the size and complexity of the administrative problem involved in the process of transferring children from the primary to the secondary stages of schooling in a situation where the school population is steadily increasing. Primary school children have to be sorted out and provided, in the words of Section 8 of the 1944 Act, with 'such variety of training and instruction as may be desirable in view of their different *ages, abilities and aptitudes*'. In the post-war period it was assumed, with no previous sociological inquiry and too little reference to medical and psychological opinion, that boys and girls are ready for transition from primary to secondary education at the age of 11+; and further that at this age they can be separated into three categories of 'ability and aptitude' namely, (1) the pupil who is interested in learning for its own sake, who can grasp an argument or follow a piece of connected reasoning; (2) the pupil whose interests and abilities lie markedly in the field of applied science or applied art, and (3) the pupil who deals more easily with concrete things than with ideas. From these assumptions in the Norwood Report of 1943 there emerged the tripartite division of secondary education— grammar, technical and modern secondary schools. There was no mention of such a system of separate schools in the 1944 Act. Whether these three types of education be conducted under one roof or in separate schools, or in a combination of two types, is a matter for the decision of each local education authority. And it is at this point that controversy breaks out, for the decision affects the happiness of many children and may create acute anxieties among both parents and children. It is worth noting that Scottish opinion, at least outside the four large cities, has rejected the tripartite division and decided for the 'omnibus' solution, because Scottish tradition has always tended in this direction.

15

Selection

Obviously the retention of the tripartite system of schools depends on the validity of the selection test, above all on the prognostic value of an I Q measured at the age of 11·0, *i.e.* on the constancy of the I Q throughout childhood and adolescence. Until the end of the war it was believed that there was a high degree of constancy in the I.Q. This belief was based on *average* scores of large groups which showed a high degree of constancy. On these results a vast administrative system of secondary school selection was elaborated. But further research has revealed that *individual* scores within these large groups were by no means constant, sometimes varying by as much as 20 points between tests separated by several years. Clearly, then to decide the educational future of children by a test at 11+ has no foundation in psychological evidence. Moreover school assessments of children's performance have shown that there may be 30 per cent of borderline cases, any one of which might be above or below the 'in' or 'out' line determination admission to a grammar school.

Recent surveys have revealed the following factors affecting selection of children for secondary education:

1. Mental growth, like physical growth, varies with individuals, speeding up at times and then slowing down.
2. Growth seems to slow down and cease earlier in persons of low intelligence and to continue longer in individuals of high intelligence.
3. Environmental influences, home circumstances or emotional stress at home or school, may affect the results of an intelligence test by as much as 20 points.
4. I Q measurements are influenced by the degree of mental stimulation experienced throughout adolescence. This factor is important. Most children leave school at 15+ or 16+ and enter jobs demanding little mental exercise for the rest of their lives; a privileged minority stay on at school and university and engage in mental activity from 17·0 onwards. Hence, says P. E. Vernon, 'education during the teens does affect the ultimate adult intelligence level. The man with full secondary and university education has on average a 12 I Q point advantage over the man who was equally intelligent at 15·0 but has had no further education since'.
5. Measurements of I Q are most reliable when made in the later rather than in the earlier years of childhood and adolescence and are then more accurate in predicting future performance.

These observations suggest that selection at 11+, even when the I Q score is supplemented by school performance and teachers' assessment, is hardly a firm foundation for deciding a child's future schooling. This constitutes one of the major arguments of those who support the comprehensive school. The Plowden Report (1967) recommends 12+ as a more suitable age for transfer from primary to secondary education.

Three Schools or One

Citizens whose educational aims are strongly influenced by social rather than by academic considerations, especially those desiring a more homogeneous society, generally support schemes for comprehensive schools in which children of all classes and widely varying abilities are educated in one large school community. They fear the emergence of an intellectual and managerial *élite* separated in training, sympathy and interest from those engaged in humbler tasks. Their opponents point to the unwieldy size of comprehensive schools and fear the lowering of the academic standards of the grammar schools when merged into the larger unit. Many local authorities are committed to the comprehensive idea; in others the dispute continues; and lack of funds arrests development in all areas. Although there are many fine new schools throughout the country tens of thousands of our children are still educated in slum schools surrounded by slums. This is particularly true of the primary schools. The Plowden Report (1967) paints a grim picture of the primary schools in our great cities.

But whatever be the final outcome of 'the comprehensive controversy', whether our brighter children are educated in separate grammar schools or in the academic streams of larger comprehensive schools, we must realize that 70 per cent of the secondary school age group do not come into this category. Here are the mass of the future citizens of our country, not the leaders but the general body of useful people who do so much of the world's work. The Newsom Report, *Half Our Future* (1963), vividly presents the problem. The spread of ability in this 70 per cent of adolescents is very great, ranging from border-line grammar school standards to that of eleven-year-olds who cannot read. Hundreds of thousands of these children are doomed to live in conditions least likely to develop the abilities and moral capacities they possess. Forty per cent of the 'Newsom' sample attended schools whose buildings were condemned as seriously defective. Most of these children come from 'slum dwellings where people of all nationalities compete for shelter', where linguistic inadequacy, disadvantages in social and physical background and poor attainments at school are part of a total pattern of deprivation: 'We simply do not know how many people are frustrated in their lives by inability to express themselves adequately; or how many never develop intellectually because they lack the words with which to think or reason'. It is not, perhaps, realised by doctors and teachers how frustrating linguistic inadequacy can be and with what a serious social handicap the child from the 'monosyllabic home' faces his teacher, his school and his world. These unpromising conditions are not improved by immigrant populations who crowd into already crowded areas and whose children have a right to the local education provided. And yet the Newsom Report presents us with a hope and a challenge: 'Today's average boys and girls are better at their books than their predecessors half a century ago. There are reasons to expect that their successors will be better still'. (Newsom, paras 49–54. For a fuller discussion see Castle, E. B.: *A Parents' Guide to Education*).

Sources of Tension

Emotional stress of some kind is an inevitable condition of growing up and is inseparable from any educational system, especially from one that aims at a fair deal for all. We do not know how far a fully comprehensive secondary system, by eliminating the tensions created by selection at 11+ would reduce the strains of schooling. It will possibly be a whole generation before selection for secondary schooling entirely disappears. In the meantime, in England and Wales, the grammar school still retains the highest esteem of the ambitious parent, and for many thousands of children selection tests are a source of nervous strain which is only increased by parental anxiety. The unsuccessful child may be depressed by a sense of personal failure because he is not living up to parental expectations. It is too easily assumed by supporters of the comprehensive school that such tensions will disappear when selection at 11+ (or 12+) no longer exists. But some form of selection *within* the school, by what is oddly called 'streaming', is bound to occur and can easily lead to similar strains, especially as children allocated to C or D streams tend to stay there for the rest of their schooldays: *i.e.* a potentially B or C child tends to accept the 'C' ness or 'D' ness of his first assessment. This tendency has stimulated a strong movement against streaming especially in primary schools where the only supporters of streaming seem to be the most conservative and the least imaginative teachers.

On a purely statistical basis present methods of selection—by intelligence and aptitude tests, tests in English and number and school report—are reasonably satisfactory. But we are forced to the view that even the most delicately devised tests will always leave a margin of error in the prognosis of a child's total educable capacity. We can be certain of the upper and lower ranges of ability but we can never hope to draw a line between those who should be in and those who should be out of any particular type of secondary schooling. Hence for some time the emotional strains involved in selection procedures will continue. Some of them will be eased by better school provision; by improved methods of selection; by the appearance of more comprehensive schools; by a more generous provision of teachers and by smaller classes; above all, by imaginative developments in the schools themselves warranted to evoke the growing capacities of boys and girls and set them on the way, through a happy and industrious childhood, to a good start in adult life. But all strain will not be removed, and moreover need not be removed, from a situation where individual ambition clashes with the impartial operation of a principle.

Paradoxically enough the vastly increased opportunities provided by free secondary education have not necessarily widened the area of parental choice. In 1930 a parent could choose his children's school if he could pay the fees for the school he liked, which few could do. In 1970 his right to choose is bound by conditions, financial, geographical and administrative. Can he choose a denominational school for his child? Yes, if there is one in his area. Can he send his child to a grammar school rather than to another type of secondary school? Not unless the child has qualified by the entrance test. These are reasonable conditions under the present system. But can a parent chooose between a bad school (*e.g.* where there is excessive use of corporal punishment) and a more enlightened one? Not unless it is within the same administrative area. Thus in the last 40 years we have moved from the undemocratic position, where secondary education was available if you could pay for it, to the more democratic but irritating situation where your children must go to the school which the local authority, not the parent, chooses. Here is a real cause of tension and grievance, for schools can vary enormously not only in academic efficiency but in cultural quality. Another area of diminished choice and of emotional stress appears at the 18+ stage. Up to the 1930s a sixth former could choose his university; in 1970, owing to the enormous pressure on university places, the university chooses its students.

Other sources of unnecessary strain among schoolchildren lie within the schools themselves. Among these may be anxiety concerning examinations, especially where the child of mediocre talent is additionally burdened with over-anxious or ambitious parents; excessive competition in the classroom (it is best that a child should compete only with his own inertia); association with pupils of greater ability; incompatibility of teacher and pupil; and the inability of a weakly or sensitive child to stand up to the rough-and-tumble of school life. On the other hand misbehaviour and poor work are as likely to result from too easy as from too difficult study. Accurate grading (often difficult in a small school) and circumstances that produce good work with a little but not too much strain, where successful effort engenders its own encouragement and establishes its own confidence, where the authority of the teacher and the freedom of the pupil are in harmony, where as many children as possible are doing things they want to do and can do, and where each child feels some responsibility for his own progress—this kind of situation is likely to produce effort without unnecessary tension in the class-room. And, what is more, problems of discipline will loom less ominously in the school.

Schools today are far happier places than they used to be because teachers are more humane, more sensitive to the total needs of children, more alert to the manifold resources of a child's energy and more willing to use them. The rod, once the normal magisterial insignia and the inseparable adjunct to learning, very often now lies mouldering in the cupboard. But it is worth noting that Britain shares the honours with Sweden in being the only two countries in Western Europe to allow corporal punishment in schools. The good teacher now knows that good discipline depends on good teaching and good personal relationships. He is prepared to give more place to practical and aesthetic activity, he more often sees 'subjects' as fields of human endeavour and brings the world into the class-room by taking his pupils out of it; he serves his pupils on the playing-field and in the countryside, and he realises, more than was ever realised before, that a school is a community of persons whose purpose is to provide the raw material of moral and social experience. The best schools are aware that the child's first need is security and that security comes from the child's association with mature and disinterested personalities. And the best teacher is he who exercises an unremitting and unsentimental care for children. But lest too rosy a picture is given of present conditions we must emphasise that we are referring only to the best teachers and the best schools. As the Plowden Report indicates there are still too many miserable school buildings housing too many deprived children and too many mediocre and indifferent teachers, to permit any complacency to enter into our views of contemporary education. We must hope that in both equipment and staffing more schools will become more like the best. Then they will be very good.

One other factor in the situation should be noted, especially by those working in that elusive area between school and home: parent-teacher co-operation improves steadily. Many a school head will agree that the younger generation of parents are less suspicious of the teacher's trade and more willing to discuss their children's problems than were parents 30 years ago. It is all to the good when home and school find themselves in partnership in the difficult job of rearing the young.

Education in Developing Countries

The aims and problems of education discussed in the foregoing pages have some relevance to similar but far more acute problems in the developing countries overseas. In the words of President Nyerere, the educational objective is 'to work ourselves out of poverty'. And this is a basic povery, unknown in the wealthy nations of the world, where the gross national product is no more than £25 a head per annum, or may be less. Half the people in the world are illiterate, half suffer from malnutrition and disease. Ignorance is a major factor in their lives. These evils are indivisible; each reacts on the other in a vicious cycle of cause and effect. To remove ignorance is to pave the way to better physical well-being, to higher food production, to better social conditions. Hence the educational aim of the under-privileged peoples is not merely to produce more people who can read and write, although these skills are basic to all human communication, but to develop systems of education that span the needs of a nation from the highest university grades through secondary and primary schooling, so that academic and technological knowledge and the humbler practical skills can be applied to the improvement of social and economic life.

There are many lions in the path. Poverty we have already noted; add to this a rapidly increasing population, sometimes at the rate of three per cent per annum, which means a doubling of population in 25 years. In some developing countries half the population is under 15·0 and half of these children are under 5·0. What this means in terms of educational planning can readily be imagined; governments are confronted with the task of providing not only for the 50 per cent of children of school age who are not in school, but for a rapidly increasing school-age population clamouring to enter classrooms and to be taught by teachers who do not exist. A poor country might provide hundreds of new schools, absorbing tens of thousands of children, but there would probably be still no more than 50 per cent of her children in school. All these backward countries are thus faced with a combined economic, educational and demographic problem, in which too many children chase too few schools and too few teachers because there is too little money. Add to this wide scale unemployment, especially among school leavers; the reluctance of young people to stay on the land where they can see only a future of rewardless toil; and the mistaken view that education brings release from the social stigma of manual work, although the great need is not for clerical workers but for skilled artisans and farmers, that middle group of workers who are the backbone of a progressive economy. Educational planners are faced with the problem of priorities thus described in the report of the Uganda Education Commission *Education in Uganda* (1963)

> 'The problem for those who plan educational policy, then, is this: when over half the nation is illiterate and the people rightly clamour for education, when teachers are in short supply and inadequately trained, when government and industry demand trained recruits, when unemployment is widespread and increasing, when the nation is poor—what policy should the government pursue? If the government decide first to educate the neglected 50 per cent it would fail to find teachers to teach them; if secondary education is neglected, the potential supply of teachers would diminish. Moreover, schools can be built in months, but it takes many years to make a teacher. Here is a real dilemma, for behind all these considerations remains the stark fact that the country cannot at present afford to make all desirable improvements in a general advance on all fronts'. (Paragraph 235.)

All these problems are being tackled bravely and intelligently by the newly independent governments. But educational planning must also include adult education, for every effort should be made to avoid the danger of skills and knowledge learned at school fading away because they have not been articulated with the needs and experiences of adult life. Most governments realise that the education of the whole community is involved. For the success of mass education, especially literacy campaigns and instruction in food production and in hygiene, depends on the intelligent co-operation of the people it aims to serve. The basic nature of co-operation between home and school is well expressed in a sentence of the Uganda Commission's report: 'No single reform in this country could have more beneficial effect on its children's education than the institution of school meals in day schools'. Too many children go hungry to school. Having had no meal since the previous night, they spend the school day listless and incapable of learning for lack of properly timed and balanced meals. As the report *Mass Education in African Society* (1944) pertinently insists: 'Just as the education of the child must lead up to the development of the adult so must schemes for adult education reach down, as it were, to join hands with the school. The plans at one level must ensure the fulfilment of activities at other levels'. In the writer's experience one of the most depressing legacies from colonial times is the comparative absence of active co-operation between the various branches of the social services—educational, medical, agricultural and social development—whose officers had failed to realise that they were in fact all engaged in a single campaign to remove ignorance, to prevent disease and to produce food. Each department is too often narrowly and busily engaged in its assumed separate sphere of activity.

Hence aims and problems of education in the underdeveloped countries must be conceived in the broadest terms. Literacy is a tool and no more; it can never be the end of education. The evil legacy of ignorance and poverty can be dispelled only by the increase of vocational skills, especially agricultural skills in countries where 90 per cent of the population will be tied to the land; by education in the laws of personal and community hygiene, especially as they apply to the enemies of health in any particular locality; by simple knowledge of biological and economic processes, especially as they affect diet and food production. But, as Guy Hunter has pointed out, what is ultimately at issue in the developing countries of the world is 'the growth of new nations, new societies of men, not merely the construction of new economies'. These new societies, it must be noted, have to do in one generation what it took centuries to evolve in the older societies of the West. Tribal institutions are still divisive; there is still the conservative drag of a pre-scientific culture; dangerous élitist trends appear in the highly educated groups—the anti-social attitude that higher education, in Nyerere's angry words, 'confers the automatic right to high salary and status'. Education, then, has another task, as true education in any country always has: to inculcate a set of simple values, a sense of personal responsibility, self-reliance, habits of co-operation, and among the highly educated few the conviction, again to use Nyerere's words, that 'further education is the training of the few in the interests of the many'.

E. B. CASTLE

Bibliography

Official Publications (H.M.S.O.)

15 to 18 (Crowther Report) 1959.
Higher Education (Robbins Report)1963.
Half Our Future (Newsom Report) 1963.
Children and their Primary Schools (Plowden Report) 1967.
Public Schools Commission, First Report, 1968.

Other Publications (for U.K.)

AYERST, D. (1967). *Understanding Schools.* London: Penguin Books.
CASTLE, E. B. (1968). *A Parents' Guide to Education.* London: Penguin Books.
FLOUD, J. E., HALSEY, A. H. and MARTIN, F. M. (1956). *Social Class and Educational Opportunity.* London: Heinemann.
GLASS, D. V. (1954). (Ed.) *Social Mobility in Britain.* London: Routledge and Kegan Paul.
HADFIELD, J. A. (1962). *Childhood and Adolescence.* London: Penguin Books.
JACKSON, B. (1964). *Streaming. An Educational System in Miniature.* London: Routledge and Kegan Paul.
PEDLEY, R. (1963). *The Comprehensive School.* London: Penguin Books.
STENHOUSE, L. (1967). *Discipline in Schools.* London: Pergamon Press.
TANNER, J. M. (1961). *Education and Physical Growth.* Oxford: Blackwell.
WALL, W. D. (1947). *The Adolescent Child.* London: Methuen.
—— (1968). *Adolescents in School and Society.* National Foundation for Educational Research.

For Tropical Countries

BEEBY, C. E. (1966). *The Quality of Education in Developing Countries.* Harvard: Univ. Press.

CASTLE, E. B. (1966). *Growing Up in East Africa.* London: Oxf. Univ. Press.

CURLE, A. (1963). *Educational Strategy for Developing Societies.* London: Tavistock.

FOSTER, P. (1965). *Education and Social Change in Ghana.* London: Routledge and Kegan Paul.

GRIFFITHS, V. L. (1953). *An Experiment in Education.* London: Longmans.

HODGKIN, R. A. (1957). *Education and Change.* London: Oxf. Univ. Press.

HUNTER, G. (1962). *The New Societies of Tropical Africa.* London: Oxf. Univ. Press.

U.N.E.S.C.O. (1949). *Fundamental Education.*

COLONIAL OFFICE, No. 186 (1944). *Mass Education in African Society.*

Education in Uganda (Castle Report) 1963.

Kenya Education Commission (Ominde Report) 1964.

19   Vocational Guidance in Britain

THE term Vocational Guidance (or Vocational Counselling in the U.S.A.) is normally reserved for the procedure used by those who spend most of their time advising on careers, who tackle the problem in a systematic fashion and the basis of whose theory and practice is a psychological one. These vocational advisers may be psychologists, or they may be youth employment officers or careers masters and mistresses in schools.

This systematic approach and procedure is fairly new in this country and owes its origin almost entirely to the National Institute of Industrial Psychology. When Dr. (now Sir Cyril) Burt became head of the Vocational Guidance Department of the Institute in 1922 he at once began to combine the practice of vocational guidance with research investigations. The practice of vocational guidance at the National Institute of Industrial Psychology incorporated certain features which, although there have been considerable modifications in detail since the 1920s, remain essentially these:

The parents, on deciding that their child needs vocational guidance, get in touch with the Institute. A vocational adviser is allocated to the case and he immediately asks for reports from the head of the school and if possible from the form teacher and the house-master. The parents, too, are asked for a full report giving health history, development, special interests and similar information. (Some very useful reporting forms, which really do help the reporter, have been developed over the years.) The child then comes to the Institute, preferably accompanied by the parents, who can enlarge on any of the material provided in their report. The boy (or girl) is interviewed at considerable length, fills in questionnaires on his interests, hobbies and preferences and is given several tests. Nowadays, and particularly as a result of the research work carried out on service men and women during the war, tests tend to be restricted to these factors: general intelligence, verbal facility, mechanical comprehension, spatial perception and attainment in English and mathematics. (Elaborate performance tests involving the use of complicated apparatus give disappointingly small additions to the material gleaned from the pencil-and-paper tests.) By this time the vocational adviser will normally be in a position to formulate and discuss with the boy some suggestions of possible jobs. The vocational adviser then drafts his report which is discussed with the boy and his parents, preferably at another visit rather than by correspondence.

The vocational adviser will have been able to form a clear, and in most cases, an accurate, picture of the child. (He will probably have found it helpful to collect his material under seven headings: physique, attainments, general intelligence, special aptitudes, interests, disposition and circumstances.) He will also have at his finger-tips or in handy references very considerable information on careers. What is just as important, and scientifically even more important, is to have a considerable body of evidence indicating which kinds of jobs are more or less suitable for people possessing certain characteristics. This no one has in any clear-cut form. There are some obvious negative indications—for example that a very shy person would probably not do well in, or enjoy, careers X, Y and Z; that people whose intelligence is below average would have to toil superhumanly to get any kind of university degree; and so on. On the positive side, as the indications tend to be less obvious they wander away from scientific validity. The nearer a person gets to being a very good all-rounder, the more difficult is the task of the vocational adviser. The validation of job standards is not an easy matter and it is scarcely surprising that comparatively little progress has been made. Two current research attempts sound hopeful. The first is to find 'critical requirements of the job' and this involves discovering the reasons for people failing in it. One could thus hope to arrive at the *relevance* of particular personal characteristics to particular jobs or groups of jobs which are psychologically similar. The second approach is to try to discover the ranges of intelligence, attainment and background of people already doing a certain job: the minimum of these indicates the minimum standard for that job. It is plain that it will take a long time to cover an important part of the occupational field when one considers the difficulties. First, there are very few research investigators. Second, firms are, understandably enough, not eager to allow psychologists to test, interview and collect detailed personality descriptions of their employees, nor are they often willing to disclose which of these employees are good, bad and indifferent at the job.

If this aspect of vocational guidance (as practised by psychologists at the National Institute of Industrial Psychology or elsewhere) is not nearly as scientific as it should be, it is fair to ask where the scientific basis of vocational guidance is to be found. There are two aspects, one global and the other highly specific, which have been validated. The global approach has been to follow up those youngsters who took vocational advice and compare their success (in terms of satisfactoriness and job satisfaction) with (*a*) that of the youngsters who did not accept the advice and (*b*) that of control groups of school-leavers who were given no tests or long inter-views but who had been given vocational advice on the usual basis of scant informa-tion. The greater success of those who, after full vocational guidance procedure, follow the advice has been clearly demonstrated by several investigations. The more specific aspect of vocational guidance which has been submitted to validation is the testing of the tests. Reputable vocational advisers use only those aptitude tests which have reasonable correlations with criteria, the criteria usually taking the form of performance in jobs which appear to require that particular aptitude.

The Youth Employment Service

Before 1948 rather less than half of those leaving English local authority schools were entitled to receive some kind of vocational guidance from the juvenile employment officers (as they were called) of the local education authority. The rest were in areas where the Department of Employment and Productivity (then called the Ministry of Labour and National Service) was responsible for this. In Scotland, only one authority (the city of Edinburgh) and in Wales only three (Cardiff, Merthyr Tydfil, and Swansea) exercised these powers; the rest of Scotland and Wales was the responsibility of the Department of Employment and Productivity.

In 1945 the committee on the juvenile employment service under the chairmanship of Sir Godfrey Ince was set up with the object of considering measures necessary to establish a comprehensive juvenile employment service and to make suggestions for a practicable scheme. The greater part of the report of this committee (generally referred to as the Ince Report) was embodied in the Employment and Training Act, 1948. The most important provisions of this Act were:

(i) Local education authorities were to be offered a last chance to take over responsibility from the Department of Employment and Productivity;
(ii) The grant to local education authorities from central funds for the running of the service was to be considerably increased;
(iii) A Central Youth Employment Executive (C.Y.E.E.) was to be set up to help, inspect and supervise the working of the service throughout the country.

In fact, as a result of the offer, many more local education authorities accepted responsibility for the Youth Employment Service (as it has come to be called) and the majority of school-leavers are now in areas covered by their vocational guidance staff.

Where the local educational authority is responsible, the youth employment officers (Y.E.Os) are members of the Director of Education's staff with offices housed in buildings of the local authority; in the Department of Employment and Productivity, the youth employment officer is a civil servant on the staff of the Exchange Manager, and his office forms part of the Employment Exchange. The youth employment officer, whether education authority or Department of Employment and Productivity, (a) reports to a local committee composed of representatives of the local education authority, employers, teachers, workpeople and others interested in the welfare of boys and girls, and (b) is helped, inspected and supervised by the Central Youth Employment Executive. The staffing of a local youth employment service is usually of the order of 1 youth employment officer for each 600 to 1000 school-leavers annually but the staff ratio is, year by year, improving. In cities, the officers are usually in one bureau, in counties they are sited at strategical places throughout the area.

The procedure, although not standardised, follows a pattern which had been advised by the Central Youth Employment Executive. The headmaster of a local education authority school sends in to the youth employment officer an estimate of the number of school-leavers that term. The Officer visits the school and gives his 'school talk' to the assembled children. He advises them to think about jobs and to discuss the matter with their parents, he runs over the kinds of jobs available—not only local jobs—and announces that he will be back to see them all individually. He may supplement his talk with visual aids, exhibitions, special talks from experts on particular jobs and may arrange visits to work places. By the time he returns to the school a few months later there has been completed by the teacher a report on each school-leaver. This report is on a standardised form and allows for these entries: a statement of the pupil's good, average, and weak subjects; a rating of general ability on a three-point scale; a statement of any positions of responsibility held and of any other achievements; a report on special aptitudes (for example, mechanical); a statement of the pupil's health (for example, vitality, obvious disabilities). The teacher is ready to supplement this orally when the youth employment officer consults him. At the interview with the child the officer may have a teacher with him and/or a parent. Some officers see the child first and have a consultation later with teacher and parent. At the interview the officer hopes, in about fifteen minutes (the average time he can allow himself), to round off the picture of the child and to come to agreed conclusions about the type of work to be sought.*

No definite vacancy—*this* job, *that* firm—is offered on this occasion; it is at a further (short) interview at the Youth Employment Bureau that the youngster is told of particular vacancies. The vacancies are obtained from employers who are, however, not obliged to notify them to the youth employment officer, nor need employers fill them via the Youth Employment Service. It will be seen that the success of the youth employment officer is to a large extent bound up with the confidence that employers have in him and this, in turn, is dependent on the efficiency which the officer has shown in the past. The employer is under no obligation to take any of those who have been selected by the youth employment officer as 'possible'; he may reject all of them and fill the vacancy from some other source.

When the school-leavers are settled in their jobs, the youth employment officer has the continuing responsibility of trying to keep track of them until they are 18. This review of progress is carried out by various methods, for example, by holding open meetings when all are invited to call in, by correspondence and by calls at their places of work (although the last is discouraged except in special circumstances.) The progress, if it can be called that, of the 'grasshopper' is, of course, constantly under review, without any special effort on the part of the youth employment officer—but neither he nor his more stable contemporary is *obliged* to use the service or to accept any vocational advice offered.

The shortcomings of the service are, in the main, due to financial restriction but some are caused by other factors. The chief limitations of the efficiency of the official vocational guidance service for school-leavers are these:

* Excellent pamphlets on careers are provided by the Central Youth Employment Executive, and youth employment officers often supplement these by compiling job-descriptions of trades and professions within their own area. The Central Youth Employment Executive also make available to youth employment officers and schools, films, film-strips, display material and the like.

1. The absence in most schools of a clear policy of, and procedure for, collating material on the child which would be useful to the vocational adviser.

2. The limitation imposed by the Employment and Training Act on the nature of the material which can be passed on to the youth employment officer. For example, the teacher is not allowed to record in writing anything about the child's personality, temperament, background, and interests.

3. The absence of test results from the standardised report form. This is not due to limitations imposed by the Act, but more to (1) above and to scepticism about the value of tests.

4. The inadequacy of the fifteen-minute interview at the school. This is basically a staffing problem and a result of the speed with which youth employment officers must operate to cover their assignments in the allotted time.

5. Until recently, the absence at the centre (C.Y.E.E.) of a research outlook. It can be argued that it is the function of the universities to carry out research but it is unfortunate that, for example, no large-scale follow-up is being sponsored by the C.Y.E.E.

6. The inadequacy of the 'coverage' of grammar schools in England and senior secondary schools in Scotland. To some extent this is due to shortage of staff in the youth employment service but it is also, in some cases at least, a reflection of the attitude of the heads of these schools to the youth employment officers.

Looking to the future, the kind of vocational guidance service required to fit the needs of our school-leavers might be outlined as follows:

1. Secondary school organisations would allow for staff and time to collate on each child material which would be relevant for vocational guidance. This material would be recorded in a systematic fashion, preferably on a cumulative record card. This would provide a useful basis for continuous educational guidance throughout the child's school career. As aids to both educational and vocational guidance, tests would be given at certain points in the child's school life (possibly at 7, 10, and 14 years) and their results recorded.

2. At the beginning of the school-leaving year a careers master or mistress would show increasing interest in the child's records, would get to know the parents and their wishes and hopes, and would have throughout the year several formal and informal interviews with the child. He would also be responsible for careers information (books, pamphlets, films) and for arranging visits to places of employment, where this is not already done for ordinary educational reasons.

3. Well before the child was due to leave, the careers teacher would have, in most cases, clear ideas about the *kind* of job for which the child appeared to be suitable. In other cases, he would have agreed with the parents, headmaster and child that the best guidance to offer would be for the youngster to remain at school, or transfer to a more specialised educational institution; in other cases again he would be doubtful about what kind of advice to offer and would present the whole picture to the youth employment officer in the hope that together they could find a solution. Whatever the stage reached by the careers teacher in his preparatory vocational guidance, the youth employment officer could best employ his limited

time at the school by briefing himself with the information garnered by the careers teacher and discussing it with him. The officer would certainly need to interview the child at school, if only to get to know him and because he has to have subsequent dealings with him; but he would not have to attempt the impossible task of assessing the child's abilities, aptitudes, interests, temperament and the like, all in fifteen minutes. The youth employment officer could thus concentrate on the important task of interpreting all the available material in terms of guidance to actual jobs.

It is only fair to say that the youth employment service is now conscious of its limitations particularly since the publication of 'The Albemarle Report' (1965) which emerged from a working party set up 'to define the main issues facing the youth employment service in the light of recent developments in education and changing needs of industry'. The recommendations, if implemented, would go far to eliminate the shortcomings of the service and would meet most of the strictures mentioned in this article. It is particularly encouraging to see an extension of guidance to older pupils, the ratio of Y.E.Os. to school leavers being markedly improved, and greater mutual respect and co-operation between schools and Y.E.Os. What is even more heartening is to see a change in the climate of opinion at the C.Y.E.E. about research; amongst other things, the C.Y.E.E. is giving energetic encouragement *and* financial backing to the development of an occupational interests guide which should help youngsters and their counsellors in arriving at occupational decisions.

Vocational Guidance at Industrial Rehabilitation Units

The Dpaertment of Employment and Productivity has 12 Industrial Rehabilitation Units (I.R.U.) in England, Scotland and Wales in or near large cities. The purpose of the Industrial Rehabilitation Unit is to provide a rehabilitation course for men and women who have been ill, injured, or unemployed for a long time. The chief activities are woodwork, engineering, arts, crafts, gardening and gymnastics; no vocational training is given. In addition to the occupational supervisors and the remedial gymnast there is a team of five who are particularly concerned with assessing the trainees' fitness for work or training. These are: the Rehabilitation Officer (who is in charge), the Medical Officer (who attends part-time), the Vocational Officer (a psychologist), the Disablement Resettlement Officer, and the Social Worker.

Soon after entering, the trainees are given two intelligence tests, and tests of arithmetic, mechanical comprehension, mechanical information and spatial perception. They are interviewed, usually in the third week, for about an hour by the vocational officer who normally has at that time reports from the medical officer, the occupational supervisor and the social worker. Towards the end of the course the recommendations for employment and training are discussed at a meeting of all five members of the team plus the Chief Occupational Supervisor. The recommendations are based on all the information available.

A recent development is to use I.R.Us. for the assessment and guidance of handicapped school leavers who are also exposed gradually to the atmosphere, techniques and discipline of work life.

Occupational Guidance Units

These have been set up in the last few years by the Department of Employment and Productivity in a dozen or so large centres of population throughout U.K. Their purpose is to give vocational guidance to men and women above the ages catered for by the youth employment service. The youngest tend to be about 20 or so and this group includes university dropouts, a luckless and bewildered group of young people sorely in need of help. Others are those who are considering not only changing their jobs but changing their careers. The occupational guidance units are manned by experienced officers of the D.E.P. who have the knowledge of the 'market' at their finger-tips and by means of long and skilful interviewing are able to help their clients to make realistic decisions about their future careers. Occupational psychologists are available at occupational guidance units for the assessment of some people.

Other Vocational Guidance Centres

Roffey Park, an independent rehabilitation centre in Sussex, and the Belmont Hospital in Surrey, are doing work similar in nature to that of the Industrial Rehabilitation Units. In Belfast there is an Adult Vocational Guidance Service privately sponsored and financed but run by psychologists.

Most university departments of psychology give a little time to vocational guidance, but only London (Birkbeck and the Institute of Psychiatry), Liverpool and Edinburgh have developed it to the point of having staff and time clearly devoted to this part of the applied field. In these four university departments vocational guidance practice is integrated with teaching and research. Research is being concentrated at present on four problems: (i) the reliability and validity of interviewing; (ii) classification of careers into psychologically realistic categories and levels; (iii) criteria of job satisfaction and satisfactoriness; (iv) the employability of the feeble-minded; (v) the assessment of occupational interests. These, together with large-sample follow-up of groups given vocational guidance within the Youth Employment Service, are the chief current research needs. Development work is also under way on (*a*) the building up of batteries of cheap and valid tests, and (*b*) job-description methods which can be easily used by youth employment officers.

Summary

Vocational guidance as a systematic procedure with a psychological basis has existed in Britain for only 40 years or so. It began with the National Institute of Industrial Psychology which continues by training courses and conferences, by research and publications, to develop its study and practice. The main elements in the procedure are these: reports from whoever is in a position to know the youngster well; tests, particularly of intelligence, vocabulary, mechanical comprehension, spatial perception and attainment in English and mathematics; questionnaires and attitude scales; interviews and, later, discussions on possible careers with parents and child; a detailed report carrying recommendations. Follow-up has shown that the overall procedure has a high validity.

The largest 'official' vocational guidance system is the Youth Employment Service, run in some cases by the local education authorities, in others by the Department of Employment and Productivity. The procedure has these characteristics: a talk to school-leavers by the youth employment officer; a call, later on, at the school to receive a report on each child; a discussion with the teacher and then short interviews. At this stage he usually formulates a general recommendation which he makes more specific when the child calls at the Youth Employment Bureau. He continues to exercise a certain measure of supervision over school-leavers until they are 18. The whole procedure could be considerably improved by the school staff playing a stronger part in the preparatory vocational guidance before the youth employment officer appears at the school.

Industrial Rehabilitation Units combine vocational guidance with rehabilitation for industrial casualties. Roffey Park and the Belmont Hospital carry out similar functions. Occupational guidance units cater for older men and women considering a change of career.

A few university departments of psychology combine vocational guidance practice with teaching, training and research.

DENIS McMAHON

Bibliography
Official Publications (H.M.S.O.)

Report of the Committee on Juvenile Employment Service (The Ince Report) (1945).
Employment and Training Act, 1948.
The Future Development of the Youth Employment Service (The Albermarle Report) 1965.
The Youth Employment Service. Central Youth Employment Executive.
Careers for Men and Women. Department of Employment and Productivity. (Pamphlets).
Choice of Careers, New Series. Central Youth Employment Executive. (Pamphlets).

Other Publications

DAWS, P. P. (1968). *A Good Start in Life*. Careers Research and Advisory Centre.
EARLE, F. M. *et al.* (1931). *Methods of Choosing a Career*. London: Harrap.
HEGINBOTHAM, H. (1951). *The Youth Employment Service*. London: Methuen.
OAKLEY, C. and MACRAE, A. (1937). *Handbook of Vocational Guidance*. London: Univ. Press.
RODGER, A. (1939). The work of the vocational adviser. In *The Study of Society*. Ed. F. C. Bartlett, *et al.* London: Kegan Paul.
—— and DAVIES, J. G. W. (1951). Vocational guidance and training. In *Chambers's Encyclopaedia*. London: Newnes.
—— (1953). Vocational guidance in Britain. In *Current Trends in British Psychology*. Ed. C. A. Mace and P. E. Vernon. London: Methuen.

20 Mental Health of the Child, the Family and the Community

Introduction: Historical Perspective

IT is almost exactly fifty years since there came into being, first in the United States, shortly after in Britain, the Child Guidance movement. Motivated by concern, the impulse to serve, and an unquestioning belief in the ultimate victory, this was a genuine 'movement' rather than a professional activity. The enemy to be conquered was no less than mental illness. The approach was a seemingly logical one, that treatment of the 'sick' adult came too late; the focus was to be childhood. That this somewhat ambitious preventive programme was not achieved is in retrospect hardly surprising. Today we should hardly attempt as much. What is remarkable is how Child Guidance has taken root, developed, withstood the inevitable phase of disillusionment, and has nurtured the growth of several professional disciplines—of child psychiatry, educational psychology, and psychiatric social work. Lacking any solid foundation of scientific knowledge these pioneers nevertheless divined the essential principle of the inter-disciplinary team, with representatives from the fields of social work, pedagogy, and medicine. In this respect, perhaps more than in any other, they were ahead of their time, giving a lead not only to general psychiatric practice but to medical practice as a whole. From the outset the focus was clearly on *the child in the family*, and the term 'Child Guidance' a misnomer. In fact, doubly so, as with experience the range of therapeutic measures developed far beyond the confines of 'guidance'. However, 'Child Guidance' it was, and if now somewhat anachronistic has served well the purpose of identifying a new professional discipline.

Although the opening of the Boston Psychopathic Clinic, the first of its kind, just antedated the first world war, it was the post-war disruption of family life on a hitherto unrecorded scale which forced attention on the newly-defined problem of 'juvenile delinquency'. Within a few years there was inaugurated in this country the East London Child Guidance Clinic, shortly afterwards the Notre Dame Child Guidance Clinic in Glasgow, and gradually thereafter clinics throughout the United States and Europe. Within a short time experience had taught that by no means all the 'problem children' were the products of 'problem families' or of 'broken homes'. Moreover anti-social behaviour was found to be but one of many forms of symptomatology. *Childhood emotional disorder*, as it came to be known, could present as a developmental lag, educational failure, nervous complaints or

446

habits, bodily symptoms, or combinations of all or any of these, and others. Though physicians in general were slow in recognising the importance of this unexplored field, it must be recorded that as early as 1911, on his appointment as director of the paediatric department in Vienna, Von Pirquet set up a psychiatric clinic for children. In Britain, another paediatrician, Hector Cameron, led the way with his book *The Nervous Child* (1946). In this he was surely influenced by his teacher, John Thomson, himself a pioneer in social paediatrics in Scotland, whose little monograph, 'Opening Doors', was addressed to the mothers of mentally handicapped children, an early exercise in what today we should term parent-counselling (Craig, 1968). The first children's psychiatrists were either paediatricians confronted with significant numbers of child patients whose disorders proved inaccessible to traditional methods of investigation and treatment, or psychiatrists who, influenced by the teaching of Sigmund Freud and Adolf Meyer, began to discard the static nosological concepts of nineteenth century psychiatry and to inquire into bio-graphical and environmental factors. Patients began to be regarded as people, not just cases, and their emotional health understandable in terms of their individual responses to previous as well as current environmental experiences. The mental health of children was seen to be important not only in relation to the health and happiness of boys and girls and their families, but to their future stability and character in adult life.

In Europe and the United States concern about the welfare of the individual child can be seen historically as a fairly recent phenomenon, and by no means the prerogative of the medical profession. Compulsory primary education, which dates from the beginning of this century, produced a new problem for educationalists, the child who did not seem to learn. Binet undertook a major survey of the abilities of Parisian school-children, and was able thereby to provide norms of performance for successive ages. Along with Simon he devised the earliest intelligence-tests which were published in 1905. It now became possible to calculate the 'intelligence quotient' and to classify school children in terms of ability—or so it seemed. With hindsight we now appreciate that 'intelligence' is too complex a phenomenon to be designated by a number or percentage, except with very careful safeguards; that the intelligence-test score is dependent on the skill and experience of the tester, the child's motivation, physical health, special sensory functions and emotional state. Today a wide range of psychological procedures are available for (*a*) various age groups—infants, toddlers, school children; and (*b*) the assessment of different aspects of the child's abilities, motor, perceptual, conceptual, etc. (see Chapter 9). These procedures are usually carried out by the *clinical or educational psychologist*.

Modern methods of teaching children with physical and mental handicap owe much to the original principles devised by an Italian physician, Dr. Maria Montessori, during the early years of this century. Well ahead of her time was her emphasis on sensory training, on the balancing of liberty and discipline in the classroom, and on the importance of health as an educational consideration. *The Montessori method* is now an established teaching method for normal young children, not only the retarded; and *remedial teaching* an important feature of many child guidance services. A parallel development in Austria and Germany was the practice of *heilpedagogie*, a form of special education emphasising the child's total personality.

The psychiatric social worker, a term which first came into use in the United States, is the modern descendant of the mental after-care worker, concerned with rehabilitation after recovery from mental illness or breakdown. It was a logical step in the direction of preventive psychiatry for some workers to focus their efforts on patients who were also parents. Others were members of the earliest clinical teams organised by Healy in his efforts to combat delinquency. The technical procedure whereby the psychiatric social worker endeavours to help clients, whether they be parents, foster-parents, child-caring personnel, or others, is termed *casework*, a combination of acceptance, support, and non-directive help.

Freud did not undertake psycho-analytic work directly with children, though he did successfully manage the psychotherapy of a child by instructing the child's father, a physician, in the appropriate technique (Jones, 1955). The development of psycho-analysis for use with children was pioneered mainly by Anna Freud and Melanie Klein. Though presenting different theoretical views and therapeutic procedures, both highlight in their work (*a*) the child's relationship with the therapist and (*b*) the therapist's understanding of the child's utterances and play. To the uninitiated it often comes as a surprise that the play-activities of young children are considered valid data for scientific observation, that the content of play is related not only to the stage of development but also to the imaginative life of the child, compounded of drives, wishes, confusions, and fears; that play, spontaneous as well as in the context of psychotherapy, has a protective or healing quality. Whether psychoanalytic theory is approved in toto, with reservations, or not at all, play as a diagnostic and therapeutic procedure with younger age-groups is now accepted practice. In a broader context, play is recognised as a healthful activity serving emotional growth. Its understanding is, therefore, a basic necessity to children's nurses, nursery-school teachers, and paediatricians.

During 1927/28 the Commonwealth Fund provided scholarships to the United States for a small group of British trainees. The provision of mental health services for children and parents, however, came slowly; by 1939 there were only 22 child guidance clinics in the United Kingdom. Again the impact of war helped to focus attention on children at risk psychologically, especially the reactions of those evacuated from the cities to children's homes, foster-families, and residential nurseries (Burlingham and Freud, 1954). As discussed in Chapter 10, the suspected harm as a result of prolonged or repeated separation of young children from their families was confirmed by first-hand experience. By 1966, 400 child guidance clinics had been established, mainly by education authorities in response to the recognition of the special educational needs of 'the maladjusted child' by the Education Act of 1944. It is doubtful whether this terminology is conducive to enlightened legislation. 'Maladjusted' is a static epithet, which begs the whole question of aetiology, and implies an inconvenient deviation from an idealised norm. While it is recognised in principle that the emotional problems of childhood are of concern to more than one discipline—as witnessed by the professional team in clinical practice—administrative responsibility remains fragmented between education and health services. A fresh opportunity for integration now presents, however, with the imminent establishment of local authority social work departments (see Chapter 17).

The development of specialised facilities for children and adolescents has lagged behind general psychiatric provision and although at the time of writing there are units in most of the teaching centres in Britain, associated with general psychiatric hospitals, paediatric hospitals (or departments) or both, the service is at an early stage of development. Out-patient consultative work, originally confined to separate clinics, is gradually being restored to its appropriate place alongside other medical specialities in general and paediatric out-patient departments. For the child who requires a period of investigation and care away from home, child psychiatric in-patient units, carefully designed and furnished to afford space and informality, have been developed for short-term admissions; for longer-stay patients medically super-vised hostels and residential homes have proved more successful. Close links are required with adult psychiatric and paediatric hospitals, with mental subnormality services, with children's and probation departments, and other social service agencies. Residential schools catering for emotionally disturbed children should have visiting children's psychiatrists. To the traditional nuclear team of psychiatric director, psychologist, and psychiatric social worker there is now being added the child psychiatric nurse, the child psychotherapist and the teacher specially trained to work with emotionally disturbed children.

The Nature and Size of the Problem

Classification of Psychiatric Disorders of Childhood and Adolescence

A classification of psychiatric disorders of childhood and adolescence must take account of the fact that we are concerned with a growing and developing individual, and also the need to see the 'patient's symptoms' in the context of family and community. A really satisfactory classification has not yet been achieved, although two separate bodies have recently attempted to do so (G.A.P., 1966; Rutter *et al.*, 1969). The essential categories are presented as follows:

Aspects of Normal Development. Many of the so-called emotional problems of young people brought for professional help prove, in retrospect, to be no more than transient or minor deviations from healthy development. Where personality is concerned it may be thought dangerous to use the term 'normal' as we may well ask 'What is normal?' What is accepted behaviour, for example, in one culture or social class may not be in another. This is why it is important that medical training should include some basic study in anthropology and sociology, as is envisaged in the recommendations of the Royal Commission on Medical Education (1968); most practising paediatricians have had to be self-educators in these fields. What is 'normal' can be judged, of course, only with reference to the accepted deviations from the mean, allowing for age and sex. Whereas the norms of psycho-motor

development are widely known, this is still by no means so of emotional development (see Chapter 10). Competence in the management of psycho-paediatric
problems calls not only for an intimate knowledge of the vicissitudes of development
throughout childhood and adolescence, but also for an understanding of the
emotional attitudes of adults in general, and parents in particular.

Stress reactions (Reactive Behaviour Disorders). This is a situation where the
child's behaviour is observed to be a reaction to environmental stress. This stress
may be persistent or episodic, and its alleviation produces an improvement, or
cure of symptoms. 'Stress' means different things at different ages. To the infant
this may be tense handling, grossly restricted nursing and fondling, or being
'battered'. For infants and toddlers separation from an adequate home is potentially
stressful. So is witnessing violence between the parents, an absentee or alcoholic
father, more than one 'mother' in competition or conflict. In the older child
'stress' may be due to unrealistic expectations from ambitious parents or teachers,
refusal to recognise the presence of a handicap, disappointment at the child's sex—
all of which may occur irrespective of social class. Mild forms of psycho-somatic
illness may be seen as stress reactions; others as psycho-neuroses; a few in association with personality disorders.

Incidence: very common; ubiquitous. Diagnosis often retrospective.

Psycho-neuroses and 'pre-neuroses'. The presenting symptoms may be
similar to those above, *e.g.* marked anxiety, persistent fears, rituals, aggressiveness,
passivity and so on, and environmental factors may be correctly identified, but their
modification, or the removal of the child from them, does not lead to improvement
or only temporarily so. The condition has become 'internalised', and psychotherapy
of some form is required.

Incidence: common. May call for observation for a time before diagnosis
emerges.

Personality disorders. A much more pervasive type of disturbance affecting
total personality, for example, the child's capacity to give and receive love (and
therefore to sustain friendships), to exert spontaneous control over his own
impulses, to work and learn in a sustained way in keeping with capacities. This
diagnosis is not usually made before 8 or 9 years though aetiological factors may have
begun to operate much earlier. Modification is always difficult and slow, sometimes
impossible, and measures may have to be limited to appropriate social and educational placement. Some delinquents belong here; a much smaller number are
symptomatic of psycho-neuroses; the majority are reactive behaviour disorders.
Diagnosis and management call for the expertise of a child psychiatric
team.

Incidence: high in association with social and cultural deprivation.

Developmental deviations. *Global*, i.e. Mental Handicap. Moderate grades
('dullness') are often idiopathic, and frequently environmental in origin, the result
of social deprivation. These children are also prone to develop reactive behaviour
disorders, psycho-neuroses, and especially personality disorders. Severe grades are
usually of organic aetiology.

Specific

Speech: dysphasia, etc.

Motor: hyperkinesis; 'clumsy child'.

Perceptual: dyslexia; visuo-motor.

Dysrhythmia, especially temporal lobe.

Investigation frequently calls for a comprehensive, multi-disciplinary, assessment team. Management is often both medical and educational, and calls for long-term supervision.

Childhood Psychoses. Markedly deviant behaviour and developmental patterns and modes of thinking and feeling often dating from the pre-school period. Early infantile autism (Kanner's syndrome) is a rare form. So also is the schizophrenic episode before puberty. Frequently psychotic and/or autistic features are seen in association with severe mental retardation.

The Causes of Psychiatric Disorder in Childhood and Adolescence

The above classification, however imperfect, may help the reader to appreciate the widely differing types of disorder under consideration, and thereby to avoid generalisations about aetiology, prognosis, or appropriate management. For convenience we may consider three causal dimensions, biological, psychological, and social.

BIOLOGICAL. This is the most clearly relevant to severe mental retardation and specific developmental disorders, and may be the result of genetic transmission, noxious factors in pregnancy, perinatal complications, or postnatal factors. In psycho-somatic disorders the role of biological factors is less obvious. Here as elsewhere the present view tends to be *dualistic, i.e.* that what we call 'disease' is the result of interaction of host and environment, a situation of complex variables. For example, it is now widely documented how often a psycho-somatic disorder starts in response to a stress situation; but that does not explain why one particular bodily system or organ is affected. Why one individual reacts with the skin, another with the bronchial tract, a third with the gastric mucosa may be explained in two quite different ways (*a*) an inherited, 'constitutional', probably genetically determined predisposition, or (*b*) a psychological conflict or personality problem related to a specific phase of early development, and with certain bodily associations.

In the childhood psychoses we can say no more at the present time than that biological factors are probably of major importance, possibly in creating the 'vulnerability' to environmental factors.

As regards the stress reactions, personality disorders and psychoneuroses, at first glance biological factors seem to play an insignificant role. Certainly social and psychological factors are paramount, but we should note the vulnerability of brain-damaged and mentally handicapped children to stress. This may mean only that these sections of the community which are 'at risk' as regards physical health and development are also the most deprived, culturally and socially.

Confronted with the individual child presenting a problem of behaviour, or attitude, or psycho-social development, we are more often than not dealing with *multifactorial causation.* This does *not* mean that all behaviour disorders of children are due to environmental factors, *e.g.* parental influences. Nor that these disorders are due entirely to inherited causes, or predispositions as yet undiscovered. We must take into account all these parameters—constitution, life experiences and present environment.

PSYCHOLOGICAL CAUSES. In Chapter 10 the emotional phases of development have been described, and attention drawn to the general agreement, irrespective of theoretical orientation, about the importance of childhood experiences on later character formation and emotional stability. The emphasis at the present time tends to be more on the quality of *continuing relationships* of the developing human being, than on the idea of a fortuitous, damaging 'happening' or *trauma*. In considering factors such as sensory deprivation, repeated or prolonged separation experiences, or exposure to inappropriate anxiety, account must be taken not only of their degree and duration, but also of the stage of the individual's development at which they occur. We are gradually mapping out *critical periods* in the human life cycle; time at which there appears to be heightened psychological vulnerability. Crucial to all the rest is the quality of relationships within the family, or extended family. Attempts are being made to delineate particular sets of circumstances (the one-parent or dominant parent family, divided child care, parental illness and so on) in the belief that later psychological disorders may be correlated with specific *family constellations*. Researches are aimed at identifying not only the noxious factors or circumstances, but also the strengthening or protective factors which allow development, despite all sorts of experience, to proceed to ordinary, healthy, well-adjusted adulthood.

SOCIAL CAUSES. This third category is clearly closely related to the other two, but is useful in describing factors in the wider field—not just individuals, or even families, but communities of families and individuals. It is hardly an original observation that in a generation with an increasingly high standard of living (though not for all), and when the physical health of the community, and of its children in particular is impressively good, emotional disorder becomes ever more a burden. Juvenile delinquency is a particular manifestation of social unease which has been considered separately in Chapter 23. It is a problem which appears to recognise no national or political frontiers, in spite of occasional propaganda statements to the contrary. Kellmer Pringle (1965) has succinctly categorised five groups of children 'at risk': (1) socially and culturally underprivileged children; (2) families where personal relationships suffer from some degree of impairment and where there is some emotional neglect; (3) families where there is a serious or irreversible physical or mental illness or a disabling handicap; (4) the child who has one parent only, be it because of illegitimacy, divorce, desertion, or death; (5) families affected by sudden and disruptive crises.

Prevalence of Childhood Emotional Disorder

The Underwood Report (1955) estimated that between 5 and 11 per cent of the chool population require psychiatric attention at some stage, and while recognising the variations in different regions, even the most conservative figure adds up to a formidable demand for expert help. In 1966, it is known that 57,000 school children in England and Wales attended child guidance clinics (Henderson, 1968). Waiting lists exist in many places indicating inadequacy of services and trained personnel. In particular, the dearth of provision for adolescents is indicated by the fact that less than 20 per cent of those attending clinics are from secondary schools. The number of children considered in need of psychiatric help depends on several factors, for example, the awareness and understanding of teachers and medical officers, their belief in and experience of the available facilities, and not least the capacity of school and child care personnel to tolerate deviant behaviour. Almost everywhere there are four times as many boys referred to clinics as girls, yet women outnumber men at adult psychiatric out-patient clinics, a trend which begins in the mid-teens. It is unlikely that there are relatively fewer schoolgirls with emotional problems than schoolboys, but probable that their symptoms present in less obvious, and less provocative forms, until adolescence.

Community Provision

The *Child Guidance Service* in the United Kingdom, as we have seen, is in the main administered by Education Authorities, and staffed primarily by Educational Psychologists whose professional background is usually that of teaching. The emphasis is on providing a *school psychological service*, with the full awareness that many of the learning and behaviour problems are of social and psychological origin. Of recent years use has progressively been made of social workers in tackling what are often family or community factors. This area of work will require to be co-ordinated with the new Social Work Departments which in Scotland (and probably in due course also in England and Wales) have replaced Children's Departments with a more comprehensive family-agency type of service. Another important area of Child Guidance work is in co-operating with the School Medical Service in the assessment of children with physical and mental handicaps, and making appropriate recommendations for special educational placement. It is widely recognised that the *quality and integration* of assessment, which frequently calls for the services of medical, surgical, audiometric, speech and other experts, leave much to be desired. Opportunities for the detection of difficulties at the nursery school level are increasingly presented, but have been taken by only a very few authorities. The main focus of work is, then, on the school population, and the helping methods employed are (1) assessment and appropriate placement; (2) remedial teaching; (3) counselling of parents; and (4) of older children; (5) psycho-therapy, mainly supportive; and (6) milieu therapy. This last, in which an environment is tuned to the needs of children with special problems of behaviour, learning, and personality, is provided by special *day and residential schools for maladjusted children*. Teachers and child care workers specialising in this field now have their own professional organisation (The Association for Workers with Maladjusted Children), and a start is being made to provide training and refresher courses. Child guidance services now widely recognise the need for skilled child psychiatric participation in many facets of their work.

The Hospital Service

A comprehensive child psychiatric service should provide (a) out-patient consultation and treatment facilities, and (b) in-patient resources for both urgent admissions and longer term observation and treatment, with some arrangements for admission of parents, especially mothers, along with the children when indicated. In centres of population these facilities may be augmented by (c) a day psychiatric hospital service (Stone, 1966). For pre-school and young children, child psychiatric services are best organised in relation to paediatric facilities, and every paediatric department or hospital should have child psychiatric resources. The Nuffield Provincial Hospital Trust has supported the establishment of new child psychiatric departments and centres. With the approaching imminent development of general-practice health-centres an important opportunity exists for building in as an integral part of the service offered, psychiatric consultation to families.

The majority of minor developmental problems and less severe stress reactions will require to be managed by family doctors, some by paediatricians, others by educational psychologists, and a great many by doctors working in child health clinics and nursery schools. During antenatal screening the detection in the expectant mother of negative or ambivalent attitudes towards the pregnancy, of inadequacy or of fear, and in the neonatal period of irrational anxiety or lack of interest in the handling of the infant—all of these present opportunities for preventive psychiatric intervention. The orientation of doctors towards community and family mental health clearly depends on appropriate emphasis on the behavioural sciences during undergraduate and postgraduate training.

INDEPENDENT AND VOLUNTARY AGENCIES have made a significant contribution in many countries. The residential, long-term care of children with (a) multiple handicaps and (b) severe disorders of personality development including psychotic disorders has been undertaken with skill and dedication by the Rudolf Steiner organisation. Barnardo's, traditionally concerned with the orphaned and the abandoned child, has begun to explore methods of providing for the emotionally disturbed child in both residential-home and boarding-school settings. Other organisations working along similar lines are the Save The Children Fund, and various Catholic orders. Short-term holiday homes for the mentally handicapped are provided by the National Association for Mental Health, and voluntary associations of Parents of Autistic Children have set in motion the establishment of schools and centres.

It is the traditional role of British voluntary effort to experiment in untried areas of communal need, and when the worth of a project is established, to exert constructive pressure on the appropriate authorities. We must be grateful that among many areas of endeavour, child and family mental health has not been ignored. At the same time it must be recorded that a great deal remains to be done in providing (1) hostels, homes and schools for mentally handicapped children, and especially (2) those with behavioural problems, and (3) with multiple handicaps; (4) facilities, day and residential, for psychotic and autistic children; (5) day centres for observation and treatment of pre-school children; and (6) facilities of all kinds, out-patient, day and residential for adolescent psychiatric patients.

But what is needed most of all is a comprehensive plan of development for hospital and community psychiatric services, including those for children and adolescents, with particular emphasis on co-ordination with the resources of the Health, Education, and Social Work departments.

The Role of the Paediatrician

The Child in Hospital

Some children, especially the under-fives and even older ones who are emotionally vulnerable, may develop disturbance as a result of admission to hospital, especially if repeated or prolonged. This is now a well established fact, and no longer a matter of controversy. Our present concern must be to minimise the potentially harmful accompaniments of hospitalisation.

Firstly, children should not be admitted to hospital if they can be effectively investigated and treated as out-patients. In the case of babies and toddlers all paediatric units should have facilities for the admission of mothers (or occasionally fathers), and where because of domestic or other reasons this is not possible, mother-substitute care should be undertaken by a member of the ward staff trained in this work. This is not simply a diversional or play programme, it is a child care function, and is essential for all age groups but especially the very young. It is quite fallacious to imagine that infants are too young to matter. Infants require gentle handling, nursing and 'conversation'; toddlers someone to know and trust, and allow to comfort; older children a confidant. In the absence of these human requirements, toys and decorated walls are an irrelevancy. Liberal arrangements for parent visiting are likewise essential but can be completely sabotaged if the senior medical or nursing staff, especially ward sisters, are not genuinely enthusiastic. It is devastating to nurses to have lectures on child development in which the dangers of sensory deprivation and separation experiences are stressed only to see these principles ignored or denigrated by their superiors on the job.

Many paediatric units now issue useful and attractive *booklets to parents** prior to the child's admission to hospital, stressing, for example, the need to explain truthfully and more than once to the child why admission is necessary; the danger of dishonest promises; the comfort from taking a favourite toy or possession to hospital, and so on. Credit must go to the Society for Welfare of Children in Hospital, a voluntary group of parents and others, for much constructive endeavour in this area.

Not nearly enough attention is paid to the *timing* of children's admission for

* *e.g.* those available from National Association for Mental Health, 39 Queen Anne Street, London. W.1.

'cold' procedures, such as elective surgery. For example where there is freedom of choice it should be possible to avoid admission coinciding with the arrival of a new baby in the family, or first attendance at school, or a recent bereavement. All that is needed is a brief preliminary enquiry to exclude inopportune timing of admission, but again this must be done by a sister, receptionist, or resident doctor who believes in the importance of such considerations. It remains a matter for concern that tonsillectomy continues to be performed in numbers that suggest a rite rather than a rational clinical procedure.

Where prolonged stay in hospital is unavoidable the caring arrangements, as advocated as long ago as 1947 by James Spence, should allow the children to live in small groups looked after by a housemother, with facilities for schooling, and a rich activities programme. The paediatrician should take a lively interest in the work of the ward teacher, nursery nurse or housemother, not only to maintain morale but to utilise clinically their observation on the abilities, interests, and behaviour of the children in their care. Evidence of cruelty and neglect often comes to light with a child's admission to hospital, not merely in the dramatic instances of the diagnosis of 'battered baby' syndrome, but, for example, where a child is not visited. In such instances the case-work skill of the medical social worker should be enlisted.

Where a hospital unit is situated in a centre of population opportunity presents for experimentation with paediatric day care, without the necessity of separation from home, and especially in the assessment of complex developmental problems.

The Handicapped Child

Recent discoveries in genetics, inborn metabolic errors, antenatal and postnatal infections, perinatal emergencies, and rhesus incompatibility have provided the paediatrician with exciting possibilities in the prevention of both physical and mental handicap. Developmental assessment, especially of infants and very young children, demands the co-ordinated skills of many different specialities, paediatric neurology, child psychiatry, clinical psychology, audiometry, genetics, biochemistry and so on. The fascination of all this new technical skill must not blind us to the absolute necessity of really effective co-ordination of services and the importance of re-sponding with equal skill and compassion to the human needs precipitated wherever handicap is diagnosed. To meet this challenge the paediatrician and the family doctor need psychiatric expertise in the management of adults as well as children; and must be familiar with the range of parental behaviour in response to grief. Apathy, depression, rage, denial, may appear as quite irrational attitudes towards the professional helper and call for skilful management. The mistaken belief still widely persists that such skills are nothing more than a blend of common humanity and common sense. In fact the effective use of empathy, support, and counselling is a clinical skill, which is not the esoteric prerogative of the psychiatrist or case worker, but given reasonable aptitude may be taught and learned. At no stage is this skill more needed than in conveying to parents the fact that a newborn child is abnormal, a task which is rightfully that of the paediatrician. This is, of course, only the first stage of continuing responsibility to the child and his family.

Psycho-social Paediatrics

The potential role of the paediatrician in this field is limitless, and this realisation is reflected in the development of what has been called 'the new paediatrics', that is the social and psychological aspect of children's medicine. Milton Senn in the United States (Solnit and Provence, 1963), and Winnicott (1958) in Britain have dedicated themselves to this theme, in its therapeutic, preventive and educational aspects. The skills which are called for in the management of the handicapped child are equally pertinent to the care of the long-term patient. Diabetes, haemophilia and heart disease, for example, all pose complex problems, and opportunities for support and guidance of child and parents. Likewise in the treatment of congenital abnormalities, extensive burns, and prolonged orthopaedic procedures, there are important considerations beyond surgical expertise. As yet, there are very few follow-up studies in any of these conditions which take account of personality development and family reactions. The care of the dying child and his family has been the subject of several studies, but the findings have yet to make a significant impact. Advances in metabolic and endocrine knowledge bring with them enormous problems, *e.g.* in relation to renal transplant and inter-sex. The opportunities for closely integrated effort between the paediatrician and child psychiatrist are manifest, and call for a fresh look at the education and training of both.

Present and Future

It is clear that the psychiatry of childhood and adolescence calls for a wide range of expertise, in psychiatry, paediatrics, developmental neurology, and psychology, and has close links with education, social work, and the law. It is equally clear that clinical facilities, however well placed, can provide only a partial solution to the problem of emotional ill-health in the young. *Prevention* must therefore be our goal, but as we have seen from the account of classification and aetiology, this must be tackled on a wide front encompassing biological, educational, and sociological fields.

In a valuable report to the World Federation for Mental Health, a study group (Gould, 1968) has recently estimated that at any one time in the United Kingdom about 10 per cent of the child population under 15 years of age are 'at risk' as regards emotional development. This means that of about a million 'at risk' children there is a hazard of (1) later emotional ill-health (2) delinquency, and (3) failure to realise innate potential in education, work, and social capacity, rightly stressed as the greatest loss to society. Caplan (1961) envisages a massive public health programme at three inter-related levels of community action. (1) *Tertiary Prevention*—the amelioration of established emotional disorder and prevention of complications. This is an integral part of clinical service. (2) *Secondary Prevention* aims at reducing the duration of mental illness by early diagnosis and treatment.

This is likewise the aim of any clinical service, but calls also for imaginative programmes of early detection as part of routine health inspections of school children and attenders at infant and nursery schools, child health centres, and even antenatal clinics. Physicians will require to be assisted in mental health screening of this kind by nurses, teachers, and welfare workers, and this means ensuring that the training curricula of these professions are geared to this end. (3) *Primary Prevention*—the promotion of mental health by the modification of pathogenic forces, biological, psychological and social. This encompasses a wide range of endeavour including genetic counselling, antenatal chromosome studies of 'at risk' pregnancies, intensive perinatal care, and effective management of paediatric emergencies likely to affect the central nervous system; marriage education programmes, skilled psychological counselling for young parents, expert screening of prospective foster-parents and adopters, recognition of 'at risk' families and effective supportive intervention at times of crisis.

Inseparable from programmes of community mental health is the need for more effective research, especially prospective developmental studies, and epidemiological surveys across communities and between the generations. The interdisciplinary team is likely to be as essential for mental health research as it has proved for clinical practice.

FREDERICK H. STONE

References

BURLINGHAM, D. and FREUD, A. (1954). *Infants without Families : the Case for and against Residential Nurseries*. London: Allen & Unwin.

CAMERON, H. (1946). *The Nervous Child*. London: Oxf. Univ. Press.

CAPLAN, G. (1961). *Prevention of Mental Disorders in Children*. London: Tavistock.

CRAIG, W. S. (1968). *John Thomson. Pioneer and Father of Scottish Paediatrics*. Edinburgh: Livingstone.

GOULD, J. (Ed.) (1968). *The Prevention of Damaging Stress in Children*. Church.

GROUP FOR THE ADVANCEMENT OF PSYCHIATRY, VI, 62 (1966). *Psychopathological Disorders in Childhood : Theoretical Considerations and a Proposed Classification*. New York.

HENDERSON, P. (1968). Changing pattern of disease and disability in schoolchildren in England and Wales. *Brit. med. J.*, 2, 259.

JONES, E. (1955). *Life and Work of Sigmund Freud*, Vol. II. London: Chatto and Windus.

KELLMER PRINGLE, M. L. (Ed.) (1965). *Investment in Children*. London: Longmans.

Report of the Committee on Maladjusted Children to the Minister of Education, (1955). London: H.M.S.O.

Report of Royal Commission on Medical Education (1968). London: H.M.S.O.

RUTTER, M. *et al.* (1969). A tri-axial classification of mental disorders in childhood. An international study, *J. Child Psychol. Psychiat.*, 10, 41.

SOLNIT, A. J. and PROVENCE, S. A. (1963). *Modern Perspectives in Child Development*. New York: International Univ. Press.

SPENCE, J. C. (1947). The care of children in hospital. *Brit. med. J.*, 1, 125.

STONE, F. H. (1966). The day care approach to emotionally disturbed children. In *Emotionally Disturbed Children*. Ed. S. M. Maxwell. Oxford: Pergamon.

WINNICOTT, D. W. (1958). *Collected Papers. Through Paediatrics to Psycho-Analysis*. London: Tavistock.

21   Health Education

The Scope of Health Education in the Promotion of Child Health

PREVENTIVE medicine and child health are indivisible and the practice of the prevention of disease and the promotion of health is seen at its optimum as applied to the age group 0–15. The development of modern paediatrics from being merely a branch of clinical medicine has made possible a public health policy which, so far, has hardly been applicable to other age groups. The improvements in the level of child health during this century have been due, not only to the control of the dangerous infectious diseases and general medical advances, but also to a raised standard of parentcraft. Charles (1953), writing as Chief Medical Officer to the Ministry of Health, stated that 'From its earliest inception the Maternal and Child Welfare Service has been educational and preventive in character . . . now the wider sphere of family health must become the concern of Medical Officers of Health, Health Visitors, and Midwives'. The same author, later (1956), reaffirmed that health education had always been the principal task of Infant Welfare Centres (now called Child Health Centres). The Cohen Committee on Health Education (1964) stated in their report that, from the evidence they had received, they were convinced that priority (in health education) must continue to be given to the education of mothers. To quote (paragraph 115 of the Report):

> 'It almost goes without saying that a healthy mother, aware of the measures required to feed an infant, to bring him into a happy home, to know if he is making normal progress and to protect him from infection, is able to give her child health which might well be denied to the children of mothers ignorant of the lessons provided by health education'.

Public health policies during the second half of the twentieth century continue to assign priorities to the needs of mothers and children and this is due to a variety of social and economic trends. The high value placed by most communities on child life owes something both to economic and psychological factors. In Britain, the child has never been so highly valued as he is today but this was not always so, as the social history of the nineteenth century reveals. Early health education may be said to have begun with the work of the sanitary pioneers—*e.g.* Chadwick, Southwood-Smith and others—who drew attention to the insanitary conditions in towns and the effect of these on mothers and children. In those days, the target of health education was the legislators and the influential who had it in their power to change conditions.

The sanitary reforms of the earlier part of the nineteenth century were followed by the setting up of special medical services to cater for mothers and children at the end of the century (see Chapter 14). By then, the vulnerability of these groups was accepted and, as pointed out above, health education was an integral part of the work of the doctors, nurses, and social workers, who staffed these services—first on a voluntary basis and later, as officials of local authorities. The Interdepartmental Committee on Physical Deterioration (1904) stated, in its Report, that there was scope for the prevention of illness and the promotion of physical and mental development in school children, and health education—although not named as such—was included in their recommendations.

These advances in public health policy were initiated at a time when children were the cause of poverty among large sections of the population in Western Europe. Now, only in under-developed communities are children still the cause of poverty. In some communities, children are still regarded as an investment for the country's economic future, apart from their value to parents in old age, and an economic motive for the preservation of child life is strong and influences governmental action. In the Western European type of civilisation and in the United States, children have acquired a value of their own and a considerable slice of the GNP is devoted to their well-being. This creates intense interest in education for parentcraft.

The work of the World Health Organisation during the last twenty years is also an important factor. Maternal and Child Health programmes enjoy high priority and it is significant that health education has been an integral part of the programme of the Organisation since its inception. All maternal and child health programmes have a health education component and, in many instances, health education teams are in the field in advance of medical and nursing teams.

The World Health Organisation has done much to promote health education in all parts of the world and it is fair to say that, even in Britain, methods and techniques now in use owe much to the experience and researches of W.H.O. health educators working in less developed paart of the world. Nine main areas of health education are recognised, applicable to the total field of public health, and first priority is given to 'The Quality of Child Care'. Amplified, this includes hygiene, immunisation, nutrition, education of the school child in human biology, and improvement of the doctor/patient relationship. The latter is not so remote from the problem of parentcraft teaching because an intelligent dialogue between parent and medical adviser is vital if advice is to be understood and followed.

Emphasis is necessarily placed on the education of the mother. In this country the study by Spence et al. (1954) on 'A Thousand Families. . . .' called forth the general comment from the research team that the single dominating factor that emerged from their survey was the quality of the maternal capacity which they claimed could compensate for poor conditions, including an indifferent or even vicious father. While accepting this, it is necessary to point out that the modern trend is to involve fathers in parentcraft teaching or, at least, to encourage them to support their wives by taking an intelligent interest in the subject.

In general, then, it may be claimed that health education has developed largely as a result of contemporary interests in child health. There are practical, as well as historical, reasons. After school children, the mothers with young children are a relatively 'captive' audience in the sense that they are dependent upon personal services rendered by doctors and health visitors who accept health education as one of their activities. In Britain, the establishment of clinical preventive services for mothers and children, from which therapeutic tasks are specifically excluded, has created a professional working environment in which health education has been positively encouraged. This was an important point mentioned by several writers during the controversy over the future of the Infant Welfare Centre (Dalzell–Ward, 1955: Reid and Reid, 1954). Reid and Reid, in a study of medical consultations held at a welfare clinic (1954), listed the questions asked by mothers seeking reassurance and commented that many of the questions asked concerned subjects which might never have arisen if the mothers had been fully instructed in various elementary matters at an early stage. To quote:

> 'It is less time-consuming to write a prescription than to deliver a lecturette but the latter, at least in the field of child welfare, is usually the more valuable'.

Modern health education also owes much to the development of the social sciences which have provided a new diagnostic tool to the study of epidemiology. It is now widely recognised that knowledge without change of behaviour has no impact on health at all. There is, naturally, an increasing preoccupation by modern health educators with studies of behaviour patterns and with the exploration of possible methods of influencing behaviour. It must be remembered, however, that health education has an even greater potential and that purely pragmatic reasons should not be allowed to prevent activities which can aim at a general improvement of the level of enlightenment of the people. This was the aim of early health educators who were, perhaps, somewhat naïve in their outlook and who lacked the skills to communicate in meaningful terms and did not discriminate in the groups to whom they communicated. The fact that they communicated mainly with people like themselves should not be cited as evidence that attempts at general public enlightenment are not worth-while. Broadly, health education—like general education—can be looked upon as a factor in social evolution and although we are unlikely—and, indeed, genetic principles forbid it—to reach the stage where generations are born with ready-made knowledge we can, at least, ensure that the future generations are born to parents who are possessed of a basic knowledge of human biology and ecology and who have been allowed to develop powers of deduction which they can then use to place this knowledge to good effect.

Specific Examples of the Value of Health Education in the Promotion of Health in Childhood

In preventive medicine there are three main aims. The highest ideal, of course, is the promotion of health but, unfortunately, too little is known about the nature of health at the present day to lay down any reasonable criteria. Schwarz (1969.)

sets out a statistical method of deciding priorities in health education showing that mortality and morbidity figures will highlight different sets of priorities. He concludes that the pattern of morbidity and mortality is the basis of any health education programme but that regional differences must be taken into account. There is also a distinction between the short term and long term programmes—the short term programme acting as a booster to reinforce the effects of the long term programme.

The study undertaken by the Kent Paediatric Society (1954), entitled 'The Epidemiology of Health'—a theme which was suggested by the late Professor John Ryle, then President of the Society—showed that although it was possible to identify 50 school children aged 11 to 12 out of a population of 1,200 school children of that age who, by all the criteria of absence of disease with, in addition, the presence of positive factors of personality and physical stamina, enjoyed perfect health, it was not so easy to detect associations between the standard of health and environmental, genetic and parental factors which were of any significance. In fact, of some 350 items in a questionnaire, statistical significance was found in about a dozen.

This study, therefore, went some length to be able to diagnose health—a novel activity for doctors—but took us very little further on methods of discovering the causes of health. However, as in the case of the 'Thousand Families' study, general non-specific and overall 'lowest-common-multiples' of health were detectable; for example the quality of home life—and this was independent of income; the attitudes of parents; the collective ambitions of the family and particularly the degree of family integration, were significant and on a statistical basis. It was also important that in this investigation positive values on the psychological, emotional, and intellectual side were of much more importance than positive values on the physical side. The unity, therefore, of body and mind and spirit, so often mentioned by people in idealistic terms, could be observed reasonably objectively in this investigation. It was the selection of the right priorities by the parents of these very healthy children that was important rather than the level of economic achievement. It was significant that the majority of these children had passed tests to receive grammar school education.

The results of this investigation support a policy of a greatly enlarged parentcraft education, taking in psychological and social factors, as well as the basic skills of general care and maintenance, promotion of nutrition and education, and protection from common danger which—up to the present—have formed the standard content of a parentcraft syllabus. However, there are two other aims of preventive medicine—namely, to prevent the incidence of illness and to detect early signs of departure from the normal and to apply some kind of corrective or remedial action. So far, evaluation of health education has been confined to these two aims.

Charlotte Naish (1954) was one of the first to assess the effects of health education, which she carried on in her own practice. The evaluation of a four-year programme of health education in the city of Aberdeen, published by MacQueen (1960), is the most ambitious study of its kind in this country.

Aims and Methods of Health Education

The World Health Organisation (1954) has defined three main aims of health education which are intended to apply to every community in the world and to all problems of public health which can be tackled by health education methods. The aims are (i) to ensure that the community looks upon health as a valued asset; (ii) to equip individuals with knowledge and skills, and to influence their attitude so that they can solve their own health problems; (iii) to promote the development of health services.

When these aims are applied to the problems of child health, it is seen that they are sufficiently wide to allow their application either in developing countries with fundamental problems of defective sanitation and meagre nutritional resources or in the highly sophisticated countries of Western Europe. The first aim of health education, to influence the community in its attitude to health, probably has been achieved when one considers the health of children, the high value placed on child health, the psychological appeal of the sick child, and the willingness of the community to invest resources in services that protect the health of children. The great interest shown in all matters concerning children is reflected in the newsworthiness of any incidents that are reported relating to children's life and wellbeing, and the column inches of press or the time devoted on television to these topics. It may be necessary, however, to influence the community in matters of detail regarding the well-being of children. It is unfortunate, for example, that an argument which is advanced against the fluoridation of water supplies suggests—erroneously—that fluoridation would benefit only children and would therefore be an extravagant measure.

Included in the second aim are such matters as personal hygiene, knowledge of nutrition, the advisability of a balance between rest and activity, basic knowledge about child development—physical, emotional and intellectual—and knowledge regarding environmental factors most likely to be favourable to the full development of the children and to the promotion of their health. Today a wide range of skills is needed in order to be effective as a parent. Some of these cannot be learned didactically—for example, the capacity to react appropriately in a family crisis, or to take appropriate action when an accident occurs in the home. Emotional crises, such as occur during the course of child education and school life, also call for skills in handling which are now recognised as coming within the ambit of education for family life. There is an increasing number of health problems which can be solved by individuals, as well as an increasing number of situations where a choice has to be made which is entirely the parents' own. The most straightforward instance of this is the case of immunisation. Immunisation against diphtheria was technically possible as early as 1921 but did not become a widespread public health measure until 1940, when it was launched by a broadcast by the then Chief Medical Officer of the Ministry of Health.

Since that time there has been a continuous public campaign on behalf of immunisation carried on by the mass media of all kinds and reinforced by the of health at the present day to lay down any reasonable criteria. Schwarz (1969) work of health visitors and individual doctors. Thus when new prophylactic measures were developed—against whooping cough, tuberculosis, poliomyelitis and, most recently, measles—there was a well-organised system of health education which already had established rapport with the public who, in turn, had been led to expect developments in immunisation. Nevertheless, in order to maintain the level of immunity necessary in the community, to prevent the return of such diseases, it is necessary to continue to urge parents to have their children immunised. It is not possible to foresee a time when health education to promote immunisation will not be necessary. As immunisation is not compulsory in Britain, it has been necessary to explain the general principles of artificial immunity and to create a feeling of confidence in the effectiveness of the measures offered, so that the campaign has been concerned with education as much as with propaganda.

The third aim of health education—to promote the health services—might seem at first-hand to apply only the developing countries. In Britain, it can be interpreted to mean the sensible and economical use of the health services by the public. The public's expectations of the different branches of the health service are still vague and there is often a considerable gap between their expectations and reality. It is probably fair to say that there is greater understanding, relatively, of the proper use of the preventive clinical services provided by local health authorities for mothers and children than there is of the general practitioner services. Surveys done on the use of child health centres appear to indicate that most mothers are fully aware of the valuable advice that can be obtained there and they do not go purely for the purchase of welfare foods. Closely allied to the proper use of health services is the question of the doctor/patient relationship, and it is understandable that W.H.O. included this in one of the nine areas of health education.

The methods used in health education can be classified into individual, group, and mass. Individual health education may, virtually, be health counselling and it is not entirely pedantic to distinguish between the two. Individual health education invariably arises from a clinical or problem situation, and the advice given is that appropriate to the individual circumstances and is not based entirely on generalisations. Group and mass health education is usually aimed at people who are symptom-free or not involved in problems at the moment, and will be based upon broad generalisations which apply to groups and communities rather than to individuals. For some years now, the kind of advice offered in group and mass health education has been based upon epidemiological information. Perhaps the most obvious situation where there might be a difference in the approach to the individual, as compared with the group, is in the field of nutrition. Modern health education aims at guiding people to a wise choice within the wide range generally available to them. In an individual case the choice may have to be made in the light of special circumstances, so that it is as important to stimulate powers of deduction as to inform.

What Kind of Information and at What Level?

A modern parent, in order to be fully effective, needs to have some ideas of the following areas of knowledge. Child development—physical, intellectual and emotional—the early detection of illness and the recognition of signs where medical or other professional help is required, nutrition, personal hygiene with an emphasis on teaching the child to care for himself, infectious diseases and the methods of prevention by immunisation. Environmental factors which are likely to affect the child's health also require understanding. Included in these are the need for cleanliness and good order in the home, the prevention of domestic accidents, enough knowledge of first-aid to enable them to arrest bleeding or to restore the air-way, and the importance of making space available for safe play. This may be summed up as general care and maintenance of the child and protection against common dangers and this suffices for the early years.

Ideally, however, we should start to train parents consciously to be health educators for their own children, and the kind of information they require should include that which can be passed on to the child as well. A good deal of what was called health education, 30 years ago, was virtually the inculcation of good personal standards. These the child should learn in his own home, although they may need to be reinforced in the early years of school. Parents must also have an idea of their child's social needs in respect of play with companions, experience of domestic activity, and experience of as many varied environments as possible—for example, on family holidays or visits to relatives. The significance of ordinary daily activities of living in the promotion of the child's normal development must be emphasised. The modern concept of parentcraft, however, goes far beyond this and parents also need to have an idea of their child's educational needs and to be able to co-operate with the schools. They should be prepared well ahead for the changes of adolescence and this involves not only an understanding of physical changes but also emotional changes and inter-relationship between parents and children in the family. So called 'sex education' should be given throughout the child's life as soon as the child begins to ask questions. Even before the child is capable of verbal communication, the mother should be helped to accept the normal sexuality in her infant as it is expressed in various ways.

At the present day, we possess a wide range of scientific information that we can employ as the content of health education for parents and children. The subject is, in fact, becoming less and less empirical as advances in epidemiology, and in the social and psychological sciences, give us more precise information on which we can predict various patterns of human behaviour and their effect upon health. Health education has fully to accept the fact that physical and mental health are indivisible and, indeed, the frequency of psychosomatic disorders in children makes it all the more important that parents should understand this. As we may assume that the majority of children are born without defect, and are endowed with the normal potential for physical and intellectual development, the major part of education for parenthood is concerned with securing an awareness of normality, a tolerance of temporary departures from normality within the usual limits and a recognition of the general principle that if the child's social and physical environment is optimum then normal development is inevitable.

It is important to avoid reliance upon unrealistic norms. Attention to this was drawn by a joint committee of the L.C.C. and the Tavistock Institute (1954). The anxiety created in mothers by the fact that their children do not weigh precisely the same amount as others, or that teeth do not appear at the right time or some other novel development occurs, is communicated to the child and can harm both of them. It is necessary to be realistic, however, in that all children will suffer from some minor illness and that the parent is the first person to make a diagnosis. This is not a diagnosis in the pathological sense, but rather a diagnosis in which the mother acts as to whether to care for the child herself, to let the incident pass, or to seek professional help. In this context the sub-clinical syndrome of 'failure-to-thrive' becomes the most sensitive index of the small child's health. For the sake of the mental health of the child and his parents, it is essential to avoid inculcating the continual fussiness which is shown by repeatedly checking the child's progress, taking his temperature and the like. Thriving and *not* thriving are the indices whereby the mother can gauge the level of health of her child. It is the task of the health educator to find ways of best communicating this idea to parents.

Parenthood provides an excellent learning situation in which ideas of human biology can be acquired which will have a general benefit to the community at large. Teaching of systematic anatomy and physiology is not desirable, even if it were possible, in the short time available for parentcraft activities. Nevertheless, there are some situations in which a simple idea of anatomy and physiology will help to understand problems which arise and ways in which they can be tackled. This was recognised, years ago, by Grantley Dick Read in his scheme for psycho-prophylaxis of childbirth, in which the simple idea of the anatomy of the gravid uterus and its mechanics during labour is taught to expectant mothers. There is circumstantial evidence that cervical rigidity, causing delay of labour, is less likely to occur in mothers who have some idea of physiology. A knowledge of this kind is also valuable in managing breast feeding successfully.

In the care of a young child there are several situations in which some idea of anatomy and physiology is helpful—in toilet training, for example, a situation which is fraught with dangers to the child's emotional development. Some aware-ness of the way in which voluntary control develops, and the role of the central nervous system in this, will help an intelligent mother to understand that voluntary control cannot be forced upon the child before development is ready for it. As a child is so prone to upper respiratory tract infection, some idea of the anatomy of the nasopharynx and middle-ear cleft is also helpful (Dalzell–Ward, 1962). Similarly, an idea of the bronchial tree and the way in which it drains its secretions is generally helpful, and not only in cases where early bronchiectasis has already developed.

Information of this kind should not be communicated in a systematic way but should be integrated with the general topic of child development and related to practical problems that may arise. A fully comprehensive course in parentcraft should incude a session on the detection of early illness and nursing of a sick child, and it is in this context that some of these anatomical and physiological principles can be included. The level of communication will be appropriate to the group and this is where educational skills are needed, both in the choice of language and in the expression of ideas which will be meaningful to the group, and also in the use of the visual aids which are indispensable.

Up to the present, few doctors have had any training in this work although a few have a natural aptitude for it and have taken advantage of increased opportunities, such as the In-Service Training Programmes which have been provided by The Central Council for Health Education during the last 20 years. Only one textbook of clinical medicine—that of Gardiner–Hill (1958)—has included guidance on rapport between doctor and patient as the background to the interpretations of clinical signs and symptoms. There are signs, however, that official opinion concerning medical education is changing, and the Report of the Royal Commission on Medical Education (1968) refers to the training of doctors in teaching methods. Health Visitors have been much better favoured in this direction as health education has been included in their basic training, and on the whole they have taken much greater advantage of the In-Service Training programmes available (Hale *et al.*, 1968).

Stages in Health Education for Child Care

In British practice the antenatal period has become a traditional one for health education activities. With increasing interest in the emotions of an expectant mother and her husband, and in the importance of these to the emotional development of their child, the content of health education in this period has gone a long way beyond the hygiene management of pregnancy, nutrition, diet, clothing, exercise, etc., and preparation for labour. A comprehensive programme of health education for the antenatal period indeed requires a team of experts. The Royal College of Midwives (1966) conducted a survey into provisions for antenatal health education, which included a study of the felt needs of expectant mothers and their husbands.

The research was carried out in two parts—the first being conducted by means of a questionnaire circulated to all maternity hospitals and units and all Local Health Authorities in England and Wales, and the second part by means of a national field survey including a number of group discussions with expectant mothers, and mothers of first babies booked for hospital delivery.

The report recognised the importance of education in preparing young people for marriage and parenthood but concluded that there was a need for considerable extension of this teaching in school. It was recommended that such education should not take the form of isolated classes in 'sex education' or 'mothercraft' but should be part of education, as a whole, and could be usefully introduced from the age of 11 onwards.

It was found that many women approached the idea of starting a family with anxiety—on account of the birth itself, about the child's forming a barrier in relationship with the husband, about producing an abnormal child—and they were often aware of their inadequacy as parents. The report recommended that whilst the normality of child-bearing should be emphasised there should be more general acceptance that such fears were both natural and widespread.

The investigation found that only just over half the women in the sample had had any teaching about sex or the birth and growth of a baby, that antenatal classes fulfil an important function in this respect, and that there is a need to advertise these classes more widely. Many of the classes referred to in the survey had been started too late in pregnancy. Diffidence on the part of many fathers could be dispelled by creating a growing awareness, through public media, of the degree to which a modern father is prepared to involve himself in his wife's pregnancy.

When confinement takes place in hospital, informal postnatal discussion groups should be arranged for mothers before they leave hospital. At these classes, practical instruction in caring for the baby at home should be given. It is significant that the field survey showed that nearly all the mothers who attended antenatal classes appreciated the knowledge that was acquired, and gained confidence in their ability—not only to cope with labour but also with the care of the baby. The practice of husbands attending antenatal classes with their wives during the first pregnancy is on the increase and this is closely related to the practice of husbands being present during labour. During the antenatal period, too, opportunities are taken for an explanation of the process of lactation and the practice of breast feeding—a subject which requires some discussion between husbands and wives—and also the general care and maintenance of the newborn infant—*i.e.* hygiene, clothes, protection against common danger, etc.

Some health educators have also wished to include mental health concepts at this time, and to give the future parents some guidance as to the emotional needs of their child. The psychoprophylaxis of childbirth has become increasingly popular in recent years, forms the interest of at least one professional association and one national voluntary body, and is necessarily an important part of antenatal health education. It must be recognised, however, that it is only a part, and the possible 6 months available during pregnancy for health education will prove to be all too short unless some balance is maintained in the content of the health education programme.

From Birth to the Age of Five Years

It is in the Child Health Centre that we find health education most highly developed in Britain (see p. 343). In an increasing number of local health authorities, the idea of the Mothers' Club (later Parents' Club) has been added to the activities of the Centre. In this way, true community participation has been ensured and the programmes of some of these Parents' Clubs are very ambitious, including the carrying out of practical projects such as the organisation of exhibitions on the subject of child welfare. Where health centres, under the National Health Service Act, have been developed, provision is made in the plans for meeting rooms and for the necessary audio-visual equipment for the carrying out of sophisticated health education programmes. It is the health visitors who are responsible for this, although they will frequently ask for the assistance of their colleagues amongst the medical officers in charge of the centre, or public health inspectors, or social workers. The health education programme at such centres includes the conventional subjects of nutrition, immunisation, dental health, clothing, and the prevention of accidents, but there is an increasing interest in behavioural problems, discipline, and in the general study of child development from a practical point of view. For example, sessions on children's play will be conducted, mainly by group discussion, so that groups of mothers can come to terms with their own attitudes towards children's play and their particular role. Problems involved in sibling relationships, preparation of children for the arrival of a new baby, the encouragement of social activities for small children—including the problems involved in friendships with children in other families—are all dealt with—mainly by group discussion—at Child Health Centres.

Mothers who take advantage of these health education activities have been found to gain in self confidence and in powers of verbal expression. By emphasis on modern methods of education, which involve participation by the group, responsibility for learning and for communication is increasingly placed upon the mother herself. The skill of the health visitor, as health educator, is becoming more and more that of an expert who creates the *environment* for learning. The learning environment in the Child Health Centre includes a large range of audio-visual aids, exhibition material and literature. Radio and television programmes can occasionally be used as topics for discussion and the invitation to personalities—local or even sometimes national—enables the outside world to make an appearance in the Centre and to refresh and re-inforce the learning situation.

HOME SAFETY is an important topic (see also p. 351). What was formerly determined by commonsense and empiricism is now illuminated by epidemiological information. The prevention of domestic accidents is a subject which is now being studied on an international plane. The establishment of a special section in the European Regional Office of the World Health Organisation on accident prevention emphasises this (W.H.O. 1957). In Britain, the setting up of the Medical Commission on Accident Prevention, under the presidency of H.R.H. The Duke of Edinburgh, offers a further encouraging stimulus for education in safety and also provides a new power house for research and ideas.

The British Medical Association (1964) surveyed non-fatal domestic accidents and showed that, of every 100 reported domestic accidents, one quarter occurred in children under 5 and nearly one sixth in school-children. Burns and scalds occurred chiefly in children under 5. Similarly, the victims of poisoning accidents were young children who had swallowed 'a variety of pills and unpalatable potions'— the latter included cleaning fluids and paint solvents. This report recommended that the first principles of home safety should be taught in the early years at school.

The hazards to children in the home are related to burning, scalding, electrocution, accidental poisoning and injuries incurred during play. Epidemiological studies, such as that of Backett (1965), have shown that it is possible to identify 'host' and environmental characteristics leading to preventive measures. The kitchen can be a particularly dangerous place but this must not be allowed to interfere with the child's acquiring domestic experience, which is now believed to be so important in his social development. The danger points in the kitchen are the cooking stoves, with handles of saucepans so handy for the child to reach, the general-purpose cupboard which may contain large quantities of medicinal tablets and corrosive fluid stored in inappropriately labelled bottles, and the various knives and other sharp cutting tools used in the preparation of food. All these objects can be used in perfect safety, or at least with the minimum of risk, provided parents have an awareness of the hazard and are prepared to take a little extra trouble to minimise it.

The practical measures involved are usually putting things out of the reach of small children, but the educational value of this can be enhanced if parents also continually train children in safe ways of using domestic equipment. It is truly said that no education should be negative and safety education should aim at producing and maintaining a high standard of skill. One of the hazards in the kitchen is the fact that so many tasks are performed apart from cooking, for example washing and ironing or even the mending of household equipment. It should be the father's responsibility to ensure that all electrical equipment used is safe, particularly wall plugs, and that no unearthed equipment is ever employed. 'Do It Yourself' enthusiasts should be restrained when it comes to highly skilled operations, such as the repair of electric switches or other fittings. No sense of pride should prevent people sending for the skilled engineer from the Electricity or Gas Board to deal with faults.

There are other domestic situations which are particularly dangerous to small children. Burns tend to occur at bedtime when the child is being undressed in front of some kind of fire. The universal introduction of flame-proof fabrics and the use of pyjamas, rather than nightdresses, for very small girls, will undoubtedly materially reduce the incidence of fatal or serious burns in the home. Fire-guards are obligatory under an Act of Parliament wherever children under the age of 7 are present in the home. Occasional National Safety Weeks have been shown to cause a great increase in the provision of fire-guards. Children's toys should not be placed so that children will reach over a fire or a heater in order to touch them. Because of the high cost of other forms of heating, paraffin heaters are very popular and particularly so with immigrant populations who may be forced to live in overcrowded conditions. Every winter, disastrous fires are reported as a result of the unwise use of these heaters which is not due, as a rule, to faulty design but to a failure of the owners to read the instructions and to comply with them.

The Royal Society for the Prevention of Accidents devotes a good deal of time to the prevention of domestic accidents and issues leaflets, posters and other material for use by local authorities and local Home Safety Committees. Medical

Officers of Health carry out surveys in their areas of domestic hazards, and organise educational campaigns. Children also need education on road safety, and one of the great tragedies is the toll of life of small children who have just entered school and who are obliged, either because their parents are unwilling or unable to accompany them to school, to 'go it alone'. Training in kerb drill is popularised by television 'fillers' produced by the Central Office of Information.

Health Education in General Practice

There is obviously a great potential for health education in general practice and this will be realised, eventually, with greater integration of the health services. The attachment of health visitors to general practices is the first step and in one practice the health visitor spends 10 per cent of her 'surgery' time in health education tasks (Fry *et al.*, 1965).

Group health education has been organised by individual family doctors and the most interesting, from the point of view of child health, is that described by Hasler (1968). In this case, the partners in the practice enlisted the co-operation of a health education officer, health visitor, midwife, and a speaker from a commercial agency to provide systematic health education in child care.

Special problems are involved in the case of immigrant families. On the one hand, there is the need to give information regarding the medico-social services available in support of the family and, on the other hand, there is a need for health education to cope with hazards to health over and above those which affect all families. In cities, in which there are large immigrant populations, welfare officers who come from the same countries as the immigrants, co-operate with the health authorities in this work. Some local health authorities have produced special leaflets printed in the languages spoken by the various immigrant groups. Great differences in customs, beliefs and attitudes to health, and the need for extreme tact, produce problems of a special character in this type of health education.

The Child at School—Preparation for Life

The position regarding health education in British schools is difficult to understand unless one is familiar with the various Education Acts which, together, mark out the historical progress of State education in this country. The freedom allowed to individual schools to decide their own curriculum is a traditional feature of British education. The Department of Education and Science advises, encourages, and inspects, but does not dictate. There is, therefore, no question of health education being imposed on any school by the Central Department, but the latter—from the days of the Board of Education—has always encouraged this activity.

Health education was first recommended by the Interdepartmental Committee on Physical Deterioration (1904) and it is closely identified with the School Health Service, which also owes its beginnings to the work of that Committee (p. 322). Official opinion is against the appearance of health education as a separate subject in the school curriculum and, although some advance has been made towards the establishment of formal curricula and even the appointment of health education specialist teachers in some secondary schools, the general picture in this country is of 'incidental' health education in which all subjects on the curriculum play their part.

Students in Colleges of Education receive special instruction in health education, however, and most colleges employ specialist lecturers in the subject. The content of the course in health education for student teachers includes the basic facts regarding the health of school children, the illnesses to which they are subject, and the preventive measures undertaken by the School Health Service in the interests of their welfare. The original aim of the course for student teachers was, to use the traditional phrase, to 'help them in the classroom'. Formerly, there was an emphasis upon the physical, sensory, and mental handicaps which might be detected by the school teacher, in the classroom, who could then ensure that the child received the necessary attention. Just as the underlying principle of the School Health Service is to take an interest in those medical conditions which may prevent the child receiving proper education, so health education from this point of view was designed in the interests of education, rather than in the interests of the child.

In addition to these subjects, students are prepared in the basic content of nutrition, personal hygiene, the effect of personal habits and choice, the prevention of accidents and, in especial, developmental features involved in adolescence. There is also a big response from students when 'main' three or four-year courses in Social Biology are offered as an alternative 'main' study. It is fair to say that the course in health education in Colleges of Education has kept pace with modern advances in preventive medicine and it now includes topical problems such as smoking, alcoholism, abuse of drugs and—of course—the almost traditional sex education which, in recent years, has been enlarged into a concept of education for interpersonal relationships. There is, necessarily, a concentration on those problems which are meaningful during school life, but there is no doubt that a good deal of the health education received in school will have a carry-over value into adult life as well. Most important is to influence the child's attitudes to his own health problems and those of the community.

The increasing interest in sociological studies in relation to education has also enlarged the scope of modern health education teaching. The study of national institutions such as the social and welfare services, as well as studies in the behavioural sciences, are now included in the course in most Colleges of Education. Unfortunately, the subject still remains eclectic and it has been difficult to secure its recognition as an academic discipline in its own right. It is encouraging, however, that, in London University, health education has been accepted as an optional subject in Part III of the Bachelor of Education Degree. The Diploma in Health Education Course, which has been organised by the University of London since 1954, accepts teachers as students. There is also a Supplementary (one year) Course for experienced teachers at the City of Birmingham College of Education.

The scope of health education in British schools is well-outlined in *A Handbook of Health Education* (1968) published by the Department of Education and Science. This is a successor to previous editions issued by the Central Department from the days when it was the Board of Education. This pamphlet, which was intended as a guide for teachers but does not lay down any syllabuses or codes of practice, covers the subject from the infant school until school-leaving age, and also at Colleges of Further Education, Colleges of Education and in Adult Education. In the infant school, health education is largely by precept and example and by guiding the child towards good personal standards of hygiene and behaviour. The organisation of the school, and provision for environmental hygiene and the care of children, is believed to be an example in itself. The infant school teacher, also, in the course of nature study lessons can begin to inculcate the general principles of the biology of living things, and there is even a growing interest in some kind of sex education in the infant school. In general, however, the work of the infant school reinforces the basic lessons in personal hygiene which should have been laid down in the home.

The social training of small children can also be regarded as a part of health education at this stage. The traditional keeping of pets in the classroom provides an early introduction, not only to sexual reproduction but also to the care of living things, their nutrition, grooming, cleanliness, general well-being, which is a model of an ecological pattern that has its application to the human race. The infant teacher's skill lies in finding learning situations and she will frequently use the family as an example—either the arrival of a new baby or the roles of mothers, fathers and relationships between siblings.

It is possible that education for mental health may begin in the infant school, as the way in which the child is aided to handle new stresses, and to make adjustments with his peer groups and to tolerate the inevitable frustrations of daily life, will prepare him for greater stresses which he will meet with in the junior and secondary school.

In the junior school, human biology can be included in the curriculum. As mentioned above, in connection with the content of health education for the parents of small children, any attempt at systematic instruction in anatomy and physiology is to be avoided. There is a growing interest in the teaching of human biology through meaningful experiences—that is, the daily events occurring in the body which reach the child's consciousness and which may cause him to ask questions. For example, the breathlessness and the pounding pulse after heavy exercise provides a learning situation for study of the heart, circulation and respiration as an integrated organic function, fundamental to homeostasis which must be regarded as the basis of normal health. Growth and reproduction, nutrition, physiology of vision, hearing, sensation, and of the central nervous system, are all suitable topics. The biological environment and its effects on health, defence against bacteria, and—it has been suggested—the phenomenon of new growth, should also be touched upon. A useful series of films (*Your Health*) made especially for junior school children, which includes all these subjects with the exception of sex education, is available from the Rank Film Library. Safety education, and the elements of first aid, are also important subjects which can be tackled in the later years of the junior school.

In view of the fact that studies of juvenile smoking show that many boys have already started by the age of 11, it is now recognised that the dangers of smoking should be tackled at the junior school stage. There may be one advantage here in that children of this age are more receptive, and more confident, of information given them by adults and the normal stage of adolescent rebellion has not yet arrived.

Dental health is also an important topic and the content should include some ideas of the structure of teeth and gums, simple ideas of the pathology of dental caries, with emphasis upon the dangers of stagnation in the mouth which can be prevented by oral hygiene. The four rules of eating nourishing meals, without snacks in between; brushing the teeth, or washing the mouth with water after meals; finishing meals whenever possible with fruit or hard root vegetables; and co-operating in dental care, should be instilled into the child continually. The school dentist, and also dental hygienists or auxiliaries, do valuable work in this field. As environment is so important in dental health, however, it is essential that parents, teachers, and school meals organisers, should be aware of the role that they can play. The vexed question of a school tuckshop is one that can only be solved by the co-operation of all concerned.

During the secondary stage of education, there should be a more deliberate preparation for adult life, including education for family life. Some Local Education Authorities have established progressive schemes for the latter subject, *e.g.* Gloucestershire Association for Family Life. In some cases, voluntary as well as statutory agencies play a part in these schemes. The School Health Service is prominent, as might be expected, but also the Churches and Marriage Guidance Councils frequently contribute. With the child's growing interest in the social scene around him, and in social institutions in which he will play a part, there comes an opportunity of relating topics such as sexual behaviour, alcohol, and the abuse of drugs, to contemporary social problems. As the pupils get older the increasing use of discussion methods is valuable. Pupils should be introduced to such institutions as the Maternal and Child Health Service, and to the National Health Service, explaining how the ordinary citizen can co-operate with the doctors and other professional people and, perhaps most significantly, what to expect of them.

Despite the sophistication of modern young people, there are still many anxieties regarding the developmental features of puberty and these require interpretation. Hollins and Dicks (1968) have published an account of what can be achieved by a male medical officer and a school nurse, working together in secondary schools. The pupils put a wide range of questions to them and it was found that people undertaking this kind of work had to be extremely resourceful and preserve a serenity in order to cope with the varying questions on every aspect of health and sexual behaviour.

Bacon (1964) has also given an account of a comprehensive scheme for health education in schools in Hampshire. He comments on the report of a Working Party to consider the subject of health education in Hampshire schools. As regards 'education for family life', this is concerned with the whole of the interpersonal relationships between husband and wife and children, child care and rearing, dietary, cooking and budgeting, home care and cleanliness, and the prevention of sickness and accidents. Bacon mentions the need to add 'health sense' to the traditional qualities fostered in schools, and he calls 'health sense' a largely sub-conscious mental state which leads people to value health in themselves and in the community of which they are a part.

The literature regarding health education in British schools reveals a growing interest and an extension of progressive policies. There is also a wide range of audio-visual material to support the teacher, or the outside lecturer, and a considerable number of books, designed to be read by the school child himself, are now available. The National Association for Maternal and Child Welfare has encouraged parentcraft teaching in girls' schools for many years, and provides an advisory service as well as an examination system. Parentcraft teaching is undertaken very largely by health visitors, who visit schools for the purpose, although in some secondary schools it is undertaken by the regular teacher who also covers the subject of health education. Parent-teacher links are widely fostered nowadays, and this provides additional opportunities for promoting health education.

There is usually a close partnership between the School Health Service and the Local Education Authority and although some teachers will claim that, ideally, all classroom teaching should be done by the regular class teacher it seems that, in the majority of schools, outside help is welcome. The corollary is that doctors and nurses should be willing to undertake special training in teaching methods. A useful compromise is to form a partnership with the regular class teacher, who virtually conducts the class and maintains the normal rapport, with the outside expert contributing the content. Health Education Officers, too, perform valuable work in schools and some of them are actually trained teachers. In some cases, however, Health Education Officers from other disciplines, such as health visiting, have built up a close rapport with all schools in the area (see also p. 361).

Discussion Methods

Since health education aims at training in decision-making, there has been a tendency—in recent years—towards the use of active discussion methods in which a simulated experience can be given to a group. This is particularly useful when decisions have to be taken in making an approach to a child where behavioural problems are concerned. Even when concerned with children at a non-verbal communication stage, it is important that parents should be faced with the actual psychological and emotional experience they would undergo in reality. It is a common event in the course of discussion when a particular question is asked— for example, how to deal with enuresis or toilet training, or how to tell small children about sexual reproduction—for someone to volunteer a statement which they believe represents the kind of action they would take.

In such a situation the use of role-playing is valuable. A person who volunteers a statement of what action they would take is invited to play the role of a parent in that actual situation, while another member or members of the group are invited to play opposing roles—for example, husband and wife, mother and son or daughter, parents and schoolteacher, and the like. The discussion leader sets the scene by describing the situation and the relationships involved and then invites the participants to role-play, without any previous scripting or rehearsal. The discussion leader stops the role-playing at a point where it is apparent that no progress is being made, or, on the other hand, that an important point has been scored. The remainder of the group are invited to make their comments and the usual practice is to ask those who criticise to volunteer to play the role themselves.

It may be necessary to have three or four consecutive episodes of role-playing, each lasting several minutes, before the group arrives at a final solution. A refinement of this technique is to tape-record the proceedings and then, on playing the tape back, to invite the group to discuss it. This technique is also useful in situations where the problems of handicapped children are concerned. It can be used in professional in-service training, for example, to analyse the problems involved in telling a mother that her child is mentally or physically handicapped when this may not be clear to her.

Group discussion has become fairly well established in health education practice, and there is some difference of view between those who believe that group dynamics should be practised and those who feel that, in view of the short time available and the essentially practical nature of the task, a structured discussion leading to a practical solution should be aimed at. For practical purposes the structured discussion is sufficient and evaluation procedures have established that this can result in a change of attitude leading to a more or less permanent change in behaviour. There is an increasing availability of audio-visual aids to introduce discussion, and the situation has now arrived when no audio-visual aids, such as films or filmstrips, would be considered to stand on their own merits but only as aids to discussion.

The range of audio-visual aids now available to the health educator extends from the simple flannelgraph—one of the earliest aids to be introduced—to the use of closed-circuit television. The flannelgraph, which can be described as a system of mobile pictures, consists of a black backcloth on which can be stuck (and moved about) coloured felt patterns representing anatomical features, statistical material, or symbols representing such basic concepts as defence against infection, the principles of immunisation, etc. Silhouettes of human beings at various ages can also be arranged and moved about to illustrate relationships.

There are many standard flannelgraph sets on the market and, in addition, many health educators design and construct their own flannelgraphs for a particular purpose. The aim in a flannelgraph is simplicity and the fewer the pieces the better. Considerable artistic skill is necessary in order to translate the intellectual concepts involved in health education into meaningful symbols. This is particularly the case in statistical material where the scales adopted have to be carefully worked out beforehand.

The filmstrip and the 'two-by-two' slide are extensively used in health education. A slide collection may be of greater value than the filmstrip as it enables a greater selection and flexibility. Slides or filmstrips accompanied by recorded sound, usually on a disc to be played on a record player, are valuable, particularly when concerned with the problem-centred approach to health education. A problem-centred approach means a study, by a group, of a particular problem of child development or behaviour or illness, problems of an emotional or sociological character, and the working out of general principles as a result of the discussions. A number of slides and filmstrips, accompanied by sound, have been produced for this type of health education and they range from toilet training to the problem of young people who have contracted venereal disease. Teaching notes are supplied with these strips and slides, and guidance is given to the discussion leader on how to initiate discussion and to ensure that sound general principles emerge, which could guide people to practical action, rather than a snap decision.

A more sophisticated development of this technique is the use of the thematic film. Originally introduced by Cohen-Séat, in France, as part of the study of depth psychology, this has now been adapted for health education purposes in this country—mainly by D. Lynton Porter (1969). A thematic film, 16 mm., black-and-white, silent, is virtually a 'movie' Thematic Apperception Test and portrays, for about 2 or 3 minutes, a fragment of a human relations problem in which the group identify themselves with the characters shown on the screen, and are given entirely visual clues for the purposes of discussion.

The tendency in health education films, now, is away from the elaborate documentary, which is extremely costly to produce and therefore tends to remain in catalogues for far too long, and towards the production of a less expensive, expendable film which does not aim at being didactic or completely comprehensive but provides material for discussion. As film is the most expensive medium used in health education, it is as well to reserve it for the task which it does best, and this may be summed up as being the demonstration of human emotion, behaviour and the sociological principles involved in health. This has been elaborated by Dalzell–Ward (1963) in respect of films designed to prevent young people from taking up smoking.

Just as the cinema was hopefully looked to in the early days of health education as a valuable medium, it is natural that television is often considered as the modern medium for health education. Both the B.B.C. and Independent channels have produced valuable series—broadcast to schoolchildren—covering a very wide range of health topics, including venereal diseases. Broadcast television is used to its greatest advantage where a discussion can be organised by a teacher or a discussion leader at the receiving point. Partnership between a health educator and a skilled professional producer has been demonstrated most appropriately in the schools broadcasting system. It is the practice of the broadcasting agencies to produce teaching notes which can be circulated in advance of the programmes and provide a guide to additional reading and to material which can be used in the classrooms.

The extension of closed-circuit television services in the major local education authorities, notably in Glasgow and London, have also made it possible for health education to be included in these schemes. Programmes for primary schools, on subjects like dental health and foot health, have been designed and transmitted to Glasgow schools in that system. The use of closed-circuit television and broadcast television also opens up the possibility of the use of video-tape recorded programmes. A new invention—E.V.R. Electronic Video Recording—will make it possible, within the near future, for master programmes to be produced in large numbers on specially prepared film which can then be used in the E.V.R. sets in schools, health clinics, and any other places where health education is carried on.

An important addition to the range of visual aids is the overhead projector. This is an instrument offering great flexibility in use; transparencies can be purchased ready-made or they can be designed by the individual health educator. It is also possible to draw and write on transparent material that can be moved along during the course of a lecture and, with practice, this instrument can be used with a most impressive panache.

Programmed learning—a development in general education, involving either simple printed programmes in booklets or the more elaborate teaching machine— has now been adapted for use in health education. There is great promise in the use of this method for individual pupil study. In some schools, it is possible to organise instruction booths, that can be used by individual pupils, in which teaching machines or learning programmes can be used in conjunction with individual slide sets, tape-recordings, and even microscope slides.

The use of exhibition techniques is also part of the modern health education scene. The criticism of exhibitions as static is no longer valid in the light of the use of modern materials and techniques. Health education exhibitions vary from large displays which might be visited by thousands of people in the course of a Health Week, or as part of some other community event—for example, an agricultural show, flower show, or civic occasion—to small, expendable 'triptych' displays which can be set up in a corner of a child health centre. Many health visitors are skilful in organising exhibitions on such subjects as dental health, foot health, immunisation, nutrition, and clothing. Small exhibitions of this kind are useful in conjunction with school medical inspections, where they can be set up in the waiting room and studied by parents and children together. Exhibitions should use colour, variety, and movement, and offer active participation—for example, the use of quizz-boards worked by electric buttons, the provision of stereoscopic exhibits that can be viewed through binoculars, etc. It is possible to produce a health exhibition in a completely contemporary style which can compare with commercial exhibitions.

Evaluation

Evaluation of health education projects is essential in order to make an economic use of resources and to measure the effectiveness of the approach. Evaluation procedures are applied to campaigns, materials and methods. The criteria of evaluation and the method adopted vary. In the planning stages of a campaign decisions as to priorities may be made, following an epidemiological study (Schwarz, 1969). When priorities and aims have been established—*e.g.* the reduction of the incidence of respiratory diseases (Dalzell–Ward, 1962)—the next stage of evaluation is an examination of the feasibility of alternative plans for organisation and methods to be adopted.

An essential measure is to establish a baseline from which to chart progress. In the case of an immunisation campaign, for example, the number of children immunised, the extent of knowledge concerning immunisation, and the attitudes of parents, would be essential data. These data would not only be a guide to the approach most likely to be effective but they would also supply criteria of success. Posters and films are evaluated by conducting testing procedures under controlled conditions. Questionnaires, inviting comments and opinions as well as recall of information, can be used or personal enquiries made by skilled interviewers. Evaluation techniques are derived from the behavioural sciences and resemble the techniques used by commercial advertisers in assessing the effectiveness of their campaigns.

In health education, the final criterion is change of behaviour which should have followed perception of information and change of attitude. Such evaluation procedures are applicable only to events that can be numerically assessed over a short period of time. Inability to demonstrate a change of behaviour should not prevent health education projects being carried on if the basis is sound scientifically— *e.g.* projects to raise the standard of mental health through human relations teaching.

Personnel and Agencies in Health Education

Health Education Officers, who are employed by well over half the Local Health Authorities in England, Wales and Scotland, are trained and experienced in the use of the techniques described above and, in addition, undertake the public relations functions that are necessary in order to create a link between the health education department, the health department, and the public. However, practical day-to-day health education is also carried on by the doctors and nurses working in the public health service, and one of the functions of the Health Education Officer is to help his colleagues to carry out such tasks by the building up of supplies of equipment, by organisation of meetings, and by the arranging of in-service training programmes. These are the arrangements made locally but, in addition, there are a number of agencies at national level in regular contact with local health authorities, with other branches of the health service, and voluntary bodies who play an important role in the organisation of health education.

The Health Education Council, which came into operation in 1968, following the recommendations of the Cohen Committee (1964), is now the central agency in England and Wales for the co-ordination of health education, for research into methods and evaluation, for the production of materials, and for the provision of training courses, both in-service training and—at a later date—basic professional training for health education specialists.

The Health Education Council has taken over the functions of the Central Council for Health Education, which had been in operation since 1927, and also those of the Ministry of Health (now the Department of Health and Social Security) in respect of national campaigns on such subjects as food hygiene, immunisation and vaccination, and the control and prevention of infectious diseases. In Scotland, the Scottish Council for Health Education is responsible for in-service training of professional people and direct services to local authorities, while a special unit in the Department of Home and Health, Scotland, is responsible for national campaigns, research, and the production of materials. In addition to these agencies, which are directly responsible to the Secretary of State, Department of Health and Social Security, or to the Secretary of State for Scotland, there are a number of voluntary bodies whose work is either directly concerned with public education, or where health education plays a part in their programme.

Thus, the National Association for Maternal and Child Welfare stimulates interest in parentcraft education in schools and conducts examinations and, through the medium of its Annual Conference and its literature, makes a substantial contribution to health education for parentcraft. Similarly, the Royal Society for the Prevention of Accidents, with a Division concerned with home-accident prevention, carries out direct education of the public through the medium of conferences, literature and consultative advice. For the handicapped child there are a number of agencies—e.g. the Spastics Society and the National Society for the Mentally Handicapped Child—part of whose work is giving advice to parents on the care of their children and also in creating a favourable climate of public opinion. These agencies, too, have produced literature. The General Dental Council has a health education section and carries out a comprehensive production programme in health education materials of all kinds. The Oral Hygiene Service— a commercially sponsored organisation—carries out a complementary function. Both these agencies, together with the British Dental Association, co-operate in the promotion of dental health through the medium of exhibitions—including mobile unit exhibitions—the production of films, and the provision of material for school teachers. Dental Health Weeks are organised by these agencies to involve the maximum amount of participation by school children. The National Association for Mental Health, which covers the entire field of mental health including the welfare of backward or maladjusted children, produces literature and gives advice and, through its conferences and meetings and training schemes for professional people, carries out health education in respect of mental health of children.

Professional training for health education in Britain is still somewhat meagre. The University of London Diploma in Health Education Course, which has been in operation since 1954, produces about 20 to 25 qualified holders of the Diploma each year, and offers an academic year's comprehensive course which includes the pedagogic sciences, the basic of public and social health, the science of communica- tion and evaluation, social anthropology and the behavioural sciences as applied to health education. Health education has been included for some years in the basic training of health visitors and, also, for doctors taking the Diploma in Public Health. The Royal College of Nursing and the Health Visitors' Association provide facilities for training and experience in health education for their students of all grades, including those taking the Health Visitor Tutor's qualifications.

A. J. DALZELL-WARD

References

BACKETT, E. M. (1965). *Domestic Accidents*, W.H.O. Public Health Papers No. 26. Geneva.

BACON, L. (1964). Health education and the schools. *Health Education Journal*, **22**, 216.

BRITISH MEDICAL ASSOCIATION (1964). *Accidents in the Home*. London: B.M.A.

CHALKE, H. D. (1962). Parents' groups in Camberwell, *Health Educational Journal*, **20**, 3.

CHARLES, J. (1953). *Annual Report of Chief Medical Officer, Ministry of Health*. London: H.M.S.O.

—— (1956). *Ibid*.

COHEN, LORD (Chairman) (1964). *Health Education*, Report of a Joint Committee of the Central and Scottish Health Services Councils. London: H.M.S.O.

DALZELL-WARD, A. J. (1955). The future of the Child Welfare Centre, *Medical Officer*, **93**, 303.

—— (1962). Health education and respiratory diseases. *Public Health*, **76**, 110.

—— (1963). The sociological film, *Scientific Film*, October.

DEPARTMENT OF EDUCATION AND SCIENCE (1968). *A Handbook of Health Education*. London: H.M.S.O.

FRY, J., DILLANE, J. B., CONNOLLY, M. M. (1965). The evolution of a health team: A successful general practitioner-health visitor association. *Brit. Med. J.*, **1**, 181.

GARDINER-HILL, H. (1958). *Clinical Involvements or the Old Firm*. London: Butterworth.

HALE, R., LOVELAND, M. K. and OWEN, G. M. (1968). *The Principles and Practice of Health Visiting*. London: Pergamon Press.

HASLER, J. C. (1968). Health education by community health team. *Brit. Med. J.*, **3**, 366.

HOLLINS, F. R. and DICKS, S. (1968). A personal relations project in senior schools. *Medical Officer*, **120**, 261.

INTERDEPARTMENTAL COMMITTEE ON PHYSICAL DETERIORATION (1904). *Report*. London: H.M.S.O.

KENT PAEDIATRIC SOCIETY (1954). *A Study in the Epidemiology of Health*.

LONDON COUNTY COUNCIL AND TAVISTOCK INSTITUTE (1954). Preventive mental health in the maternity and child welfare services. *Medical Officer*, **92**, 303.

MACQUEEN, I. A. G. (1960). Evaluation of a scheme of health education. *Medical Officer*, **103**, 295.

NAISH, C. (1954). An experiment in family practice within the National Health Service. *Lancet*, **1**, 1342.

PORTER, D. L. (1969). *Behaviour and Its Analysis through Thematic Film*. Proceedings of Royal Society of Health Congress, Eastbourne.

REID, J. J. A. and REID, M. (1954). Medical consultations at a group of child welfare clinics. *Medical Officer*, **91**, 273.

Report of Royal Commission on Medical Education (1968). London: H.M.S.O.

ROYAL COLLEGE OF MIDWIVES (1966). *Preparation for Parenthood*.

SCHWARZ, K. (1969). Health education and child health. *Health Education Journal*, **28**, 34.

SOCIETY OF MEDICAL OFFICERS OF HEALTH—MATERNAL AND CHILD HEALTH GROUP (1955). Memorandum on the future of the Child Welfare Centre. *Public Health*, **48**, 51.

SPENCE, J., WALTON, W. S., MILLER, F. J. W. and COURT, S. D. M. (1954). *A Thousand Families in Newcastle upon Tyne*. London: Oxf. Univ. Press.

WORLD HEALTH ORGANISATION (1954). Expert committee on health education of the public. First Report. W.H.O. Technical Report Series No. 89, Geneva.

—— (1957). *Accidents in Childhood*. W.H.O. Technical Report Series No. 118, Geneva.

22　The Reproductive Years

A FEATURE of obstetric practice in the United Kingdom over the past 10 or 12 years has been the sudden, dramatic change in the pattern of pregnancy among young teenagers. Between 1948 and 1955 some 200 girls aged 13 to 15 years had babies in England and Wales each year but over the period 1956 to 1966 the number has risen from 269 to 1,288 (Table 18). There is no sign of any levelling off in these

TABLE 18

Maternities in England and Wales in Girls aged 13 to 15 years.
Registrar-General's Annual Statistical Review (England and Wales)

	1948	1949	1950	1951	1952	1953	1954	1955	1956
15 years	176	169	176	167	176	170	155	185	208
14 years	37	31	39	25	36	46	33	40	56
13 years	1	3	6	4	5	10	5	8	5

	1957	1958	1959	1960	1961	1962	1963	1964	1965	1966
15 years	243	309	393	601	731	929	984	901	970	1,068
14 years	45	62	78	98	133	192	174	172	170	193
13 years	9	10	10	15	23	19	22	15	23	27

figures and this is contrary to the overall birth rate which has been falling since 1964 (Fig. 83). Presumably the newer forms of birth control (and their greater availability) are now having a significant effect on the pregnancy rate throughout most of the community but these younger girls are a notable exception.

So far as numbers are concerned it is the 15-year-old who poses the major problem. Figures 84 and 85 show that not only have the numbers increased but also the proportion of girls aged 15 who become pregnant each year has risen from 0.8 to 3·28 per 1,000 over the period 1956 to 1966. (The disproportionate rise in number of pregnancies beginning in 1961 and the subsequent fall in 1964 reflect events of 15 years previously when there was a sudden rise in the number of births immediately following the war.)

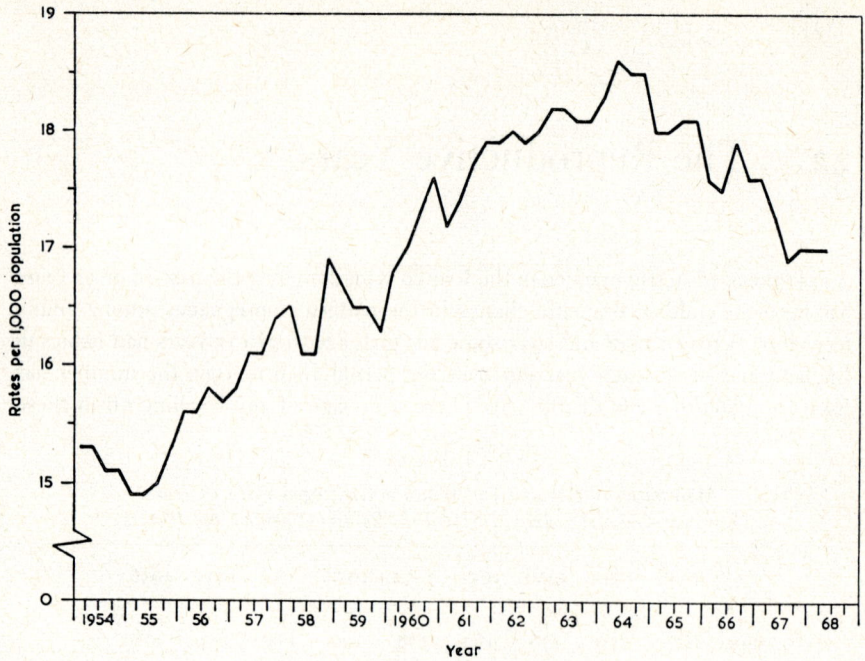

FIG. 83. Birth rate for England and Wales, 1954–68.

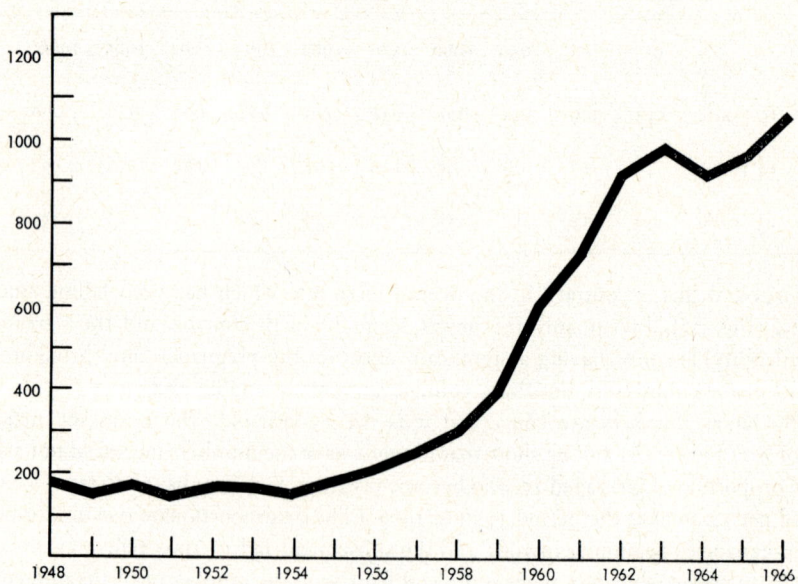

FIG. 84. Number of pregnancies per year in girls aged 15 in England and Wales.

It is difficult to understand or grasp the significance of the interest that has centred increasingly on teenagers these past 10 years or to evaluate the exploitation of the 'teenage market' by the press, magazines, radio, television, cinema and theatre. The steady rise in the number and proportion of young girls who become pregnant each year is one of the few objective measurements that can be applied to this situation and the trend is alarming. In part, at least, the increase may be due to the steady fall in the age of the menarche in western countries over the past 100 years—in 1850 the average age at which girls had their first period was

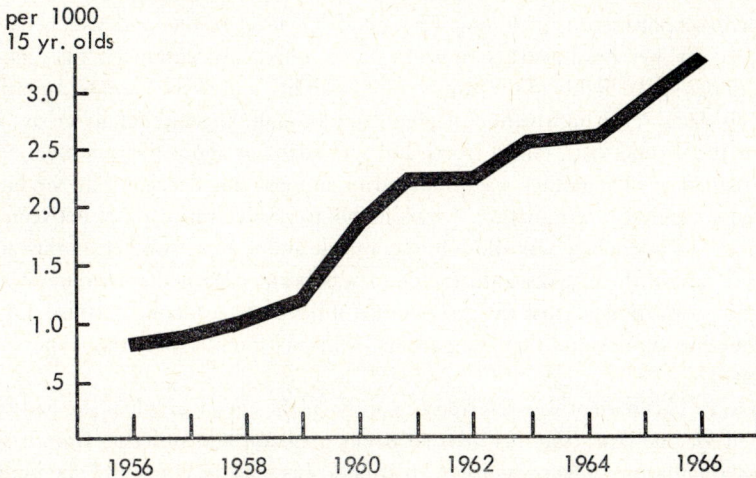

Fig. 85. Proportion of girls aged 15 who became pregnant each year in England and Wales in 1956 to 1966.

17 years; now it is 12½ years. But there are other considerations which relate closely to the society we live in and to the values we place on personal behaviour and on personal relationships. Our society is increasingly permissive with free love, promiscuity and sex play portrayed openly in magazines, on radio and television, in films and on the stage. It can fairly be argued that the glamour of these situations is played up; the tragic consequences are either ignored or played down. A heavy duty lies on editors and producers to set and maintain high standards and be the arbiters of good personal and social behaviour. Another important contributory factor is the earlier financial independence of the young—it could be that they achieve independence before they are mature enough to accept it and that an increasing incidence of pregnancy in girls under 16 is part of the price that has to be paid for this earlier independence—a heavy price indeed. Inevitably at some stage something must be done to reverse this upward trend but the change will be neither sudden nor dramatic and it may take a generation or two before society addresses itself seriously to this problem.

The national figures are disquieting but tell nothing of the personal and family tragedies faced by many of these young girls and their parents not only at the time of the pregnancy but afterwards. The case histories of four patients seen either in the Princess Mary Maternity Hospital or the Royal Victoria Infirmary over the past few years bring out some of the dynamic issues that can stem from pregnancy at this early age.

Case 1. I first saw this girl at the age of 15 when she was four months pregnant but found it difficult to obtain a coherent history for she was disinclined to talk about the pregnancy or what it meant to her. Her mother, who was with her, described how the girl had become more and more withdrawn over the past two months and would now scarcely speak to other members of the family. She had an excellent school record, including very good 'O' level results and had been encouraged by her headmistress to work for a university entrance. The general practitioner spoke highly of the family, of its stability and of the parents' ambitions for their daughter. Confirmation of pregnancy brought an acute family crisis. The girl, at the second visit, talked freely and was adamant about the continuation of the pregnancy. Her mother was prepared to support this decision but the father pressed strongly for termination. I was unable to resolve this conflict between the parents. The pregnancy was allowed to continue and the girl and her mother went south to stay with relatives until the child was born. I learned subsequently that adoption was arranged, that the girl in spite of her early academic promise did not continue her studies and that the parents, some six months after this experience, separated.

Case 2. This patient was referred to see me at the age of 22 when she had been married for one year. She was then 10 weeks pregnant and suffering from hyperemesis gravidarum. The response to treatment was unsatisfactory and she became increasingly introspective and lost a great deal of weight. After three weeks she suddenly confided privately to me that she had had an illegitimate pregnancy terminated several years previously as a teenager still at school. She had kept this information from her husband and this was now weighing heavily on her mind. After talking to me her condition did improve but rapidly deteriorated a week later. Concern about his wife brought the husband to see me and to my surprise he told me that he knew of his wife's earlier pregnancy but as she had never mentioned it throughout their courtship and marriage he had carefully avoided the subject. I suggested that he speak at once to his wife and a tearful meeting followed but her condition improved and the pregnancy was subsequently uncomplicated. So far as I can assess the marriage continues securely and the patient has since had a second child.

Case 3. After three years of marriage this patient was referred to the infertility clinic because she had had two abortions at 14 and 16 weeks. She was anxious to have a child. On examination I found a deep laceration of the cervix on the right side extending almost into the fornix. At the end of the consultation she told me in private conversation that she had had a pregnancy terminated by dilatation and curettage at the age of 15. Shortly after marriage, before the first abortion, she had told her husband of the illegitimate pregnancy and she did not think this had altered his affection for her. The laceration was duly repaired and a third abortion occurred eight months after the operation. A year later she passed from my clinical care but by this time she was increasingly aware of her husband's resentment that she was unable to have a child and he was openly blaming this failure on her pre-nuptial therapeutic abortion. When I last saw her she was deeply concerned about the future of her marriage.

Case 4. At the age of 15 this patient went into labour 19 days after the expected date of delivery. All arrangements had been made for adoption of the baby. After 14 hours in labour the cervix became fully dilated and at the same time time a slow fetal heart rate and meconium staining of the liquor were noted. She was known to have some transverse contraction of the pelvis (true conjugate 4·5 in., widest transverse diameter 4·6 in.). The leading point of the fetal head was just below the level of the ischial spines and the greatest diameter of the head was in the pelvic inlet. A difficult decision had to be made between forceps delivery or caesarean section—the vaginal route was chosen. The delivery was more difficult than had been anticipated and the baby required considerable resuscitation. The baby weighed 3·8 kg. (8 lbs. 5 oz.) and showed signs of neurological disturbance during the neonatal period. Arrangements for adoption had to be cancelled. Two months after delivery there was still evidence of neurological disturbance but at 9 months a paediatrician found no evidence of residual damage and arrangements were made for the child's adoption.

Personal and Medical Consequences

Depending upon the girl and upon her family background there may be any reaction to pregnancy from complete, untroubled acceptance to total rejection and emotional breakdown. Each case is different. Again it is important to remember possible long term effects of the pregnancy. Too often the girl's formal education ceases abruptly and this is especially unfortunate when she is intellectually able and thinking in terms of higher education. Few schools make any special arrangements for these girls.

The view is widely held that these young girls have fewer complications in pregnancy and labour and this is substantially true. From the obstetric viewpoint they are not a great worry—a slightly increased risk of pre-eclamptic toxaemia (Claman and Bell, 1964; Semmens, 1965; Lewis and Nash, 1967; Utian, 1967) and a tendency to produce underweight babies (Hulka and Schaaf, 1963; Semmens and McGlamory, 1960; Stine *et al.*, 1964). In the occasional case there may be an element of disproportion (especially if the girl is very young or of small stature). Here the obstetrician must be very careful not to allow the girl's age to stand in the way of operative delivery if there are reasonable indications for interference. There is an understandable temptation for the obstetrician, in the face of difficult labour, to place more risk than he normally would upon the baby and an already difficult situation can be aggravated as in case 4.

In the individual case therapeutic abortion may appear to be the immediate and obvious answer to a distressing problem (under the new Abortion Act there were 92 abortions carried out on girls under 16 during the period April 27th to July 2nd 1968 (Registrar General's Quarterly Return for England and Wales)) but examples of later physical and psychological sequelae are not unusual. The cervix in a girl of 14 or 15 tends to be small and firm and dilatation, no matter how carefully performed, can result in laceration with heavy bleeding at the time and cervical incompetence in later pregnancies (see case 3). Again, though it may not be immediately apparent, the young girl may suffer considerable psychological trauma which may have a profound effect on her future happiness in marriage. In any society there is a special need to protect the young and the emphasis should be upon the avoidance of pregnancy rather than upon therapeutic abortion. First priority must be wider recognition of the alarming rise in the number of pregnancies among young teenagers. There must follow a careful re-appraisal of parental responsibility and of the widespread permissiveness which is now a feature of our society.

Table 18 and Figs. 84 and 85 are reproduced from the *Lancet* by permission of the editor.

J. K. RUSSELL

References

CLAMAN, A. D. and BELL, H. M. (1964). Pregnancy in the very young teen-ager. *Amer. J. Obstet. Gynec.*, **90**, 350.

HULKA, J. F. and SCHAAF, J. T. (1964). Obstetrics in adolescents. *Obstet. Gynec.*, **23**, 678.

LEWIS, B. V. and NASH, P. J. (1967). Pregnancy in patients under 16 years. *Brit. med. J.*, **2**, 733.

Registrar-General's Quarterly Return for England and Wales (2nd Quarter, 1968). London: H.M.S.O.

SEMMENS, J. P. and McGLAMORY, J. C. (1960). Teen-age pregnancies. *Obstet. Gynec.*, **16**, 31.

—— (1965). Implications of teen-age pregnancy. *Ibid.*, **26**, 77.

STINE, O. C., RIDER, R. V. and SWEENEY, E. (1964). School leaving due to pregnancy. *Amer. J. publ. Hlth.*, **54**, 1.

UTIAN, W. H. (1967). Obstetrical implications of pregnancy in primigravidae aged 16 years or less. *Brit. med. J.*, **2**, 734.

23   Children in Trouble

IN this chapter it is proposed first to consider some of the biological, physical, psychological and social factors contributing to antisocial behaviour or a need to protect children through court action. This leads on to views about socialisation and punishment. These are followed by a brief review of trends in juvenile delinquency. And finally consideration is given to services for children at risk, including the juvenile courts themselves, and the range of treatment available both before and after a court appearance.

Biological, Physical, Psychological and Social Factors
Contributing to Antisocial Behaviour

Criminological research in the last 70 or more years has discredited simple explanations of criminal behaviour and shown the complex interrelation of different factors which precipitates such behaviour in a predisposed person of given age and sex in given circumstances at a certain moment in time. It is now recognised that there is no one all-sufficient cause of delinquency, which indeed reflects a 'complex continuing interaction between a developing biological organism and its physical, psychological and social environment'.

Biological and Physical Factors

Lombroso's theory of inherited criminal types characterised by certain physical stigmata such as thick ear lobes is long since discarded.

The German psychiatrist, Kretschmer, endeavoured to discover the complex relationships between mental disorder and different types of physique and character. He distinguished three main constitutional types: the leptosome, characterised by long, thin limbs; the athletic, with strongly developed musculature; and the pyknic, small and rotund type. He was primarily interested in correlations between these physical types and various forms of mental illness. His typology, bearing in mind all his own reservations, has also been applied in criminological research. It does not attempt to predict who will become delinquent but what crimes they are likely to commit, and when in the criminal life curve, if they do so. Sheldon's somatotyping is similar to Kretschmer's, though his terminology is different, and he relies on standardised photographs rather than verbal descriptions. The Gluecks in their classic study *Unravelling Juvenile Delinquency* (1950) found, using Sheldon's techniques, that 60 per cent of 500 delinquent boys were mesomorphs (athletics) as against 30 per cent in the matched control group of non-delinquent boys.

Gibbens (1963) in his study of borstal boys, using Sheldon's techniques, found 'an exceptional concentration of mesomorphic (muscular) physique'. Genetic studies of the XYY syndrome may also show a significant association with aggressive behaviour.

In these and other studies a high degree of physical defects and disabilities has been found amongst delinquents. Ferguson (1952) found that of all the boys who left school in Glasgow in one year the delinquency rate between 8 and 18 was significantly higher if the boy's height was below 56 in. at 14 than if it was above; in addition, twice as many of the small boys had more than one conviction. These may be part of a cluster of adverse family and social factors or delinquency may be a means of compensating for physical defects.

Various research studies have tried to clarify the relations between premature birth, brain damage, epilepsy or other neurological conditions and delinquency. The results seem to show 'that even minor degrees of neurological disease, injury, or congenital abnormality are liable to exaggerate the effects of an adverse environment or of underlying defects of personality; but that in the absence of these additional factors even very serious injuries may not produce any permanent deterioration in behaviour' (West, 1967). Recent results show that young schoolboys who are delinquent or troublesome are significantly more careless than others in psycho-motor tests.

Most present day children are much healthier, better nourished and better housed and clothed than those of a generation ago. It is worth pondering the relation, in adolescence in particular, between greater physical vigour, more leisure, more mobility, and delinquency. The increasing gap between the onset of puberty and psychological independence is also significant.

Psychological Factors

The psychogenic elements in delinquent and wayward behaviour are comprised of as yet unclear constitutional elements in personality types, coupled with the life experience of the individual, particularly in his family setting. There are, for example, innate differences in intelligence but the development of intelligence is affected by family experience, especially linguistic and other stimulus or the lack of it, in the early years. Eysenck and others have also found apparently innate differences in the ease with which conditioned responses can be established and the degree of their persistence. This is related to introvert-extrovert personality types; in turn extroversion 'is associated with mesomorphic physique, slow conditioning, low aspiration, low reaction to stress, low sedation threshold and low persistence' (West, 1967).

Recent research studies, using carefully matched control groups, show little difference in the intelligence of delinquents and non-delinquents unless this is also associated with cultural and emotional deprivation. But delinquents are commonly found to be significantly more retarded educationally.

There is some clinical evidence of developmental abnormality in psychopaths. The commonly accepted characteristics of the psychopath are: inability to relate to others, disregard of social standards, apparent absence of guilt feelings or ability to learn from experience, emotional immaturity manifested in impulsive actions, inability to postpone gratification and lack of foresight. This general failure to mature is of course found in less extreme form in those not labelled psychopathic. It is both consequence and cause of disordered family life. It may well be that brain damage predisposes to psychopathy in some and less serious manifestations in others.

Inadequate personalities, who form a large part of the adult male prison population, show lack of drive and general purpose. They are also prone to marriage breakdown. No doubt they contribute as inadequate, passive fathers to the genesis of juvenile delinquency.

Emotional immaturity, coupled with low frustration tolerance and sometimes high aggression, are perhaps the commonest factors in delinquency. These in turn can be shown to stem from inadequacies in child rearing. The common elements here seem to be indifferent, cruel or rejecting parents or discontinuity of loving relationship with parents or parental figures. This may take various forms, including lack of a parent and inadequate substitute care; discontinuities of care at crucial developmental stages, for example, being in and out of hospital, or a children's home or foster home; having a parent who is absent from time to time on account of desertion or physical illness or mental disorder or imprisonment; living in or being removed from a home broken by death, desertion or separation. The effects of these violent disjunctions of experience, or other crises, are related to the age of the child, the quality of mothering experienced before or during separation, and their duration and frequency. So far as emotional development is concerned, they may seriously affect the child's capacity to receive and give love, his sense of security and of personal identity, and therefore his capacity to mature emotionally, to control his hostile aggressive impulses and to form other than shallow relationships with others. They may also increase his guilt feelings or else lead to a strong reaction formation against both anxiety and guilt. They are likely to make it more difficult for the child to internalise consistent standards of social behaviour because he is subjected to inconsistencies.

Lack of loving parental care and of training in adequate standards of social behaviour is significantly associated with juvenile delinquency and other wayward behaviour. The well established interrelated concomitants are: poverty, unemployment, large families, ignorance about infant and child care, poor diet, poor housing and passive, neglectful or careless parents.

The effect in psycho-analytic terms of inadequate nurture leading to response to stress by crime rather than neurosis is: relatively unmodified instincts, a weak ego unable to divert instinctual energy into socially acceptable behaviour, and an undeveloped super-ego (Friedlander, 1947). Delinquents commonly show lower frustration tolerance and are likely to react aggressively. Frustration may spring from a sense of injustice, whether rational or leading to projection onto others in order to make one's own motives acceptable. This is a familiar characteristic of young offenders and their families. The antisocial character has early in life failed to develop a strong super-ego and thus he remains at an immature level of development, unable to tolerate frustration, resentful of authority, restless, self-centred and unable to postpone gratification of his wishes. He forms shallow attachment to others. Sociometric studies show that such children are not popular with other children at school. There is another, though probably smaller, group of children whose delinquency is related to their low self-esteem, anxiety and depression. They are more likely to commit solitary offences.

Many normal children also commit offences; sometimes because they are responding to delinquent social values; sometimes as a reaction to a crisis situation like a family bereavement or an impending examination; sometimes as an isolated lapse from parental standards; sometimes because they are tough youngsters in a tough neighbourhood but neither emotionally disturbed nor maladjusted.

Mannheim (1965) summarises as follows the various classifications of reasons why a child steals: '(a) Because he wants to use the article for his own enjoyment, which seems the most "normal" case; or (b) because he wants to hoard it, which betrays some complications; or (c) because he wants to give it away to buy with it love, security, response, recognition; or (d) for the thrill of stealing (new experience); or (e) because he wishes to test somebody's affection, notably that of his parents . . . or (f) because he has given up hope and only wishes to spite and hurt. . . .'

In adolescence any of the foregoing factors may become more acute, in addition to the development of strong homo- or hetero-sexual interests. Adolescents, particularly those from an insecure background, go through a period of rebellion against authority and adult values, whether within or outside the family, often as part of the necessary process of finding their own identity. This is accompanied by dependence-independence conflicts and swings from childish to adult behaviour and from over-confidence to loss of confidence and depression. Weak or rigid fathers or over-possessive or too indulgent mothers often precipitate adolescent rebellion, delinquency or maladjustment.

Relations with the father are particularly important at this time: good, even though ambivalent, relations help the boy or girl to use freedom without repudiation of controls, whereas fathers who are too strict, rigid, punitive, permissive, inadequate or not there at all may lead to violent repudiation of authority in general. It is not of course suggested that family conflict or rejection is the sole cause of adolescent rebellion, or of the opposite reaction—retreat into isolation or drug dependence.

Most adolescents find understanding, acceptance and common values in a peer group at the gregarious stage before they start serious courtship. For some these may be delinquent groups, increasingly coupled with drug taking as means of getting new experiences and excitement. A small minority, whether middle or working class, leave home and become rootless in big cities. Many others survive and settle down in their 20's.

Adolescent girls may become delinquent, primarily through shoplifting in large stores, often successfully but also often unaware of store detectives or closed circuit television. They are, however, more likely to engage in sex adventures, sometimes (in addition to normal sex drives) in search of that human closeness, affection and sense of mattering to someone that has been missing at home. They are frequently afflicted by an imbalance between their physical development and their emotional or intellectual maturity. They often run away from home after a series of rows, especially with their fathers, and are for a period out of work. A number make for London, from so far away as Glasgow, with the help of lifts from lorry drivers. When they arrive in a city they are sometimes befriended and protected by men or by prostitutes, sometimes not. Some go to the police for help when they become destitute and frightened, others may be detected in the streets, cafes or night clubs. Some are thankful to go home, others refuse to do so and come before the juvenile court.

Social Factors

It is obvious from what has been said about psychological factors predisposing to delinquent or wayward behaviour that these are usually mixed with social factors, though this does not cast light on the relative proportions in the individual that lead to anti-social behaviour. In some conformist milieux the puzzle may be why an individual becomes delinquent, but in an antisocial sub-culture the problem is why some do not, or else become law-abiding adults after some juvenile escapades. It is equally surprising why some young people exposed to considerable emotional damage yet survive without serious impairment of their mental health.

Theories of delinquent sub-cultures (including gangs) are primarily associated with such American sociologists as Miller, Cohen, Cloward and Ohlin, Sutherland and others. Excellent analytical summaries may be found in Mannheim (1965), Downes (1966) and West (1967). The main empirical studies in this country relate to Liverpool (Mays, 1959), Bristol (Spencer, 1964), 'Radby' (Sprott, 1954), Croydon (Morris, 1957), Cardiff (Wilson, 1962) and Stepney (Downes, 1966). These have all concentrated on neighbourhoods or new housing estates with high delinquency rates. Their findings show certain strong similarities and have produced partial validation of some elements in American theories, though there are considerable differences between the crime situation in the United States and this country.

Social class distribution is significant. Morris (1957) found in his study of Croydon that of young delinquents on probation or committed to approved schools in 1952, 1 case in 3,003 came from the Registrar-General's head of household occupational class II (skilled workers), 1 in 380 from class III (semi-skilled), and 1 in 187 from class V (unskilled and casual workers). Other enquiries confirm this over-representation of social class V. But it must be remembered that a cluster of other factors is also operative for many of those in social class V. For a high proportion the family income is both low and erratic (though occasionally with a high total family income); they are often poorly housed, overcrowded and living in bad neighbourhoods; they may react by indifference or aggression to a situation

17

where there is little hope of betterment, and thus antisocial behaviour is transmitted from one generation to another. Indeed it is almost impossible to disentangle the influence of a poor neighbourhood from that of family pathology. Large family size, which is significantly related to delinquency, is also interrelated with over-crowding, poor nutrition, insufficient emotional or physical nurture or parental training, street play and responsibility for younger siblings.

The Liverpool, 'Radby', Croydon, Tower Hamlets and Cardiff studies all show 'rough' areas in working class districts with a much higher concentration of juvenile delinquency and its concomitants than in the 'respectable' areas. These may be nearby streets or parts of new housing estates in the same working class neighbourhoods. For example, Power (1967) found in the 300 census enumeration districts of Tower Hamlets an annual boy delinquency range varying from 12 per cent to 1 per cent. One boy in 4 in the whole area was likely to be found guilty of an offence by the time he was 17 but in the black spots this rose to 50 per cent. There are marked differences in codes of conduct, values and behaviour between the respectable and the rough families. The roughs see nothing wrong with stealing and no reason to change their behaviour about it, they are not ambitious, have little independence or sense of privacy, their family relationships are apt to be unstable and their ideas of hygiene and nutrition primitive.

The respectable have many middle class characteristics, striving for better status or more possessions, showing respect for the property of others, disciplining children and requiring of them good standards of behaviour and educational achievement. Naturally there are many families between these two extremes. In any event, the delinquency prone families do not account for more than a proportion of children in trouble. Many others come from more comfortable and apparently secure homes where predominantly psychological factors may predispose to or precipitate delinquency. Single court appearances may be primarily related to the neighbourhood and the school but multiple appearances usually indicate deep-seated family problems. These often have nothing to do with materially poor conditions but relate to family conflict, lack of emotional warmth, too great pressures on children to succeed, or driving ambition for higher material standards or social status. In any event, it is the home with chronic family conflict which produces the worst social misfits, whether these are delinquent or neurotic, or both.

Moreover, in trying to understand the social factors in delinquency it is necessary to study the school as well as the family, neighbourhood and peer group. The Social Medicine Research Unit found that in the 20 secondary modern schools in Tower Hamlets the annual average delinquency rate per 100 boys aged 11 to 14 varied from 0.7 per cent to 7.8 per cent. This was not explicable in relation to whether the boys lived in high or low delinquency districts. For example, one school had a 3 per cent delinquency rate from high delinquency districts and 4 per cent from low delinquency districts, while another school had a 25 per cent delinquency rate from each. In other words, one school was protecting boys from delinquency while in the other they were at risk (Power et al., 1967). These pre-liminary findings suggest that individual schools may play a significant part, for better or worse, in social education and that much more research is needed to clarify the reasons for these differences.

Finally, it is necessary to remember that juvenile delinquency is not a certain outcome of faulty upbringing or a poor environment: it is simply one of several ways in which emotional immaturity or poor socialisation may be manifested. For example, the more criminal adolescent behaviour in this country seems to be due rather to arbitrary or indifferent parents in neighbourhoods where there is an anti-authority code of roughness and daring than to the class conflicts which American studies stress. Gangs characterised by rules, criminal aims, stable membership, accepted leaders, gang warfare, and the like, are rare here other than in transient form. Groups of boys may either be composed of friends and relations or be loose antisocial groups: they may be noisy, aggressive, impulsively delinquent and sometimes destructive but they do not primarily exist for delinquent purposes. Teddy boys, mods and rockers and beatniks—all with distinctive forms of dress and hair style—are different forms of adolescent group, characterised either by aggression or drug taking, and essentially means of finding 'togetherness' and identification. These and other adolescent groups of both sexes are, it has been suggested by various observers, ways of getting status and some sense of belonging, romance, emotional release and excitement (sometimes including violence) in a drab world of uncongenial work and dreary surroundings. Downes (1966) suggests that those who leave the tedium of a drill-sergeant type of secondary modern school for similar tedium in semi-skilled and easily changed jobs only retain their sanity by spontaneity, irrepressibility and rule-breaking. In other words, some social delinquency is an essentially healthy reaction to over-conformist demands without countervailing opportunities of reward; especially where there is little change of advancement in work, and no interest in the job other than the money it produces. Money and leisure both become important because they are the means of escape to excitement, glamour, romance and 'kicks'.

The working class 'corner boy' obviously has more leisure than his contemporary, the 'college boy' who continues to study at school or college: he may have more spending money too. Indeed teenagers are a largely classless group so far as 'pop' records, scooters, coffee bars and hair styles and, increasingly, drug taking are concerned. In many localities mobility has made relationships more impersonal, thus the wider social controls and supports become loosened and there are fewer accepted and socially enforced standards of behaviour. In our society there are no *rites de passage*, no clear transition from childhood to adulthood. Young people's earnings are often high but their status ill-defined in a society where increasingly the possession of material goods is the criterion of success. Some young people in trouble seek to acquire more and more of these, perhaps thereby bolstering up their feelings of adulthood and self-worth and trying to compensate for poverty of human relationships. Or they identify with rebellious peers rather than with their fathers and other authority figures and accept an antisocial scale of values. Others contract out and become beatniks or drug takers. For boys, scooters or cars apparently fulfil needs for proof of masculinity, the thrill of speed and the discharge of aggression. If they are too young to hold a licence or unable or unwilling to hire-purchase their own car or scooter, there is always someone else's handy and a group of two or three may go off together and drive until the petrol gives out or they have an accident or are spotted by the police.

Socialisation, Control and Punishment

The traditional role of courts is to punish and the very term 'children in trouble' suggests punishment. It is therefore necessary to look at some aspects of this extremely complex concept, which in any event is often loosely used with different meanings. The popular usage centres on punishment in its deterrent or retributive aspects as deprivation or damage to someone for a wrong done by him, whether this is transgressing parental prohibitions or committing an antisocial action.

All social groups, from the simplest to the largest and most complex, exercise various controls over their members to ensure conformity to cultural norms and values. This is true of the family or the adolescent peer group as well as the neighbourhood and the nation. Socialisation into a culture or sub-culture is thus a continuous process, with unperceived pressures to conform, and with controls and punishment normally only visibly exerted where failure becomes noticeable. Group disapproval and exclusion are powerful means of securing the desired standards. The law is a form of social control both to protect the innocent and to punish the guilty. So far as children and young people are concerned, efforts are increasingly made to control and socialise without negative punishment.

All punishment is directed to changing behaviour through experience of the unpleasant consequences of certain actions. This is known in learning theory terms as 'negative reinforcement'. It has two aspects in popular attitudes, the first a feeling that some balance has been upset which must be put right, an eye for an eye and a tooth for a tooth, *i.e.* doing something to redress the past; the second is deterrence, inflicting unpleasant consequences which it is thought will not only deter the troublemaker from similar future actions but also others who perceive the consequences of such behaviour. These are deep-seated impulses in human nature: the troublemaker has often given vent to the repressed desires of others and must be made to suffer for their guilt, projected onto him as moral indignation. At the same time, the deterrent theory of punishment rests upon the discredited assumption that all wayward human actions are rationally motivated and within conscious control: he knew it was wrong to act as he did, he was free to choose and he chose wrong, therefore it is only just that he should be punished.

This assumption is made by those parents who impute an adult time sense and adult capacities for distinguishing between good and bad conduct to small children. But, as Professor Ellis said in the chapter on punishment in earlier editions of this book, 'Described in adult terms, it may be said that the infant is normally greedy, self-centred, uncontrolled both physically and emotionally, aggressive, destructive, sexually curious and exhibitionist, and with no respect for personal property. When speech has been acquired, phantasy is so confused with fact that for some considerable time there is little conception of 'truth' in the adult sense.' In short, the baby is an embryo delinquent and maybe the puzzle is why law-abiding citizens in time emerge from such beginnings rather than why a minority become children in trouble. The processes of socialisation take place for normal children primarily in response to loving parents and a desire to please them. This is a response of love and a defence against frightening and as yet unregulated ambivalent feelings of love and hate. Piaget (1932) traced in children of different ages the growth of the concept from the earliest stage of acceptance that certain behaviour is wrong because it is forbidden to the later internalisation of general standards of conduct.

What matters for the child's satisfactory development is dependable love and consistency of discipline, indeed inconsistent parental discipline is a major predictor of delinquency proneness. This includes arbitrary alternations between laxity and punishment or disagreement between parents about discipline, the one being lax and the other harsh, with the lax partner often shielding the child with lies and evasions from the harsh one. Similar, though less damaging, consequences may be suffered by schoolchildren in circumstances where the standards of the home, the school, the play group, the neighbourhood and the mass media conflict with each other. The family (including sibling) standards will usually be more powerful than the others. Children's reactions will also differ where there is conflict between these different standards. The classic example is of course the difference in some areas between the school's standard of morality and behaviour and that of the home, the neighbourhood and the street play group. Where the gap is not too wide some children will come to terms with different behaviour required in different situations, others will reject or be indifferent to one standard and internalise the other, others yet will be left confused about all standards of behaviour and remain at the immature stage of personality development characteristic of antisocial characters. Naturally a close relationship with one person, whether parent, other relative, teacher or friend, over a sufficient period will substantially affect the particular code of behaviour emotionally accepted by the child. The processes of socialisation and control thus differ according to the age of the child and possible conflicts between different standards.

A new element enters in at adolescence with problems of being neither child nor adult, of a sudden increase in spending money, and coping with the change from school to the harsher and often dull world of work. The adolescent's urgent need to conform to the standards of the immediate peer group, to be like everyone else, to experiment with ways of living, together with an often intense interest in the opposite sex, coupled with increased independence and freedom of choice, make all the processes of socialisation, control and punishment more complex at this stage. There is generally a greater or lesser degree of rebellion against or emergence from parental controls. To quote Professor Ellis again, 'It cannot be too strongly emphasised that the delinquent in this case is often obeying rules and standards of his own group which to his mind are more compelling than those laid down by a larger society in which he feels his place is unimportant and to which he feels little direct loyalty.'

The great complexity of socialisation and control in relation to children and adolescents makes us much less sure than formerly about the role of punishment. Control as such is essential. The child whose parents do not exercise consistent control and discipline is less likely to develop the necessary internal controls. But punishment as a means of enforcing desired conduct is a separable issue. Learning theory and common sense suggest that both positive and negative reinforcement are necessary to the internalisation of any desired behaviour. Either approval or disapproval should follow quickly from the act in question, not be out of proportion to it, and be reasonably certain. Severe punishment but uncertainty of detection teaches greater skill in avoiding detection, while most children have not yet discovered that virtue unaccompanied by approval is its own reward.

It is often said that working class parents punish by physical means and middle class parents by temporary withdrawal of love (see chap. 13). 'Conditional love', indifference, over-indulgence, playing on children's fears, or excessive physical punishment are all damaging. Indeed in extreme cases they can result in hostile antisocial character formation or neurotic disorders.

Teachers play a large part in socialisation. They can reinforce the sense of confidence, security and desire to learn which a child brings from a good home. They can do a good deal to redress the balance by creating a more secure milieu and warmth and acceptance for a child from a home where there is too little or too erratic love or poor social standards. As has been said, they will find it much more difficult to make real relationships with children in districts whose standards are markedly different from their own. 'Lack of verbal skill and lack of parental desire for education make it difficult for school teachers, as representatives of an alien culture, to compete with the boy's contemporaries as a main source of influence in school days . . .' (Gibbens 1963). But the onus is largely on the school to discover how to bridge the gap. Many schools, including some for delinquent children, have successfully abolished corporal punishment. Punishment is both unjust and stupid for antisocial children who have had too much already or are reacting to parental indifference or to lack of parents. It is also unjust to punish children whose educational failure is due to low intelligence, lack of comprehension, undetected physical defect or lack of concentration due to emotional causes. Punishment by sarcasm, ridicule or other verbal insensitivity can be destructive to a child's confidence, and thus further stultify his capacity to learn. Large classes and bad working conditions often drive all but the best teachers into using negative means of maintaining discipline, particularly where they are faced with persistent misbehaviour by groups of children, defiance, breaches of school rules and damage to equipment, or else by passivity, boredom and lack of interest or initiative. Thus the ill-behaved and sometimes truanting child often experiences hostility from teachers rather than the skilled assessment and special teaching and work with his family which, as has been said earlier, is usually needed. Some truancy and delinquency is indeed a reaction to stress at school or in the home. The remedy is to locate and lessen the stress not to punish the child. A 'don't care' attitude to punishment is often a protection against and reaction to lack of parental affection. Here again punishment is inappropriate. The attention-seeking child, who even seems to provoke punishment, is usually trying to awaken response in a parent or parent substitute on the basis that even a negative response is better than indifference. 'Testing out' behaviour is also aimed at discovering the reality of a relationship. All this is not to deny that there are tough youngsters who sometimes need firm though not punitive control for their own sake and that of others. It is not easy to do this by non-physical means when physical violence is part of their way of life.

All that has been said makes it clear that those who impose controls or punishment should be aware of their own motives. This is especially necessary where sex offences, cruelty, neglect or violence are concerned. All these arouse strong retributive emotions which can obscure the need to understand causation and treat accordingly. Such understanding may indicate more drastic and long-term treatment measures than retribution, an eye for an eye or a tooth for a tooth. This creates a problem in juvenile courts where increasingly the attempt is to treat rather than to punish. This is an alien concept to most parents and children, whose views of human motivation are very different from those of psychiatrists and whose sense of justice is based upon a tariff system: an absolute or conditional discharge or a small fine or perhaps probation for the first offence, a stiffer fine, probation or an attendance centre order for the second, and, hopefully, subsequent offences; and only being 'put away' in the last resort when all else has failed. In short, treatment for disturbed relationships and behaviour, especially if it is 'only talking', is still an alien concept. Bridging this gap without outraging a child and his family's sense of justice is no easy task. It is also essential to remember that punishment itself is subjective: it only becomes punishment if it is experienced as such by the person at the receiving end. Thus to send a disturbed child away from home to a residential school may seem to one the extreme of punishment and to another a blessed release from an intolerable situation.

Most older children and adolescents understand restitution in the form of making good damage done, provided the restitution is directly related to the damage to, say, a stolen cycle, and that the amount does not take months to repay.

A few children in trouble are obsessed by guilt feelings which they seek to relieve by committing easily detected offences. The punishment they court will only temporarily relieve the guilt without touching its cause. Such 'offenders from a sense of guilt' naturally need psychiatric assessment and treatment. They are not to be confused with conflict-ridden children, usually timid and over-sensitive, who act out their conflicts; nor with those whose delinquent or wayward behaviour is a cry for help in a situation of, to them, intolerable pressure.

Trends in Juvenile Delinquency

Delinquency is a legal definition not a clinical or sociological concept. It ranges from riding a bicycle without lights to homicide and also embraces a wide diversity of children from the normal to the psychiatrically disturbed. The contributory factors are diverse and as yet not well understood. Treatment also tends to be based upon principles of punishment and deterrence, increasingly mixed with efforts at reform, with the difficulty that causation is complex and not easily amenable to change, assessment is far from perfect and comparatively little is known about what will deter or reform in the individual case. Moreover we are unsure whether concepts that derive from notions of moral judgment are as relevant as the more scientific non-judgmental attitudes of child guidance clinics, assuming that the aim of both courts and clinics is to help children and adults to become more able to accept social controls and to exercise choice in a responsible way. Children in trouble with the law are those who for various reasons are conspicuously failing to do this, whose parents are unwilling or unable to help them sufficiently and on whose behalf society has decided to intervene, for both their sake and that of the community. Down to the mid-nineteenth century the emphasis was almost wholly on the protection of the community: now the protection and reclamation of the child is given at least equal importance. Opinions differ as to which in the last resort should be given priority, though some deny a conflict. For instance, the White Paper *Children in Trouble* (1967) says: 'It has become increasingly clear that social control of harmful behaviour in the young, and social measures to help and protect the young, are not distinct and separate processes'.

Juvenile delinquency is more frequent in urban than rural areas and is predominantly a male phenomenon: only about 7 per cent of the offences found proved in any given year are committed by girls, though the actual percentage varies with age. The reasons for this are little understood, except that boys are more physically active and aggressive than girls. 'It has been pointed out with some justification that troublesome boys go in for crime, whereas troublesome girls merely go with boys' (West, 1967). Gibbens (1961) suggests that 'the girls tend to nurse their grievances and anxieties until adolescence, when they emerge suddenly in wayward or sexually promiscuous behaviour. One of the many problems in prevention is that, whatever is done for the boys, there will continue to be a number of girls who draw little attention to themselves until they emerge in adult life as the rejecting or unstable mothers of the next generation's delinquents'. The commonest offences by boys up to around the age of 14 are stealing and sometimes in addition breaking into enclosed premises. After 14 they tend to change from the adventurous offences to the 'proving' offences of rowdyism, malicious damage and taking and driving away cars and scooters. Delinquent adolescent girls typically go on shoplifting expeditions, either singly or in little groups.*

The criminal statistics seem to indicate an alarming increase in youthful offences per 100,000 of the population in the age group since 1938, though some of this is due to alterations in the law, some to changes in methods of detection, some to differences in police policies, some to a greater public willingness to report cases,

---

* For a valuable recent study of social and psychological factors see John and Valerie Cowie and Eliot Slater, *Delinquency in Girls*, Heinemann, 1968.

some to more open-counter shops and some to the steep rise in the number of motor vehicles on the roads.

Although the number of juvenile offenders has gone up very considerably since 1938 their percentage to offenders of all ages has remained fairly constant. It was 35·8 per cent in 1938 and 28·8 per cent in 1965. Apart from the peak at 14, the biggest increase has been in the 17 to 21 age group. Thereafter the rates per 100,000 population in the age groups fall dramatically from 35·4 per cent for boys of 14 to 4·2 per cent for men between 40 to 49 (1965 figures). Serious though youthful thefts, destructiveness and violence may be, it is also the long term trends that matter, whether the young offender becomes the adult criminal. Here the available evidence indicates that, although some of the most serious crimes of violence are committed by those under 21, the majority of youthful offenders do not become adult criminals. Delinquency indeed largely consists of offences against property committed by boys. The offences of teenage violence are largely group fights or rowdyism round dance halls, cafes and cinemas. The younger the delinquent when he is first convicted the more likely he is to commit further offences. About 50 per cent of the boys who appear before juvenile courts come back at least a second time and 25 per cent three or more times. It is important to detect these 'at risk' children and concentrate more effective treatment resources on them early. Ferguson and Cunnison's study of Glasgow schoolboys (1956) demonstrates, like other similar studies, that the bulge of delinquency and proneness to reconviction persists up to the age of 18. Delinquency is thus to a large extent a self-limiting complaint which attacks boys rather than girls. We do not know to what extent the successes claimed by various forms of treatment are really due to the subject beginning to recover from the attack. But comparatively few continue and become adult recidivists. The aggressive youthful offender tends to settle down in the 20's with marriage and family responsibilities, though we do not know why this happens. Conversely many adult recidivists have no record of convictions as juveniles. They tend to be inadequate, solitary men who have probably got by with sufficient protection in childhood and youth but prove unable to meet the demands of adult life.

Much delinquency, from petty larceny to sex offences, is under-reported. Various studies show the actual percentage of delinquents in the general population to be very much higher than the criminal statistics suggest. The percentage of boys appearing before a court before their eighteenth birthday ranges from over 12 per cent in some districts to over 45 per cent in others. But these percentages are very much higher for undetected delinquencies admitted by boys to research workers. One group of 180 boys of 15 to 17 admitted to 69,468 offences, mainly larcenies and traffic offences, of which 90 per cent were undetected. Juvenile delinquents who appear before the courts thus represent an unknown proportion of the total and their characteristics may or may not differ from deviants in general. These findings suggest that much delinquency is 'normal' being regarded as scrounging, winning, nicking, or borrowing, rather than theft. Middle class parents are likely to take a more disapproving attitude towards property offences but these, when detected, are more likely to be dealt with within the family, or the school. Many offences which require education, like fiddling income tax returns and firms' expenses, or embezzlement or false pretences, are not normally youthful offences. The fascinating question remains whether young delinquents are on the whole more likely to become law-abiding citizens if they are detected and treated as children in trouble or if they escape detection and being so labelled and dealt with.

Drug taking is increasing rapidly amongst both boys and girls, sometimes while they are still at school. Their number far exceeds the figures of those found guilty of being in illegal possession of certain 'soft' or 'hard' drugs. In many towns there are drug risks in some schools, coffee bars and youth clubs. There are many groups of young people who take soft drugs, mainly marijuana, amphetamines or barbiturates. They speak of feelings of exultation, of belonging, of release from inadequacy, shyness, and difficulties in making relationships, of escape from depression or anxiety or other personality problems, and of a greater sense of freedom and adequacy. Individuals say they start because everyone is doing it, for curiosity, for kicks, for a new experience. Some are fairly stable members of delinquent groups in their locality. Others may be adolescents from a rather narrow middle class background who have become alienated from their parents' way of life and values. Sometimes they drift away from home and join other rootless young people.

There is much controversy as to whether soft drugs are necessarily harmful with a serious risk of the youngster become 'hooked' on hard drugs (primarily heroin) or whether this happens for social and personality reasons.* Once addicted, a boy or girl may become alienated from family and friends. At this stage it is vital to help and support the family and that the youngster should experience personal friendship as well as being helped to accept treatment. There has been an acute shortage of treatment facilities, both out- and in-patient, in clinics and hospitals; this is beginning to be remedied as more treatment centres are opened. But many youngsters revert to drug taking after hospital treatment through lack of prolonged rehabilitation and aftercare to support and re-educate them. Recovery from either drug or alcohol addiction seems to be closely related to the social setting to which the addict returns and the amount of individual help and encouragement he receives.

Psychiatrists and others concerned with delinquent and wayward youth agree that there has been an increase in the number of seriously disturbed children and adolescents, both boys and girls, whose violent, bizarre or suicidal behaviour or persistent absconding or drug taking disrupts any ordinary children's home, approved school or hostel. But this may represent a constant proportion of the increased number of children appearing before the juvenile courts, while it may also indicate better services rather than an actual increase in the incidence of psychiatric disturbance.

Children and adolescents brought before juvenile courts as being in need of care nearly always present serious problems on account of their family and social circumstances and often because of the interrelation between these and their own

* See for example, the report of the Wootton Committee (1969) *Cannabis*, London, H.M.S.O.

personality problems. Many young people charged with offences present no great problem and the prognosis is good but compulsory care proceedings are usually the end of the road after other services have failed to help sufficiently or when there has been a family crisis, sometimes leading to an illegitimate pregnancy, to running away from home, or to cruelty or neglect.

Identification, Assessment and Treatment of Children at Risk

Research casts light on some children in certain families and social circumstances who will be more at risk than others. This suggests that more resources should be concentrated on help to such children as early as possible; though children in trouble are only part of a larger group of children in need of special care for the sake of their mental health. Moreover some children who become neurotic or delinquent may do so as a result of a precipitating crisis or temptation rather than clearly predisposing circumstances.

The known facts about high risk neighbourhoods have led to a few experiments in extra provision for educational priority areas as recommended in the Plowden Report (1967). There are further plans for comprehensive government-sponsored community development projects in areas of special need with a concentration of 'high need' families. Pioneer experiments like the Bristol Survey (Spencer, 1964), Avenues Unlimited (1967), the Sparkbrook Association (Rex and Moore, 1967) and others suggest that it is essential to use community development methods to arouse the active interest and co-operation of local people in decision making and implementation of plans to improve the environment and raise their own standards. Most parents want to do their best for their children but may be too overwhelmed, incompetent or lacking in confidence or ability to be able to do so. Any comprehensive plans for children at risk must therefore include the parents rather than still further usurping their function. Some of the pioneer family advice centres set up by Children's departments soon made this discovery (Leissner, 1967). It has been made in other forms by those running play centres, including those for culturally deprived children (Wilson 1966).

The most specific legal requirement to help children at risk is contained in section I of the Children and Young Persons Act, 1963. There is no uniformity of provision by Children's departments under this section: some have barely begun to implement it, while others are experimenting with play groups, holidays, home helps, efforts to keep the family together when the mother has died or deserted, help in cash or kind, and almost anything else that may be appropriate in individual circumstances to prevent children from having to be received into care or appearing before a juvenile court.

Children Under Five

The Children's departments and health visitors (who are increasingly working with general practitioners) and child health centres are the main sources for detection of children under 5 who are at risk. The means of help include support of many kinds from family planning, budgeting or practical advice about child care to parent counselling for mothers and fathers who are incompetent, rejecting, frustrated or overwhelmed. Perhaps the largest proportion of this latter group are the very immature, those of low intelligence and those whose own life experience makes them incapable of loving and reasonably efficient parenthood. A high concentration of such adverse factors as high infant mortality rates, frequent admission to hospital and reception into care is found amongst children in large families of unskilled manual workers. They also include mentally disordered parents. The children of unmarried or unsupported mothers are also often at risk because their mothers cannot cope with a combination of caring for them, work, loneliness and difficulties with landladies.

Unfortunately many small children at risk are not taken to child health centres and otherwise remain undetected until a drama or a tragedy brings them before a juvenile court in need of care. They include the classic cases of physical neglect, dirt, lack of clothing, insufficient food. These incompetent parents may be affectionate and can sometimes be helped with much support on family service unit lines to keep their home together. Sometimes the mother has gone out, leaving the children alone in physical danger or emotional distress; or the mother has deserted and the father has tried to look after the children, asking a neighbour to 'drop in' when he is at work rather than seeking help from the social services for fear his children will be taken away from him. Ill-treatment of children includes not only indifference and neglect but also the battered children whose apparent proneness to accidents has made a hospital suspicious when X-rays reveal mended but unreported fractures. Abandoned children are also sometimes brought before a juvenile court, though this is unnecessary as the local authority Children's department can receive them into care under Section I of the Children Act, 1948.

Children of School Age

Once children start going to school, the education system should be the first line of defence and detection through teachers, psychologists, education welfare officers and the school health service.

The three main sources for the socialisation of children are the family, the neighbourhood and the school. The first two initiate them into the local culture and standards of behaviour. These may or may not be synonymous with the standards of morals and conduct upheld by the school. Schools which demand standards directly opposed to those of home and neighbourhood may precipitate truancy or delinquency as an escape from an intolerable conflict of demands.

Some teachers say they can 'spot the troublemakers' from the primary school stage, though others deny this. The Gluecks' famous prediction tables have validated various factors, of which the family cohesiveness and the quality of maternal supervision and discipline are the most important, as high risk predictors from about the age of six. Stott's Bristol Social Adjustment Guide (1958) has also proved effective in spotting incipient delinquency on the basis of certain behaviour in class. What matters is not only identification, whether on tested prediction studies or individual hunches, but what follows from it. Sometimes to identify a child as a potential troublemaker merely results in a self-fulfilling prophesy instead of a comprehensive and skilled assessment of the child, his family and his circumstances with a view to providing help suited to his and his family's needs. Such children should be assessed wherever possible by a psychiatrist or educational psychologist. They are often emotionally and culturally deprived, aggressive and hostile. They need skilled education and socialisation in small classes, coupled with other means of compensation for what their families and neighbourhood are unable to provide. At the same time, long-term social work support to the family, including material help where necessary, may result in lessened tensions, insecurity and failure of communication.

Appropriate action by schools and Children's or Social Work departments indeed depends on accurate assessment of the individual child showing early signs of delinquency or waywardness. This skilled assessment for the purpose of deciding upon appropriate action is all the more necessary since youthful delinquency can occur in children who run the gamut from the healthy and normal to the severely maladjusted. It is as ill-judged to suggest psychotherapy for a child whose standards are formed round delinquent family values as it is to punish a rejected child who is symbolically stealing love from his mother's purse or the family larder.

Early detection or preventive action is also more likely where classes are small enough and teachers sufficiently interested and well informed to encourage children to talk to them about their doings and the things that trouble them. There is, for example, a familiar connection between illness or death or the birth of a new baby or the mother's or father's re-marriage and delinquency. If children were able to talk out their anxieties, sorrows and hostilities naturally and quickly these might less frequently explode in forms that add fuel to the fire.

Fortunately many schools nowadays actively encourage parents to visit the school, talk with teachers and get to know what they are trying to achieve with the children: unfortunately the parents of troublesome and troubled children are the ones least likely to do so. This may be due to ignorance, distrust of 'them', feeling tongue-tied and awkward, or plain indifference or hostility. Sometimes such parents only have contact with the school through 'the school board man' because of the children's non-attendance. It is all too common to discover in the juvenile court disturbances of behaviour that could have been detected and dealt with at some much earlier stage, but nothing was done because no one noticed or at any rate took action. What is several people's or services' responsibility is often no-one's, particularly where troublesome children are concerned. As the Seebohm Report says: 'The present state of knowledge (particularly of what tends to produce persistent offenders), is not sufficient to enable anyone to say with confidence how effective particular measures are in preventing children developing obvious social needs which cannot be met. But that does not excuse the community from trying, by the best means available, to prevent trouble arising. Some of the means may be so obviously right on general grounds of humanity (for instance the provision of better housing and better social care for the under fives) that there is everything to be said for pressing ahead with them even though knowledge of their exact beneficial effects may be lacking. Common sense suggests that measures which look promising should be tried and systematically evaluated.'

Some schools are appointing as school counsellors teachers who are specially designated to help children who need or want to talk about things that are bothering them. Some school counsellors are trained teachers who have also taken a course in counselling. The Seebohm Report suggests that social workers on the staff of the proposed social service departments should be attached to schools.

It is agreed that truanting from school is in itself a danger signal. What a child does when he truants is a clue to the cause: if he is with several other children they may be truanting because neither they nor their families think going to school really matters; or girls may be kept at home to help; both girls and boys may be finding the educational pressures too high; school phobia or withdrawal is another aspect of non-attendance with a different cause. Kahn and Nursten (1968) sum up non-attendance thus: 'A truant is usually thought of as a child who is absent from school without his parents' or the school's permission, although there is another type of truant who is kept at home by his parents because the child can be of some direct help by his presence within the family. Either the child or the parents can initiate absence from school. If it is the child who starts it, unknown to the parent, it can be called truancy; if it is the parent who openly encourages the child to stay away, it can be called school withdrawal. Both are social problems. By contrast, the child with school phobia may want to go to school, but he finds that he *cannot*. He is suffering from an emotional problem, based on acute anxiety at the thought of leaving home. It is because he fears leaving home that he cannot go to school. In fact, school phobia is a misleading term as it is only the result of another problem, the source of which is the tie between parent and child and its ensuing conflicts. These brief definitions show that the social problem of truancy and the emotional and pathological problem of school phobia are very different.' At present few school welfare officers are trained either to detect or to handle the more complex cases of truancy.

In some areas cases of school refusal may be referred either to a child guidance clinic or to the Children's department (in Scotland the Social Work department). It is unfortunately common for cases of non-attendance at school only to come before the juvenile courts after a series of warnings to the parents, and sometimes after they have been fined in the adult court, but without any real diagnostic assessment having been made of the reasons why the child is truanting. Moreover the trouble has often continued for a considerable time, with the result that it is all the more difficult to re-establish the habit of going to school as well as detecting and attempting to deal with the underlying causes. Remedial teaching is also likely to be needed. Obviously children who truant with others for a bit of excitement may also steal, indeed young delinquents often have a record of truancy.

No general information is available about the extent to which the schools, the children's service and the police deal with children known to be in trouble without bringing them before a juvenile court. It is often suggested that the small number of middle class children charged with offences does not necessarily indicate respect for the law but rather police unwillingness to charge, coupled with a common expectation that the school and the family will deal effectively with the situation. Some, notably Baroness Wootton, argue that it would be better for all children in trouble to be dealt with within the education system. Others think that the school has no particular expertise in this, that such children are often regarded as a nuisance and that beyond a certain point schools as such are not equipped to understand or treat them and their families. Children in trouble cannot be effectively helped without involving their families and usually not without also trying to bring about favourable changes in their spare time activities, their attitudes and the companions with whom they associate. This calls for extended and imaginative provision, including experimental use of group therapy.

The part played by the police is affected by local community attitudes and by the policy in different police forces. In certain cities in England and Scotland there are police juvenile liaison schemes. In some of these, specially selected officers may with the parents' agreement regularly visit the home of a child who is giving trouble, has committed a minor offence, or is out of parental control, or is an adolescent in bad company or moral danger. Formal cautioning at a police station is fairly widely used. In many districts the police have friendly contacts with youth clubs and schools, often giving talks on some aspect of the law, especially road safety and traffic offences.

In favour of preventive work by the police, it is argued that they often know a neighbourhood and its cross currents extremely well, that they can communicate with children and their parents more effectively than middle class teachers and social workers, that they embody the social controls which children must learn to observe, and that a quick police caution or regular visits to the home are often more effective than the long drawn out ordeal of a court appearance. Moreover, shopkeepers and others are more willing to report juvenile thefts if they know these will be dealt with quickly by the police rather than entailing long waits in court. On the other hand, it is argued that the police may have punitive attitudes and too clear-cut and simple views of human behaviour, that they are insufficiently trained to detect the difference between naughty boys from ordinary families and severely disturbed family relationships, so that they may actually worsen a situation by warnings and admonitions or trying to do the work for which probation and child care officers are trained, and in any event thereby postponing systematic assessment and treatment.*

The relation between juvenile delinquency and broken homes or homes where there is marital conflict, large families, poverty, overcrowding or other stress, suggests the need for much more adequate services in terms of time, resources, universality and skill than are at present available. This also applies to the personal social services in general. As the Seebohm Report says 'The need for a more unified provision of personal social services has been made plain by growing

* For an interesting account of a training course in Scotland see Mack, J. A. (1968). *Police Juvenile Liaison—Practice and Evaluation*, School of Social Study, University of Glasgow.

knowledge and experience. There is a realisation that it is essential to look beyond the immediate symptoms of social distress to the underlying problems. These frequently prove to be complicated and the outcome of a variety of influences. In many cases people who need help cannot be treated effectively unless this is recognised. Their difficulties do not arise in a social vacuum; they are, have been, or need to be involved in a network of relationships, in social situations. The family and the community are seen as the contexts in which problems arise and in which most of them have to be resolved or contained.'

The doctor's surgery is one of the key points for early detection of conflict, disturbed family relationships or other stress but there is inadequate liaison at present between the family doctor and the local authority services. There have been a few experimental attachments of social workers to general practice teams (Goldberg *et al.*, 1968) and the Seebohm Report recommends that these should be extended. Children who show incipient signs of disturbance or backwardness in school or whose physical defects may be contributing to wayward behaviour may be referred to the school health service and sometimes from there to a child guidance clinic. Unfortunately some families most in need of help are those least likely to keep appointments.

As has been said, 14 is the peak age for stealing and related offences, *i.e.* one year before the school leaving age. It is sometimes suggested that for many boredom and for some anxiety about leaving school are connected with this.

Adolescents at Risk

Once boys and girls have left school there is no universal comprehensive service ot meet their needs and to which they will readily turn. The youth service itself is inadequate in the range and sometimes the quality of its provision. Many young people may be in the streets because there is no club for them to join. The youth employment service often takes great pains with youths who register with a Youth Employment Bureau and constantly change their jobs but its powers and its staff are limited.

Workers with unattached youth and those working with young drug takers have shed light on the extent to which some young people are alienated and adrift or may be turned out of their homes periodically. It is strange that we provide no comprehensive social care services for the two most vulnerable groups, the under fives and those of 15 years upwards, both of whom are at the maximum points of emotional, physical and mental development.

Pioneer projects include the appointment of unattached workers to mix with street corner groups (Morse, 1965: Goetschius and Tash, 1967), or experimental coffee bars and clubs (Biven and Holden 1966). The purpose of the first is to meet alienated young people on their own ground and of the second to provide meeting places that would attract them. Such projects try to demonstrate that the workers want to know and make a relationship with young people who are rejected by most adults. This relationship may lead some young people to seek counselling help that might result in their breaking out of the vicious spiral of unhappy, hostile children who often grow into antisocial adults and who as parents cannot give to their children the security they have never experienced themselves. These imaginative projects are suggesting hopeful new methods but their number is pitifully inadequate to the need. Moreover, because they impose enormous strains on the staff regular psychiatric consultation is essential.

Juvenile Courts and Children's Hearings

The juvenile court system began with the Children Act, 1908. The Social Work (Scotland) Act, 1968, embodies in law changes in attitude which are as revolutionary as those which took children out of the adult courts 60 years ago. It was preceded by a number of reports and White Papers (see Chapter 17). Perhaps the dominant notes in all the controversy and discussion have been a desire to spare children the stigma of criminality; a feeling that when 95 per cent plead guilty to the charge, court hearings are frequently superfluous; a desire to encourage the more active participation of parents; and a belief that agreement about desirable action could often be reached without a court appearance. All these issues, particularly the last one, are naturally controversial.

Some hold strongly that children have a right to a court appearance as a safeguard against being wrongfully accused and subjected to intervention in their lives, and that decisions about compulsory action, particularly being sent away from home, should only be made by a court. Others reply that innocence or guilt is not so relevant as whether intervention is needed in order to give additional help and support to some children and their families. They also point out that adults frequently interfere in children's lives without their consent and that to be sent away to a boarding school for social reasons is basically no different from being sent to a boarding school for educational reasons or to a residential special school for health reasons. All are agreed that where the child or his parents contest the reasons for his appearance or where they do not agree to the proposed treatment the case should be heard in a court of law within the rules of evidence.

There is also general agreement about the need for a sieve or series of sieves to catch the child at risk of becoming delinquent or who has begun to get himself into trouble, in order to forestall a court appearance. Everyone also agrees about the importance of much more effective interaction between the school, the home and the community, including school counselling and, at an early stage, skilled assessment of the reasons for truancy. Most people at least pay lip service to the need for more play groups, camps, youth clubs, vocational guidance and counselling services for young people. The two sieves closest to the juvenile court or children's hearing are the police juvenile liaison schemes and the powers and duties of local authority Children's or Social Work departments under Section I of the Children and Young Persons Act, 1963. The different official policies for England and Wales and for Scotland are united in intention to strengthen these first lines of defence. Indeed in each it is proposed to change the whole balance so that instead of some children in trouble being dealt with by the police or the social services who would otherwise come before the courts, the main weight of responsibility will rest upon these services and only a minority of children who cannot be helped without a court order for their own welfare and the protection of the community will come before the courts.

In England and Wales, when the Children and Young Persons Act, 1969, comes into operation, such cases will continue to be heard in the existing juvenile courts, which will also continue to hear charges against young people between their fourteenth and seventeenth birthdays. All juvenile court magistrates will be selected by the Lord Chancellor for inclusion on the juvenile court panels. Magistrates are already required to undergo some training. In Scotland the juvenile courts will be abolished after 1970 and all cases will be heard by children's hearings, constituted from children's panels whose members will be appointed by the Secretary of State for Scotland. Both juvenile courts and children's hearings consist of three members, of whom one must be a woman and one the chairman.

The revolutionary consequence of these administrative and legal changes is that in time there should be early identification of children with social or emotional handicap, assessment at properly staffed and equipped assessment centres, and planning and action on a variety of fronts to lessen the social disabilities that beset them and their families and to provide any specific treatment they may need. This day is not yet but at least we are clearer about aims, even if paucity of knowledge and resources still limit their achievement. When the Children and Young Persons Act comes into full operation the age of criminal responsibility will be 14 (England and Wales). Below that age all cases (except homicide) will be heard as care proceedings. In Scotland the age is to be 16 (though the Lord Advocate may decide that certain serious cases shall be heard in the Sheriff's Court or the High Court). The commission of an offence will be one of the grounds on which a child will be alleged to be in need of compulsory measures of care. Others will be that he is in moral danger or his proper development is being avoidably prevented, or he is neglected or ill-treated, or beyond his parents' control, or not receiving efficient full-time education. It will be necessary for the person bringing the case to prove not only one of these circumstances but also that the child is unlikely to receive the care or control he needs unless the court or the children's hearing makes an order.

These will be those cases where the efforts of the Children's or Social Work department or the police have not been successful or where it is initially evident 'that voluntary help would not be enough—because for example, the child and his family are not willing to co-operate, or deny the need for any intervention, or because despite their intention to co-operate the family are too infirm of purpose to do so effectively'.

The arrangements for bringing children before the court or the hearing are the same in intention though administratively different. In Scotland an official called a Reporter, appointed by the local authority, is responsible for arranging children's hearings and also for investigating every case referred to him by the police or the local authority or any other source. He may, after investigation, either decide that no further action is required and so inform the child and his parents, or refer the case to the local authority for advice, guidance and assistance, or, if he thinks the child needs compulsory care, arrange a hearing and get reports on the child's social background. He also ensures that the decisions of the hearing are carried out and periodically reviewed.

The child's parents have both the right and duty to be present at every stage of a hearing. This also applies to the juvenile courts in England and Wales. A court or hearing may also ask either the child or his parents to withdraw if it wishes to speak to either in the absence of the other. The Reporters are given considerable powers in relation to access to and the conduct of children's hearings. In England and Wales there will be a different system. Care proceedings will be brought by the police, the local authority or 'other authorized person'. Young people between the age of criminal responsibility and 17 may only be charged with an offence by a 'qualified informant' (the local authority, the police or an officer of the Crown) and if the case cannot be adequately dealt with by for example the parents, the school, the Children's department, a police caution, or care proceedings. In any event, the local authority must be consulted and, unless urgent action is necessary, information will be sought from those who know the youngster and his family before action is taken. The factors likely to be taken into account would include the gravity of the offence, or on the contrary that there is not very much wrong and a court appearance and a fine or other deterrent will probably be sufficient; or if the offence was committed with someone else who is to be prosecuted; or if it is known that action without the backing of a court order is not likely to succeed.

In care proceedings the court will hear all the relevant circumstances from the witnesses and the child and his parents and then decide whether or not the case is proved and also whether it is necessary to make an order. At a children's hearing the chairman will explain to the child and his parents the grounds for the referral of the case. If they agree with these the hearing will proceed. If they do not agree the referral may either be discharged or the case be sent to the Sheriff (sitting in chambers) for a finding on the facts. The Sheriff after hearing the case can either dismiss it or, if he decides that the grounds for the referral have been established, return it for a further children's hearing to decide what action will be in the best interests of the child.

Any wise juvenile court will try to include the child and his parents in discussions about the action that should follow from the court appearance. They must in any event be told the main points in the school, probation, Children's department, psychiatric or other reports received by the court. They are less likely to co-operate if they feel that arbitrary decisions have been made without their own views being taken into account. But if the alternatives and the reasons for preferring one decision to another are discussed with them they will often agree, even to removal from home, except perhaps in those neighbourhoods where this is the final calamity. Nonetheless, juvenile courts have power to make orders without the agreement of the parties concerned and sometimes must do so. There is a right of appeal to a higher court. In Scotland if the child and his parents accept the hearing's decision it will become binding but if not they can appeal to the Sheriff against the decision. He will either confirm the decision or, if he decides that it was not justified, remit the case back for a further hearing or else discharge it.

The effect of these new provisions is that two different systems will be in operation in Britain, the one based on decisions which are only binding with the child and his parents' consent, the other based on decisions that are binding without consent. Some say the consent will be Hobson's choice, that it is harmful to a child to hear his parents consent to his being 'put away' and that if they do not agree and the case goes to the Sheriff this will merely drag out the proceedings unnecessarily, when under the juvenile court system one tribunal can gain co-operation or exercise compulsion. In any event, it should only be necessary to bring cases to court where consent to treatment or control would not be forthcoming otherwise. On the other side it is argued that the children's hearings will be a more effective means of involving parents and children in facing bad behaviour, their own responsibilities in relation to it, and discussion about the causes of such behaviour and what effort and support are needed by and for the family to enable it to function better. It is also suggested that if a child is sent away from home without the family having a part in the decision this faces him with their powerlessness to protect him from 'them' and reinforces the belief that this is a punishment for his wrong doing rather than a positive measure to help him overcome his difficulties, however much he may dislike this.

In the 1970's we shall have in Britain two divergent systems with the same aim. It is greatly to be hoped that from their beginning inbuilt research and evaluation will enable us in time to learn what in each system is more and what less effective in helping children and families in trouble and thus also protecting the community.

As important as the nature of the tribunal is the way in which it conducts its proceedings. The children's hearings are presumably free from many of the legal formalities so confusing to children and parents in the juvenile courts: yet it is essential to emphasise dignity, order and a fair and impartial hearing. It is essential for any tribunal to have sufficient time to hear each case without a sense of rush and without children, their parents and others having to wait for hours in crowded waiting rooms. It is also important that the magistrates or panel should be able to communicate with children and their parents. This can be difficult when the proceedings are formal and members of the tribunal are predominantly middle class and children and their parents predominantly working class, with different linguistic codes, and often a different standard of values and behaviour. This reinforces a lively sense of the gap between 'them' and 'us' and the duty to protect 'our Johnny' from 'them', coupled with belief in the tariff system in relation to offences and punishment. Moreover, most parents and children do not expect that a court will listen to them, try to understand them as individuals, and think their point of view important. They may only be able to put into words concrete happenings rather than intangible relationships; and in any event, working class values and norms—like middle class ones—differ considerably even within one district. Bridging these gaps, particularly when most people are anxious, some truculent and others only wanting to get it over and done with, poses problems which have as yet only begun to be identified.

It is obvious that juvenile court magistrates and members of children's panels should not only be chosen for their ability to understand and communicate with a variety of young people in trouble and their parents but also that they should have systematic and 'live' training in this and in the complex causation of wayward behaviour, as well as in necessary elements of the law. It is envisaged that in future there will be much closer and more systematic consultation than in the past between magistrates or panel members, the local authority, the police and the probation service and voluntary organisations, both about individual cases and about general provision for children in trouble.

Assessment and Prediction

The new arrangements presuppose that children who are actually or potentially in trouble will be known to and be systematically assessed by the education and children's services, and sometimes by psychiatrists, psychologists, general practitioners and the police. As things are this is not a valid assumption because of our lack of resources for comprehensive assessment, planning and reassessment in the light of changing circumstances. It would be disastrous if the alternative to action by the juvenile court were no action or less effective action. The courts at present receive assessment reports from probation officers, the school and sometimes from the Children's department and a psychiatrist. Often these different assessments are made in isolation from each other and sometimes under artificial conditions. At present the most consistent attempts at classification are made at classifying approved schools but this is a late stage and classification is only effective if a wide range of treatment is available suited to very different needs.

Forms of Treatment

The range of decisions available to juvenile courts or children's hearings is to be reduced but the variety of treatment facilities increased. For children up to 14 (16 in Scotland) there will be the alternatives of supervision, intermediate treatment, binding over the parents for the children's good behaviour (England and Wales), or a care order or a hospital or guardianship order under the Mental Health Act, 1959. Juvenile courts will in addition continue to be able to fine young people found guilty of offences (14 to 17), require them to pay damages or costs, or discharge them absolutely or conditionally. Remand homes and approved schools as such are to be abolished. They will be used as part of a more flexible system for observation and residential treatment. Attendance centres and detention centres will also by degrees cease to be available.

In England and Wales residential treatment will be by way of a care order to the local authority. This will enable the Children's department to use whatever is the best available residential institution for the particular child or place him in a foster home or try him back in his own home as seems best in changing circumstances. A care order will last till the age of 18 (in certain circumstances 19). It may be revoked by the court on the application of the local authority, the child or his parents, at any time if it thinks this desirable.

The Scottish system is rather different in that the children's hearing is required to review each order for supervision or residential treatment at least once a year, or at the request of the local authority, or (at an interval of not less than 3 months) a child, or his parents may request a review of the order. The children's hearing may continue, vary or terminate an order. No child is subject to supervision (which may include a residential provision) longer than is necessary in his interest.

Supervision Orders

In future only supervision not probation orders will be made for any young person under 17. In Scotland probation officers are now part of the local authority Social Work department. In England and Wales the separate probation and aftercare service will continue. Supervision orders for children under 14 are to be to the local authority Children's department unless a probation officer is already working with the family; between 14 and 17 an order may be made either to the local authority or a probation officer (England and Wales). In Scotland all such orders will be to the Social Work department. Many children placed under supervision will already be known to the Children's or Social Work department and the order will thus be a more formal continuance of casework already started with them and their families. This should be based upon as accurate as possible an assessment of all the elements in the situation which contribute to the child's antisocial or disturbed behaviour, whether in himself, the family relationships, the school or the neighbourhood. The aim should be to make an effective relationship with the child and his family, both for support and control, using professional understanding and competence to help bring about changes in ability to function better. This will naturally include working closely with the school and other social services and related professions. The range of children and young people under supervision varies from the normal to the most severely disturbed or antisocial. The very fact of dealing with many children in trouble outside the courts or hearings will mean that it is only the most difficult cases whom we know least how to treat or control constructively who will be subject to supervision orders.

Conditions may be inserted in a supervision order. These may include living with a named person, receiving some form of intermediate treatment (see below) or treatment for his mental condition.

Intermediate Treatment

This is the new title to be given to various forms of treatment as part of a supervision order but which do not entail long-term removal from home. The first category will consist of short residence or participation in some activity for a total of up to 30 days in each year. It could include evenings or weekends in some recreational activity or work project or social service or adventure training. The second category will entail residence for not more than a total of 90 days in a year at a specified place.

Intermediate treatment is intended for children who can be helped by casework in their homes but who also need a short period or periods away for fresh and stimulating experience and better human relationships. Existing examples are the attendance centres run on Saturdays by the police (these are to be remodelled and become part of the general provision), outward bound courses and the Duke of Edinburgh's award scheme. Northorpe Hall is an imaginative experiment in which delinquent boys between 9 and 13 are offered the opportunity of spending a weekend a month in groups of 9 or 10 at a house near Leeds where the staff give them an experience of happy, friendly, family life with plenty of interests and activity. There is simultaneous casework with the family. The various new forms of intermediate treatment are largely based on the premise that much delinquency results from boredom, social ineptitude and a poor social and physical environment. Many delinquents steal in little groups or take other people's cars or scooters for the excitement as well as because they may suffer from thin or damaging human relationships.

The twofold aim is thus to give young people richer and more varied experience and excitement by legitimate means, and in close contact with interested and helpful adults. The principle applies to all ages from pre-school play groups to projects for adolescents.

Residential Provision

The intention of new legislation is that the range of residential provision shall be extended and freed from the entrance requirement that now separates approved schools and remand homes from the rest. Thus it will all be potentially available to any child needing care whether or not he has been in trouble with the law or found to be in need of care. These institutions are to be comprehensively named community homes. Residential schools for maladjusted and educationally sub-normal children will remain part of special educational provision. Aftercare will it is hoped be more comprehensive and continue as long as necessary after the compulsory period ends.

Those who need residential provision range from abandoned, battered or neglected children to young people convicted of violent crime, in need of treatment for mental disorder or 'hooked' on hard drugs. Many children committed to the care of local authorities are boarded out with foster parents, while efforts are made to keep in touch with the families of all children, where possible to allow them home for holidays, and to return them home 'on trial' when it seems likely that they may be able to remain at home.

Under the Children and Young Persons Act, 1969, children's regional planning committees have been set up. They will develop a full range of observation, assessment and residential facilities (including hostels) for children and young people in co-operation with the health and education services and voluntary organisations. Some of the present approved schools will become ordinary boarding schools, others may concentrate on social education or provide secure accommodation or other special provision for children or young people who are severely disturbed or antisocial. Effective residential provision for children in trouble will mean facing the enormous task of accurately assessing the needs of individual children, determining the right grouping for different community homes, providing a stimulating regime and, most important and difficult of all, helping 'to produce satisfactory personal relationships for . . . boys and girls and . . . (to help them) to gain satisfaction from their own identity as people, as potentially productive men and women' (Miller, 1968). This requires staff adequate in numbers, trained to understand the needs of disturbed children and young people and with the warmth and maturity to offer them a stable relationship, which some will test out to the uttermost. All community homes should be essentially therapeutic communities in whatever form is appropriate to the age and needs of the children, though some will cater for those who need this under security conditions.

Residential treatment for severely disturbed young people between the ages of 12 and 19 needing psychiatric treatment will be provided jointly by the Home Office and the Department of Health and Social Security in Youth Treatment Centres.

Conclusion

From all that has been said, it is obvious that a very wide range of services and facilities is needed to help children in trouble, that many of these, like better housing or smaller school classes or more play groups or better provision for adolescents, are necessary for all young people. And that services should be organised to provide both comprehensive assessment and continuity of care so long as it is needed. It is equally obvious that these services can only be effective if more and better qualified staff of all kinds with the right personalities are available. This applies to teachers, social workers, psychologists and psychiatrists, and with special force to the staff of residential institutions. All are in short supply and in particular those able to communicate with disturbed youngsters and to withstand the enormous strain of working with them.

Lastly, the gaps in our knowledge are obvious. There is need for far more research, controlled experiment and evaluation if we are to find ways of lessening the number of today's children in trouble who will in time repeat the pattern with their children, and if we are to discover how to improve the environment and lessen the social stresses which help to produce delinquent, antisocial, maladjusted or inadequate personalities.

EILEEN L. YOUNGHUSBAND

Note. The Local Authority Social Services Bill at present (Summer 1970) before Parliament provides for the amalgamation in new social service departments of the present children's and welfare departments and certain other local authority functions in England and Wales.

References

AVENUES UNLIMITED (1967). *Technical Summary of the Second Project Report.*

BIVEN, B. and HOLDEN, H. M. (1966). Informal youth work in a cafe setting. *Howard J. Penology*, **12**, 1.

Children and their Primary Schools (1967). London: H.M.S.O. (The Plowden report).

Children in Trouble (1967). London: H.M.S.O.

DOWNES, D. M. (1966). *The Delinquent Solution.* London: Routledge.

FERGUSON, T. (1952). *The Young Delinquent and his Social Setting.* London: Oxf. Univ. Press.

—— and CUNNISON, J. (1956). *In Their Early Twenties.* London: Oxf. Univ. Press.

FRIEDLANDER, K. (1947). *The Psychoanalytical Approach to Juvenile Delinquency.* London: Routledge.

GIBBENS, T. C. N. (1961). *Trends in Juvenile Delinquency.* Publ. Hlth Papers No. 5. Geneva: W.H.O.

—— (1963). *Psychiatric Studies of Borstal Lads.* Maudsley Monographs No. 11. London: Oxf. Univ. Press.

GLUECK, S. and GLUECK, E. (1950). *Unravelling Juvenile Delinquency.* Harvard: Oxf. Univ. Press.

GOETSCHIUS, G. W. and TASH, M. J. (1967). *Working with Unattached Youth.* London: Routledge.

GOLDBERG, E. M., NEILL, J., SPEKE, B. M. and FAULKNER, H. C. (1968). Social work in general practice. *Lancet*, **2**, 552.

KAHN, J. H. and NURSTEN, J. P. (1968). *Unwillingly to School.* 2nd ed. London: Pergamon.

LEISSNER, A. (1967). *Family Advice Services: Studies in Child Development.* London: Longmans.

MANNHEIM, H. (1965). *Comparative Criminology.* London: Routledge.

MAYS, J. B. (1959). *On the Threshold of Delinquency.* Liverpool: Univ. Press.

MILLER, D. (1968). Schools for young offenders. *Howard J. Penology*, **14**, 231.

MORRIS, T. (1957). *The Criminal Area.* London: Routledge.

MORSE, M. (1965). *The Unattached.* London: Penguin books.

PIAGET, J. (1932). *The Moral Judgment of the Child.* London: Routledge.

POWER, M. (1967). Epidemiological studies of delinquency. *J. Med. Women's Fed.*, **49**, 4.

POWER, M. J., ALDERSON, M. R., PHILLIPSON, C. M., SHOENBERG, E. and MORRIS, J. N. (1967). Delinquent schools? *New Society*, **10**, 542.

Report of the Committee on Local Authority and Allied Personal Social Services. Cmnd 3703. London: H.M.S.O. (The Seebohm report).

REX, J. and MOORE, R. (1967). *Race, Community and Conflict: A Study of Sparkbrook.* London: Oxf. Univ. Press.

Social Work and the Community (1967). London: H.M.S.O.

SPENCER, J. (1964). *Stress and Release on an Urban Estate.* London: Tavistock.

SPROTT, W. J. H. (1954). *The Social Background of Delinquency.* Nottingham: Univ. Press.

STOTT, D. H. (1958). *The Social Adjustment of Children.* London: Univ. Press.

WEST, D. J. (1967). *The Young Offender.* London: Duckworth.

WILSON, H. (1962). *Delinquency and Child Neglect.* London: Allen & Unwin.

—— (1966). Pre-school training of culturally deprived children. *Howard J. Penology*, **12**, 1.

24   Child Health in the Tropics

THE tropical areas of the world today are faced with problems affecting their childhood populations which extend far beyond those of exposure to a particular climate. For the most part, the tropics represent developing but still very poor areas where the standard of life of the great majority of the indigenous population forms a striking contrast to that of the small minority who have achieved the highest levels of education and living; the contrast is not only between urban and rural populations, since the worst living conditions may be found in slum areas surrounding modern cities. Although tropical communities and cultures have through the centuries been subjected to change, occasioned principally by invasion, famine, and epidemic disease, new factors operating during the present century (and particularly during the past 25 years) have accelerated change to an unprecedented extent. Political emancipation coupled with the emergence of ruling and professional classes familiar with the European, American or Russian systems of education are resulting in pressures from within which are more irresistible and more radical than moulding from without. The construction of roads and the introduction of air and motor transport have been responsible not only for expansion of trade but also for migration and detribalisation. Probably the most important factor, however, in upsetting the equilibrium between reproduction and survival has been the spread of Western medicine. Although hygiene has lagged behind therapy, and many set-backs have occurred from failure to overcome prejudice or to understand local custom (Dorolle, 1953), modern methods of prophylaxis and treatment are becoming increasingly accepted. Thus in yaws areas, the dramatic effect of intravenous arsenic on the primary and secondary lesions created confidence in the potency of intravenous injections, which has been followed by the even more impressive results of antibiotics.

When to therapy is added prophylaxis, including vaccination against smallpox, yellow fever and plague, control of malaria and sleeping sickness, and the provision of uncontaminated water supplies, it will be realised that a factor of enormous weight and potential has been thrown into the balance. It is, of course, true that the medical services are as yet far from adequate and in many areas rudimentary and that global malaria-control alone will continue to tax their resources for years to come. But what is most significant is that the medical and sanitary services have already had a profound effect on population and survival and that their further development has been given high priority by communities which have achieved or are approaching self-government.

Before considering the specific problems of child health in the tropics, therefore, it is essential to recognise that the fundamental issue is not the comparatively simple one of reducing infant and maternal mortality or of safeguarding the health of the schoolchild. It is rather that of achieving a stable balance between the increasing chances of survival and the food available to support the population. In most countries half of all deaths are children whose survival would lead in time to famine as the population quickly outgrows food production (Fox, 1966). Sons are much needed in many populations for religious, defence, food-growing or wage-earning reasons and child-bearing and rearing continues until at least one son is beyond the years of greatest danger. Parents are unlikely therefore to heed appeals to exercise self-discipline or practise birth control until they witness a generation arise whose survival to maturity is so good that large families are no longer necessary. Death control must accompany or even precede birth control. It is unlikely, however, that poor and densely populated countries can so balance the two programmes that nutrition will improve. Oral contraception is likely to be too expensive for the many millions whose annual income can provide protection for only two or three months in addition to buying the bare necessities of survival. The necessity for limitation of population by contraception is being faced realistically in India, and has been accepted as a matter of social policy. For the maximum benefit to the childhood population to be achieved, however, it is important that contraception should be linked with intelligent family planning and the suitable spacing of pregnancies. It is then obvious that the principal paediatric effort in developing countries will be in the direction of community rather than individual health (Jelliffe, 1965).

Agriculture and Diet

Agriculture and husbandry are so closely related to the staple diet that they must be considered as forming an essential background to the problems of child health. Although there will be major differences between one tropical area and another, the occurrence of a wet season characterised by torrential rains and lush growth followed by a dry season during much of which food production is minimal, provides common problems. The heavy rains are apt to result in soil erosion wherever the land has been cleared of trees, and roads may become impassable for wheeled traffic. (It is significant that there is no indigenous wheel found in the culture of tropical Africa, and that the majority of market produce is still transported on foot). The dry season is marked by enervating heat, dust, flies, and shortage of water, whilst pests and village fires make heavy inroads on stored harvest. Owing to the depredation of parasitic and other diseases, the raising of livestock is precarious throughout the tropics, whilst religious belief or local custom may exclude any or all animals as articles of diet or militate against the improvement of existing stock. Thus the pig is banned as unclean by Moslem communities. The Hindu religion, which regards the cow as sacred, not only necessitates an almost exclusively vegetarian diet for the majority but results in an enormous cattle-population of India which consumes much of the available food and contributes very little milk.

In tropical West Africa, the extensive trypanosome belt is largely devoid of cattle (though attempts are being made to introduce stock immune to sleeping sickness); little of the meat and none of the milk produced in northern Nigeria is available for the southern areas. Indeed, the nomad habits of the Fulani herdsmen in the north make them as much a liability as an asset owing to the destruction of crops which follows their wanderings, and so far have made the economic utilisation of milk, *e.g.* by drying, impracticable on any major scale.

It may be said that, with certain exceptions, meat contributes little to the staple diet in tropical areas, since even when stock can be successfully reared (*e.g.* pigs in Thailand and goats in many areas) the meat tends to become a cash product beyond the means of the average peasant or the animals are regarded as capital which is not readily expended. What is of even greater importance in considering the health of the infant and young child is the almost universal lack of milk. Even where milk is or could be available, there is frequently a strong prejudice against its use. This is perhaps understandable in view of the very great likelihood of milk being infected at source or becoming contaminated, although the traditional practice of the Hindu is to boil milk before consuming it. In recent years the ponderous water-buffalo in India has been recognised as a better source than the cow of rich milk (about 33 calories per fl. oz.). This animal seems also to be resistant to tuberculosis. The Kaira milk co-operative in Gujarat State has made good use of foreign aid to provide a very large and effective organisation by which bulk carriers bring in buffalo milk for pasteurisation and rail distribution to points as remote as Bombay. The plant also makes ghee, butter, dried milk powder and baby foods. This is an excellent example of foreign money* making possible the import not of foreign food (which would tend to prevent local development of the food industry) but of efficient plant to establish a very large milk industry entirely comparable with those in developed countries and using local labour from village hut to the manager. The stunting effect on local development of supplying un-limited milk powder from abroad has been described by Najjar (1965).

In contrast to those communities depending almost exclusively on tilling soil which is yearly being washed away, river and coastal dwellers have tended to base their economy on fishing. The liberal inclusion of fish in their diet is commonly recognisable at an early age in the physique of the children. Whereas young children weaned on to an exclusively vegetable diet tend to develop large protuberant abdo-mens (accentuating the commonly seen umbilical hernia) children in fish-eating communities do not. There is also suggestive evidence that both childhood and terminal stature is greater amongst fish-eaters than in those areas where foods with high protein content are scarce. It is possible that improved transport and methods of preservation may in time render fish a valuable supplement to the diet of populations living at a distance from sea or river, whilst in some rice-growing areas 'fish-farming' on the flooded rice-fields has been introduced with the same purpose.

At the present time, food production in the developing areas is being faced as a

* Some of the plant was presented by Scottish farmers.

world problem by co-operation between local governments and the United Nations working through the Food and Agriculture Organisation (FAO). The provision of expert advisers, agricultural equipment, and training of local personnel has been accepted as a responsibility by the richer nations, and there is no doubt that real progress is being made through international co-operation and mutual aid. But without minimising the present achievements or future possibilities of development of the tropical areas, it is extremely dubious whether food production is in fact keeping pace with population or is within measurable distance of doing so. Calder

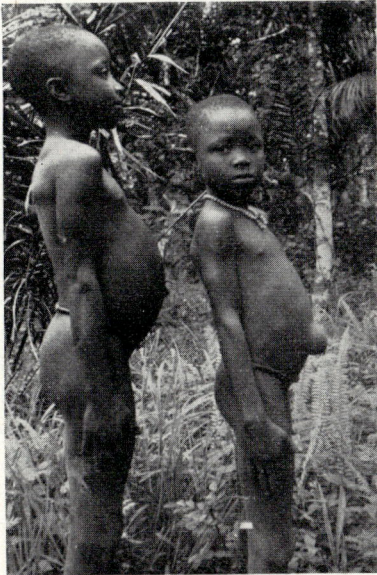

FIG. 86. West African children from a village where the staple diet is cassava, showing abdominal distension and umbilical hernia.

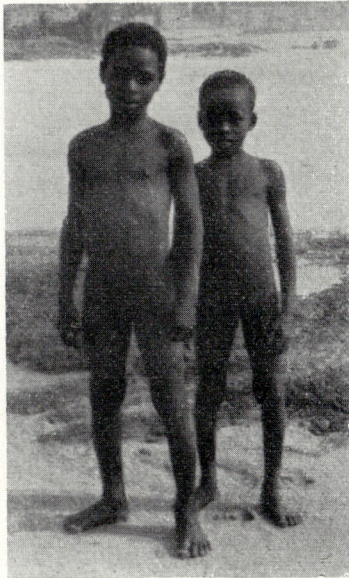

FIG. 87. West African children from a fishing community, showing good physique contrasting with Fig. 86.

(1954), who wrote with enthusiasm on the prospects of development, also stated, 'Seventy per cent of the Asian peoples depend on rice as their staple diet and, while the population has increased by over 10 per cent since the outbreak of the Second World War, the rice production is no greater, and in India considerably less, than in 1939'. This difference in tempo between control of disease (and hence increase in population) and increased agricultural production is partly accounted for by a greater reluctance to accept new agricultural methods, systems of land tenure, and dietetic habits than to accept Western medicine. Partly also, it stems from the fact that control of epidemic disease is in many areas a necessary precursor of agricultural or other development (a lesson learnt from the construction of the Panama canal, which was only possible after the area had been cleared of yellow fever). This inevitably leads to a time lag between the operation of the medical services and the increased productivity which may follow. Unfortunately, also, visiting foreign experts have not always been fully aware of local conditions, customs, and religious beliefs before advising on major undertakings, and a number of costly failures have taught the necessity for local co-operation.

Apart from an increase in the staple diet, however, there are undoubtedly potential sources of food in many areas which are not fully utilised. Williams (1954), in discussing the real needs of the developing countries, has stressed the role played by ignorance as a cause of malnutrition. De Silva (1951) has also emphasised that in Ceylon malnutrition is due more to poverty than to shortage of food. In tropical Africa there are many potential foods which are either taboo or not eaten from ignorance of their value, whilst others are squandered owing to difficulties of transport or preservation. Much information about the value of both animal and vegetable protein is available from such tables as those of McCance and Widdowson (1960), Platt (1962) and Gopalan and Balasubramanian (1963). The last is particularly helpful because it describes each foodstuff in a number of Indian languages so that identification is easy. A survey of foods available in the area and reference to the above tables will indicate how the needs (Davidson and Passmore, 1969) may be met or how the position may be improved by the introduction of a food which has been shown to be palatable and within the financial resources of the common man and his family. Palatability must be stressed and if children are to welcome the diet, new tastes may need to be blended with old ones. Thus a familiar meal of plantain may be fortified by mixing into it a ground nut gravy. Soya bean is often rejected unless it can be presented in disguise. The same need for palatable presentation arises when Bengal grain is offered to a population which has not experienced it before. The agriculturist's approach to the problem is well described by Najjar (1965).

Since major increases in food production may take many years to achieve, the immediate necessity is for the existing resources to be fully utilised and for wastage to be reduced to a minimum. This can only be brought about by education at every level, designed to render the particular population concerned best able to be self-supporting and self-sufficient. It must be remembered that an educational system suitable for an industrial population in a temperate climate may be largely inappropriate for one which has tropical problems to face and a completely different culture. There is an obvious danger in allowing the principles of fundamental education to be lost in the rapid expansion of elementary education with an acute shortage of fully trained teachers, whilst literacy itself is too often regarded simply as the road towards black-coated employment and away from manual labour or craftsmanship.

Environmental Sanitation

While adequate nutrition may be regarded as a basic need of any human community, nutrition is closely linked with environmental sanitation and the control of infectious disease. In the developing countries, much of the value of

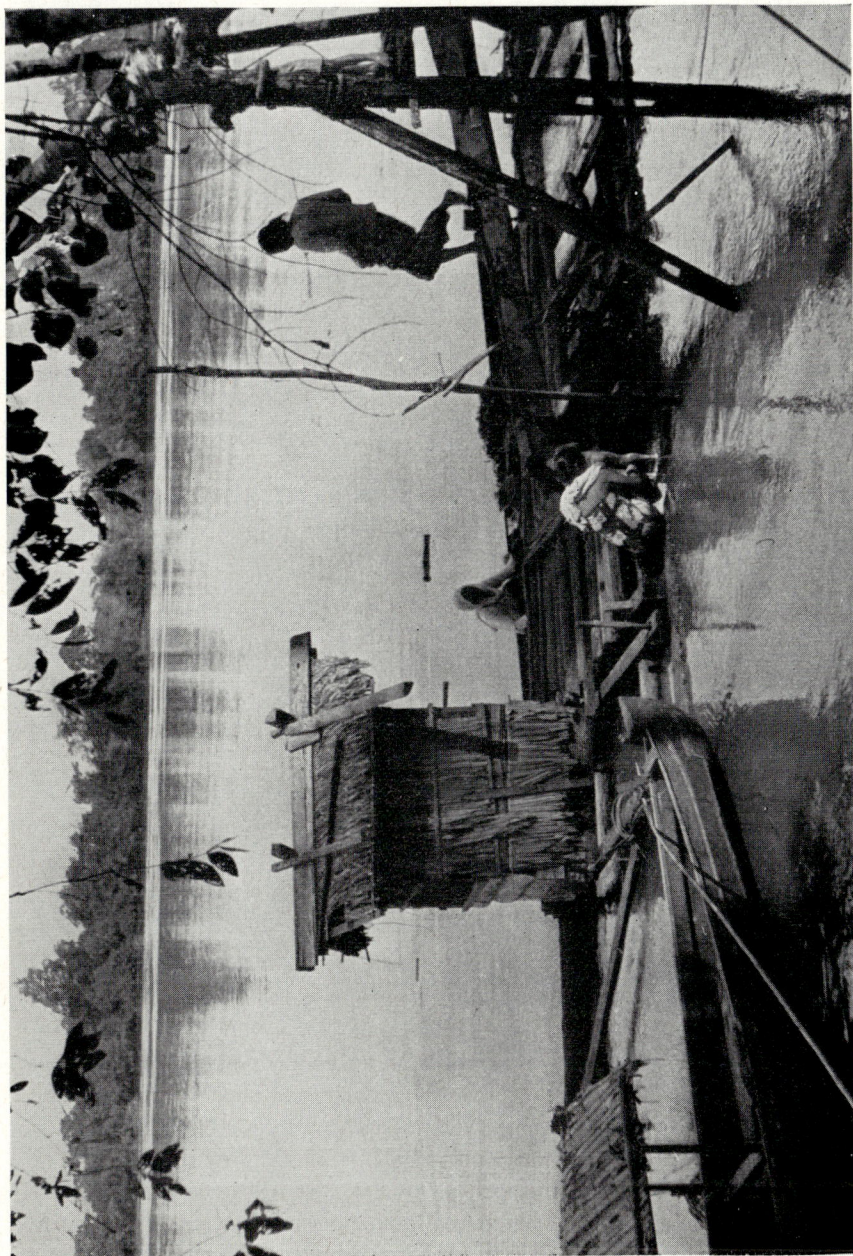

FIG. 88. Environmental sanitation in Indonesia. The small hut serves as latrine, bedroom and store for fishing nets. All transport in this area is by canoe and the river is infested with crocodiles.

the limited food available is lost as the direct result of intestinal parasitic infestation and of the diarrhoeal disorders. These in turn are primarily the result of insanitary disposal of excreta, and of the contamination of soil and water. In South East Asia it is common to see the same canal, or even stagnant water, being used indiscriminately as latrine, laundry, bath and drinking reservoir.

Of the more important intestinal parasites, *Ascaris lumbricoides*, hook-worm and whipworm are spread by the ova escaping in the stools and becoming infective in contaminated soil; in the case of *Strongyloides stercoralis* the larvae are passed. Infestation with *Ascaris* and whipworm occurs by ingestion of contaminated food and water, whilst the larvae of hook-worm and *Strongyloides* cause infestation by

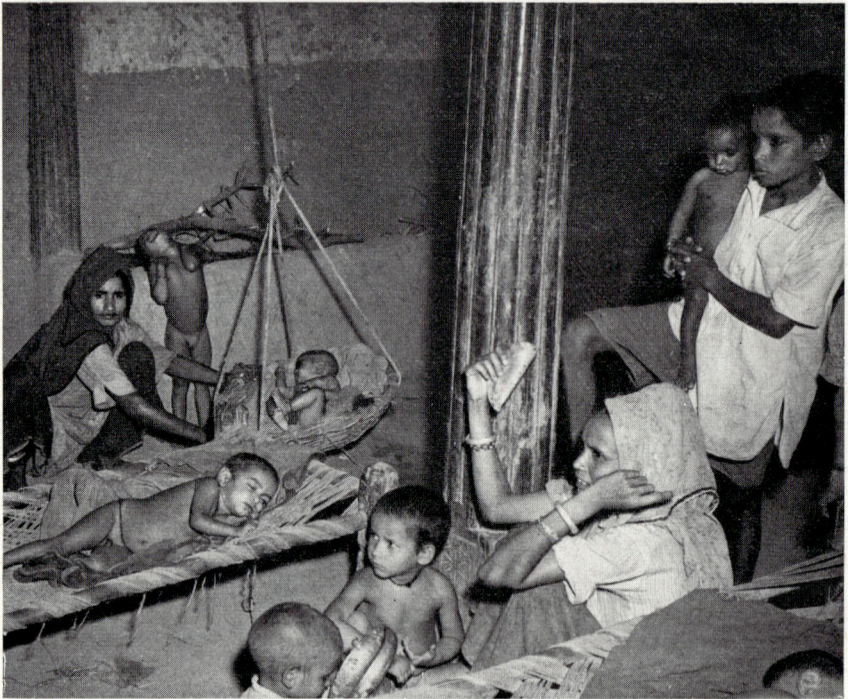

Fig. 89. Overcrowding in an Indian home.

penetration of the intact skin, as may occur when children are walking barefoot on infected ground. Whilst children are probably the greatest sufferers and principal source of spread, the problem of intestinal parasitic infestation is essentially one affecting the whole community and can only be satisfactorily solved by health education leading to sanitary disposal of excreta. Many hospitals in developing countries maintain a very high standard of sanitation but there are others where conditions are so bad that the staff may abandon all pretence at maintaining simple cleanliness. Failure to provide effectively controlled lavatories for the patient and his circle of relatives or to supply and maintain the simplest hand-washing facilities leads to indiscriminate defaecation in the hospital grounds. Infection is then spread by soiled hands and by flies which commute between the grounds and the overcrowded hospital. Health education of relatives under such conditions is unlikely to inspire them to improve sanitation in their own town or village.

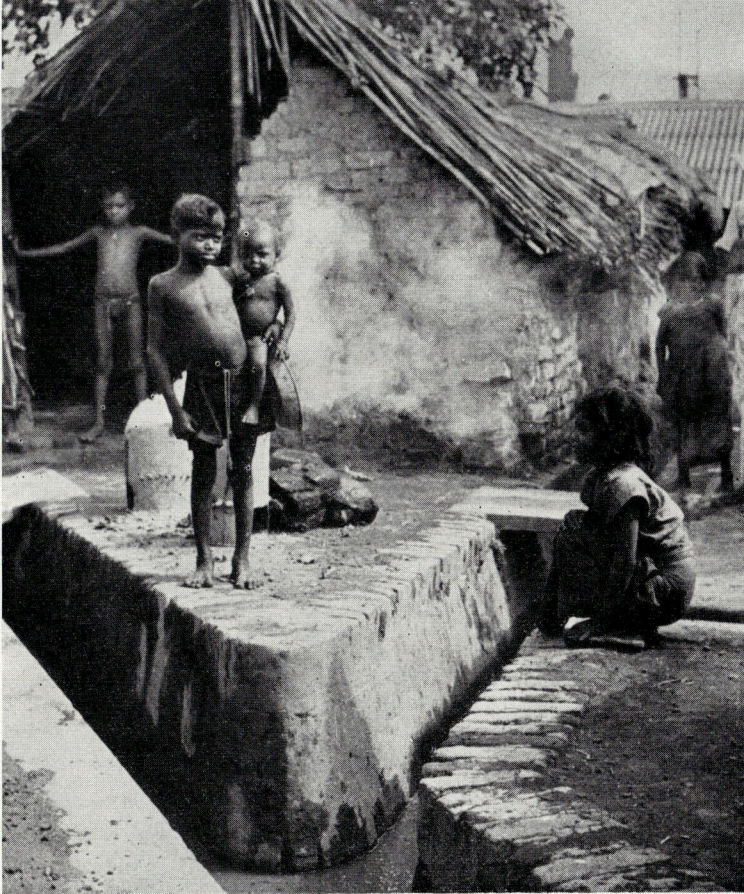

FIG. 90. Slum conditions in Calcutta. Children sit around open sewers.

Bilharziasis, which involves the liver, viscera, and genito-urinary tract or rectum, and causes very great disability in children in endemic areas, is transmitted by bathing in infected water which harbours the intermediate host (a mollusc). The ova are excreted in the stools or urine. Whilst personal hygiene plays an essential part in control of the disease, the provision of piped water for bathing and the use of molluscicides to destroy the intermediate host in natural waters are also important methods of attack.

The diarrhoeal disorders, of which *Shigella* infection is now probably the chief

18

pathogenic agent in adults and children, account for a major part of the infantile mortality in many areas, and for high morbidity in childhood throughout the tropics. (In the study of protein malnutrition in children under 5 in southern India, it was found that 25 per cent of those examined had a history of recurrent diarrhoea, and that approximately 15 per cent were suffering from diarrhoea at the time of the examination). In prevention, objectives must include not only the

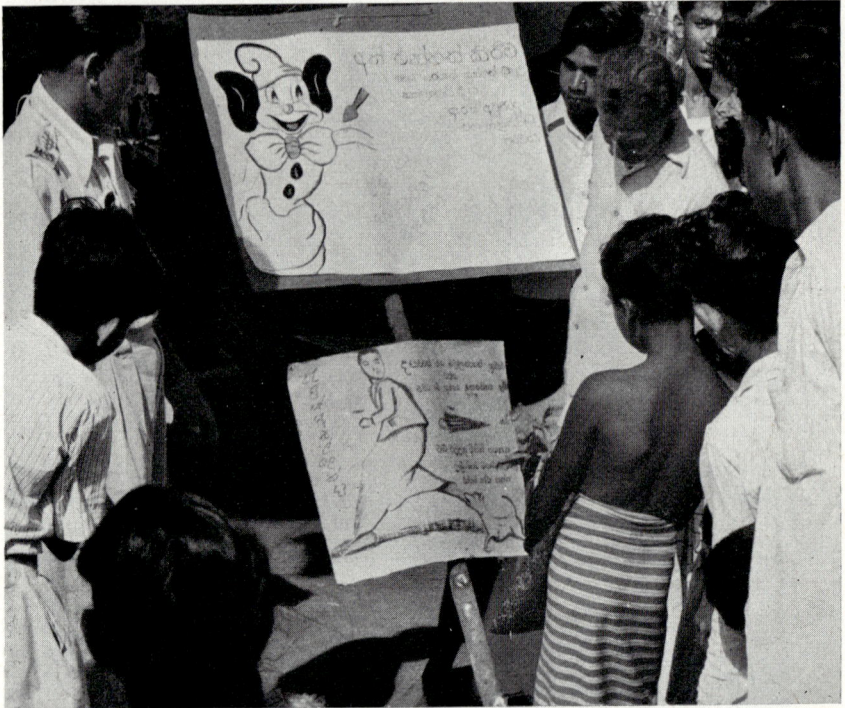

Fig. 91. Street corner health education in Ceylon. Posters explain the need for vaccination against typhoid, smallpox and rabies in order to attract volunteers to the tent where a public health nurse carries out vaccinations (WHO/Photo 5406).

safe disposal of excreta, but also the provision of easily-accessible piped water, reduction of the fly-index, and improved standards of food handling.

Overcrowding. Overcrowding in the home, commonly associated with inadequate ventilation, is a major factor in the spread of infectious and contagious disease, and is seen at its worst in the larger cities. The nidus of childhood infection is most commonly found within the family, and in the case of pulmonary tuberculosis, usually in an adult with whom the child is in close contact. The crowding together of large families including adults and children of all ages is particularly favourable to the spread of tuberculosis, and this is in fact one of the most widespread and lethal diseases of developing countries.

Infant Mortality

It is only possible to speak in general terms of the infant mortality in many tropical areas owing to the paucity of reliable vital statistics. Figures available for the more populous and developed areas, where registration of births and deaths may be effected with some approach to accuracy, can certainly not be taken as applying to remote and forest areas where the population may be almost wholly illiterate, infant deaths are regarded with fatalism, and the desirability of recording them in no way understood. In such areas, we are largely dependent for information on isolated field studies carried out by trained observers able to study small and stationary communities, observing each woman of child-bearing age over the necessary period, and recording the result of each pregnancy. In one such study by Harding (1948) in Sierra Leone, the infant mortality rate was found to be 417 ± 48 per 1,000 live births in one year which was marked neither by famine nor major epidemic disease. Onabamiro (1949) reviewed the information then available for West Africa, and various authors (*e.g.* Jelliffe, 1952) have estimated that from 300 to 500 of every 1,000 live-born babies die in infancy. If 'infancy' is taken as the first 5 years of life rather than the first year only, this is probably still largely true in some areas. Even the official figures applying to the capital cities of the West African territories where medical and social services tend to be concentrated, are still excessively high by modern standards. Whilst West Africa is here taken as an example, comparable data suggest a similar overall picture in other tropical areas such as South America, and it must be remembered that floods or epidemic disease may produce peak years in mortality which are now seldom seen in temperate climates.

It is probably no exaggeration to say that in some of the tropical areas of the world, the mortality of infants and children under 5 years of age is at least 6 to 10 times as high as it is amongst the most developed nations.

Causes of death, illness and disability. If it is difficult to discover the number of deaths it is much more difficult to ascertain the cause. Registration of the dead does not necessarily specify diagnosis which is often no more than symptomatic, *e.g.* diarrhoea, convulsions, coma, fever. Even in teaching hospitals diagnosis may be entirely unsupported by radiological, biochemical or microbiological evidence while in much of the developing world autopsy is refused for one reason or another. The absence of accurate diagnosis among the teeming rural population (80 per cent of more than 500,000,000 people in India) implies that statistics drawn from teaching centres are unlikely to reflect accurately the nation's problem. By taking a clearly defined rural area and another urban one and by recording births, illnesses and causes of death in childhood as accurately as possible, sufficient knowledge can be gained of the top ten health problems to permit the preparation of a programme aimed both at prevention and treatment of as many of them as possible within the available budget. In considering the causes of the extremely high mortality during the first 5 years of life, it is advisable to break it down into age groups although there are insufficient data to assess at all accurately the relative contribution of each period. It may be borne in mind, however, that in the countries where a rapid fall has occurred in infant and childhood mortalities during the present century, the greatest absolute decrease has been in deaths under one year, but the greatest relative decrease in deaths in the age group one to five years. It is certainly true of the tropical areas that (as in Britain in the nineteenth century) the greatest number of deaths occurs during the first year, but that an immense saving of life could be effected in the age group one to five years. It is also generally true that where there is a high infant mortality rate, the stillbirth rate is also high and that this helps to make the fetal wastage still more excessive.

Neonatal and birth-deaths. Infant deaths which are the direct result of delivery are essentially an obstetric problem, and in most areas the obstetric services are expanding rapidly through the setting-up of village maternity units and the training of midwives, though local religious practice, *e.g.* purdah, may militate against institutional delivery. On the other hand, where the obstetric services are readily accepted, accommodation is apt to become so overcrowded that discharge on the first or second day after delivery results in many preventable infant deaths. In units where it has been possible to aim at retaining mother and infant until the cord has separated, the practice appears to have been amply justified.

Since the great majority of deliveries are still domiciliary, there remains an immense field not only for expansion of the supervisory services but also for general education of women in hygiene and infant care. It is still not very uncommon for cases of obstructed labour to reach hospital when the mother is almost moribund, or where sepsis has occurred through interference and the introduction of septic material into the vagina. Female circumcision,* with consequent cicatrisation, is said to account for a significant number of difficult deliveries in areas where it is a usual practice.

Neonatal deaths which are not the direct result of delivery will also be influenced to a great extent by local custom. Where delivery takes place on the mud floor of a hut and the cord is cut with an instrument that has not been sterilised, there is a common risk of umbilical sepsis or tetanus. The likelihood of neonatal tetanus occurring is increased when mud or dung is used for dressing the cord, and there is no doubt that in many areas tetanus is an important cause of neonatal death (Jelliffe, 1951).

The practice of forcing fluid, *e.g.* by cupping the hand round the infant's face and pouring a stream of water over the nose and mouth, or of immersing the infant's head in water shortly after birth (as amongst the Fulani), is liable to lead to suffocation or inhalation pneumonia, and the same applies to forcing 'pap' into the mouth of the newborn. (A belief exists amongst some West African tribes that colostrum is dangerous, and the infant is kept from the breast for three or

---

* Female circumcision, which is sometimes performed in infancy but more commonly at puberty, may consist of clitorectomy alone or with extensive excision of the labia minora and incision of the vulva. It is still practised in many parts of Africa, and carries the common risks of sepsis and haemorrhage in addition to those of later scarring. An account of the rite in Sierra Leone is given by Gervis (1952).

more days after birth.) In some parts of India gastro-enteritis occurs in the new-born in spite of breast-feeding. This may be due in part to the practice of giving the infant a piece of cotton rag soaked in sugar water to suck during the first few days until lactation is established. The solution may be enjoyed by the baby and it is certainly very attractive to flies.

Amongst many unsophisticated populations there is a natural prejudice against gross congenital deformities, and affected infants rarely survive. (A curious exception in Southern Nigeria is albinism, which is relatively common, although it provides a handicap in a tropical climate.) In some communities there still exists a strong prejudice against twins and multiple births, and in others considerably less care is taken in ensuring the survival of female than of male infants.

With regard to congenital malaria, it is known that parasites can pass the placental barrier and cause death within the first 3 days, and this has been demon-strated in the case of infants of European mothers delivered in the tropics. The present evidence suggests, however, that true congenital malaria is rare (Covell, 1950), though infection shortly after birth may (if sufficiently heavy) overcome any existing congenital immunity.

During the latter part of the first month of life, bacterial and parasitic infections play an increasingly important role in causing death from respiratory and diarrhoeal disorders.

Postnatal deaths and morbidity. During the first year, the almost universal practice of breast-feeding in unsophisticated communities provides some protection against the diarrhoeal disorders, though these nevertheless carry a substantial mortality, and rank with respiratory infections as one of the major causes of death. Despite breast-feeding, worm infestation becomes increasingly common during the first year. Whilst ascaris infestation seldom endangers life, except occasionally by causing obstruction, it is undoubtedly a contributory factor in causing digestive and nutritional disorders. (The role of hookworm infestation in causing anaemia in infancy and early childhood is probably related both to the actual load of parasites carried and to the basic nutrition of the child, since an iron-deficient diet will render adequate compensation for blood-loss difficult or impossible.) Of the common childhood diseases, pertussis and measles take a much higher toll of infant life than they now do in temperate climates. The infant during the first year is exposed to the infections prevalent in the particular area, *e.g.* malaria, smallpox, meningococcal meningitis, dysentery, trypanosomiasis, etc. While these are responsible for a high mortality in the younger age groups the problems are primarily those of general control. The reaction to the first infection with malaria appears to vary widely with individual immunity. Bruce-Chwatt (1952) has described five types of response by newly infected infants, varying from severe loss of weight and inability of the young organism to cope with the infection, to a mini-mal reaction with normal weight-gain (which he regards as high inherited tolerance to the malarial parasite). During the first 3 months of life the infection rate was found to be lower than might be expected from the length of exposure in a highly endemic area, but by the age of 12 months, over 80 per cent of the infants studied had become infected (Fig. 92). Nutritional marasmus occurs in the first year when breast and supplementary feeding are inadequate. Vitamin deficiency, including infantile beri-beri, may occur at this age.

Later infancy and early childhood. (One to five years.) Whilst the nutrition of the young infant is commonly safeguarded by breast-feeding, nutritional disorders account for a high mortality and morbidity when the age of weaning is reached. Although it is usual for breast-feeding to be continued for two years or more, lactation is often inadequate in quantity rather than quality after the first

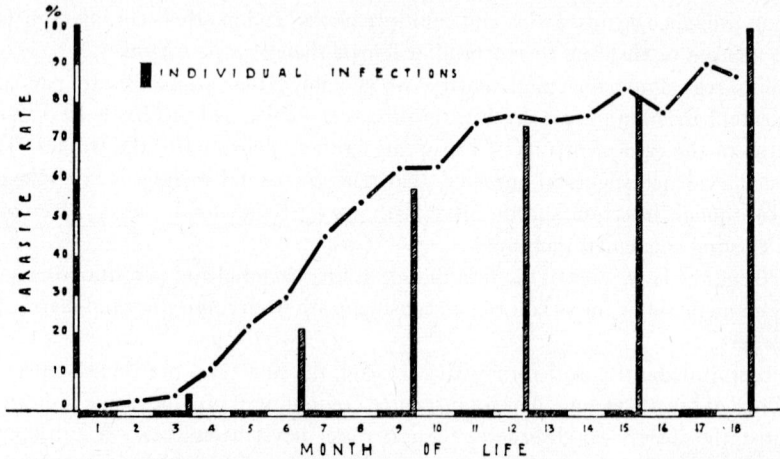

FIG. 92. Parasite rates as random samples of all examinations and as individual infections in 138 African infants (from Bruce-Chwatt, L. J., 1952, *Ann. trop. Med. Parasitol.*).

year. During the period of supplementary feeding, *i.e.* when soft solids are being given in addition to the breast, even a small amount of breast-milk may protect the infant against severe protein deficiency, which is often precipitated when the infant is completely weaned. Semi-solid food, *e.g.* premasticated plantain, millet porridge, or cornflour, is given at a variable age depending on local custom and staple diet, but as a general rule there is little attempt to provide food suitable for the infant, whilst the toddler is almost wholly dependent on the adult diet. Although there are exceptions, the infant commonly receives little or no milk after lactation is exhausted, and where the staple diet is a vegetarian one his diet may be grossly deficient in first-class protein. It must be emphasised, however, that there are wide variations in the nutritive values of plant proteins, and increased attention is being focussed on the use of locally available plant proteins in infant and child feeding. Thus in Central America a protein-rich preparation, Incaparina (consisting of 38 per cent cottonseed flour, 29 per cent corn meal, 29 per cent sorghum, 3 per cent Torula yeast, 1 per cent calcium carbonate and vitamin A at 20,000 i.u./lb.) has been produced by the Institute of Nutrition of Central America and Panama. It superficially resembles the maize gruel in common use, and has been successfully marketed on a commercial basis.

KWASHIORKOR, the vernacular name applied to a nutritional disease first described in Ghana by Williams (1933, 1935), is a condition occurring particularly in this age group. It is now more correctly regarded as part of a spectrum designated 'Protein-calorie malnutrition', a term which describes a clinical and biochemical disorder ranging from nutritional marasmus to kwashiorkor through

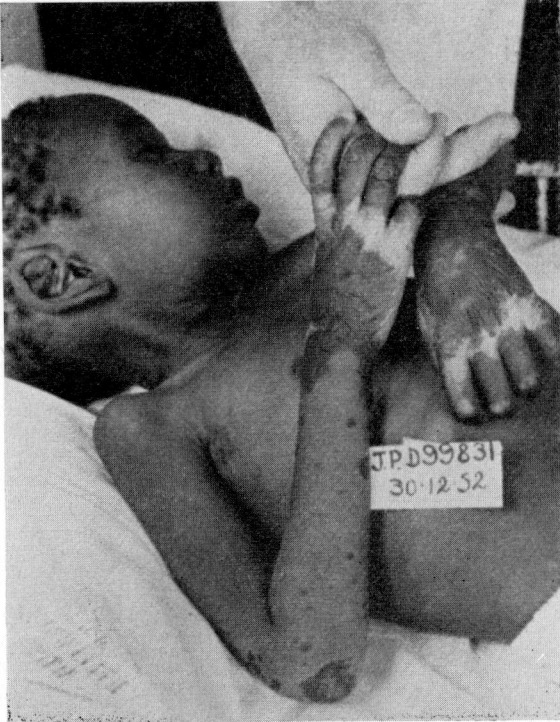

FIG. 93. Kwashiorkor.

shades of marasmic kwashiorkor. It is characterised by failure to thrive and retardation of growth; apathy, anorexia, and misery; and by loss of normal pigmentation of the hair and skin. The hair, which in dark-skinned races is normally of crisp texture and deeply pigmented, becomes fine, silky, and reddish-grey or even silvery in colour, whilst the skin loses the normal dark gloss that is characteristic of the healthy infant. In addition, a variety of dermatoses occur, of which a crazy-pavement rash on the lower legs, napkin area, back or abdomen is the most characteristic. Oedema is a classical feature of the disease, and may mask the true degree of wasting. The liver undergoes fatty or fibrotic changes, and there is atrophy of the pancreas and intestines. Fatal cases frequently show evidence of associated respiratory infection. In South East Asia, kwashiorkor is often associated also with evidence of vitamin A deficiency, though this is not an integral part of the syndrome.

If untreated, the disease in severe form carries a high mortality, but the description 'malignant malnutrition' is not now generally regarded as acceptable, since many cases can be saved by treatment with calcium caseinate or, when it is unavailable, by skimmed milk. The latter system of feeding, however, may cause diarrhoea because of temporary lactase deficiency in the bowel. The exact relationship of kwashiorkor to hepatic degeneration with or without oedema in older subjects, which is widespread in the tropics, is still debatable, but it is probable that protein deficiency is at least one common aetiological factor in both groups.

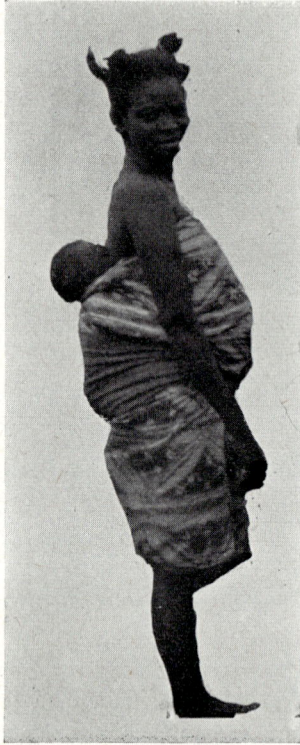

FIG. 94. The young infant in Africa is commonly carried on the back and breast-fed on demand.

Kwashiorkor has been observed in almost all countries where protein deficiency is at all common. Whilst these are not exclusively tropical, they include Ghana, Nigeria, the Congo, Uganda, Kenya, South Africa, West Indies, Cuba, India, Indo-China, Thailand, Indonesia, Ceylon and Malaysia. The disease, which as a world problem is less common than nutritional marasmus, occurs (1) in the age group in which protein requirements are high and (2) amongst peoples whose diet is deficient in protein-rich food and where the ratio of protein to carbohydrate foods is low (Trowell, 1954). It is seen particularly but not exclusively where the staple diet is maize or tropical roots such as cassava or manioc which are deficient in methionine and the disease is often accompanied or probably precipitated by infection. The importance of measles has been stressed by Morley (1968). Kwashior-kor is a preventable disease and provides an important index of protein-deficiency attacking a particularly vulnerable age-group. Where kwashiorkor is common, every severe case is likely to be associated with a number of mild cases, and evidence of protein deficiency will also be found in the adult population, particularly in pregnant and nursing mothers.

OTHER HAZARDS. During the one to five year period, the young child commonly experiences a profound change in the mother-child relationship and increased exposure to risks of every kind. Whereas the young infant is commonly carried on the mother's back and breast-fed on demand, the older infant is often delegated to a small sister, whilst the toddler is left to a much greater extent to fend for himself, particularly when he has been succeeded by another baby. The picture of the malnourished 'deposed child' of 3 or 4 beside the healthy baby at the breast is a familiar one. At the same time his mobility exposes him to greater environmental risks under conditions of primitive sanitation and hygiene. Apart from threadworm infestation, *Ascaris lumbricoides* is the most ubiquitous type of worm infestation in the tropics, and is commonly acquired in early childhood. Where hookworm or schistosomiasis is endemic the child is likely to become infected from contaminated soil or water. In malarial areas the infection rate reaches its peak incidence. (The 'spleen-rate' in this age group is often used as a rough index of malarial infection of the community, and serves this purpose in endemic areas although it should be borne in mind that the spleen enlarges readily in early childhood from causes other than malaria.) The mortality and morbidity from malaria in infancy and early childhood in the tropics are still high, and where the disease is holendemic the adults who survive represent a 'salted' community where immunity has fought a more or less successful battle with infection. There is also evidence that malarial infection in childhood is a contributory factor in producing the liver damage which is almost universal in many areas, and that chronic malaria and malnutrition are together responsible for the greatest loss of work potential in the underdeveloped territories. In 1952 it was estimated that the total annual number of cases of human malaria averaged 350 million, with a mean mortality of one per cent, a substantial proportion of which occurred in infancy and childhood. A relationship between malaria and childhood nephrosis has been suggested. Since the intro-duction of modern insecticides and house-spraying, the disease has been eradicated in a number of countries and others are progressing toward this state. The emer-gence of resistant mosquitoes and parasites, however, has further qualified the previous cautious optimism.

Later Childhood

Although the older child is subject to the common risks of the area in which he lives, including infection, malnutrition, and trauma, there is no doubt that the mortality between 5 years and adulthood is very much less than in infancy and early childhood. To an increasing extent, boys of school age are coming under supervision which makes both treatment and prophylaxis more feasible. In the case of girls, where education in the basic principles of health, diet and infant hygiene is most needed if major progress is to be effected, there has been much more apathy or active hostility to bringing them into the educational system. Even in areas where elementary education is being demanded, it is often found that the school population includes only one girl to every ten or more boys (Fig. 105). In Moslem communities and others where purdah is practised, there is particular

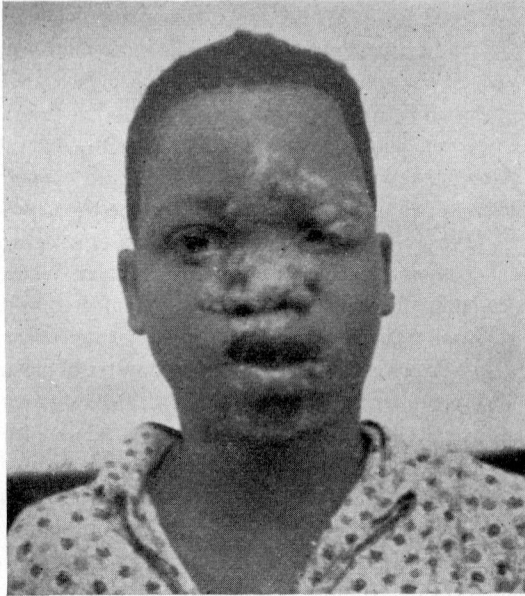

Fig. 95. Facial yaws in a Nigerian boy of 13 years.

difficulty in bringing education to girls of school age and even more so in training older girls to form the nucleus of the teaching, health visiting, nursing and other professions in which their co-operation is most needed. Many experienced workers feel that the spread of female education (which should be directed in the first instance to fitting girls for intelligent motherhood rather than for purely academic posts) is a fundamental step which must be taken if tropical countries are to develop further.

The health problems of the child of school age are, as has been mentioned, essentially those of the community in which he lives but two conditions which can be attacked intensively in this age group call for special mention.

Yaws, of which the geographical distribution is shown in Fig. 97, is essentially a disease of tropical and near-tropical areas. It is due to infection with a treponeme (*Treponema pertenue*) which has many affinities with *Treponema pallidum*, the causative organism of syphilis. The infection is not, however, venereally acquired, and the consensus of opinion is that infection takes place at the site of an abrasion by contact with infected material, usually by direct body-contact. Studies in Jamaica (Chambers, 1938; Turner and Saunders, 1935) indicate that the peak incidence of primary infection is in the second 5 years of life, and that the commonest site is on the lower extremities (which are most liable to minor trauma when children are walking unshod through the bush). The crowding together of naked

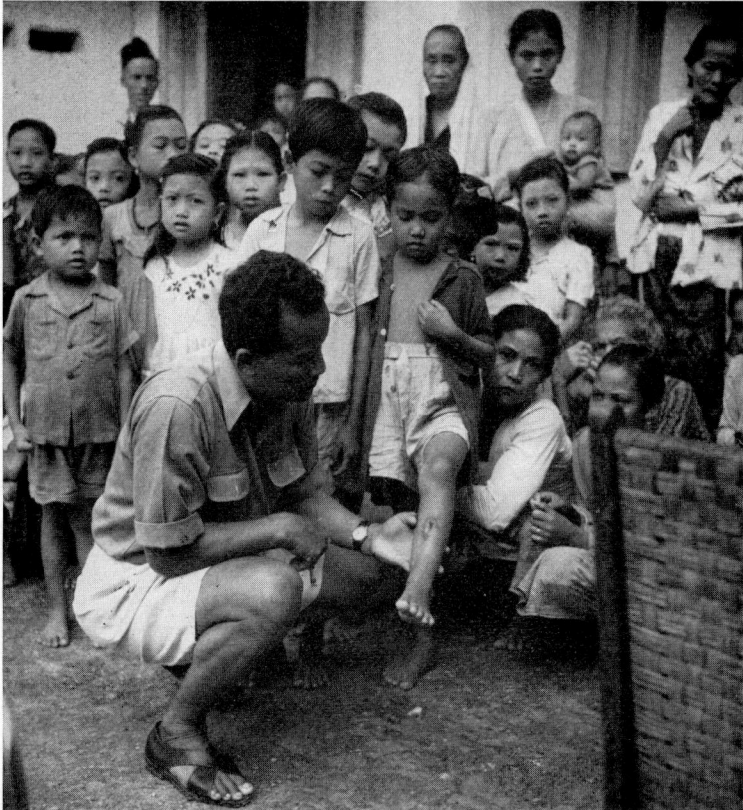

FIG. 96. Indonesian yaws eradication team visiting one of the smaller islands. The population was systematically examined and cases of yaws treated with a single injection of PAM. In 10 years, 34 million people were examined and 5·5 million infected persons treated.

children on the floor of a hut at night is particularly likely to spread infection, whilst in the case of breast-fed infants a mother-child infection may pass in either direction although the condition is not congenitally acquired. The incubation period is thought to be 3 to 4 weeks.

After a variable period the primary infection is followed by secondary lesions, which include the characteristic 'framboesial' eruptions, and maculopapular and pustular rashes. Since the disease is not painful at this stage, and does not interfere with normal activity, children are often not brought for treatment whilst the

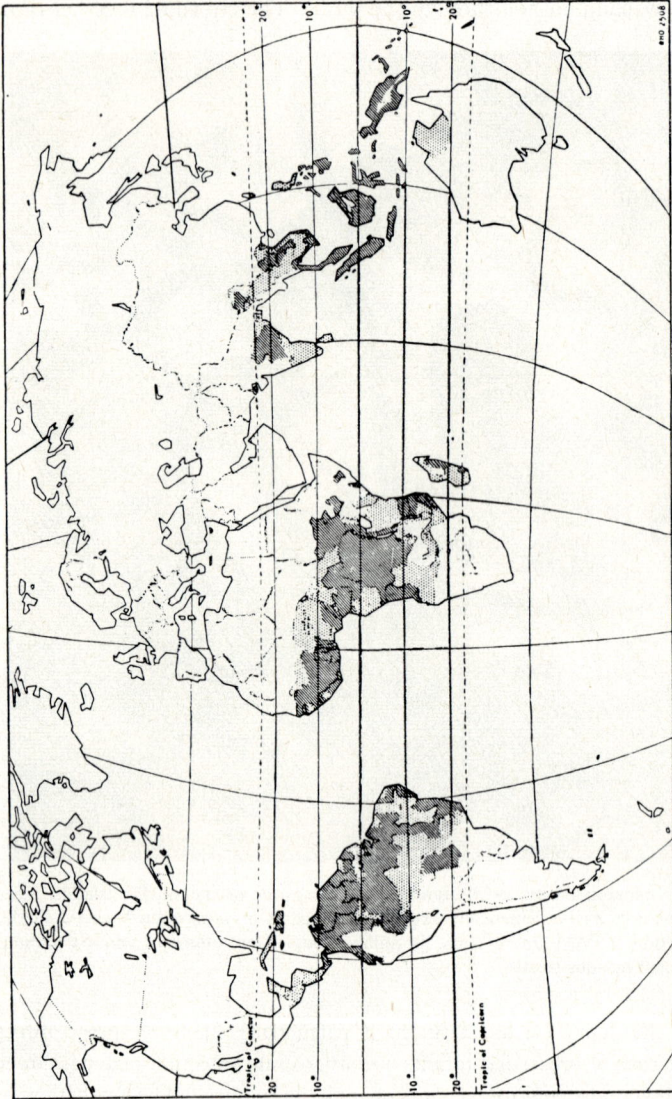

FIG. 97. The yaws areas of the world. Darkly shaded areas—yaws widely prevalent. Stippled areas —yaws known to be present. (*Courtesy of W.H.O.*)

condition is still infective and readily curable. Indeed, in some areas yaws is regarded as almost inevitable, and children may even be deliberately infected.

The tertiary lesions are likely to appear in later childhood or easily adult life, are liable to be intensely painful and cause extensive destruction of superficial tissues with great deformity. Whilst not a killing disease, tertiary yaws is certainly responsible for great disability and suffering throughout the tropics.

Some indication of the magnitude of the yaws problem in Africa alone was given by Hackett who stated in 1954: 'In the area of Africa in which yaws is endemic, the total population is about 103 million, the total annual sick attendance is 24 million (about 23 per cent) and yaws attendance is 1·32 million, that is about 5 per cent of the total sick attendance or about 1 per cent of the total population. These figures can be safely regarded as under-estimates.' In Indonesia, when the anti-yaws campaign was started in 1950, approximately 15 per cent of the population was infected.

Yaws is most effectively attacked in the primary and secondary stages, since early treatment can result in complete cure and at the same time eradicate sources of infection. When repeated injections of intravenous arsenic provided the best method of treatment available, it was often found that the rapid disappearance of primary and secondary superficial lesions resulted in many patients failing to complete an adequate course of treatment and subsequently relapsing. More recently, using penicillin, large-scale anti-yaws campaigns have been carried out under the guidance of W.H.O., supplies being provided by the United Nations International Children's Emergency Fund (U.N.I.C.E.F.). Treated areas include Haiti, Indonesia, Thailand and the Philippine Islands. With the long-acting penicillin preparations now available, control or local eradication of the disease is at least possible by intensive mass treatment, provided that the methods of the initial campaign can be consolidated into the health services of the area.

Endemic goitre. The geographical distribution of endemic goitre (Fig. 98) is widely different from that of yaws, and is not limited to tropical areas. It represents, in contrast, a world problem which has largely been solved in the more advanced areas but is still practically untouched in affected parts of the tropics. In these areas, thyroid enlargement may be evident in 50 per cent or more of girls of school age and a relatively lower percentage of boys. It is often present in infancy or early childhood, and several members of a family may be affected (Fig. 99). The condition tends to become more severe in succeeding generations, and the relationship to endemic cretinism and also to associated deaf-mutism is well recognised. Although the aetiology is complex and various dietetic factors, faecal contamination of water supply, etc., have been introduced into the picture, it has been repeatedly shown that there is a close relationship between a high local incidence of endemic goitre and low iodine-content of water (and hence of vegetables grown from it). This has been demonstrated in Nigeria and Ceylon by Wilson (1954a), who also emphasised the importance of geological formation and the 'leaching' effect of tropical rain.

Prophylaxis is readily undertaken in those countries where refined salt is used,

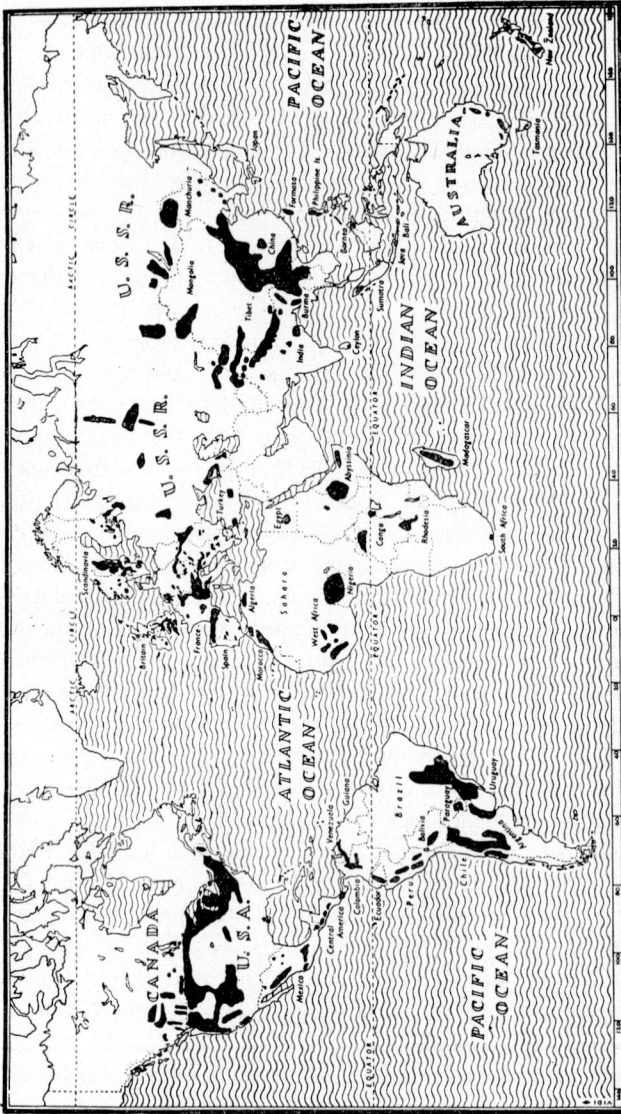

FIG. 98. The goitre areas of the world. (*Courtesy of the Chilean Iodine Research Bureau*).

and where large-scale iodisation of such salt can be effected before distribution. For this purpose, potassium iodide in a proportion of 10 mg. per kg. has been found effective in temperate climates, and has served to eradicate endemic goitre in many areas. In northern India and in the tropics generally, however, the problem of prophylaxis is much less simple since populations generally are used to eating crude salt produced by evaporation of sea or salt-lake water, burning of vegetable matter, or mining of local rock salt, and often with a negligible iodine-content. The practical difficulties of iodising this on the spot are formidable, whilst a change in age-old dietetic habit, *e.g.* to the use of pre-treated refined salt, is apt to meet with

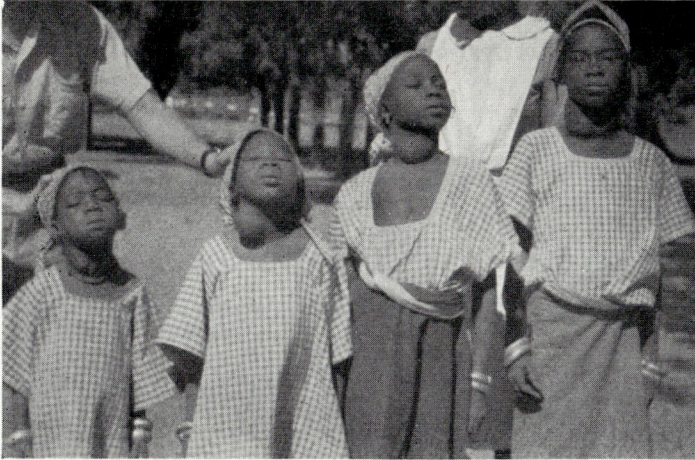

FIG. 99. Endemic goitre affecting four sisters (Northern Nigeria).

great opposition. Furthermore, potassium iodide is unstable under tropical conditions, and treated salt rapidly loses its iodine-content from the action of humidity, heat, and storage. Potassium iodate, which is much more stable than iodide, is equally effective in prophylaxis and can be added in suitable dosage to either salt or flour without toxic effect (Study Group on Endemic Goitre, 1953). Whilst this represents an important advance, the problems of effective distribution still have largely to be overcome.

Folklore and Child Health

Good medicine demands a study of local beliefs and customs and every chance of learning about these should be taken, preferably before launching a preventive and curative service if this is to avoid failure and ridicule. Thus although the child before puberty is, in general, subject to comparatively few restrictions compared with the adolescent or adult, survival is often prejudiced even before birth by local custom relating to pregnancy and parturition. Trant (1954) in describing some of the numerous food-taboos current in East Africa points out that deprivation falls particularly heavily on the pregnant woman since she must not only avoid the foods which are generally taboo to women (which may include eggs, fowls, mutton, pork, milk and fish) but also observe further restrictions for fear of damaging the fetus or prejudicing her confinement. The extreme degrees of anaemia of pregnancy which are common in most tropical areas are often largely attributable to local custom, which may insist that the foods of higher nutritional value are reserved for men or sold as a cash crop and that pregnancy (far from necessitating a better diet) is essentially a period of prohibitions.*

In almost all primitive communities, parturition and the puerperium are surrounded with a variety of rituals, some of which are innocuous (*e.g.* disposal of the placenta or cord, ritual purification after childbirth) whilst others may directly affect the survival of the child (Thompson, 1966). The risks of sepsis or tetanus are common to all types of home delivery where no precautions are taken to guard against them, but are enormously increased when obstructed labour leads to unskilled interference. In many communities the cord is not cut until the placenta is delivered, and whilst this will have no adverse effect in a normal delivery, prolonged retention of the placenta may be responsible for the death of the child. Cutting and dressing the cord (which have already been referred to in relation to neonatal tetanus) are effected in various ways, and the cord may either be tied with fibre or thread or (particularly when torn, bitten or cut with a blunt instrument such as a stone or bamboo knife) left untied. The risks of haemorrhage from the cord are, of course, greater when a sharp instrument is used.

Whilst in some nomadic communities the mother is expected to return to full activity almost immediately after delivery, the puerperium is often a time of more or less prolonged seclusion until ritual purification has been effected. Thus in some West African tribes the mother has to remain in the hut in which she was delivered for a fixed number of days, or on a mud couch under which a fire is kept continuously burning. In many communities wives and girls (and even nurses) are seriously undervalued. Thus a man who can readily find a new wife may take no action to make life easier for the present one in pregnancy and parturition. Should she urgently need blood transfusion her husband may very well decline to donate the blood because this is believed to have serious effects on virility and fertility. Similarly daughters are likely to be fed on what the sons have left although one does not need to go as far as the developing world of the tropics to see males receive the lion's share. Even medical students in some such countries, although able to regurgitate to their examiners their teaching about erythropoiesis, reproduction, the relative food needs of male and female and the merit of immunisation or the dangers of tetanus and of rabies, may decline to participate personally in any of them. And their teachers may be as guilty. This is a field for the convinced and the courageous to set a public example.

* There is evidence that the African newborn infant is smaller than the European or North American, *e.g.* an average birth-weight of 6 lb. 5 oz. in Ibadan (Walker, 1950) as compared with an average of over $7\frac{1}{4}$ lb. shown from recent American and British studies, a difference which is significant even allowing for differences in sampling. Although it has been argued that smaller birth size reduces the risks of difficult delivery, there is nothing to be said in favour of the low-protein, iron-deficient diets often enforced on pregnant women in the tropics.

Reference has already been made to the common practices of withholding the breast for the first three days, *i.e.* until colostrum is replaced by milk, the forcing of fluid or pap on the newborn, the universality of breast feeding and its duration, weaning habits, and the close mother-child relationship during early infancy. Where polygamy is practised, the older infant will very early become one of a group of younger children within the compound and a little later within the village. Whilst the tie to one or other parent remains (depending to some extent on whether the community is patrilineal or matrilineal), the child is very soon aware that he is part of a family group that is not limited to his parents, brothers and sisters. It is, for instance, quite common in some communities for a crying child to be picked up by any woman in the compound and given the breast as a comforter. If the mother dies during the child's infancy, he may be suckled by an aunt or grandmother, though sometimes there is a strong prejudice against such an 'ill-luck' infant and he will be allowed to die.

This conception of the extended family group, with its associated loyalties and taboos, is fundamental to the structure of unsophisticated societies, and is emphasised in the initiation ceremonies which commonly accompany the approach of puberty, betrothal, the payment of bride-price, and marriage. Where, as at present, the existing structure is liable to be broken by migration and detribalisation, formal education, or the impact of alien influences, there is a very real danger of a chaotic interregnum before fresh loyalties and responsibilities are firmly established.

The transition from 'primitive' to formal education is one which has potential dangers which must be clearly recognised if they are to be overcome. Thus the child in an unsophisticated community is primarily learning by direct imitation of his parents and elders, who are his teachers and whom he will admire for the possession of skills which he is anxious to acquire. The boy will be given by his father increasing responsibilities, *e.g.* herding, helping with house or canoe building, inclusion in fishing or hunting expeditions, whilst much of his play activity will be directed to fitting him to these ends. The girl will learn from her mother, and from an early age will be required to care for a younger baby, carry a pot of water balanced on her head, learn planting, grinding corn, cooking and the agricultural pursuits undertaken by the women of the tribe. Fortes (1938) who gave a detailed analysis of both play and economic activities among Tallensi children, found that the beginning of dichotomy in work and play was seen in the 3 to 6 year olds and that the dichotomy was well established by the age of 12. Their whole education was thus directed to fitting them for the traditional occupations of men and women of their tribe.

With the introduction of formal education, the child no longer learns from parents but from a professional teacher who is concerned with academic disciplines having little or no relationship to the customs of the child's home or tribe. He is acquiring skills which his father and elders probably do not possess, and which he may easily come to regard as superior to skilled craftsmanship or manual labour of any kind. If he returns to his own village, he may find himself a social misfit in the traditional structure of the community, unwilling to accept the authority of the elders and unfitted to take on the occupation of his father. As in any society, only a limited proportion of children will be really fitted to proceed to higher academic education, and there is at present an urgent need for the provision of technical education and apprenticeship.

It should be emphasised that these difficulties arising from the introduction of formal education apply essentially to the period of transition through which many of the tropical countries are passing, and will largely disappear when literacy has

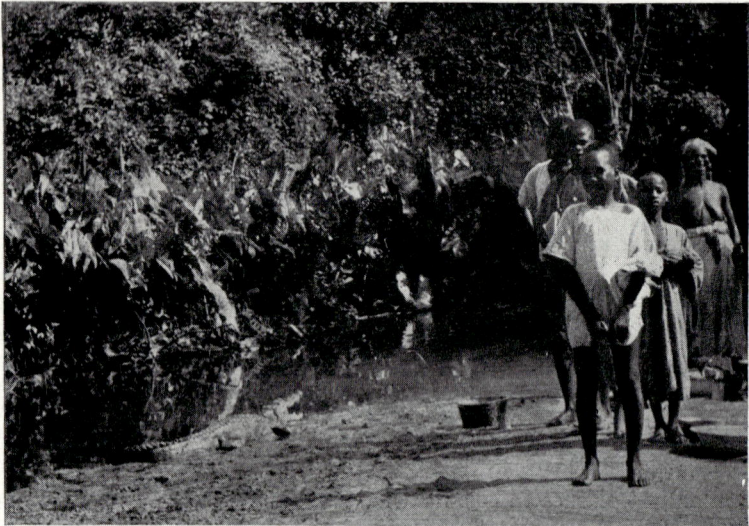

FIG. 100. Crocodile pool used for washing and drinking, and believed to increase fertility. On the left, a young crocodile lies asleep, undisturbed by the villagers. (The Gambia).

become general for more than a generation. This will, however, involve profound modifications in the whole structure of society and the period of change during which new disciplines are replacing the old is bound to cause some disharmony and discontent.

Although it is impossible to do more than illustrate a few of the innumerable ways in which traditional custom will affect child health, mention must be made of the vast subject of indigenous 'medicine'. The word 'medicine' is often used rather loosely to cover both magical and religious practices and also forms of therapy based on the use of active drugs (the distinction not always being wholly clear even in temperate climates). In the developing areas of the tropics the great majority of children who now attend school (and almost all those who do not) will already have been brought in contact with deeply-held concepts of health and disease which are logically almost wholly irreconcilable with those of Western medicine. Thus a crocodile-infested water-hole may be preferred as a source of drinking water to a piped water supply on the grounds that the former increases fertility, or a well feared lest it should have pierced the vein of an underlying dragon; whilst almost every disease or calamity is liable to be attributed to the breaking of a taboo, the anger of Gods or demons, or the malevolent influence of a particular individual. Measles, for example, may be ascribed in India to the work of a deity and may not be discussed, let alone treated along Western lines. It is against this background of early-childhood belief and training that the results of later education in health and hygiene must be viewed. Whilst many health projects have broken down from failure to discover or compromise with local belief or from the active hostility of medicinemen, it is now almost equally common to find two opposing systems of medicine accepted simultaneously or consecutively. Where indigenous medicine involves the propitiation of outraged deities or ancestors, or homoeopathic magic, and Western medicine the use of chemotherapy, the patient may come to no harm in consequence of what might be described as psychosomatic treatment. But where, as is often the case, the armamentarium of the practitioner includes drugs (usually of vegetable origin) with strong pharmacological action, e.g. emetics, purgatives, vermifuges, vesicants, and abortifacients, dual therapy may be lethal. Indeed, these active preparations themselves carry much greater risks in infancy and early childhood than in later life, owing to the entire lack of control of potency and dosage. The semi-mystical belief in the value of frequent purgation of small children is not, of course, limited to the tropics, but it is there more liable to initiate intractable and fatal diarrhoea: whilst the West African custom of treating infants with enemas (blown through a small calabash, and containing a variety of irritants) may produce sloughing of the rectum and gangrene. In Nigeria a compound of tobacco leaves and cow's urine is commonly used in treatment—a mixture which among other things produces profound hypoglycaemia in babies and small children. But although many traditional practices may be dangerous or disastrous, it is too common a mistake to dismiss indigenous medicine without attempting either to understand or evaluate it. It is salutary to remember that fashions come and go in Western medicine, which is still far from exact science, and that this applies particularly to the treatment of children.

Medicine, hygiene, nursing, agriculture and education in tropical countries are now to an increasing extent becoming the responsibility of those who, whilst themselves nationals of these countries, have been trained in a European culture. These workers are faced with the supremely difficult task of selecting what is fundamental and universally applicable in western civilisation, and distinguishing this from what is the result of purely local circumstance, economy and environment. On their success in applying essentials whilst retaining as much as possible of what is best in their own indigenous cultures will depend the future progress of the countries.

Infant and Child Health Services

The question immediately arises as to whether the structure of the child health services in Europe and North America is wholly applicable to tropical areas.

Obviously it is impossible to create from nothing and with slender resources a complete health service for children. It must grow slowly as the population can afford it: but such populations should learn from Sir Winston Churchill who at the height of the 1939–45 War stated in a radio broadcast 'There is no finer investment in any community than putting milk into babies'. Nor is there much point in creating a service with foreign money unless the country has developed the educational and financial requirements to maintain it when the source of money dries up.

Medical graduates find little to attract them and their dependents in poor and insanitary villages after 6 or more years on a college campus. Though 80 or more per cent of the population live in such surroundings remote from city life, as in India, at least as high a percentage of medical graduates settle down in the great centres of population where they may be better remunerated and where domestic, educational and social opportunities exist. These doctors may be induced in future to relinquish their private work in the towns at least for a few years but inducements must be given to compensate them. Even then it will be difficult to induce (rather than to direct) a young graduate with a general training to go to a village health centre, possibly with his wife and young family. It will be even more difficult to find enough specialised paediatricians to work in such conditions. The paediatrician or general physician must visit and study the area and its paediatric problems and will then head and direct a team of medical assistants and nurses but child-birth and the new baby's first few days or weeks may remain in the hands of village mid-wives for some time yet. It is imperative therefore that all such staff should have training appropriate to their task and should seek new methods designed to yield a better service at limited cost.

It is also essential that both undergraduate and postgraduate educational pro-grammes should emphasise indigenous paediatric problems and how best they can be prevented or cured with the simplest and cheapest means. A village doctor need know little or nothing about Maple Syrup Urine Disease (taught to him at a western university) provided that he efficiently recognises malaria, hookworm or tuberculous meningitis and knows how to prevent and treat them. Indeed, not only their studies but their undergraduate and postgraduate examinations should be directed toward ensuring this (British Paediatric Association Report, 1968: *British Medical Journal*, 1968: *Lancet*, 1968).

Pilot projects can be mounted to provide a service for a few small and easily defined rural and urban areas, which will give information about the basic social, nutritional and infective problems of the child population. A simple plan of preven-tion and treatment can then be implemented at reasonable cost, from which further projects can be launched in time. Thus regular recording of weight on a simple chart such as that provided by Glaxo for use in West Africa is most helpful. Weight progress will be watched with special care in babies who are vulnerable for such reasons as multiparity, multiple pregnancy, illegitimacy, female sex, malfor-mation, maternal death, exceptional poverty, etc.

The organisation of preventive and simple treatment clinics demands much thought about their site, expense, staff and equipment. The bigger centres may be small hospitals with ability to marshal parents and patients into some kind of order and to select from them those whose need is immediate. Parents may have a long wait but this can be used to provide health education in an entertaining way. A village clinic should be sited at the most convenient point for the people whom it serves and may be held in a modest building constructed according to a well-considered national plan. Where this is unavailable then a hut or the shade of a great tree may be enough. Such clinics should attract mothers and children because they are treated nicely, because the simple audio-visual aids are fun, because they see that clinic-supervised children are healthier and happier and because the clinic offers cures as well as simple health education. When the doctor, aide or nurse talks sufficiently loudly to one mother that all the others can hear, one interview may be shared by many. The clinic should not be too rigid about the age of children attending. Thus when mother brings the new baby along it is very useful to see and examine the older child who has been displaced from the breast or an older one perhaps who has fever or a cough or anaemia.

When the child goes to school he or she—and it is important to include the girls—may receive much health education from the school teacher whose training included it. Such information can be taken home and disseminated among friends (my own children attending an Indian school at the ages of 11 and 8 years were well taught about the cause and prevention of malaria and about the available sources of vitamins).

Linkage of maternity and child-welfare services was in Britain a logical development in the early stages of the health services, but with increasing specialisation a dichotomy developed between obstetrics and child care: thus, although the midwife is trained in care of the newborn, she often has little experience of supervising the infant beyond this period. For midwives working in developing countries the district-nurse-midwife might well serve as a model. A proper training in child health and some knowledge of disease in infancy and childhood is essential since the linkage between the two services is likely to remain a very close one, particularly in rural areas. Tetanus is a good example of how mortality may be reduced by obstetric-paediatric co-operation. Neonatal tetanus has such an abysmal prognosis that prevention is essential. This can be achieved by an obstetric service (including the village midwife) which uses a sterile technique of occluding the umbilical cord, the material being issued in simple sealed packets. Immunisation of the mother with toxoid in pregnancy is also effective by conferring temporary passive protection on the fetus.

Child health clinics. In considering the expansion of infant welfare services in the tropics, it should be clearly borne in mind that in Europe the need for infant clinics and schools for mothers arose primarily from the widespread employment of women in industry and the consequent decline in breast-feeding during the latter part of the nineteenth century. The French *Gouttes de Lait*, the British infant welfare centres, and the American well-baby clinics were all in the first instance designed to reduce the high infant mortality of artificially fed infants during the first year of life. Indeed, the American movement was originally concerned largely with the provision of clean milk suitably modified for infant feeding at low cost. As the services have developed, the European clinics have attempted to encourage breast-feeding (though after 50 years of propaganda less than 20 per cent of women in Britain breast-feed their infants to the age of 6 months); 'safe' milk has been made generally available, and emphasis has been placed on the routine use of vitamin supplements in the prophylaxis of rickets and scurvy. In the case of breast-fed infants, weaning is usually recommended at 6 to 9 months on the assumption that

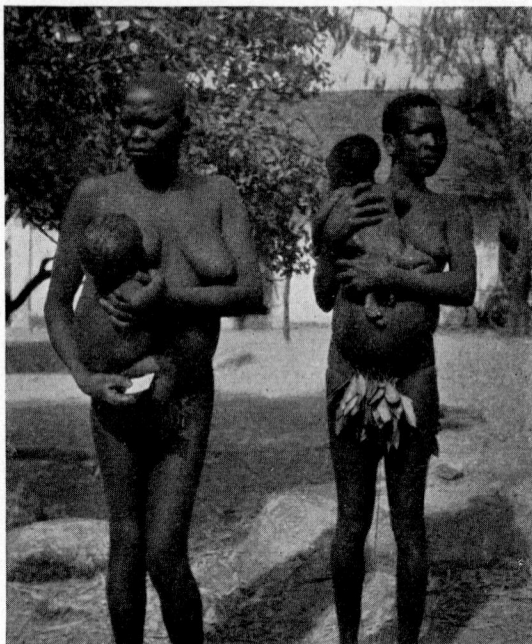

FIG. 101. Women of one of the most primitive African tribes attending an infant welfare clinic. When no clothes are worn, the infant is commonly carried on the hip or in a raw-hide sling on the back.

safe dried cow's milk will subsequently be available, and that appropriate mixed feeding has been started. Child health clinics have not been designed for the treatment of any except feeding disorders and minor ailments, again on the assumption that facilities for treatment of illness are readily available elsewhere.

In the tropics the position may be fundamentally different. Not only is breast-feeding accepted as the normal procedure, at least in rural areas, but the supply of 'safe' cow's milk is often negligible. The deficiency diseases against which prophylaxis should be primarily directed are those prevalent in the particular area. Thus xerophthalmia, infantile beri-beri or kwashiorkor may be found to be a greater local hazard than scurvy, which is rare in the tropics and particularly so in breast-fed infants. Again, the medical services as a whole are not so comprehensive that 'preventive' clinics which do not undertake treatment are likely to be generally accepted or understood, at least at the present time.

Clinics in a tropical area are most likely to be successful if the medical officer or nurse responsible is prepared to unlearn a considerable amount of the practice designed for European countries, and to make a detailed study of local conditions, including the staple diet and food prices. It appears unprofitable to concentrate too exclusively on the technique of breast-feeding during the first months of life, when

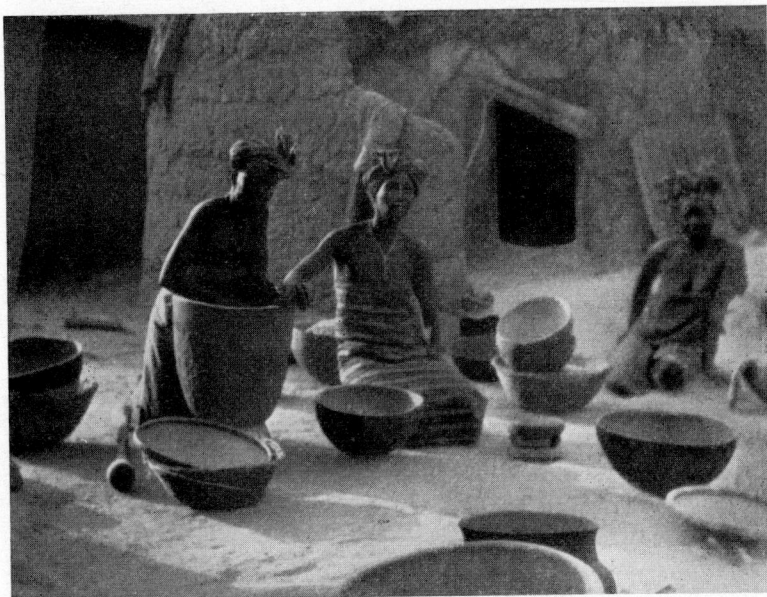

FIG. 102. Polygamous household in Northern Nigeria. The three wives have separate huts but share a common compound. The children had, at the time of this photograph, been taken to the village infant welfare clinic by the father (see Fig. 103).

the age of introduction of mixed feeding, the technique, and a detailed consideration of the local foods available (though often not utilised) and their preparation are of much greater importance. Early weaning from the breast (as distinct from the introduction of supplementary feeding) is apt to deprive the infant of a small but valuable supplement of protein during the first part of the second year. (It should also be remembered that in polygamous communities the nursing mother usually does not cohabit with the husband during lactation, and that if the infant is taken off the breast before the customary time a second pregnancy is likely to follow prematurely.)

Demonstrations of cooking and infant hygiene are invaluable as for example at the Mwanamugimu Clinic at Makerere, Uganda. Two main groups of parents attend. The first consists of mothers with their kwashiorkor children. Resident at the Clinic for some time, the mother learns about the good foods which are manifestly making her child better from day to day. She learns that these foods are within her purse and her husband's agricultural skill. Records at the Clinic show where cases are coming from and a team may go there and invite fathers, mothers and children to attend the Clinic for some days. Father learns about producing good protein foods, mother learns how to cook and give them and the child gets better day by day. This Clinic receives financial aid but its influence must grow out into the community and it is hoped it will continue until this kind of education is no longer required. Health visiting is probably the most valuable of all child health

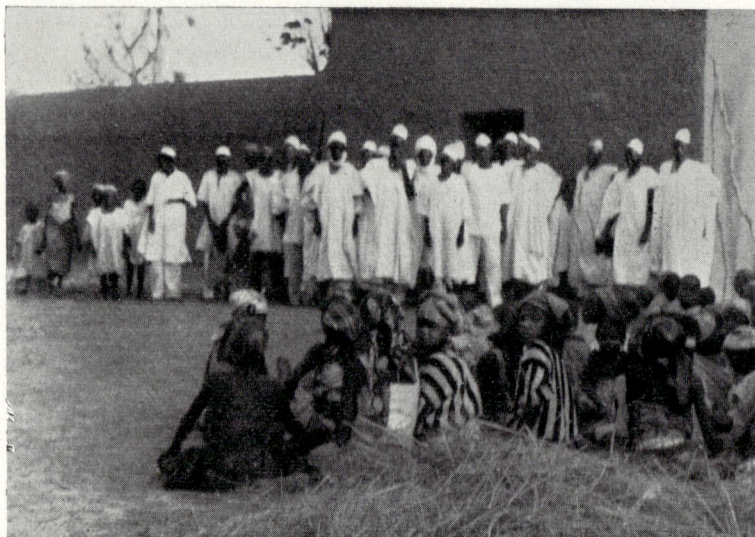

FIG. 103. Children and fathers at a village clinic in Northern Nigeria.

activities, and though time consuming and extravagant of personnel it should be the aim to develop this service wherever possible. Enormous clinics alone are very apt to defeat their own object since paediatrics, more than any other branch of medicine, depends essentially on gaining the confidence and co-operation of the individual mother.

The amount of medical treatment actually given in the clinic must depend to a large extent on its situation. In rural areas, where it is likely to be based on a health centre or maternity unit, it will probably be necessary to treat all childhood ailments which do not necessitate transfer to hospital. If it is practicable to include a small number of 'observation cots' in such a unit, where sick infants can be retained during the day for observation, test-weighing, rehydration or treatment, it will be found that hospital admission can often be avoided and the mother instructed in home-care. Where the clinic is based on a hospital, the clinic tends to become a sieve for the out-patient department, minor treatments being given by the nursing sister whilst more severe ailments are passed on for medical care. It is only in the large urban areas, where hospital treatment is readily available elsewhere, that independent clinics devoted exclusively to prophylaxis and the teaching of mothercraft are likely to be found practicable. In some of these clinics, the attendance of older schoolgirls has been found valuable both in promoting health education and in recruiting helpers.

Moslem communities will continue to provide a unique problem in child health work so long as purdah is strictly observed. Whilst purdah-clinics held after dark may provide a partial solution, the extent to which they are used will depend largely on home visiting and persuasion. To clinics held during the day, infants are apt to be brought by sisters little older than themselves or by their fathers (Fig. 103). There is a great need for women medical officers and health visitors in Moslem areas, but often extreme difficulty in promoting female education and so recruiting trained personnel from the indigenous community.

The pre-school child. Whereas in Britain the child of 2 to 5 years is reached by a variety of agencies other than the child health clinic, *e.g.* the general practitioner, health visitor, day nursery and nursery school, in many tropical areas almost all these are unavailable. Since this age group is highly vulnerable and often the most neglected, it is particularly important that clinics should encourage attendance until the toddler is safely established on an adequate solid diet, and that mothers should be urged to bring up the older child for inspection when the new infant is born or at any time if the former is failing to thrive. The aims and organisation of an 'Under-Fives Clinic' in Nigeria are well described by Morley (1966). A similar system 'The Ankole Pre-school Protection Programme' has been reported by Cook (1967).

In some of the larger cities it is found that many three to five-year-olds are decanted on to the street when the mothers set off for market in the morning, and left with little food and no supervision until late in the day. Conditions here might be improved at relatively small cost by the institution of toddler's playgrounds where small children could be left in safety, and some general supervision exercised.

School medical service. As a long-term policy, the general aims of the European school medical services are equally applicable to the tropics, *viz.* the provision of general inspection of all schoolchildren at intervals throughout their school life, consultation clinics for cases specially referred, reference of more severe disabilities to hospital, treatment of minor ailments, and health education. It would be unrealistic to minimise the difficulties of full achievement of these aims in rural areas, but the fact that an increasing number of children of school age are being brought into the educational system and are under the general supervision of adults whose teachers' training can and should include a modicum of health education, provides a structure through which the health of the schoolchild can to some extent be safeguarded. At the present time a great deal can be done through the teachers by giving them some instruction (including visual aids) in the recognition of diseases common in their area and by advice regarding diet. This latter applies particularly to residential schools, where economy or graft may result in the appearance of deficiency diseases.

The particular medical problems of the schoolchild will, of course, differ widely from those in Britain. Thus yaws or fungus infections of the skin may prove the major contagious condition in a particular area, whilst parasitic infestation or malaria may be so widely disseminated as to represent an almost universal hazard. And yet western-trained doctors may so copy their teachers that school health

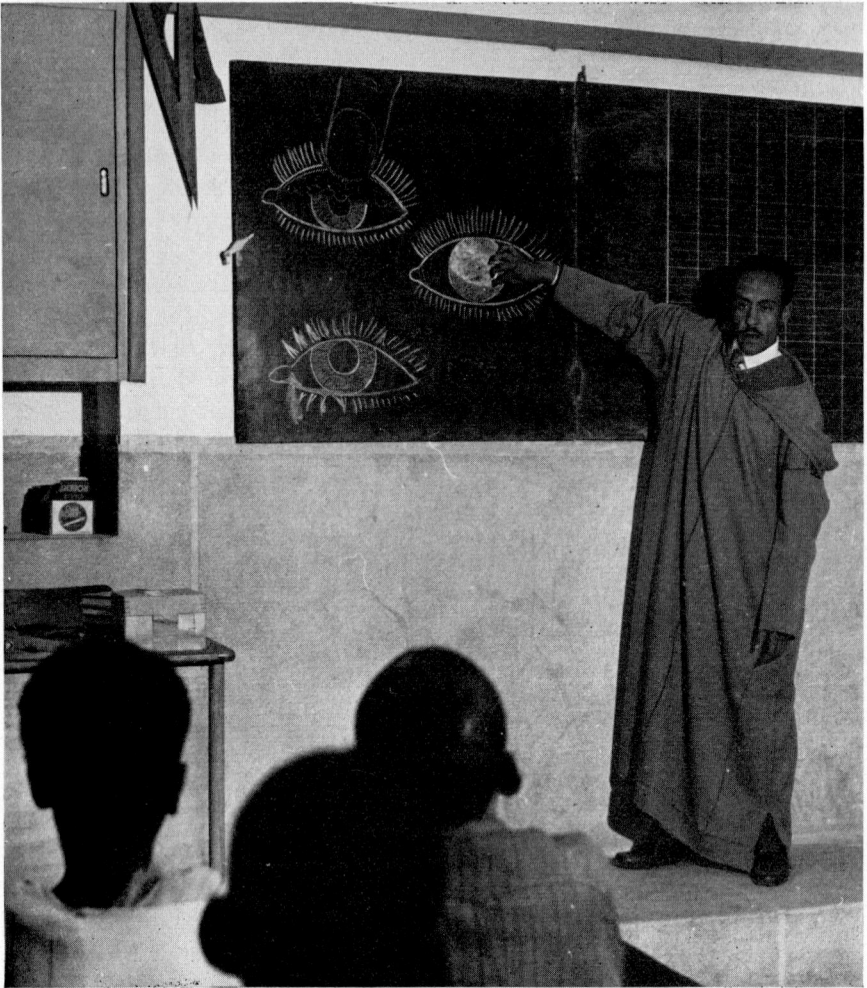

FIGS. 104 and 105. Health education and treatment of infective eye diseases are carried out in a village school in Southern Morocco (from W.H.O. film 'Open your Eyes').

cards often bear the comment 'Advise T's and A' rather than 'Nutritional anaemia'.

In general, although the health and physique of schoolchildren often compare very favourably with those of the youngest age groups, the schools have a most important part to play in improving standards of hygiene, *e.g.* in teaching the use of latrines, the dangers of infected water, the necessity for early treatment of infectious disease, and indirectly in improving diet. Thus one of the major problems of the tropics is the alternation of 'fat and lean periods' corresponding with wet and dry seasons. In residential schools a more or less consistent diet is possible throughout the year, and in day-schools where it is a common practice for children to obtain a mid-day snack from street traders, the type of food sold can be supervised and improved (Wilson, 1954b). Even the provision of a mid-day school meal

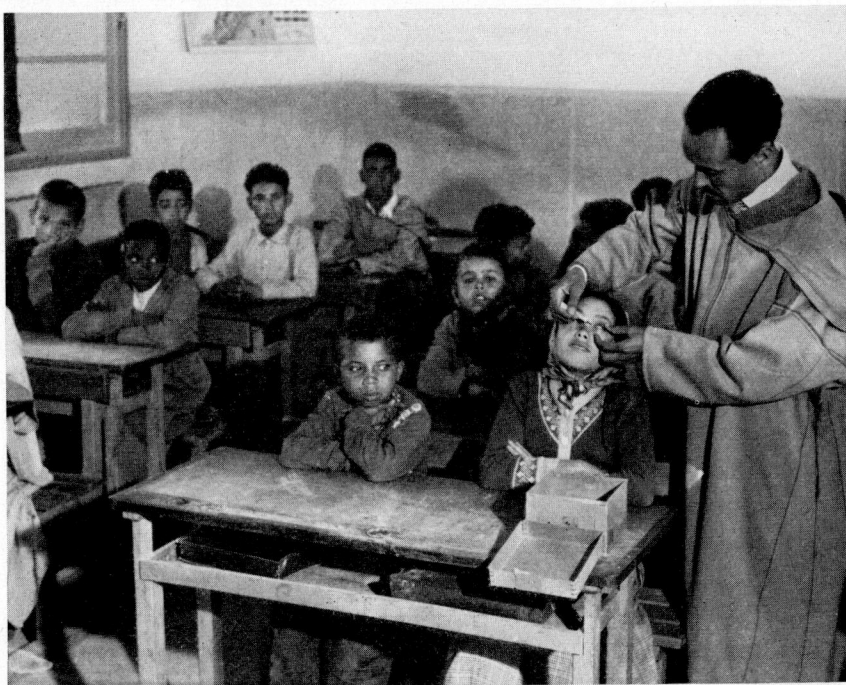

FIG. 105

at cost price has been found practicable in some day-schools, and this beginning of a school meals service offers immense possibilities. A health survey of primary schools in Uganda and an approach to health education are well described by Brown and Wilks (1966).

The Future

With regard to the control of disease, there is good reason to hope that large areas of the tropics will, within a relatively short time, be cleared of many of the diseases which have held back their development for centuries. It has been pointed out (Chaudhuri, 1954) that many so-called 'tropical' diseases, e.g. plague, cholera, dysentery, leprosy, malaria, yellow fever and smallpox, flourished in Europe or North America at no very remote date. With the vastly improved modern methods of attack, the difficulties, though great in tropical areas, are not insuperable, provided that the peoples of the countries concerned are firmly convinced of the importance of the undertakings. This is a large proviso, but the Indian Five Year Plan is already showing what can be done when major schemes have the backing of the electorate and the support of W.H.O. and U.N.I.C.E.F. Thus parts of India, which had been abandoned to jungle a thousand years ago on account of malaria, have not only been cleared of malaria but are rapidly being brought under cultivation with the aid of F.A.O. Tuberculosis, though still one of the major killing

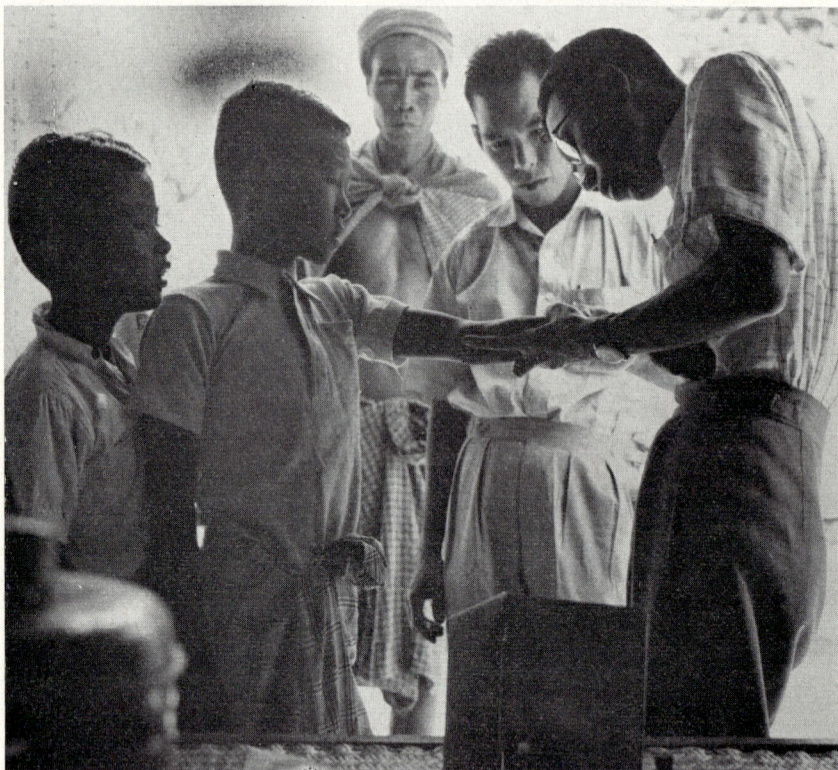

FIG. 106. Burmese health assistant carrying out tuberculin test preparatory to BCG vaccination.

diseases of tropical areas, is being attacked as a world problem. BCG vaccination programmes have been carried out in 64 countries with the assistance of W.H.O., U.N.I.C.E.F. and I.T.C., and represent one of the largest international health programmes of the century.

Many other examples in different parts of the tropics could be cited. But the bleak fact remains that control of disease leads rapidly to increase in population, and that productivity must increase even more rapidly if the present low standards of living are to be effectively improved.

Little has been said here of the great amount that has already been done in tropical countries—the building of modern hospitals, clinics, schools, technical colleges and universities, or the real progress that has been made in agriculture.

It would have been equally possible, though perhaps more misleading, to draw illustrations entirely from these sources. But the major child health problems of the tropical areas lie not amongst that minority of children who are receiving education, diet, and medical attention of high quality, but amongst the great majority who are not. (It should be emphasised that the distinction is not altogether one of urban versus rural populations, since in many of the larger cities the living conditions in the slums are very much worse than in most villages; nevertheless the social services tend to be concentrated in the more densely populated areas, and the remoter areas have often remained remarkably primitive.) The present picture is one of extreme contrasts—some of the existing institutions being more than a thousand years in advance of cultures existing side by side. The child who is required to hurdle over the centuries in a single lifetime, reaching a modern university from a primitive village community and from there going on to shoulder responsibilities of democratic government or administration which call for integrity, vision, and balanced judgment, is being faced with a phenomenally heavy task. It is not surprising that there have been failures, but rather that successful progress has already been so great.

J. W. FARQUHAR

References

BRITISH MEDICAL JOURNAL (1968). *Paediatric Teaching for Overseas.* 2, 465.

BRITISH PAEDIATRIC ASSOCIATION (1968). *Report of the Overseas Committee.* London.

BROWN, R. E. and WILKS, N. E. (1966). Health survey in Ugandan primary schools. *Trop. Geogr. Med.,* 18, 183.

BRUCE-CHWATT, L. J. (1952). Malaria in African infants and children in Southern Nigeria. *Ann. trop. Med. Parasitol.,* 46, 173.

BURGESS, A. and DEAN, R. F. A. (Ed.) (1962). *Malnutrition and Food Habits.* London: Tavistock Publ.

CALDER, R. (1954). *Men Against the Jungle.* London: Allen & Unwin.

CHAMBERS, H. D. (1938). *Yaws (framboesia Tropica).* London: Churchill.

CHAUDHURI, R. N. (1954). Tropical medicine: past, present and future. *Brit. med. J.,* 2, 423.

COOK, R. (1967). *The Ankole Pre-school Protection Programme.* Copies may be had from Dr. W. M. U. Moffat, P.O. Box 221, Mbarara, Uganda.

COVELL, G. (1950). Malaria. *Trop. Dis. Bull.,* 47, 1147.

DAVIDSON, L. S. P. and PASSMORE, R. (1969). *Human Nutrition and Dietetics.* 4th ed. Edinburgh: Livingstone.

DEAN, R. F. A. (1953). Med. Res. Counc., Spec. Rep. Ser. No. 279. London: H.M.S.O.

DE SILVA, C. C. (1951). Whither medicine in Ceylon? *J. Ceylon Br. Brit. med. Ass.,* 46, 47.

DOROLLE, P. (1953). Ethnology and health problems. *Chron. Wld. Hlth. Org.,* 7, 355.

FORTES, M. (1938). *Social and Psychological Aspects of Education in Taleland.* Supplement to Africa, 9.

FOX, SIR T. (1966). The multiplication of man or Noah's new Flood. *Lancet,* 2, 1238.

GERVIS, P. (1952). *Sierra Leone Story.* London: Cassell.

GOPALAN, C. and BALASUBRAMANIAN, S. C. (1963). *The Nutritive Value of Indian Foods and the Planning of Satisfactory Diets.* 6th ed. Spec. Rep. Ser. No. 42. Indian Counc. Med. Res.

HACKETT, C. J. (1954). Extent and nature of the yaws problem in Africa. *Bull. Wld. Hlth. Org.*, 8, 129.

HARDING, R. D. (1948). A note on some vital statistics of a primitive peasant community in Sierra Leone. *Population Studies*, 2, 373.

JELLIFFE, D. B. (1950). Tetanus neonatorum. *Arch. Dis. Childh.*, 25, 190.

—— (1951). The African child. *Trans. Roy. Soc. trop. Med. Hyg.*, 46, 13.

—— (1965). Paediatric practice in tropical regions. *Lancet*, 2, 229.

LANCET (1968). *Developing Paediatricians.* 2, 862.

LAURIE, W. (1954). Survey before service. *Lancet*, 2, 801.

McCANCE, R. A. and WIDDOWSON, E. M. (1960). *The Composition of Foods.* Spec. Rep. Ser. No. 297. London: H.M.S.O.

MORLEY, D. (1966). The under-fives clinic. In *Medical Care in Developing Countries.* Ed. M. King. Nairobi: Oxf. Univ. Press.

—— (1968). Severe measles in the tropics. *Brit. med. J.*, 1, 297 and 363.

NAJJAR, H. (1965). An agriculturalist's approach. In *Protecting the Pre-school Child.* Ed. P. György and A. Burgess. London: Tavistock Publ.

ONABAMIRO, S. D. (1949). *Why Our Children Die: Causes and Prevention of Infant Mortality in West Africa.* London.

PLATT, B. S. (1962). *Tables of Representative Values of Foods Commonly Used in Tropical Countries.* Spec. Rep. Ser. No. 302. London: H.M.S.O.

THOMPSON, B. (1966). The first fourteen days of some West African babies. *Lancet*, 2, 40.

TRANT, H. (1954). Food taboos in East Africa. *Lancet*, 2, 703.

TROWELL, H. C. (1954). Rpt. Inter-African Conf. Nutrition, 45. London: H.M.S.O.

TURNER, T. B. and SAUNDERS, G. M. (1935). Yaws in Jamaica. *Amer. J. Hyg.*, 21, 483.

VAUCEL, M. A. (1953). Le pian dans les territoires Africains Français. *Bull. Wld. Hlth. Org.*, 8, 183.

WALKER, A. H. C. (1950). quoted by Jelliffe, D. B. (1951). *loc. cit.*

WILLIAMS, C. D. (1933). Nutritional disease of childhood associated with maize diet. *Arch. Dis. Childh.*, 8, 423.

—— (1935). Kwashiorkor. *Lancet*, 2, 1151.

—— (1954). Self-help and nutrition. *Ibid.*, 1, 323.

WILSON, D. C. (1954a). Goitre in Ceylon and Nigeria. *Brit. J. Nutrit.*, 8, 90.

—— (1954b). Nutrition of schoolgirls in Northern Nigeria. *Ibid.*, 8, 83.

Bibliography

ACHAR, S. T. and BENJAMIN, V. (1953). Observations on nutritional dystrophy. *Ind. J. Child Hlth.*, 1, 1.

BLACKLOCK, M. (1936). Certain aspects of the welfare of women and children in the colonies. *Ann. trop. Med. Parasitol.*, 30.

COLONIAL OFFICE. *Annual Reports of the Colonial Research Councils and Committees.* London: H.M.S.O.

ELLIS, R. W. B. (1950). Age of puberty in the tropics. *Brit. med. J.*, 1, 85.

FORDE, D. (Ed.) (1950). *Ethnographic Survey of Africa: Western Africa.* Parts I–IV. Internat. African Inst., London.

GELFAND, M. (1964). *Witch Doctor.* London: Harvill Press.

GYÖRGY, P. and BURGESS, A. (1965). *Protecting the Pre-school Child.* London: Tavistock Publ.

HACKETT, C. J. (1946). The clinical course of Yaws in Lango, Uganda. *Trans. Roy. Soc. trop. Med. Hyg.*, 40, 206.

JELLIFFE, D. B. (1952). The African child. *Trans. Roy. Soc. trop. Med. Hyg.*, 46, 13.

KING, M. (1966). *Medical Care in Developing Countries.* Nairobi: Oxf. Univ. Press.

MEAD, M. (1931). *Growing Up in New Guinea*. London.
—— (Ed.) (1955). *Cultural Patterns and Technical Change*. New York: U.N.E.S.C.O.
PASSMORE, R. (1951). Famine in India. *Lancet*, **2**, 303.
P.E.P. (1954). *World Population and Resources*. No. 362 of Planning. London.
—— (1955). *Population Policies in India and Japan*. No. 378 of Planning. London.
PHILLIPS, A. (Ed.) (1953). *Survey of African Marriage and Family Life*. Internat. African Inst., London.
PLOSS, H. H., BARTELS, M. and BARTELS, P. *Woman*. Eng. trans. Ed. E. J. Dingwall, 3 vols. (Contains numerous references to the earlier literature *re* pregnancy, parturition, weaning, puberty, etc.)
Report of the Inter-African (CCTA) Conference on Nutrition (1952). *Malnutrition in African Mothers, Infants, and Young Children*. London: H.M.S.O.
RITCHIE, J. A. S. (1950). *Teaching Better Nutrition: A Study of Approaches and Techniques*. Washington: F.A.O.
TROWELL, H. C., DAVIES, J. N. P. and DEAN, R. F. A. (1952). Kwashiorkor: clinical picture, pathology, and differential diagnosis. *Brit. med. J.*, **2**, 798.
—— and JELLIFFE, D. B. (1958). *Diseases of Children in the Subtropics and Tropics*. London: Arnold.
UNITED NATIONS (1954). *Report on the International Definition and Measurement of Standard of Living*. New York.

World Health Organisation Publications (Geneva)

BROCK, J. F. and AUTRET, M. (1952). *Kwashiorkor in Africa*. W.H.O. monogr. No. 8.
BRUCE-CHWATT, L. G. (1956). Chemotherapy in relation to possibilities of malaria eradication in tropical Africa. *Bull. Wld. Hlth. Org.*, **15**, 852.
DEAN, R. F. A. (1953). Treatment and prevention of kwashiorkor. *Bull. Wld. Hlth. Org.*, **9**, 767.
DIRECTOR-GENERAL, W.H.O. (1959). *Review of BCG Vaccination Programmes*. Off. Rec. W.H.O. 96.
DOROLLE, P. (1953). World health and economic development. *Chron. Wld. Hlth. Org.*, **7**, 274.
HILL, K. R. *et al.* (1951). *Atlas of Framboesia*. W.H.O. monogr. No. 5.
JELLIFFE, D. B. (1955). *Infant Nutrition in the Tropics and Subtropics*. W.H.O. monogr. No. 29.
PAMPANA, E. J. (1954). Changing strategy in malaria control. *Bull. Wld. Hlth. Org.*, **11**, 513.
RAO, K. S., SWAMINATHAN, M. C., SWARAP, S. and PATWARDHAN, V. N. (1959). Protein malnutrition in South India. *Bull. Wld. Hlth. Org.*, **20**, 603.
REPORT (1958). *Expert Committee on Training of Health Personnel in Health Education of the Public*. Techn. Rep. Series, 156.
SYMPOSIUM (1953). First international symposium on yaws control. *Bull. Wld. Hlth. Org.*, **8**, Nos. 1, 2, 3.
—— (1953). Control of epidemic goitre. *Ibid.*, **9**, 171, 309.
W.H.O. (1958). *The First Ten Years of the World Health Organisation*. Geneva.
—— (1965). *The W.H.O. Programme in Nutrition, 1948–1964*. *Chron. Wld. Hlth. Org.*, **19**, 387, 429, 467.
YEKUTIEL, P. (1959). Epidemiological methods used in the study of infantile diarrhoea in Israel. *Bull. Wld. Hlth. Org.*, **21**, 374.

Appendix
Synopsis of Legislation

REGISTRATION OF BIRTHS, STILLBIRTHS AND DEATHS.

NOTIFICATION OF BIRTHS.

CHILDREN AND YOUNG PERSONS ACTS, 1933–69.

CHILDREN AND YOUNG PERSONS (SCOT.) ACTS, 1937 et seq.

CHILDREN ACTS, 1948, 1958.

MATRIMONIAL PROCEEDINGS (CHILDREN) ACT, 1958.

ADOPTION ACT, 1958.

NURSERIES AND CHILD-MINDERS REGULATION ACT, 1948, AMENDED AND EXTENDED, 1968.

SOCIAL WORK (SCOT.) ACT, 1968.

EDUCATION ACTS, 1944–68.

EDUCATION (SCOT.) ACTS, 1962–69.

EMPLOYMENT AND TRAINING ACT, 1948.

CONSUMER PROTECTION ACT, 1961.

FAMILY ALLOWANCES AND NATIONAL INSURANCE ACT, 1967.

TATTOOING OF MINORS ACT, 1969.

This synopsis of legislation dealing with various aspects of the child is designed to give a broad picture of the most important acts and their relevant provisions. For details the reader must refer to the original Acts.

Registration of Births, Stillbirths and Deaths

ENGLAND AND WALES. BIRTHS AND DEATHS REGISTRATION ACT, 1953. (*a*) Each live birth must be registered within 42 days of its occurrence with the registrar of the registration sub-district in which it occurs. Provision is made for the registration of a living exposed or abandoned newborn infant. (*b*) The Registrar-General may order the re-registration as legitimate of the birth of a person whose birth has been registered as illegitimate if the parents subsequently marry. (*c*) Each stillbirth must be registered, as for a live birth, but under the Population (Statistics) Act, 1960, the person giving information to registrar must deliver to him a certificate giving the cause of the stillbirth and estimated duration of pregnancy, signed by a registered medical practitioner or qualified midwife, or make a declaration that infant was stillborn and neither doctor's nor midwife's certificate could be obtained. (*d*) Each death must be registered within 5 days of its occurrence.

By regulations made under the Welsh Language Act, 1967, from January, 1968, births in Wales and Monmouthshire may be registered in Welsh as well as in English.

SCOTLAND. REGISTRATION OF BIRTHS, DEATHS AND MARRIAGES (SCOT.) ACT, 1965. (*a*) Each live birth must be registered within 21 days of its occurrence with registrar of area in which birth occurred or with registrar of area of usual domicile of mother. Provision made, as in England, for registration of living exposed or abandoned newborn infant. (*b*) An illegitimate birth, registered by the mother, may be re-registered as legitimate after application to the Registrar-General for Scotland. (*c*) Procedure relating to stillbirths similar to that in England. (*d*) Each death must be registered within 8 days of its occurrence.

Notification of Births

ENGLAND AND WALES. THE PUBLIC HEALTH ACT, 1936, AND PUBLIC HEALTH (NOTIFICATION OF BIRTHS) ACT, 1965. The original Notification of Births Act, 1907, and the Notification of Births (Extension) Act, 1915, were repealed by and incorporated in the 1936 Act. Every birth, live or still, must be notified on a prescribed form and enclosed in a prepaid addressed envelope to the medical officer of health of the area in which the child was born, by the father if residing at the house at the time of the birth and by any person in attendance upon the mother at the time or within 6 hours of the birth. Notification must be made within 36 hours of the birth. In practice, notification is invariably made by the doctor or midwife in attendance. Supplies of notification forms and prepaid addressed envelopes are issued through local health departments to doctors and midwives.

SCOTLAND. NOTIFICATION OF BIRTHS ACT, 1907, NOTIFICATION OF BIRTHS (EXTENSION) ACT, 1915, PUBLIC HEALTH (NOTIFICATION OF BIRTHS) ACT, 1965. The terms of these Acts are the same as for England and Wales.

N.B. In both England and Scotland, no birth is required to be notified if the duration of pregnancy was less than 28 weeks, but the birth of a live-born child must be *registered* regardless of the duration of pregnancy.

A stillbirth is defined as 'any child which has issued forth from its mother after the twenty-eighth week of pregnancy and which did not at any time after being completely expelled from its mother breathe or show any other signs of life'.

Acts Relating to the Protection of Persons Under 18 Years

ENGLAND AND WALES. CHILDREN AND YOUNG PERSONS ACTS, 1933–69. For certain parts of these Acts, a 'child' is any person under 14 years; a 'young person' is one over 14 but under 17 years.

Welfare powers of local authorities. This section, introduced by the 1963 Act, requires a local authority to make available such advice, guidance, and assistance including in exceptional circumstances cash, as may promote the welfare of children, in this section defined as those under 18 years, by diminishing the need to receive them into or keep them in care or to bring them before a juvenile court. To achieve this a local authority may make arrangements with voluntary organisations with such facilities for advising, guiding and assisting. Local authority must report to Secretary of State annually on provisions made for these facilities.

Prevention of cruelty and exposure to moral or physical danger. It is an offence wilfully to neglect or ill-treat a child or young person under 16, in a manner likely to cause suffering or injury to health. Provision is made against: seduction of girls under 16; residence of persons under 16 in brothels; causing persons under 16 to beg; giving intoxicating liquor to children under 5 (except for medicinal purposes); the presence of children under 14 in the bars of licensed premises; the sale of tobacco to persons under 16; acceptance of pawns or purchases of old metal from the young; exposing children under 12 to risk of burning; failure to provide for safety of children at entertainments.

Employment. It is illegal to employ any child under 13. Hours of employment of older children are limited within certain hours of the day. No child shall be employed to lift, carry or move anything so heavy as to be likely to injure him. No person under 17 can engage or be employed in street trading, and no person under 18 can take part in street trading on Sundays save under stated conditions. Any person under 16 taking part in an entertainment for which a charge is made, or film or broadcast, must be licensed to do so by the local authority; a child under 13 may be licensed to perform in an entertainment under strictly limited conditions, *e.g.* the part he is to act cannot be taken except by a child of about his age. Local authority empowered to license those who are between 12 and 16 and being trained for performances of a dangerous nature.

Care and other treatment of juveniles through court proceedings. This part of the Children and Young Persons Act, 1969, will be largely operative from 1st October, 1970.

'Care' includes protection and guidance; 'Control' includes discipline.

The court concerned in such proceedings is the juvenile court, from the deliberations of which the public are excluded but accredited newspaper reporters are permitted to attend. No newspaper report of any proceedings in such court may include any information or pictures that may lead to identification of any child or young person, a protection extended also to a child or young person involved in any other court proceedings and this protection covers sound and television broadcasts. A parent or guardian may be required to attend a court when a child or young person is brought before it. The age of criminal responsibility, currently 10 years, will be progressively raised to 14 years by orders of the Secretary of State. With special exceptions young persons must be tried summarily but this does not apply to homicide.

A juvenile court must proceed to make an order if it is satisfied with regard to any juvenile brought before it that: (*a*) his proper development is being prevented or neglected, or his health avoidably impaired or neglected, or he is being ill-treated; or, (b) the court or another court has found that that condition obtained in another member of the juvenile's household; or, (c) he is exposed to moral danger; or, (d) he is beyond parental control; or, (e) being of compulsory school age, he is not receiving appropriate efficient full-time education; or, (f) he is guilty of an offence excluding homicide; *and also* he is in need of care or control necessitating the court making an order.

Court orders are of five kinds: (1) requiring parent or guardian to exercise proper care and control of child or young person; (2) supervision order where juvenile is usually allowed to stay at home but under surveillance of an appointed supervisor; (3) care order where juvenile is removed from his home and boarded-out or placed in a community home; (4) hospital order under Mental Health Act, 1959, for juvenile requiring psychiatric treatment; (5) guardianship order under Mental Health Act.

Formal care proceedings in respect of any young person may be brought by a qualified informant (local authority, police constable, inspector of N.S.P.C.C.) who reasonably believes that the juvenile is 'in need of care or control' and only by a court order can such care or control be exercised. The informant must notify the local authority and probation service of his intention to bring court proceedings and the local authority and probation service must provide court with certain information relating to home surroundings, school record, health and character of juvenile to assist the court's deliberations. Formal court proceedings may not, however, be necessary if the informant believes that an alleged offence can be dealt with satisfactorily by a parent, teacher, or other person, or by means of a caution from a police officer, or through the exercise of powers of the local authority or other body not involved in court proceedings. In criminal proceedings, juvenile courts have powers to make any of the five orders (supra), together with absolute discharge, conditional discharge, payment of damages, enforcing a detention centre or attendance centre order.

Community Homes. The 1969 Act provides for a single system of 'community homes' instead of the present pattern of children's homes, hostels, reception centres, remand homes and approved schools. The legal status of these institutions will change as children's regional planning committees have agreed on plans and begun to put them into effect. The initial steps to implement this part of the Act date from December, 1969.

Local authorities in combination must appoint children's regional planning committees to cover areas approved by the Secretary of State. Regional planning committees must prepare plans for community homes for their areas and submit these for approval by the Secretary of State. As far as any existing voluntary homes are concerned, they may be included in the regional plan and may fall into two kinds, *viz.*, (a) controlled community homes where the management, equipment and maintenance of the homes will be the responsibility of one of the local authorities in the region and which will have a two-thirds representation on the body of managers; and, (b) assisted community homes where the above matters will be the responsibility of the voluntary body and the relevant local authority will have a one-third representation on the body of managers. The Secretary of State may make regulations regarding the conduct of community homes and for securing the welfare of children accommodated in them. Community homes will be subject to inspection by officers of the Home Office.

Research. Secretary of State and local authorities are empowered to undertake research in matters pertaining to these and other Acts, including the Children Act, 1948, and Adoption Acts.

SCOTLAND. CHILDREN AND YOUNG PERSONS (SCOT.) ACTS, 1937 *et seq*. In the Social Work (Scot.) Act, 1968 (vide infra), there is an important part (Part III) dealing with new and radical compulsory powers for the care and treatment of children who have committed offences or who otherwise stand in need of care for specified reasons. However, certain provisions of the existing Children and Young Persons (Scot.) Acts remain in operation but with important differences compared with those legislative measures operative in England and Wales. Such differences include: it is an offence to expose a child under 7 years to risk of burning. Any reference in the Acts to the Secretary of State means in Scotland a reference to the Secretary of State for Scotland.

ENGLAND AND WALES. CHILDREN ACT, 1948, as amended by the Children and Young Persons Acts, 1963–9. The Act makes provision for the care or welfare, up to the age of 18 and, in certain cases, further periods, of boys and girls when they are without parents or have been lost or abandoned by, or are living away from their parents, or when their parents are unfit or unable to take care of them, and in certain other circumstances.

Provision of care for orphaned or deserted children, etc. It is the duty of a local authority to receive into its care any child under 17 who is without parents or guardian, has been abandoned or lost, or whose parents or guardian are prevented, permanently or temporarily, from providing him with a normal home life, provided that the intervention of the local authority is deemed necessary in the interests of the child. The duty to receive such a child is placed on the local authority in whose area the child is found, but the local authority of area of his domicile may receive the child or provide for his maintenance. The local authority must look after the child till he is 18, if his welfare so demands, but must return him to his parents if they so desire and if this is in the interests of the child, or if the authority can arrange for his care by parents, relatives or friends.

Assumption of parental rights. A local authority may, in respect of any child already in its care, by resolution assume parental rights if the parent's or guardian's whereabouts remain unknown for at least 12 months; or he suffers from any mental disorder rendering him unfit to care for the child; or he has so persistently failed without reasonable cause to discharge the obligations of a parent or guardian as to be unfit to have the care of the child. If parent or guardian objects he can apply to a court. It is an offence to harbour or conceal a child in care of a local authority after its assumption of parental rights. Under the Children and Young Persons Acts, a court may prescribe the most suitable means of caring for a person (in case of a person brought before it) and may commit him to the care of a local authority under a 'care' order.

Provision of suitable accommodation. A local authority must provide suitable accommodation and maintenance for the children in its care either by boarding them out, placing them in community homes or in voluntary homes whose managers are willing to receive them, or by making other arrangements deemed appropriate by the authority. Secretary of State is empowered to make regulations concerning boarding-out, community homes, etc., and concerning accommodation, equipment, medical care, and religious instruction. Community home accommodation may also be provided under a regional plan by a local authority for persons over school age and under 21. Financial aid may also be given by an authority for the education and training of persons between 17 and 21 when such persons had been in the care of the local authority at the age of 17. Similarly, local authority may visit, advise and befriend any person who so desires this and who was in the authority's care up to the age of 17.

Liability to contribute to maintenance of child in care. Parents, putative father, or mother are liable to make financial contributions towards a child's care up to 16. Thereafter, if the child is in wholetime remunerative employment he is liable to make contributions. Parents must keep in touch with the authority when their child is in care, and the authority may assist them financially to enable them to visit their child.

Voluntary homes. Voluntary homes which are supported wholly or partially by voluntary contributions may remain outside the community homes system (1969 Act) but must be regulated and registered by the Secretary of State (through the Children's Department of the Home Office). Refusal or cancellation of registration may be appealed against. Grants may be made by the Secretary of State and by local authorities to voluntary bodies dealing with deprived children. A local authority is required to cause children in voluntary homes in its area to be visited by an authorised officer from the children's department. Such an officer may also visit any voluntary home outside the area of that local authority to see children in that home who are in the authority's care.

Administration. The Act also deals with its administration, *i.e.* central supervision and local execution.

ENGLAND AND WALES. CHILDREN ACT, 1958, as amended by the Children and Young Persons Act, 1969. An Act concerned with ensuring the well-being of foster-children by local authorities. A foster-child is defined as one below school-leaving age whose care and maintenance are undertaken by a person who is not a relative or guardian. Certain exceptions are specified but the definition includes children residing for periods over 2 weeks during school holidays at independent and private boarding schools.

A person proposing to take a foster-child must notify the local authority in writing of his intention not less than 2 weeks and not more than 4 weeks before receiving the child but if received in an emergency, notice must be given within 48 hours of receiving child. Written notice must specify proposed date of taking child or date of having taken him, and situation of premises where child is to be kept and must, if local authority requires, give name, sex, date and place of birth of child and name and address of every person who is parent, guardian, or from whom child is to be received. Any change of address must be notified at least 2 weeks but not more than 4 weeks before change, or within 48 hours of change if this took place in an emergency. Death of foster-child must be notified within 48 hours of the event both to the local authority and to the person from whom the child was received. In case of removal, name and address of person to whom child was removed may be required by local authority. Certain requirements may be imposed on keeping foster-children, *i.e.* number, age, sex, accommodation, fire precautions, medical arrangements, record keeping, and number, qualifications and experience of any staff engaged to look after children, and persons may be prohibited from receiving foster-children if such persons or their premises are unsuitable.

These child protection provisions apply until foster-child returns to his parent or guardian or reaches the age of 18 or lives elsewhere than with the foster-parents when he reaches school-leaving age.

SCOTLAND. The Act applies subject to amendments by the Social Work (Scot.) Act, 1968. These amendments include the transfer of supervision of foster-children to the social work department of the local authority which may arrange for the children to be visited by an officer of the department to give such advice as to care and maintenance as is considered necessary. A 'foster-child' is defined as 'a child below the upper limit of the compulsory school age whose care is undertaken for a period of more than six days beginning with the day on which the child is received into that care'. Exceptions to this definition are specified.

ENGLAND AND WALES. MATRIMONIAL PROCEEDINGS (CHILDREN) ACT, 1958. An Act extending powers of courts to make orders regarding children in connection with proceedings between husband and wife, and to require arrangements regarding children to be made to the court's satisfaction before it makes a decree in such proceedings.

A court may, before granting any decree, if it is impracticable or undesirable for a child, legitimate or illegitimate or adopted, under 16 years, to be entrusted to either of the parties to the marriage or to any other individual, commit such child to the care of the local authority until he is 18 years old or committal order is revoked. If child is committed to care of an independent person, he may be supervised by a probation or children's officer.

SCOTLAND. Provisions are similar, but before the court proceeds to grant a decree it may require a report to be made as to the arrangements for the future care and upbringing of any children by a local authority or other person appointed by the court.

Adoption

ENGLAND, WALES AND SCOTLAND. ADOPTION ACT, 1958. This Act improved and consolidated previous enactments relating to child adoption in the three countries.

An 'infant' is defined as any person under 21 but does not include a person who is or has been married. Provision is made for the granting of adoption orders by the High Court, county court and juvenile court in England and Wales, and the Court of Session and sheriff court in Scotland. Court procedure is governed by Adoption Rules and in Scotland by Acts of Sederunt of Court of Session. Adoption orders cannot be made unless:

(*a*) *Application to adopt an infant has been made in the prescribed way and certain age and residential qualifications of adopters are fulfilled.* The prospective adopter, or one of the applicants in a joint application of spouses, is 25 years old, or is 21 years old and a relative of the infant, or is the mother or father of the infant. The adopter(s) and infant must reside in England, or in Scotland for Scottish adoptions. Provision is made for domiciled but non-resident Britons to adopt an infant as well as for foreigners to do so.

(*b*) *Consent to the adoption has been given by the infant's parent or guardian.* Attendance of parents or guardian is not necessary at the court but written, witnessed consent must be produced. In case of mother of an infant written consent cannot be given until infant is at least 6 weeks old. Court may dispense with consent in certain circumstances.

(*c*) *Adoption will be to the benefit of the child*, and the court shall have regard to the health of the applicant(s) and give due consideration to the wishes of the infant if of such age and understanding. In Scotland, child's consent to his adoption must be obtained if he is over 14 years old or if a girl is over 12 years old.

(*d*) *Infant has been continuously in the care and possession of the applicant(s) for at least the previous 3 consecutive months to the application.*

(*e*) *Applicant(s) have at least 3 months before the date of the order notified the local authority of area of their residence of their intention to adopt the infant.* No period, however, before the infant is 6 weeks old can count in this 3 months period of supervision by the local authority—children's department in England and Wales, social work department in Scotland (under Social Work (Scot.) Act, 1968).

Instead of granting an adoption order, a court may, in certain circumstances, grant an interim order not exceeding a period of 2 years. Payments between contracting parties prior to an adoption are prohibited and restrictions are placed on advertisements relating to adoption.

A recent Act, the Succession (Scot.) Act, 1964, confers on adopted child the right to or interest in property of adoptive parent(s), thus bringing the adopted child into line with the inheritance law in England and Wales. Automatic inheritance does not, however, obtain in the three countries for such circumstances as titles, etc.

Adoption societies, which must be voluntary bodies, must be registered with the local authority, which is entitled to inspect their books. Regulations govern the conduct of adoption societies. Local authorities are empowered to make and participate in adoption arrangements whether the infants are in the care of the authorities or not.

A child placed with a view to his adoption is called a 'protected child' and is: (1) one under school-leaving age who is placed by a stranger (or third party) with a person who is not a parent, guardian or relative of the infant but who proposes to adopt him, or (2) one for whom notice of intention to adopt has been given to the local authority. Protected children are supervised by the local authority under provisions similar to those obtaining for foster-children under the Children Act, 1958, and these provisions apply until either (*a*) an adoption order is granted in respect of a protected child or (*b*) he attains the age of 18 years, whichever first occurs.

Under the Adoption Act, 1960, applicable to England and Wales only, where any person legitimated under the Legitimacy Act, 1959, had been adopted by his father and mother before that Act became operative, the court granting the adoption order may, on application by any of the parties concerned, revoke the order. A similar procedure exists in Scotland under a recent Act, the Legitimation (Scot.) Act, 1968.

Nurseries and Child-Minders

NURSERIES AND CHILD-MINDERS REGULATION ACT, 1948, amended by the HEALTH SERVICES AND PUBLIC HEALTH ACT, 1968. These Acts provide for the regulation of certain nurseries and of persons who for reward receive into their homes children to look after them. The Acts are applicable to England and Wales and to Scotland.

Nurseries. Premises not wholly or mainly used as private dwellings where children are received to be looked after for the day or for 2 hours or longer in a day, or for any longer period not exceeding 6 days.

Child-Minders. Persons who for reward receive into their own homes children under 5 years of age to be looked after for the day or for 2 hours or longer in a day, or for any longer period not exceeding 6 days.

A local health authority (in Scotland under the Social Work (Scot.) Act, 1968, a local authority) must keep registers, open to public inspection, of all premises and persons (nurseries and child-minders) in its area. Any person proposing to receive children as defined under nurseries and minders must apply for registration to the local health authority (local authority in Scotland). The authority must by order specify the maximum number of children to be admitted and require that precautions be taken to ensure the safety of the children and against their exposure to infection. Requirements may also be imposed regarding—number, qualifications and experience of those persons looking after the children; repairs and alterations to premises which may be required; equipment required and safety measures necessary and their maintenance; adequacy of feeding arrangements and dietary; medical care and supervision of the children; keeping of proper registers and records.

It is an offence for an unregistered person for reward to look after in her own home one or more children, to whom she is not related, for 2 hours or longer in any day or for any longer period not exceeding 6 days.

Certificates of registration must specify situation of premises to which, or name and address of person to whom, registration relates and any requirements imposed by the authority. Any change of circumstances must be reported to the authority. There are powers to refuse and to cancel registrations. Authorised persons have power of entry to premises to inspect them, the children received there, arrangements for their welfare, and any records required to be kept. Schools and nursery schools provided by local education authorities or assisted by them, hospitals and premises where child life protection enactments apply are exempted from registration under these Acts. In the Local Authority Social Services Bill (1970) the proposal is made that registration and supervision of private nurseries and childminders be transferred to social service departments of local authorities.

Social Work (Scotland) Act, 1968

An important Act to make further provision for promoting social welfare. It consolidates with amendments certain enactments relating to the care and protection of children, restricts the prosecution of children for offences, establishes children's panels to provide children's hearings in the case of children requiring compulsory measures of care, and also deals with other matters.

The Act has two main aspects, social and administrative. Socially, it is designed to offer flexibility in response to social needs. Administratively, it simplifies the structure by bringing together four services, hitherto separate, which were closely connected, *viz.* for probation of offenders, for deprived children, for welfare of aged and disabled, and for mental health. The Act states that the Secretary of State for Scotland has power to bring the Act into operation on a single 'appointed date' or on 'different dates . . . for different purposes of this Act'. The appointed date was 17 November, 1969, for operation of the general provisions of the Act: those parts dealing with children requiring compulsory measures of care were deferred till 1970. Thus the provisions of the Children and Young Persons (Scot.) Act, 1937, as amended, dealing *inter alia* with juvenile courts, etc., remained in operation for a time. From November, 1969, children's departments of local authorities were absorbed into the social work departments and ceased to exist as separate entities.

Central administration rests with the Secretary of State for Scotland acting through the Social Work Services Group within the Scottish Education Department.

Duties of Local Authorities. Councils of counties and large burghs must establish social work committees and appoint executive officers, after consultation with the Secretary of State, called directors of social work. The functions of the social work department of a local authority must include the provisions of: (1) this Act; (2) Nurseries and Child-Minders Regulation Act, 1948, as amended (1968); (3) Mental Health (Scot.) Act, 1960, local authorities' functions except ascertainment of mental deficiency; (4) National Health Service (Scot.) Act, 1947, those local health authority functions relating to care and after-care of sick *except* medical, dental or nursing care or health visiting, but including home help service; (5) Children Act, 1958, as amended by this Act, dealing with care and supervision of foster-children; (6) Matrimonial Proceedings (Children) Act, 1958; (7) Adoption Act, 1958; (8) other related Acts.

Welfare powers. This Act repeats the provisions of the Children and Young Persons Act, 1963, dealing with promotion of social welfare by making available advice, guidance and assistance including where appropriate assistance in kind or in cash.

Orphan and deserted children, etc. A local authority has functions similar to those of the Children Act, 1948, now repealed, in respect of provision for care of orphans, deserted children, and others. Parental rights may be assumed in certain instances. It is the duty of local authority wherever possible and desirable to return a child to his parents, or guardian, relative or friend. The best interests of the child in the care of a local authority must be furthered and opportunity afforded to him for his proper development.

Children in need of compulsory measures of care. Under this part of the Act, a child is defined as: one who has not attained the age of 16 years; one over 16 but under 18 in respect of whom a supervision requirement of a children's hearing is in force; one whose case has been referred to a children's hearing.

Conditions where compulsory care is required are defined: (*a*) beyond parental control; (*b*) exposed to moral danger or falling into bad associations; (*c*) lack of parental care likely to cause unnecessary suffering or impair child's health or development; (*d*) child against whom certain offences have been committed; (*f*) failure to attend school; (*g*) committing of an offence; (*h*) case has been referred to a children's hearing.

Children's panels will be set up in local authority areas, and conditions of appointment of members of panel are defined. Three members from panel sit together and constitute a children's hearing and conduct of children's hearings will be controlled by regulations. A 'reporter' must be appointed by the local authority to arrange children's hearings, investigate cases, decide what action is necessary including arrangements for holding children's hearings, attendance of child at such if deemed necessary or desirable. Parents have right of attendance at hearings. If child needs compulsory care, hearing may (1) place child under supervision; or (2) place him in an appropriate residential establishment, provided either by the local authority or by a voluntary body. Right of appeal to sheriff exists against decisions of hearing. Publication of proceedings of hearings is prohibited. Residential establishments are defined as establishments managed by a local authority, voluntary organisation or any other person, which provides residential accommodation for the purposes of this Act, whether for reward or not. Such residential establishments will be controlled by regulations.

Education Acts

ENGLAND AND WALES. EDUCATION ACTS, 1944–68. The principal Act is the Education Act, 1944, amended and supplemented by other Acts, in particular, the Mental Health Act, 1959, Criminal Justice Act, 1967, and Public Expenditure and

Receipts Act, 1968. These Acts reform the law relating to education, provide for a Secretary of State for Education and Science and a Department of Education and Science, make comprehensive provision for primary, secondary and further education, define the duties of an education authority, and with the regulations made under the Acts contain the fundamental legislation relating to the medical and dental care of schoolchildren.

System of public education. The system of public education must be organised in three progressive stages, *viz.* (*a*) primary; full-time education for pupils below the age of 10 years and 6 months; (*b*) secondary: full-time education for pupils over 10 years and 6 months and under 19; (*c*) further: full-time or part-time education for those over compulsory school-leaving age, and certain leisure time activities.

Compulsory school age. Compulsory school age means any age between 5 and 15 years; the upper limit may be raised by Order in Council. The upper age limit for pupils registered at special schools is 16.

Provision for and attendance at educational establishments. An education authority must secure adequate provision of educational facilities in its area and this includes provision of nursery schools and classes for pupils between 2 and 5 years. The parent of every child of compulsory school age must cause him to receive efficient, full-time education suitable to his age, ability and aptitude, either by regular attendance at school or by other means. Sickness is deemed a reasonable excuse for absence from school. Transport to and from school may be provided by education authorities.

Provision of milk and meals. A local education authority must establish a School Meals Service for the provision of milk and dinners for pupils. The authority may, if it thinks fit, provide other meals and refreshments. The duty to provide free milk shall only apply to primary schools and special schools (from August, 1968).

Recreational facilities. An education authority must provide facilities for recreation, social and physical training and may, with the Secretary of State's approval, maintain and manage or assist with the maintenance and management of camps, holiday classes, playing fields and other places; may also organise games, expeditions and other activities.

Provision of clothing. An education authority may provide clothing for a pupil attending any school maintained by the authority and the parent may be required to pay for or contribute towards the cost incurred.

Cleanliness. An education authority may, by written notice, authorise a medical officer to cause examinations to be made of the person and clothing of pupils at all schools maintained by it. Any such examination must be made by a person authorised by the authority. If the person or clothing of any pupil is verminous or foul, notice may be served on the parent requiring that the pupil and his clothing be cleansed within a specified period. If the authority's medical officer considers the cleansing to be inadequate, he may make an order for it to be carried out under arrangements provided by the authority (*e.g.* at a cleansing station). If a pupil again becomes verminous or foul, parent liable to a fine if condition proved due to neglect. Pupil may be excluded from school by a medical officer during cleansing period. Girls must be examined and/or cleansed by a qualified medical practitioner or woman authorised for that purpose.

Part-time employment. An education authority has power to prohibit or restrict the employment of a child if he is thereby rendered unfit to profit fully from the education provided.

School health and dental services. An education authority must provide for medical inspection, which can be enforced, and for treatment which cannot be enforced and must be free. The Secretary of State may make regulations as to the conduct of medical inspections and examinations, and as to special qualifications or experience of medical officers. Every medical officer employed by a local education authority to ascertain which children in its area should be sent to special schools for educationally subnormal children must have been approved for the purpose by the Secretary of State.

Provision is also made for a comprehensive dental service.

Handicapped pupils. The Secretary of State must define the several categories of children requiring special educational treatment as handicapped pupils. It is the duty of a local education authority to ascertain which children in its area require special educational treatment. A formal procedure is laid down for securing the medical examination for this purpose of any child who has attained the age of two years, and parents have a right to be present at such examination. If authority decides that a child needs special treatment, it has a duty to provide it either at an ordinary school or a special school or otherwise, unless parents themselves can make suitable arrangements.

Children unsuitable for education at school owing to a disability of mind. The Mental Health Act, 1959, and the Criminal Justice Act, 1967, amended previous Education Act provisions relating to 'ineducable' children. It is the duty of every local education authority to ascertain what children in its area are suffering from a disability of mind of such nature or extent as to make them unsuitable for education at school and it may, by written notice sent by an officer authorised by the authority to do so, require a parent to submit any child attaining the age of 2 years to medical examination at which parent is entitled to be present. Failure to comply with this demand renders parent liable to fine. If such child is found unsuitable for attendance at school the authority may cause this decision to be recorded and furnish local health authority with a report on the child's condition, but parent has opportunity to appeal to the Secretary of State against the proposed decision. Notice of decision to parent shall include statement of functions of local health authority regarding arrangements for treatment, care or training of child. Local health authority has power to compel attendance at training centres for such children and provide transport where necessary. Procedure is also laid down for reviewing a decision later at the instance of parent, local health authority or body responsible for management of institution where child is under care, and for cancelling decision if child is then found capable of receiving education at school. Any report issued to a local health authority under this paragraph must contain appropriate records and information relating to the child.

School-leavers requiring care from local health authorities. Children leaving school who, because of mental handicap, are in the opinion of the local education authority in need of care and guidance from the local health authority will continue to receive this following the informal passage of information between the two authorities, and not, as formerly, by statutory report.

Compulsory submission to medical examination. Where a medical examination will assist the Secretary of State to determine any question raised under the Education Acts, he has power to enforce such examination.

SCOTLAND. EDUCATION (SCOT.) ACTS, 1962–69. These Acts consolidate the enactments relating to education in Scotland. They run along similar lines to those governing education in England and Wales but with some important points of difference in sections relating to child health.

Absence from school. Sickness is deemed a reasonable excuse for absence from school but when this excuse is advanced an education authority has the right to enforce examination of the pupil by the school medical officer.

Cleanliness. Examinations to ensure cleanliness of pupils must be carried out by the education authority's medical officer or by a person authorised by him.

School hygiene. Part of the work of the medical officers of an education authority shall be to inspect and report from time to time on educational premises, furnishings and equipment, and to have special regard to the heating, lighting and ventilation, and the sanitary arrangements obtaining in these premises.

Handicapped pupils. The Secretary of State for Scotland may define the several categories of handicapped pupils. Provision is made for the compulsory ascertainment of handicapped children who have attained the age of 5 years and power is given for the ascertainment of those under 5 years. Parents must be informed of results of the ascertainment after the child has undergone both a medical and a psychological examination and of the special education to be provided and have the right of appeal to the Secretary of State for Scotland. The education authority must provide appropriate special education in special schools or by other means approved by the Secretary of State. An education authority must regularly review cases undergoing special education and a parent can demand such a review under certain conditions. This review must include fresh medical and psychological examinations. After review the authority may revoke decision regarding special education and return child to ordinary school or require continuation of special education. Special schools include special classes, child guidance clinics and occupational centres. An authority may establish a child guidance service to study handicapped, backward and difficult pupils.

Children unsuitable for education or training in a special school owing to a disability of mind. As in England, provision is made for the compulsory ascertainment of children unsuitable for education at school but with the following differences: (*a*) the compulsory age of ascertainment is 5 years, but power is given to education authorities to ascertain handicapped children under 5 years of age; and (*b*) occupational centres being classified as special schools are provided by local education authorities in Scotland.

Hence a child unsuitable for education at school includes one who is incapable of benefiting even at an occupational centre, and so must be reported to the local authority (under Social Work (Scot.) Act, 1968, the social work department) which must provide for suitable training facilities and compel attendance, arranging transport where necessary.

School-leavers requiring care from local authorities. Where it appears that a child, by reason of mental deficiency, may benefit from local authority services (under Social Work (Scot.) Act, 1968, services provided by social work department) on leaving school, the local education authority must inform parent and local authority of this fact not earlier than 6 months nor later than 1 month prior to child ceasing to be of school age. Any report issued to the local authority under this and the foregoing paragraph must contain appropriate records and information relating to the child.

Employment and Training

ENGLAND AND WALES, SCOTLAND. EMPLOYMENT AND TRAINING ACT, 1948. An Act to make provision for employment exchanges and services and for training in employment.

Youth employment services. These may be provided by an education authority in accordance with arrangements approved by the Ministry of Labour or directly by the Ministry of Labour itself. They are for the benefit of persons under the age of 18 years or over that age if still attending school. Information to be made available to the service is limited to particulars of health, ability, attainments and aptitudes; there is restriction of disclosure of such particulars but parents have right to see such records as are submitted to the service.

General control of the service is vested in the Central Youth Employment Executive, a body which is composed of officers of the Ministry of Labour, Department of Education and Science and Scottish Education Department and which is responsible to the Minister of Labour. (There is an excellent review of the work of the Youth Employment Service, 1965–68 (1968, H.M.S.O.)).

Consumer Protection

ENGLAND AND WALES, SCOTLAND. CONSUMER PROTECTION ACT, 1961. This Act is designed to protect consumers by prescribing regulations as to safety requirements of certain goods. Regulations were made in 1952 and 1960, under appropriate Acts, relating to safety of heating appliances such as electric and gas heaters, and of oil burners, and these regulations remain operative under this Act which repealed the two previous Acts. Further regulations are: Children's Nightdresses Regulations, 1964, requiring materials used to be of low flammability; Nightdresses (Safety) Regulations, 1966, extending scope of 1964 Regulations; Oil Heaters Regulations, 1966, amending previous regulations; Stands for Carry-cots (Safety) Regulations, 1966, prescribe certain safety requirements; Toys (Safety) Regulations, 1967, prohibiting use of celluloid, controlling lead and other metals in paints used for toymaking. By the Rag, Flock and Other Filling Materials Regulations, 1961 and 1965, toy-filling material must comply with prescribed standards of cleanliness.

It is an offence to sell, let under hire-purchase agreement or offer on hire specified goods not complying with their relevant regulations. Local authority can authorise in writing any of its officers to test, including purchase in order to test, any goods or their component parts to which regulations apply, to ascertain if specified requirements are complied with.

Family Allowances

ENGLAND AND WALES, SCOTLAND. FAMILY ALLOWANCES AND NATIONAL INSURANCE ACT, 1967. Under this Act, the Secretary of State for Social Services is required to pay weekly to every family an allowance in respect of each child under the age limits, *after* the first. Eighteen shillings are payable for the second child and twenty shillings for each subsequent child. A child is under the age limits: up to minimum school-leaving age (presently 15), *and* during any period before his nineteenth birthday if he is receiving full-time instruction in a school, college or university, or can qualify as an apprentice, or while schooling or apprenticeship is interrupted because of illness, *and* during any period before the sixteenth birthday while unable to work because of prolonged illness or disability. A child can qualify as an apprentice while undergoing full-time training for any trade, business, profession, etc., and earning not more than £2 per week after deduction of certain expenses. Ordinarily, allowances are payable to the mother but they may be paid to either parent.

Tattooing

TATTOOING OF MINORS ACT, 1969. It is an offence, punishable by fine, to tattoo any person under 18 years except when such is performed for medical reasons by a registered medical practitioner or one working under his direction. Tattoo is defined as 'insertion into the skin of any colouring material designed to leave a permanent mark'.

H. P. TAIT

Index

Index